MEDICAL MICROBIOLOGY

Cedric A Mims BSc, MD, FRCPath
Emeritus Professor, Department of Microbiology
Guy's Hospital Medical School
London, UK

John HL Playfair MB, BChir, PhD, DSc
Professor and Head, Department of Immunology
University College & Middlesex School of Medicine
London, UK

Ivan M Roitt MA, DSc, HON MRCP (LOND), FRCPath, FRS
Director, Institute of Biomedical Sciences
University College & Middlesex School of Medicine
London, UK

Derek Wakelin PhD, DSc, FIBiol
Professor, Department of Zoology
University of Nottingham
Nottingham, UK

Rosamund Williams PhD, FRCPath
Director of Biological Sciences
Lepetit Research Center
Gerenzano, Italy

with a contribution from
Roy M Anderson FRS
Professor and Head, Department of Biology
Imperial College of Science, Technology and Medicine
London, UK

M Mosby
St. Louis Baltimore Boston Chicago London Philadelphia Sydney Toronto

Project Manager	Claire Hooper
Design and Illustration	Catherine Duffy
	Jane Brown
Cover Illustration	Mark Willey
Linework	Marion Tasker
Production	Susan Bishop
Index	Nina Boyd
Publisher	Fiona Foley

A Slide Atlas of Medical Microbiology, based on the contents of
this book, is available. In the slide atlas format, the material is
split into volumes, each of which is presented in a binder,
together with numbered 35mm slides of each illustration. Further
information is available from the publishers.

Copyright © Mosby Europe Limited.
Published in 1993 by Mosby Europe Limited.

Typeset on Apple Macintosh®
Text set in New Baskerville; legends set in Helvetica
Colour reproduction by Bright Arts Hong Kong
Produced by Mandarin Offset. Printed and bound in Hong Kong

ISBN: 0 397 44631 4

Cataloging-in-Publication Data:
Catalogue records for this book are available from the US Library
of Congress and British Library

CIP catalogue records for this book are available from the US
Library of Congress and British Library.

For full details of Mosby Europe Limited titles please write to
Mosby Europe Limited, Brook House, 2–16 Torrington Place,
London WC1E 7LT, England.

PREFACE

This is a brand new type of medical microbiology text-book. Most existing medical microbiology textbooks are organized along traditional lines, taking each microbe in turn and describing the diseases they cause almost as an afterthought. Our approach takes into account the changes that are currently taking place in the teaching of medical microbiology in medical schools world-wide, and is geared towards making the subject more accessible and relevant to clinical practice. In the first two sections of the book we describe infectious diseases in terms of the conflict between the host and the parasite. Immunology plays a central role in this conflict, as a given microbe can infect and cause disease only if it can survive in the face of the multitude of immune and other defences brought into play by the host. At the same time we have paid the necessary attention to core medical microbiology, giving in the third section a full factual, clinically based account of infectious diseases. In this section we have employed the 'systems' approach to classification whereby infections are classified according to the particular organ system involved, so putting the study of infectious disease into a clinically relevant context. We have placed particular emphasis on pathogenesis and control, and, because of the steady, satisfying progress towards understanding infectious disease at the molecular level, we have referred to molecular mechanisms wherever possible. Although prevention and treatment of different infections is outlined in each chapter of section three, section four contains chapters specifically devoted to these topics. This section also contains a chapter, kindly supplied by Professor Roy Anderson, on the increasingly important subject of epidemiology. Finally, for easy reference, detailed information on medically important microorganisms and microbiological procedures are gathered together in a comprehensive appendix at the back of the book. The text is illustrated, expanded and enlivened by a profusion of full-colour pictures, diagrams and tables, the quality of which makes the slide atlas which accompanies this book an indispensible aid to teachers of medical microbiology.

CM, JHLP, IMR, DW, RW
London 1993

ACKNOWLEDGEMENTS

We wish to express our appreciation of the generosity of many collegues throughout the world who supplied illustrative material, particularly W Edmund Farrar, Martin J Wood, John A Innes, Hugh Tubbs, James S Bingham, Ralph Muller, John R Baker and Dilip K Banerjee. We would like to thank the library of The Wellcome Institute for the History of Medicine for providing portrait photographs for the historical profiles. We are also grateful to David Jarvis for his invaluable help in compiling the Appendix, and Professor John Oxford for his advice on the cover illustration.

Finally, we are indebted to our enterprising publishers for their faith in us, particularly to Fiona Foley, for her sustained support and encouragement. We would also like to thank Claire Hooper, our ever helpful and resourceful project manager, and Catherine Duffy and Jane Brown, our extremely talented design team.

CM, JHLP, IMR, DW, RW
London 1993

CONTENTS

section *1*

THE ADVERSARIES

part 1 **The Microbes**

1 MICROBES AND PARASITES

Contents

INTRODUCTION: WHAT IS MICROBIOLOGY?

Microbiology is sometimes defined as the biology of micro-scopic organisms, its subject being the 'microbes'. Traditionally, clinical microbiology has been concerned with organisms responsible for the major infectious dis-eases of man – and his domestic animals – whose size makes them invisible to the naked eye. It is not surprising that the range of organisms included has reflected those diseases which have been (or continue to be) of greatest importance in those countries where the scientific and clin-ical discipline of microbiology developed, notably Europe and the USA. So the term 'microbes' has usually been applied in a restricted fashion, primarily to viruses, bacteria and related organisms; sometimes fungi and protozoans ('parasites') have also been included, as relatively minor contributors, but in general they have been treated as the subjects of other disciplines (mycology and parasitology).

Although there can be no argument that viruses and bacteria are the most numerous and most important pathogens, the conventional distinction between these as 'microbes' and the other infectious agents we know loosely as 'parasites' is essentially arbitrary, not least because the criterion of microscopic visibility cannot be applied rigidly (Fig. 1.1). Perhaps we should remember that the first 'microbe' to be associated with a specific clinical condition was a parasitic worm – the nematode *Trichinella spiralis*, whose larval stages are just visible to the naked eye (though microscopy is needed for certain identification).

Trichinella spiralis, first identified in 1835 by Paget and Owen, was causally related to the disease trichinellosis in the 1860s. On the grounds of both history and physical size this parasite might be expected to feature in textbooks of microbiology, but it rarely does, instead it is found most often in textbooks of parasitology.

The clinical significance of trichinellosis is minor, and it would be unrealistic to expect the organism or the disease to receive detailed treatment in a standard microbiological text, but the absence of *T. spiralis* and other parasites reflects another characteristic of existing books which the present volume seeks to change. With some exceptions,

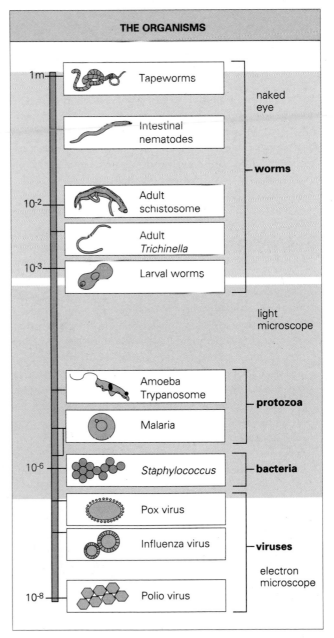

Fig. 1.1 Relative sizes of the organisms covered in this book.

microbiology texts deal with infectious organisms as agents of disease in isolation – isolated both from other infectious organisms and from the biological context in which they live and in which disease is caused. It is certainly convenient to list and deal with organisms by taxonomic category, to summarize the disease which they cause, and to review the forms of prophylaxis available, but this approach produces a static picture of what is a dynamic host–pathogen relationship. Host response can be discussed in terms of pathological signs and symptoms, and in terms of immunoprophylaxis, but it is better treated as the manifestation of the complex interplay between two organisms – host and parasite; without this dimension a distorted view of infectious disease results. It simply is not true that microbe + host = disease, and clinicians are well aware of this. Insights into understanding the reasons why it is not the case, and the events which may make it the case, are equally as important as the identification of infectious organisms and a knowledge of their chemo- and immunoprophylaxis.

THE NEED FOR A NEW APPROACH TO MICROBIOLOGY

We believe that it is time to reconsider our approaches to microbiology – in terms of the organisms that might usefully be considered within a textbook, and also in terms of the contexts in which they, and the diseases they cause, are discussed. There are many reasons for having reached this conclusion, the most important being:

- A comprehensive understanding now exists of the biological bases of infection, disease, host–microbe (and host–parasite) interactions, and the epidemiology of infectious disease. It is important for students to be aware of this understanding so that they can grasp the connections between infection and disease, within both individuals and communities, and be able to use this knowledge in novel and changing clinical situations.
- There is now a realization that the host's response to infection is a coordinated and subtle interplay involving the mechanisms of both innate and acquired resistance, and that these mechanisms are expressed regardless of the nature and identity of the pathogen involved. Our present understanding of the ways these mechanisms are stimulated and the ways in which they act is very sophisticated. We can now see that infection is a conflict between two organisms, with the outcome (resistance or disease) critically dependent upon molecular interactions. Again, it is essential to understand the basis of this host–pathogen interplay, if the processes of disease and disease control are to be interpreted correctly.

In addition two other factors have helped to mould our concept of microbiology, and our opinion that a broader view is needed to provide a firm basis for clinical and scientific practice:

- There is an increasing prevalence of a wide variety of opportunistic infections in patients who are immunosuppressed. Immunosuppressive therapies are now more common, as are diseases in which the immune system is compromised, notably, of course, AIDS (Fig. 1.2).

OPPORTUNISTIC INFECTIONS IN IMMUNOSUPPRESSION	
immunosuppression affecting:	opportunistic infections
B lymphocytes and antibody production	enteroviruses *Streptococcus* *Haemophilus* *Neisseria* *Staphylococcus* *Giardia* *Pneumocystis*
T lymphocytes and cell-mediated immunity	herpes *Cytomegalovirus* *Listeria* *Mycobacterium* *Candida* *Aspergillus* *Cryptococcus* *Pneumocystis* *Strongyloides*
B and T lymphocytes	as above, plus rubella varicella

Fig. 1.2 Organisms associated with opportunistic infections in immunosuppressed patients.

- In the West, recent years have seen a renewed interest in tropical medicine. Clinicians now see many tourists who have been exposed to the quite different spectrum of infectious agents that is found in tropical countries. There is also greater public concern over the health problems of the developing world (Fig. 1.3).

These factors point towards the need for a text that has a dual function. Firstly, it should provide a more inclusive treatment of the organisms responsible for infectious disease. Secondly, the purely clinical/laboratory approach to microbiology should be replaced with an approach that will stress the biological context in which clinical/laboratory studies are to be undertaken.

The approach we have adopted in this book is to look at microbiology from the viewpoint of the conflicts inherent in all host–parasite relationships. We first describe the adversaries, the infectious organisms on the one hand, and the innate and adaptive defence mechanisms of the host on the other. The outcome of the conflicts between the two is then amplified and discussed system-by-system. Rather than taking each organism, or each disease manifestation in turn, we look at the major environments available for infectious organisms in the human body, the respiratory system, the gut, the urinary tract, the blood, the CNS and so on. The organisms which invade and establish in each of these are examined in terms of the pathological responses they provoke. Finally, we look at how the conflicts we have described can be controlled or eliminated, both at the level of the individual patient and

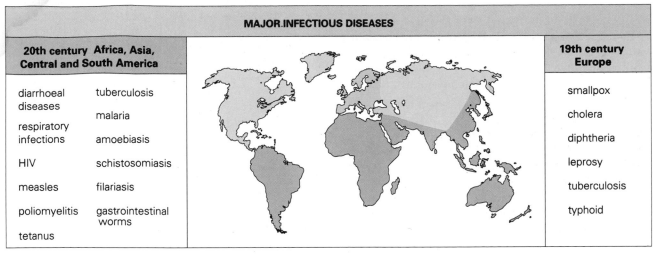

MAJOR INFECTIOUS DISEASES		
20th century Africa, Asia, Central and South America		**19th century Europe**
diarrhoeal diseases	tuberculosis	smallpox
respiratory infections	malaria	cholera
	amoebiasis	diphtheria
HIV	schistosomiasis	leprosy
measles	filariasis	tuberculosis
poliomyelitis	gastrointestinal worms	typhoid
tetanus		

Fig. 1.3 Infectious diseases responsible for major mortality and morbidity.

at the level of the community. We hope that such an approach will provide the reader with a dynamic view of host–parasite interactions and allow them to develop a more creative understanding of infection and disease.

THE VARIETIES OF MICROBES

Procaryotes and eucaryotes

A number of important and distinctive biological characteristics must be taken account when considering any organism in relation to infectious disease. One of those is the way in which the organism is constructed, particularly the way in which genetic material and cellular components are organized.

Viruses are not cells. They have genetic material – DNA or RNA – but lack cell membranes, cytoplasm and the machinery for synthesizing macromolecules, depending instead on host cells for this process. Conventional viruses have their genetic material packed in capsules. Some organisms related to viruses are even simpler in their organization. The unconventional 'slow' viruses (scrapie/Kuru group) appear to lack nucleic acid and consist only of proteinaceous infectious particles. All other organisms have a cellular organization, with bodies of single cells (most 'microbes') or of many cells. Each cell has genetic material – DNA– cytoplasm with synthetic machinery, and is bounded by a cell membrane. Two major divisions exist in the cellular organisms, the procaryotes (the bacteria) and the eucaryotes (all other organisms).

There are many differences between the two divisions (Fig. 1.4). One of the most striking is the absence of a distinct nucleus in procaryotes. Their DNA, in the form of a single, circular chromosome, is not contained in a nuclear membrane; additional DNA is carried in small plasmids. Transcription and translation from the genetic information can be carried out simultaneously. In eucaryotes DNA is carried on several chromosomes, contained within a nucleus and separated from the cytoplasm by a nuclear membrane. Transcription of DNA requires formation of messenger RNA (mRNA), and movement of mRNA out of the nucleus into the cytoplasm is necessary

before translation on ribosomes can occur. Whereas the cytoplasm of eucaryotes is rich in membrane-bound organelles (mitochondria, endoplasmic reticulum, Golgi apparatus, lysosomes) these do not occur in procaryotes. Another important difference between procaryotes and the majority of eucaryotes is that, in the first, the cell membrane (plasma membrane) is covered by a thick, protective cell wall. In Gram-positive bacteria this wall,

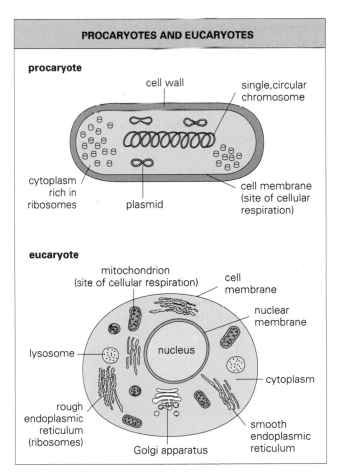

PROCARYOTES AND EUCARYOTES

procaryote

cell wall
single, circular chromosome
cytoplasm rich in ribosomes
plasmid
cell membrane (site of cellular respiration)

eucaryote

mitochondrion (site of cellular respiration)
cell membrane
nuclear membrane
lysosome
nucleus
cytoplasm
rough endoplasmic reticulum (ribosomes)
Golgi apparatus
smooth endoplasmic reticulum

Fig. 1.4 Procaryote and eucaryote cells. The major features of cellular organization are shown diagrammatically.

made of peptidoglycan, forms the external surface of the cell; in Gram-negatives there is an additional outer layer, rich in lipopolysaccharides. These layers play an important role in protecting the cell against the immune system, and against chemotherapeutic agents. They also confer antigenicity and play an important role in stimulating certain pathological responses.

Micro- and macroparasites

Identification of 'microbes' purely in terms of size and visibility distracts attention from other important characteristics. Organisms traditionally regarded as microbes are certainly small, but more significantly they can all replicate within the host. A single microbe can, theoretically, multiply to produce a very large number of progeny, thus causing an overwhelming infection. Other organisms, although microscopic in size, do not have this ability: one infectious stage matures into one reproductive stage and the resulting progeny leave the host to continue the cycle. In both clinical and epidemiological terms there is therefore an important distinction between *micro*parasites, replicating within the host (viruses, bacteria, protozoans, fungi), and *macro*parasites (worms, arthropods), where the level of infection is determined by the numbers of organisms that enter the body. Of course the boundary between micro- and macroparasites is not always a sharp one. In some macroparasites the progeny do remain within the host and infections can lead to the build-up of overwhelming numbers. *Trichinella* is one example of this type of parasite, *Strongyloides stercoralis* (another roundworm), some filarial nematodes and *Sarcoptes scabiei* (the itch mite) are others. Nevertheless, for most practical purposes, the division based on ability to replicate is helpful and informative.

Absolute size has other biologically significant implications for the host–pathogen relationship, which cut across the divisions between micro- and macroparasites. Perhaps the most important of these is the relative size of a pathogen and its host's cells. Organisms that are small enough have the ability to live inside cells and by doing so, they establish a quite different biological relationship with the host, one that influences both disease and control.

LIVING INSIDE OR OUTSIDE CELLS: THE CHOICE AND THE CONSEQUENCES

The basis of all host–pathogen relationships is the exploitation by one organism (the pathogen) of the environment provided by another (the host). The nature and degree of exploitation varies from relationship to relationship, but the pathogen's primary requirement is a supply of metabolic materials from the host, whether provided in the form of nutrients or (as in the case of viruses) in the form of nuclear synthetic machinery. The reliance of viruses upon host synthetic machinery requires an obligatory intracellular habit; viruses *must* live within host cells (Fig. 1.5). Some other groups of pathogens (*Chlamydia, Rickettsia*) can also live only within cells, but in the remaining groups different species have adopted either the intracellular or the extracellular habit (in a few cases both). Intracellular organisms take their metabolic requirements directly from the pool of

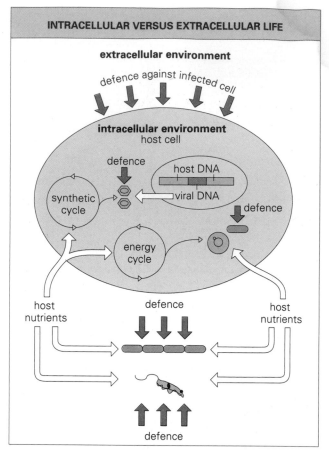

Fig. 1.5 Living inside or outside cells - the choice and the consequences. Organisms living within cells can parasitize nutrient supplies directly, as well as utilizing the energy and synthetic cycles of the cell. Viruses utilize host DNA and host synthetic machinery. Within the cell host defences do operate, but the range of options is limited; defences may kill the cell. Organisms living outside cells metabolize independently and are exposed to the full range of host defence mechanisms.

nutrients available in the cell itself, extracellular organisms from the nutrients present in tissue fluids or, occasionally, by feeding directly on host cells (for example *Entamoeba histolytica*, the organisms associated with amoebic dysentery). Macroparasites are almost always extracellular (though *Trichinella* is intracellular); many feed by ingestion and digestion of host cells, but others can take up nutrients directly from tissue fluids or intestinal contents.

Intracellular life

As will be discussed in greater detail in Section 1, Part 2, the adoption of the intracellular habit poses problems for the host which are qualitatively different from those posed by extracellular organisms. Pathogens that live within cells are, to a great degree, protected against many of the host's defence mechanisms whilst they remain there, particularly against the action of specific antibodies. Control of these infections depends therefore on the activities of short-range mediators or of cytotoxic agents, but a consequence of the latter may be the concomitant destruction of both the pathogen and the host cell, leading to tissue damage. This problem of targeting activity against the pathogen

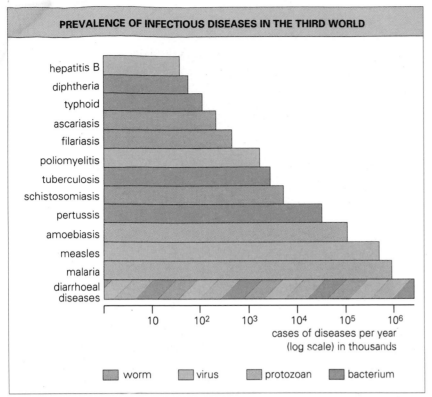

Fig. 1.6 Prevalence of diseases caused by infectious organisms in Africa, Asia and Central and South America. Data from Warren and Mahmoud, 1985.

when it lives within a vulnerable cell also arises in the use of drugs or antibiotics; selective action against the pathogen, leaving the host cell intact, is difficult to achieve. Even more problematical is the fact that many intracellular pathogens live inside the very cells that express the host's immune and inflammatory systems and thus they depress the host's defensive abilities. For example, a variety of viral, bacterial and protozoan pathogens live inside macrophages, and several viruses, including HIV, are specific for lymphocytes.

Intracellular life has many advantages for the pathogen, of which escape from host surveillance and anti microbial defences are two of the most important. However, no organism can be wholly intracellular at all times: if it is to replicate successfully transmission must occur between the host's cells and this inevitably involves some exposure, however brief, to the extracellular environment. As far as the host is concerned this extracellular phase in the development of the pathogen provides an opportunity to control infection, through defence mechanisms such as phagocytosis, antibody and complement. However, transmission between cells usually involves destruction of the initially infected cell and so contributes to tissue damage and general host pathology.

Extracellular life

Extracellular organisms are faced by constraints on their survival and development which are qualitatively different from these experienced by intracellular organisms. The most important of these are continuous exposure to components of the host's defence mechanisms, particularly antibody, complement and phagocytic cells. Living outside cells does however provide greater opportunitites for growth reproduction and dissemination than living within cells.

The characteristics of extracellular organisms lead to

pathological consequences quite different from those associated with intracellular species. These are seen most dramatically in the macroparasites, whose sheer physical size, reproductive capacity and mobility may result in extensive destruction of host tissues. The ability to spread rapidly through extracellular fluids, or to move rapidly over surfaces, also results in widespread infections being established within a relatively short time, although rapid dissemination of infection also occurs with some viruses. The rapid colonization of the entire mucosal surface of the small bowel by *Vibrio cholerae* is a good example. Successful host defence against extracellular parasites often involves problems which differ from those involved in defence against intracellular infections. These are most acute when macroparasites are concerned, because their size often renders them insusceptible to defence mechanisms that can be used against smaller organisms.

SUMMARY

We intend to provide a comprehensive cover of the organisms which cause infectious disease in man. The organisms described and discussed will therefore range from the viruses to the worms, a very considerable spread in terms of size and organizational level (arthropods will also be included in their capacity as vectors). Clearly not all the organisms included are comparable in their perceived clinical importance, although details of their prevalence (or the prevalence of diseases associated with them) may reveal a picture that is at variance with customary views of microbiological significance (Fig. 1.6). So in this book, although we will continue to place the greatest emphasis upon viral and bacterial infections, we will also emphasize infections caused by protozoa, fungi, worms and arthropods.

Further Reading ————————————————————————————————

Warren KS, Mahmoud AAF, eds. *Tropical geographical medicine*. New York: McGraw-Hill, 1985.

Mims CA. *The pathogenesis of infectious disease*. 3rd edn. London: Academic Press, 1987.

2 THE HOST–PARASITE RELATIONSHIP

INTRODUCTION

Tackling microbiology solely in terms of the identification and treatment of disease-causing organisms has the disadvantage that their biological context is distorted. A purely clinical and functional approach can convey the mistaken impression that pathogens form discrete and readily defined categories quite distinct from related, but non-pathogenic, organisms. In fact, pathogenesis is not the normal and inevitable consequence of host–microbe associations but depends on many other factors influencing the outcome of a particular association. In the study of the microbiological basis of infectious disease, host–microbe associations should be placed firmly in the context of other interspecific associations, whatever their characteristics or outcome.

SYMBIOTIC ASSOCIATIONS

All living animals are used as habitats by other organisms; no animal, however simple, is exempt from such invasion – even protozoans have their own flora and fauna. Animal evolution, the development of larger, more complex and better regulated bodies, has provided a greater number and variety of habitats for other organisms to colonize. The most complex and best regulated bodies, those of warm-blooded birds and mammals (including man), provide the most nutritious, favourable and diverse environments, and these groups of animals are the most heavily colonized.

All associations in which one species lives in or on the body of another can be grouped under a single heading – 'symbiosis' (literally 'living together'). This term has no overtones of benefit or harm, but includes a wide diversity of associations. In the past, attempts have been made to categorize types of association very specifically, but these have been doomed to failure because all associations form part of a continuum (Fig. 2.1). Three broad categories, based on the relative degrees of benefit obtained by each partner from the association, can conveniently be identified: commensalism, mutualism and parasitism.

Commensalism, mutualism and parasitism are categories of convenience

None of these categories is restricted to any particular taxonomic group. Indeed some organisms can be fitted into each of these categories depending upon the circumstances in which they live (Fig. 2.2).

Commensalism

At its simplest, a commensal association is one in which one species of organism uses the body of a larger species as its physical environment, and may make use of that environment to acquire nutrient materials.

Human beings support a very extensive commensal microbial flora on the skin, in the mouth and in the alimentary canal, as do all animals. The majority of these microbes are bacteria, and their relationship with the host may be highly specialized, with specific attachment mechanisms and precise environmental requirements. Normally the microbes are harmless, but they can become harmful if their environmental conditions change in some way (e.g. *Bacteroides, Escherichia coli, Entamoeba, Staphylococcus aureus*). Conversely, the presence of commensal microbes can benefit the host, by preventing colonization by more pathogenic species (as is well documented for the intestinal flora), and by producing metabolites that are directly used by the host (e.g. the bacteria and protozoa in the ruminant stomach). It follows that the normal definition of commensalism is one of convenience only: clearly the association can grade into either mutualism or parasitism.

Mutualism

Mutualistic relationships are characterized by reciprocal benefit between the two organisms involved. Frequently the relationship is obligatory for at least one member, and it may be so for both.

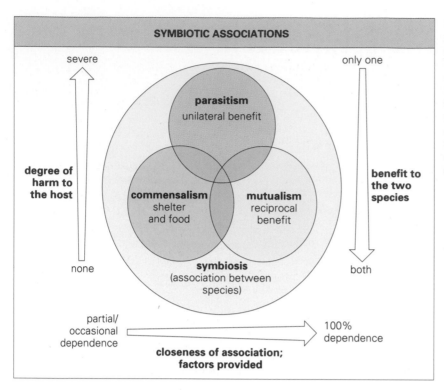

SYMBIOTIC ASSOCIATIONS

severe

only one

parasitism
unilateral benefit

degree of harm to the host

benefit to the two species

commensalism
shelter and food

mutualism
reciprocal benefit

both

symbiosis
(association between species)

partial/ occasional dependence

100% dependence

closeness of association; factors provided

Fig. 2.1 The relationships between symbiotic associations. Most species are independent of other species or rely on them only temporarily for food (predators and their prey, for example). Some species form closer associations termed 'symbioses'. Three major categories can be seen – commensalism, parasitism and mutualism, but each merges with the other; no definition separates one absolutely from the others.

CATEGORIES OF ASSOCIATION

Commensalism – large intestine of man

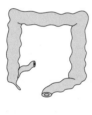

Bacteroides spp:

Host provides total environment – surface, temperature, pH, nutrition, anaerobic. Bacteria ferment digested food; host may use some fermentation products. Present in large numbers [10^{10}/g] but usually harmless; may become pathogenic if tissues damaged (surgery), if gut changes (antibiotics) or immunity reduced.

Parasitism – large intestine of man

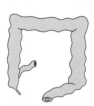

Entamoeba histolytica:

Host provides total environment (as above). Protozoan feeds on intestinal mucosa, causes formation of ulcers and dysentery, but can live as harmless commensal, feeding on digested food material.

Mutualism – rumen of cattle

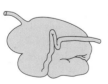

Bacteroides spp:

Host provides total environment (as above). Bacteria decompose cellulose or starch from host food, reduce to volatile fatty acids and gases. Host takes up acids across rumen wall, providing major energy sources.

Fig. 2.2 Examples of commensalism, parasitism and mutualism. The first two examples show how difficult it is to categorize any organism as entirely harmless, entirely harmful or entirely beneficial.

Clear-cut examples of mutualism are to be found in the bacterial and protozoal populations living in the stomachs of domestic ruminants. These organisms play an essential rôle in the digestion and utilization of cellulose, receiving in return both the environment and the nutritional requirements essential for their survival. Nevertheless, the dividing line between commensalism and mutualism can be hard to draw. For example, in man there is abundant evidence that good health and resistance to colonization by pathogens can depend upon the integrity of the normal commensal enteric bacteria (see Chapter 3), many of which are highly specialized for life in the human intestine, but there certainly is no strict mutual dependence in this relationship.

Parasitism

Classic definitions of parasitism state that the relationship is not only one-sided in its benefits to the parasite, but is also positively harmful to the host.

Certainly parasites do benefit from the association, being provided with their physico-chemical environment, food, respiratory and other metabolic needs and, often, the signals that regulate their developmental cycles. Equally, many parasites are certainly harmful to their hosts, but to some extent this is a view coloured by human and veterinary clinical medicine, and by the results of laboratory experimentation. In fact many 'parasites' establish quite innocuous associations with their natural hosts and are not at all pathogenic under normal circumstances (i.e. in their natural host when this is in good health); the rabies virus is one such example. This state of 'balanced pathogenicity' is generally, though not universally, accepted as being the outcome of selective pressures acting upon a relationship over a long period of evolutionary time. 'Balanced pathogenicity' may simply reflect selection of an increased level of genetically determined resistance in the

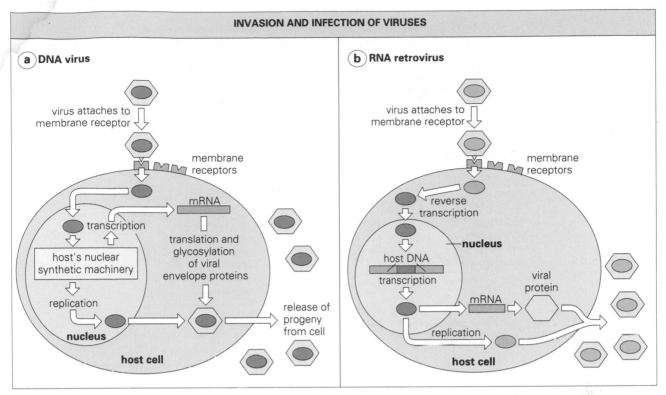

INVASION AND INFECTION OF VIRUSES

a) DNA virus

virus attaches to membrane receptor

membrane receptors

transcription

mRNA

host's nuclear synthetic machinery

translation and glycosylation of viral envelope proteins

replication

nucleus

release of progeny from cell

host cell

b) RNA retrovirus

virus attaches to membrane receptor

membrane receptors

reverse transcription

nucleus

host DNA

transcription

mRNA

viral protein

replication

host cell

Fig. 2.3 How DNA and RNA viruses invade and infect cells. a) DNA viruses such as the herpes viruses have their own DNA, and use only the host's cellular machinery to make more DNA and more virus protein and glycoprotein. These are then reassembled into new virus particles before they are released from the cell. b) RNA retroviruses (e.g. HIV) first make viral DNA, using their reverse transcriptase, insert this DNA into the host's genetic material so that viral RNA can be transcribed and then translate some of the RNA into virus protein. The viral protein and RNA are then reassembled into new particles and released.

host population. Alternatively, it may be the evolutionary norm, and 'unbalanced pathogenicity' simply the consequence of organisms becoming established in 'unnatural' (i.e. new) hosts.

So, like the other categories of symbiosis, parasitism is impossible to define exclusively, except in the context of clear-cut and highly pathogenic organisms. The belief that 'harmfulness' is a necessary characteristic of a parasite is difficult to sustain in any broader view, and the reasons for this are discussed in more detail below.

THE CHARACTERISTICS OF PARASITISM

Parasitism as a way of life has been adopted by many different groups of organisms. Some groups, such as viruses, are by their nature exclusively parasitic (see below), but the majority include both parasitic and free-living representatives. Parasites occur in all animals, from the simplest to the most complex, and are an almost inevitable accompaniment of organized animal existence. We can see, then, that parasitism has been an evolutionary success; as a way of life it must confer very considerable advantages.

Metabolic, nutritional and reproductive advantages

The most obvious advantage of parasitism is metabolic. The parasite is provided by the host with a variety of metabolic requirements, at no energy cost to itself, so it can devote a large proportion of its own resources to replication or

reproduction. This one-sided metabolic relationship shows a broad spectrum of dependence both within and between the various groups of parasites. Some parasites are totally dependent on the host, others only partly so.

At one extreme of the 'dependency' spectrum are the viruses. They possess the genetic information required for production of new viruses but none of the cellular machinery necessary to transcribe or translate this information, to assemble new virus particles, or to produce the energy for these processes. The host provides not only the basic building blocks for production of new viruses, but also the synthetic machinery and the energy to fuel this machinery (Fig. 2.3). Retroviruses go one stage further in dependence, inserting their own genetic information into the host cell DNA in order to parasitize the transcription process. Viruses therefore represent the ultimate parasitic condition and are qualitatively different from all other parasites in the nature of their relationship with the host.

The basis for the fundamental difference between viruses and other parasites is the difference between virus organization and the cellular organization possessed by all other procaryotic and eucaryotic parasites. Non-viral parasites have their own cellular machinery and multi-enzyme systems for independent metabolic activity and macromolecular synthesis (see Chapter 1). The degree to which they rely upon the host for their nutritional requirements varies very considerably and follows no consistent phylogenetic pattern, nor does it follow that smaller parasites tend to be more dependent – some of the largest parasites, the

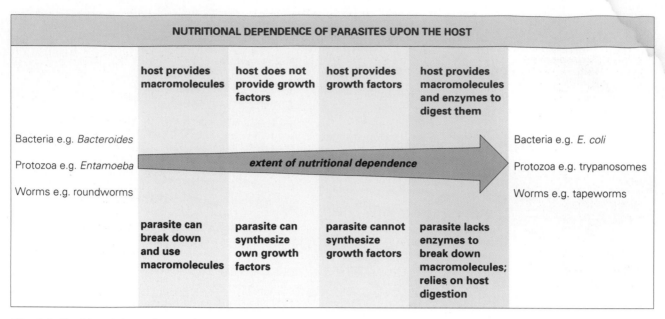

Fig. 2.4 Nutritional dependence of parasites upon the host.

tapeworms, are wholly reliant upon the host's digestive machinery to provide their nutritional needs (Fig. 2.4). All, of course, receive their nutrition from the host, but whereas some utilize macromolecular material (proteins, polysaccharides) of host origin, and digest it using their own enzyme systems, others rely on the host for the process of digestion as well, being able to take up only low molecular weight materials (amino acids, monosaccharides). Nutritional dependence may also include the provision by the host of growth factors that the parasite is unable to synthesize itself (see Fig. 2.4). All internal parasites rely upon the host's respiratory and transport systems to provide oxygen, although some respire anaerobically either in a facultative or obligate manner.

The very considerable advantage which parasitism confers, in reproductive terms, places a premium upon coordination of parasite development with the availability of suitable hosts. Indeed, one of the characteristic features of parasites is that their development may be controlled in part or completely by the host; the parasite has lost the ability to initiate or to regulate its own development (Fig. 2.5). At its simplest, host control is limited to the provision of the cell-surface molecules necessary for parasite attachment and internalization. Many parasites, from viruses to protozoa, rely on the recognition of such molecular signals for their entry into host cells, and this process provides the trigger for their replicative or reproductive cycles. Other parasites, primarily the eucaryotes, require a more comprehensive and sophisticated host signal, often a complex of host signals, to initiate and regulate their entire developmental cycle. The complexity of the signal required for development is one of the factors which determines the specificity of the host–parasite relationship. Where the availability of one of the signals is such that parasite development can occur only in one species, host specificity is high. Where many host species are capable of providing the necessary signals for a parasite, its development can be at least initiated in a wide spectrum of species, i.e. specificity is low.

Parasitism does have disadvantages

The most obvious disadvantage of parasitism (Fig. 2.6) has its basis in the coordination of parasite development by the host. No development is possible in the absence of a suitable host, and many parasites will die if no host becomes available. For this reason, several adaptations have evolved to promote a prolonged survival: virus particles, bacterial spores, protozoan cysts and worm eggs are all designed to maximize survival in the outside world, in order to increase the chances of successful host contact. The prolific replication of parasites is another device to achieve the same end. Nevertheless, where parasites fail to make contact with a host, their powers of survival are necessarily limited. Adaptation to host signals can thus have a reproductive cost, i.e. the loss of many potential parasites.

THE EVOLUTION OF PARASITISM

The facts that such a wide phylogenetic range of organisms is parasitic and that every group of animals is subject to invasion by parasites, lead to the conclusion that the development of parasitism as a way of life must have occurred at an early stage in evolution and at frequent intervals thereafter. How this process occurred is not fully understood and it may well have been different in different groups of organisms. In many, parasitism most probably arose as a consequence of accidental contacts between organism and host. Some contacts would have resulted in prolonged survival, though many would not have done so initially, and under favourable nutritional circumstances prolonged survival would have been associated with enhanced replication, giving the organism a selective advantage within the environment.

CONTROL OF PARASITIC DEVELOPMENT BY THE HOST		
stage in development of host–parasite relationship	nature of host control of parasite development	example of parasite
Entry into host body	activation signal to release infective stages	protozoan cysts
Recognition of host cells	cell membrane receptors	viruses, protozoa, bacteria
Recognition of host tissues	environmental cues (pH, redox state, $[CO_2]$, bile)	protozoa, worms
Migration through host body	environmental cues (pH, redox state, $[CO_2]$, bile)	worms
Initiation of replication or sexual reproduction	intracellular signals	viruses, bacteria, protozoa
	environmental cues (hormones, metabolites, immune effectors)	bacteria, protozoa, worms
Release from host or transmission to new host	host behaviour, host death	all parasites

Fig. 2.5 Coordination of parasite life cycles by host signals.

ADVANTAGES AND DISADVANTAGES OF PARASITISM	
advantages	disadvantages
protection from external environment	exposure to resistance mechanisms in host
provision of nuclear and cellular synthetic machinery	loss of genetic and synthetic independence
availability of metabolic requirements, especially nutritional	loss of nutritional and metabolic independence
diversion of resources into reproduction	dependence on host to control development
increase reproductive output	contact with new hosts is essential for survival of progeny
opportunity for growth and replication, i.e. to increase biomass	death of host means (usually) death of parasite

Fig. 2.6 The advantages and disadvantages of parasitism.

Bacterial parasites evolved via accidental contact

In the case of bacteria, it is easy to see how accidental contact in environments rich in free-living bacteria could lead to the successful colonization of the gastrointestinal tract and external orifices. Initially the organisms concerned would have had to be facultative parasites, capable of life both within or outside host organisms (many pathogenic bacteria still have this property, e.g. *Legionella*), but selective pressures would have forced others into obligatory

parasitism. Such a pathway is of course essentially speculative, but the close relationship of enteric bacteria such as *Escherichia coli* with free-living, photosynthetic purple bacteria gives it weight.

Many bacteria and related parasites of man and other mammals may have originated via the route of accidental contact, but it is clear that others have become adapted to these hosts after initially becoming parasitic in other species. The most obvious route by which this has taken place is through blood-feeding arthropods, as their parasites have ready access to the tissues of the animals on which the arthropods feed.

Moving into host cells

Bacteria that became parasitic by accidental contact would, at first, have lived outside host cells, but there would have been advantages in becoming intracellular. The evolution of the intracellular habit would have required further modifications to enable survival within host cells, but it could easily have been initiated by passive phagocytic uptake. Subsequent survival of the microbe would have been fortuitous and due to it having surface or metabolic properties that prevented digestion and destruction by the host cell. The success of intracellular life can be measured not only by the large number of bacteria that have adopted this habit, but also by the extent to which some organisms have integrated their biology with that of the host cell. The end-point of such integration is perhaps to be seen in the evolution of the eucaryote mitochondrion, which is widely seen as being the product of symbiotically associated heterotrophic purple bacteria (Fig. 2.7).

The pathway of virus evolution is uncertain

Clearly, parasitism by bacteria, which are undoubtedly ancient organisms (they can be traced back 3–5 billion years in the fossil record), depended upon the subsequent evolution of higher organisms to act as hosts. Whether the

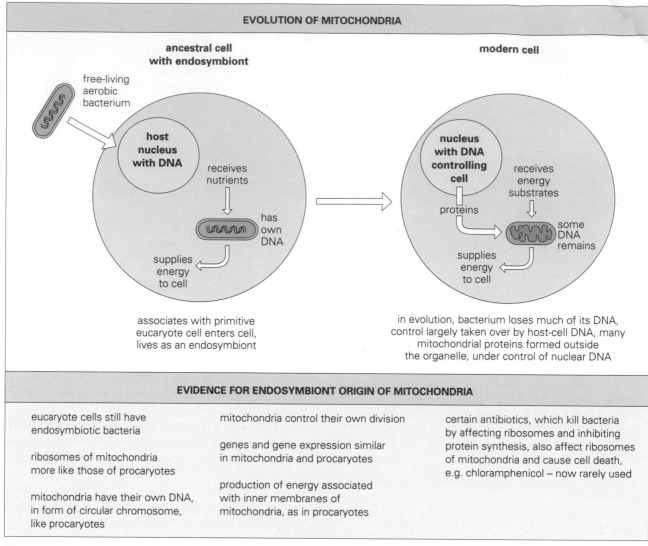

Fig. 2.7 The evolution of mitochondria. Many lines of evidence suggest that mitochondria of modern eucaryote cells evolved from bacteria that established symbiotic (mutualistic) relationships with ancestral cells.

same is true of viruses is open to question, and is dependent upon whether viruses are primarily or secondarily simple (Fig. 2.8). If viruses are seen as having evolved from cellular ancestors by a process of secondary simplification then parasitism must have evolved at some point long after the evolution of procaryotes and eucaryotes. If viruses are primitively non-cellular then it is possible that they became parasitic at a very early stage in the evolution of cellular life, at some point when, because of environmental change, independent existence became impossible. A third alternative is that viruses were never anything other than fragments of the nuclear material of other organisms and have, in effect, always been parasitic. Modern viruses may, in fact, have arisen by all three pathways.

Eucaryote parasites evolved via accidental contact

The evolution of parasitism by eucaryotes is likely to have arisen much as it may have done in procaryotes, i.e. through accidental contact and via blood-feeding arthropods (Fig. 2.9). Examples can be found among both protozoan and

worm parasites to support this view. Among the protozoa are free-living amoebae (*Naegleria* sp.) that can opportunistically invade man and cause severe, sometimes fatal, disease. There are several species of nematode worms that can live either as parasites or as free-living organisms, *Strongyloides stercoralis* being the most important in man. It is likely that trypanosomes (the protozoans responsible for sleeping sickness) were primarily adapted as parasites of blood-feeding flies and only secondarily become established as parasites of mammals.

PARASITES HAVE TO ADAPT TO HOST RESPONSES

We can view the evolution of parasitism and the adaptations necessary for life within the body of another animal as being exactly analogous to the adaptations necessary for life within any other specialized habitat: the environment for which parasites are adapted is merely one of the many to which organisms have become adapted in evolution (comparable with life in soil, freshwater, salt water,

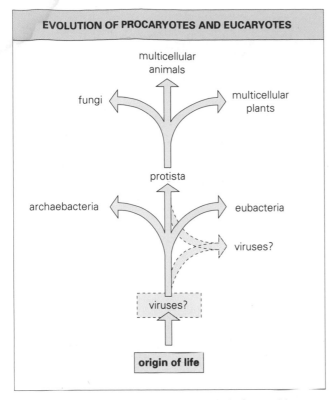

Fig. 2.8 The evolution of organisms and of parasitism. A scheme to show the possible evolution of the major groups of procaryotes and eucaryotes. The evolutionary position of viruses is unknown, they may have preceded the cellular forms of life or may be derived from them.

decaying material and so on). Such a viewpoint has some fruitful consequences, but it is always necessary to remember that in one major respect parasitism is qualitatively different from any other specialist mode of life. This difference arises from the fact that the environment in which a parasite lives, the body of the host, is not passive; on the contrary it is capable of active response to the presence of the parasite.

The attractiveness of animal bodies as environments for exploitation by parasites means that hosts are under continual pressures from infection and these pressures are increased when hosts live close together, live in insanitary conditions, or live in climates which favour the survival of parasite stages in the external world. Pressure of infection has been a major selective influence in evolution, and there is little doubt that it has been largely responsible for the development of the sophisticated inflammatory and immune responses that we see in man and in other mammals. In evolutionary terms all infection has its costs to the host because it diverts valuable resources from the activities of survival and reproduction; there has therefore been pressure to develop means of overcoming infection whether or not it causes disease. Of course, this is not the focus of clinical microbiology, which legitimately places emphasis on the costs of infection in terms of frank disease, but it should be remembered because it explains more fully the nature of the continuing battle between host and parasite – the former attempting to contain or destroy, the latter attempting to evade or suppress.

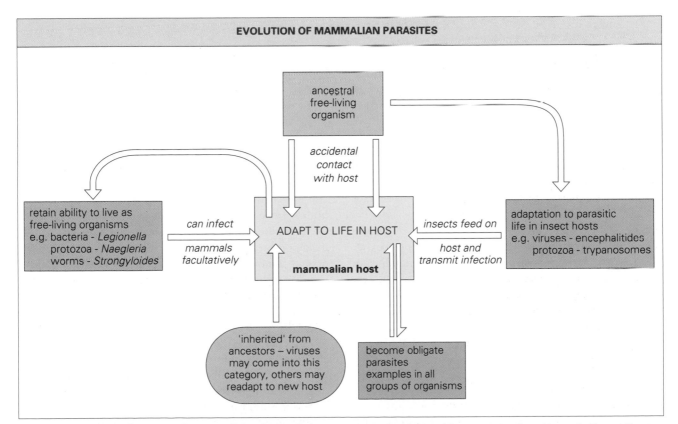

Fig. 2.9 Evolution of present-day parasites of mammals (including man). Most have probably come from free-living ancestral organisms or readapted to mammals after becoming parasites in other vertebrates. Some have been transmitted from blood-feeding insects and other arthropods, adapting to parasitize the mammal as well. Some viruses at least may have been inherited in a genetic sense, i.e. entering the host with inherited DNA.

Parasites are therefore faced not only with the problems of surviving within the environment they experience initially, but of surviving in that environment as it changes adaptively in ways likely to be deleterious to the parasite. In man and other mammals, the inflammatory and immune responses that follow the establishment of infection are the most important means by which the host can control infections by those organisms able to penetrate its natural barriers and survive within its body. These responses represent formidable obstacles to the continued survival of parasites, forcing them to evolve strategies to cope with deleterious changes in their environment. The successful parasite, therefore, is one that can cope with or evade the host's response in one of the ways shown in figure 2.10.

All of these adaptations are known to exist within different groups of parasites and they are well documented in the case of some of the major pathogens of man. Indeed their existence is often the reason why such organisms are major pathogens. Nevertheless, transmission and survival of many parasites depends upon the existence of particularly susceptible host individuals to provide a continuing reservoir of infective stages.

CHANGES IN PARASITES CREATE NEW PROBLEMS FOR HOSTS

From what has been said above, it can be appreciated that there is no such thing as a static host–parasite relationship, and that concepts of immutable 'pathogenicity' or 'harmlessness' cannot be justified. Each relationship is an 'arms race', changes in one member being countered by changes in the other. Quite subtle changes in either can completely change the balance of the relationship, towards greater or lesser pathogenicity for example.

Perhaps the most important contemporary illustration of this situation is that underlying the dramatic and explosive appearance of HIV infections in man (Fig. 2.11). Although there is still debate, a current view is that this group of viruses was originally restricted to non-human primates, but that some changes in the virus has permitted extensive infections in man. Of a different nature, but relevant to the general theme, is the acquisition of drug resistance in bacteria and protozoa (Fig. 2.12). Although the underlying genetic and metabolic changes do not by themselves influence pathogenicity, the expression of such changes in the face of intense and selective chemotherapy certainly does so.

HOSTS ADAPT TO CHANGES IN PARASITES

Changes in the host, as well as the parasite, can also alter the balance of a host–parasite relationship. A particularly dramatic example is the intense selection for resistant genotypes in rabbit populations exposed to the myxomatosis virus, which took place concurrently with selection for reduced pathogenicity in the virus itself (see Chapter 10). Because of man's long generation time there are no exactly equivalent examples, but in the context of evolutionary time there have

EVASION STRATEGIES	
strategy	**example**
Elicit minimal response	herpes simplex–survives in host cells for long periods in a latent stage–no pathology
Evade effects of response	mycobacteria–survive unharmed in granulomatous response designed to localize and destroy infection
Depress host's response	HIV–destroys T cells Malaria–depresses immune responsiveness
Antigenic change	viruses, spirochaetes, trypanosomes–all change target antigens so host response is ineffective
Rapid replication	viruses, bacteria, protozoa–producing acute infections before recovery and immunity
Survival in weakly-responsive individuals	genetic heterogeneity in host population means some individuals respond weakly or not at all, allowing organism to reproduce freely; examples in all groups

Fig. 2.10 Evasion strategies of parasites.

been major selective influences on human populations, prompting changes to permit survival in the face of life-threatening infections. A good example is the selective pressure exerted by falciparum malaria, which has been responsible for the persistence of many alleles associated with hemoglobinopathies (e.g. sickle cell hemoglobin): although these abnormalities are, to a varying degree, detrimental they are associated with resistance to infection.

Social and behavioural changes can be almost as important as genetic changes in altering host–parasite relations, both positively and negatively (Fig. 2.13). Although many bacterial infections of the intestinal tract have diminished in importance with changes in human lifestyle, there are other contemporary microbiological problems of man in the developed Western world whose onset can be traced directly to sociological, environmental and even medical change (see Fig. 2.2). A particularly good example is disease arising from domestication of pets (e.g. toxoplasmosis), because it illustrates perfectly the fact that human freedom from some infections arises primarily because of lack of contact with the organisms and not from any degree of innate resistance to the establishment of the infection itself. Diseases arising from contact with infected animals or animal products (zoonotic infections) constitute a constant threat, one that can be realized by behavioural or environmental changes which alter established patterns of human–animal contact.

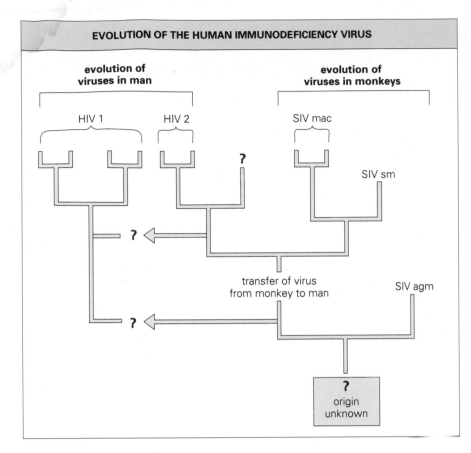

Fig. 2.11 The evolution of the HIV from its simian ancestor. A hypothetical evolutionary tree showing relationships of immunodeficiency viruses from monkeys (SIV: mac, macaque; sm, sooty mangabey; agm, African green monkey) to human immunodeficiency viruses 1 and 2 (HIV 1 and 2). It is not known how the original transfer of virus from monkeys to man took place. The rapid rate of mutation during retrovirus replication could explain the subsequent diversification of HIV in man, the different degrees of virulence and, possibly, the speed at which infections have spread.

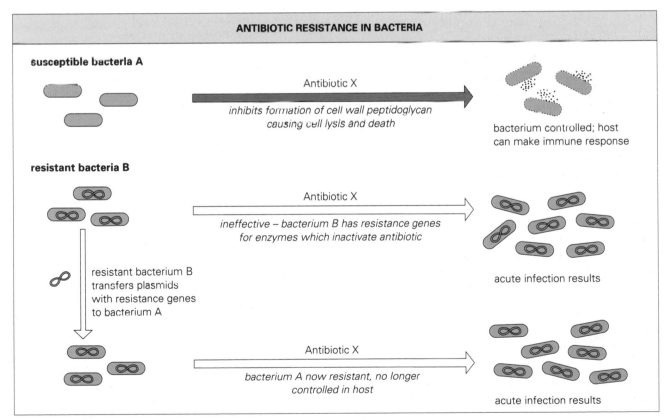

Fig. 2.12 Antibiotic resistance in bacteria. The activity of many antibiotics can be blocked by bacterial enzymes, coded for by genes located on cytoplasmic DNA in plasmids. The ability of bacteria to transfer plasmids between individual organisms means that strains or species previously susceptible to an antibiotic can acquire the ability to produce such enzymes, and so gain antibiotic resistance directly from resistant organisms. These newly resistant forms are then differentially selected under antibiotic treatment, the susceptible individuals being deleted from the population.

SOCIAL AND BEHAVIORAL CHANGES AND INFECTIOUS DISEASES		
	the causes	the results
Living	altered environments e.g. air conditioning	water used in cooling systems provides suitable growth conditions for *Legionella* bacteria spread in aerosols
Food	changes in food production and food handling practices	intensive husbandry under antibiotic protection leads to drug-resistant bacteria in animal products deep-freeze storage, fast-food production and inadequate cooking allows bacteria and toxins to enter body (e.g. *Listeria*, *Salmonella*)
Medicine	routine use of antibiotics in medicine	emergence of antibiotic-resistant bacteria as hazards to hospitalized patients (e.g. multiply-resistant *Staphylococcus aureus*)
	routine use of immunosuppressive therapy	development of opportunistic infections in patients with reduced resistance (e.g. *Pseudomonas*, *Candida*, *Pneumocystis*)
Sex	altered sexual habits	promiscuity increases transmission of sexually transmitted diseases (e.g. gonorrhoea, genital herpes, AIDS)
Water	breakdown of filtration systems overuse of limited water supplies	transmission of animal infections through contaminants leading to diarrhoeal and other infections (e.g. cryptosporidiosis, giardiasis, leptospirosis)
Pets	increase in ownership of pets, particularly exotic species	transmission of animal infections, through contamination (e.g. *Chlamydia*, *Salmonella*, *Toxoplasma*, *Toxocara*)
Travel	increased frequency of journeys to tropical and subtropical countries	exposure to organisms and vectors not found in country of origin (e.g. malaria, viral encephalitides)

Fig. 2.13 Lifestyle changes and infectious disease.

SUMMARY

Clinical microbiology will remain a field concentrated upon the identification and treatment of the major infectious diseases. It will continue, therefore, to be concerned primarily with viruses and bacteria, and will deal with these organisms in the contexts of the diseases that they cause. However, there are serious limitations in a view of microbiology that does not go beyond these priorities. Changes in medical practice, in human behaviour, in international relationships and, not least, in infectious organisms create a situation in which a wider spectrum of infectious organisms needs to be considered and a wider view of host–parasite relationships developed. Increasingly sophisticated and automated diagnostic procedures will make it as important to understand the bases of infection, resistance and pathology as it is to be able to identify organisms and prescribe appropriate prophylaxis. Such understanding, though exercised in a clinical context, must have its origin in the biological context of host–parasite relationships and in the dynamic conflict between two species, of which frank disease is merely one of the possible outcomes.

Further Reading

Mims CA. *The pathogenesis of infectious disease.* 3rd edn. London: Academic Press, 1987.

Christie AB. *Infectious diseases: epidemiology and clinical practice.* 4th edn. Edinburgh: Churchill Livingstone, 1987.

Burnet FM, White DO. *The natural history of infectious disease.* 4th edn. Cambridge: Cambridge University Press, 1972.

3 THE ORGANISMS

Contents

INTRODUCTION

Infectious diseases are caused by organisms belonging to a very wide range of different taxonomic groups. Each of these groups has its own system of classification, making it possible to identify and categorize the organisms concerned. Here, we will use these systems of classification as a convenient means of introducing the major pathogens (Fig. 3.1), all of which are discussed in detail in later chapters.

SYSTEMS OF CLASSIFICATION

The commonest classificatory system used in biology is based on the binomial system, which was established by the 18th century scientist Linnaeus. The fundamental unit of the system is the 'species', a group of similar, inter-breeding organisms, which in turn are grouped into a 'genus', a group of closely related but non-interbreeding species. Thus, each organism is identified by two names, indicating the 'genus' and the 'species' respectively. For example, the species to which humans belong is *Homo sapiens*. Although there are no other living species in the genus *Homo*, our close ancestors belonged to this genus.

In the hierarchical system of classification, related species and genera are put together into progressively broader and more inclusive categories, the final category being that of 'kingdom' (Fig. 3.2). The entire living world is divided up into a number of different kingdoms; we will be concerned with four of these – Eubacteria, Protista, Fungi and Animalia, as well as with the viruses, which do not fit into this scheme (Fig. 3.3).

CLASSIFICATION OF MAJOR PATHOGENS					
	viruses	**bacteria**	**fungi**	**protozoa**	**worms**
nucleic acids	DNA or RNA	DNA and RNA	DNA and RNA	DNA and RNA	DNA and RNA
nuclear membrane	no	no	yes	yes	yes
external cell wall	no	yes (usually) rigid peptidoglycan	yes rigid chitin	no	no
antibiotic sensitivity	no	yes	no	some	no
replication/ reproduction	within host cells	within and outside host cells by binary fission	within and outside host cells by binary fission and sexually	within and outside host cells by binary fission and sexually	outside host cells, sexually

Fig. 3.1 Characteristics of the major groups of organisms that cause infectious diseases.

CLASSIFICATION OF EUCARYOTIC ORGANISMS		
	Entamoeba histolytica	*Homo sapiens*
Species	*histolytica*	*sapiens*
Genus	*Entamoeba*	*Homo*
Family	Endamoebidae	Hominidae
Order	Euamoebida	Primates
Class	Lobosea	Mammalia
Phylum	Sarcodina	Chordata
Kingdom	Protista	Animalia

Fig. 3.2 The hierarchical system used to classify Eucaryotes.

Hierarchical classifications are meant to show the evolutionary relationships between the organisms. The lower the category (e.g. genus, family) the more recent the connection in evolution. The higher categories reflect more distant connections, but nevertheless show basic, fundamental similarities of structure and organization. These relationships are more easily determined in the eucaryotes than in the procaryotes and viruses because the range of characteristics available for classification is greater. However, modern techniques which allow comparisons between organisms to be made at the molecular level (i.e. in proteins, RNA and DNA) have made it possible to establish evolutionary relationships in these latter groups as well.

Classification of bacteria and viruses

The hierarchical system is used uniformly for eucaryotes, but not for procaryotes and viruses. A basic difficulty here is the concept of species, for which conventional criteria are less easy, or impossible, to use. Classification of bacteria is a mixture of easily determined practical characteristics (size, shape, colour, staining properties, respiration, reproduction) and of more sophisticated analysis of immunological and biochemical criteria. The former can be used to divide the organisms into conventional taxonomic groupings, as shown for the Gram-positive bacteria in figure 3.4 (see also Chapter 18). Bacteria are then classified below the species level in several different ways. Correct identification at this level is often vital in order to differentiate pathogenic from non-pathogenic forms and to allow correct treatment. For some bacteria the important sub-species groups are identified on the basis of immunological properties of their structural antigens. Cell wall, flagellar and capsule antigens are used in tests with specific antisera to define serogroups and serotypes (e.g. in salmonellae, streptococci, shigellae, *E. coli*). In others, biochemical characteristics are used to define other subspecies groupings (biotypes, strains, groups). For example certain strains of *Staphylococcus aureus* release a β-haemolysin (causing red blood cells to lyse) while others

EVOLUTIONARY RELATIONSHIPS OF KINGDOMS TO WHICH PATHOGENS BELONG
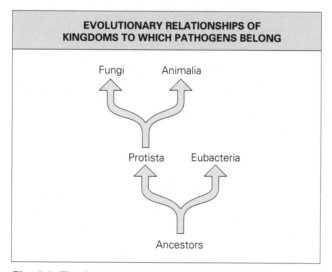

Fig. 3.3 The four kingdoms to which infectious organisms belong.

HOW BACTERIA ARE CLASSIFIED					
staining	**shape**	**respiration**	**shape/reproduction**	**genus**	**species**
Gram-positive	cocci	aerobic	clusters	*Staphylococcus*	S. aureus
			chains/pairs	*Streptococcus*	S. pyogenes
		anaerobic		*Peptococcus*	P. magnus
	bacilli	aerobic	sporing	*Bacillus*	B. anthracis
			non-sporing	*Listeria*	L. monocytogenes
		anaerobic	sporing	*Clostridium*	C. tetani
			non-sporing	*Propionibacterium*	P. acnes

Fig. 3.4 The characteristics used to classify bacteria, using Gram-positive bacteria as an example.

do not. Some streptococci release only β-haemolysins, some release both α and β, and others only α . Production of other toxins is also important in differentiating between groups, as in *E. coli*. Bacteria can also be classified below species level by their susceptibility to particular bacteriophage viruses. Phage typing is used for example in differentiating between isolates of *Staphylococcus aureus*, *Vibrio cholerae* and *Salmonella typhi*.

All expressed (i.e. phenotypic) characteristics of bacteria (as of all organisms) reflect the existence and operation of particular genes, so that direct genetic approaches can also be used in identification and classification. These include measuring total genome size (the molecular weight of the DNA present), determining the amount of the bases guanine and cytosine in the DNA, and using specific probes to identify particular sequences of DNA in the genome.

Classification of viruses is similar to that of bacteria, in that only the lower classificatory categories are used, but in general it departs even more from the system used for eucaryotes. The categories include the family and, sometimes, the genus, but the species is not used in the way that it is in other systems. In addition the names employed are much simpler than the Latin or Greek derivatives used for other organisms. Groupings are based on characteristics such as the type of nucleic acid present (DNA or RNA), the symmetry of the virus particle (icosahedral, helical or complex), the presence or absence of an external envelope, and so on, as shown for the DNA viruses in figure 3.5. As with bacteria, the equivalents of subspecies categories are used, and indeed are more easily determined than species could be, given the peculiar biological characteristics of viruses. These categories include serotypes, strains, variants, isolates etc., and are determined primarily by serological reactivity of virus material. The influenza virus, for example, can be considered as the equivalent of a genus containing three types (A,B,C). Identification of type can be carried out using the stable nucleoprotein antigen, which differs between the three types. The neuraminidase and haemagglutinin antigens are not stable and show variation within types. Characterization of these antigens in an isolate enables the particular variant to be identified (see Chapter 22). A further example is seen in adenoviruses, where the various antigens associated with a component of the capsid can be used to define groups, types and finer subdivisions.

The purposes of classification and identification

The differences between the classificatory systems used for bacteria and viruses, and those used for eucaryotes, reflects the intensely practical nature of classical microbiology as well as the practical difficulties in establishing reliable criteria for identification. In a clinical setting prompt identification of organisms is necessary so that diagnoses can be made and appropriate treatments advised. For a more complete understanding of host–parasite interactions, however, not only should the identity of an organism be known, but as much as possible of its general biology; useful predictions can then be made about the consequences of infection. For these reasons we have included outline classifications of the important pathogens, accompanied by accounts of their structure (gross and microscopic), modes of life, molecular biology, biochemistry, replication and reproduction, in the Appendix. In the present chapter we will emphasize those aspects of the cellular and molecular biology of the major groups of parasites which determine their interactions with the host, and thus the outcome of infection.

THE VIRUSES

Viruses infect every form of life, from bacteria, fungi and plants, to animals and man. They differ from all other infectious organisms in their structure and biology, particularly in the ways in which they reproduce. Although they carry conventional genetic information in their DNA or RNA, they lack the synthetic machinery necessary for this information to be processed into new virus material. A

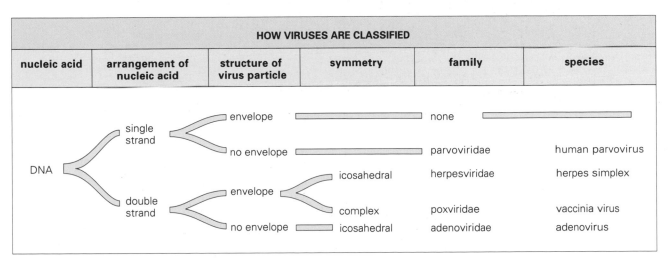

Fig. 3.5 The characteristics used to classify viruses, using DNA viruses as an example.

virus by itself is metabolically inert – it can replicate only after infection of a host cell, when it can parasitize the host's ability to transcribe and/or translate genetic information. In this process the preinfection structure of the virus is dismantled to release the genetic material. Multiple copies of this material are then synthesized and these are packaged into protein coats to produce new virus.

Viruses range in size from very small (poliovirus at 30nm), to quite large (vaccinia virus at 400 nm is as big as small bacteria; Fig. 3.6.). Their organization varies considerably between the different groups, but there are some general characteristics common to all. The genetic material, in the form of single-stranded (ss) or double-stranded (ds), linear or circular RNA or DNA, is contained within a capsule or capsid, made up of a number of individual protein molecules (capsomeres). The complete unit of nucleic acid and capsid is called the 'nucleocapsid', and often has a distinctive symmetry depending on the ways in which the individual capsomeres are assembled (Fig. 3.7). Symmetry can be icosahedral, helical or complex. In many cases the entire 'virus particle' or 'virion' consists only of a nucleocapsid. In others the virion consists of the nucleocapsid surrounded by an outer envelope or membrane (Fig. 3.8). This is generally a lipid bilayer of host cell origin, into which virus proteins and glycoproteins are inserted.

As it is the outer surface of the virus particle, whether nucleocapsid or envelope, which first makes contact with the membrane of the host cell, its structure and properties are of vital importance in understanding the process of infection. In general, naked (envelope-free) viruses are resistant and survive well in the outside world; they may also be bile resistant allowing infection through the alimentary canal. Enveloped viruses are more susceptible to environmental factors such as drying, gastric acidity and bile. These differences in susceptibility influence the ways in which these viruses can be transmitted.

Infection of host cells can be considered as a series of stages, each of which will be described separately below.

VIRUS MORPHOLOGY, VARIETY AND SIZE	
non-enveloped DNA virus	**enveloped DNA viruses**
parvovirus	herpes virus
adenovirus	poxvirus
non-enveloped RNA virus	**enveloped RNA viruses**
poliovirus	retrovirus (HIV)
rotavirus	paramyxovirus
scale: 1cm = 100nm	

Fig. 3.6 Examples of virus morphology, variety and size.

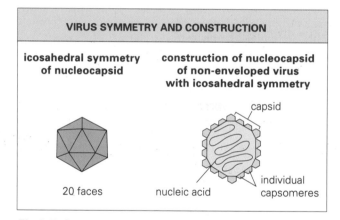

Fig 3.7 Symmetry and construction of the viral nucleocapsid.

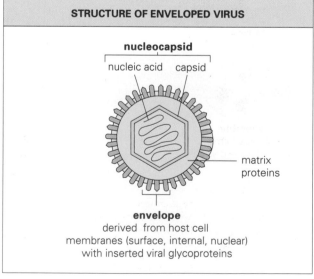

Fig. 3.8 Construction of an enveloped virus.

Infection of host cells

Attachment and penetration

Virus particles are transmitted to and enter the body of the host in a variety of ways (Fig. 3.9; see also Chapter 11). The commonest forms of transmission are via inhaled droplets (rhinovirus), in food and water (hepatitis A), direct transfer from other infected hosts (HIV), and bites of vector arthropods (yellow fever). Given the random nature of these processes, it is clear that many viruses will come into contact with hosts in which they do not normally (or cannot) develop. However viruses, like all pathogens, show host specificity, usually infecting only one or a restricted range of host species. The initial basis of specificity is the ability of the virus particle to attach to the host cell (Fig. 3.10).

The process of attachment to or adsorption by a host cell depends first upon the operation of general intermolecular forces, then upon more specific interactions between the molecules of the nucleocapsid (in naked viruses) or the virus membrane (in enveloped viruses) and the molecules of the host cell membrane. In many cases there has to be a specific interaction with a particular host molecule, which therefore acts as a receptor. Influenza virus, for example, attaches by its haemagglutinin to a glycoprotein (sialic acid) found on cells of mucous membranes as well as on red blood cells; other examples are given in figure 3.11. Attachment to the receptor is followed by entry into the host cell. After fusion of viral and host membranes, or uptake into a phagosome, the virus particle is carried into the cytoplasm across the plasma membrane (Fig. 3.12). At this stage, the envelope and/or the capsid are shed and the viral nucleic acids released.

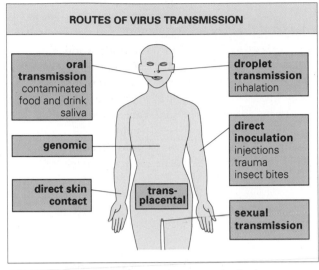

ROUTES OF VIRUS TRANSMISSION

oral transmission contaminated food and drink saliva

droplet transmission inhalation

direct inoculation injections trauma insect bites

genomic

direct skin contact

trans-placental

sexual transmission

Fig 3.9 Routes by which viruses enter the body.

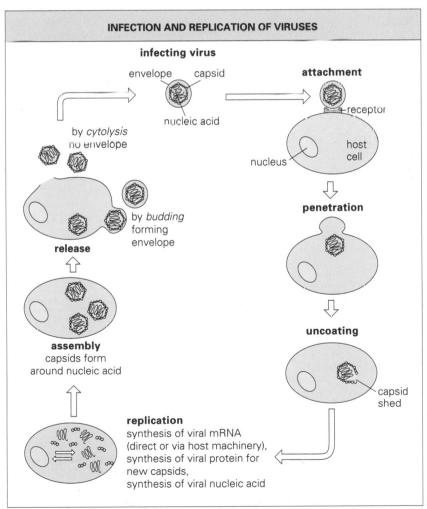

INFECTION AND REPLICATION OF VIRUSES

infecting virus

envelope   capsid

attachment

nucleic acid

receptor

by *cytolysis* no envelope

nucleus

host cell

by *budding* forming envelope

penetration

release

assembly capsids form around nucleic acid

uncoating

capsid shed

replication synthesis of viral mRNA (direct or via host machinery), synthesis of viral protein for new capsids, synthesis of viral nucleic acid

Fig. 3.10 Stages in the infection and replication of a virus.

CELL MEMBRANE RECEPTORS FOR VIRUSES	
virus	**receptor molecule**
influenza	sialic acid on glycoproteins, including the glycophorin A molecule
rabies	acetylcholine receptor
HIV	CD4 molecule on T cells
Epstein–Barr	C3d receptor on B cells
vaccinia	epidermal growth factor receptor
reovirus type 3	β-adrenergic hormone receptor
encephalomyocarditis	glycophorin A molecule
rhinovirus	intercellular adhesion molecule-1 (ICAM-1)

Fig. 3.11 Molecules used by viruses in attaching to host cells.

The virus is now no longer infective: this 'eclipse phase' persists until new complete virus particles reform after replication. The way in which replication occurs is determined by the nature of the nucleic acid concerned.

Replication

Synthesis of viral messenger RNA

Viruses contain either DNA or RNA, never both. The nucleic acids are present as single or double strands in a linear (DNA/RNA) or circular (DNA) form. The total genetic information (genome) of the virus may be carried on a single molecule of nucleic acid or on several molecules. With this diversity it is not surprising that the process of replication in the host cell is also diverse. In viruses containing DNA, messenger RNA (mRNA) can be formed using the host's own RNA polymerase to transcribe directly from the viral DNA. The RNA of viruses cannot be transcribed in this way, as host polymerases do not work from RNA molecules. If transcription is necessary, the virus has to provide its own polymerases. These may be carried in the nucleocapsid, as one of the few other molecules present, or may be synthesized after infection.

RNA viruses produce mRNA by several different routes (Fig. 3.13). In double-stranded (ds) RNA viruses, one strand is first transcribed by viral polymerase into mRNA. In single-stranded (ss) RNA viruses there are three distinct routes to the formation of mRNA. Where the single strand has the positive sense (+ve) configuration, i.e. has the same base sequence as that required for translation, it can be used directly as mRNA. Where the strand has the negative sense (-ve) configuration it must first be transcribed, using viral polymerase, into a positive sense strand, which can then act as mRNA. Retroviruses follow a completely different route. Their positive sense ssRNA is first made

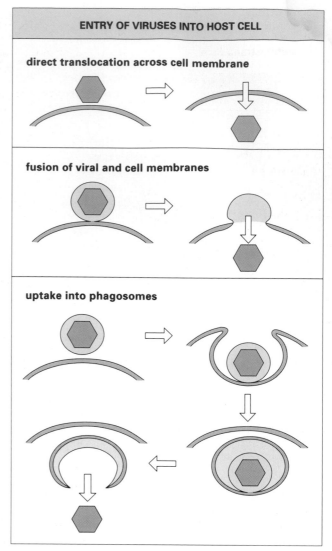

Fig. 3.12 Three ways in which viruses enter host cells.

into a negative sense ssDNA, using the viral reverse transcriptase enzyme carried in the nucleocapsid. Double-stranded DNA is then formed, which enters the nucleus and becomes integrated into the host genome. This integrated viral DNA is then transcribed by host polymerase into mRNA.

Translation of viral messenger RNA

Once viral mRNA has been formed, translation occurs in the host cytoplasm, using host ribosomes to synthesize viral proteins (Fig. 3.14). Viral mRNA, which is usually 'monocistronic' (i.e. has a single coding region) can displace host mRNA from ribosomes so that viral products are synthesized preferentially. In the early phase, the proteins produced (enzymes, regulatory molecules) are those that will allow subsequent replication of viral nucleic acids; in the later phase, the proteins necessary for the formation of the capsid are produced.

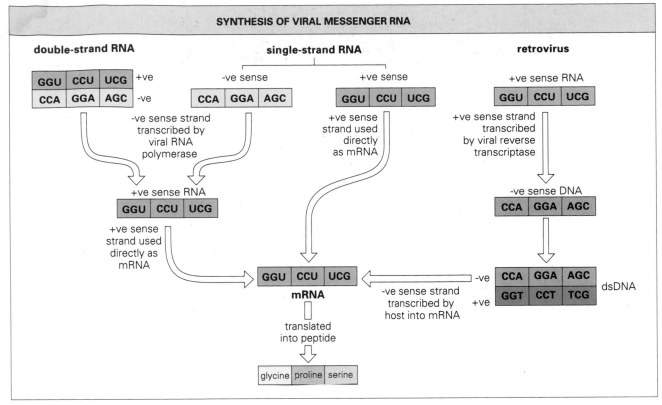

Fig. 3.13 The ways in which genomic RNA of RNA viruses is transcribed into messenger RNA prior to translation into proteins.

In viruses where the genome is contained within a single nucleic acid molecule, translation produces a large multifunctional protein, a polyprotein, which is then cleaved enzymatically to produce a number of distinct proteins. In viruses where the genome is distributed over a number of molecules, several mRNAs are produced, each being translated into separate proteins. After translation the proteins may be glycosylated, again using host enzymes.

Replication of viral nucleic acid

In addition to producing molecules for the formation of new capsids, the virus must replicate its nucleic acid to provide genetic material for packaging into these capsids. The way in which this is done again varies considerably. In positive sense, single-strand RNA viruses such as the poliovirus, a polymerase translated from viral mRNA produces negative-sense RNA from the positive sense template, which is then repeatedly transcribed into more positive strands. Further cycles of transcription then occur, resulting in the production of very large numbers of positive strands, which are packaged into new particles using structural proteins translated earlier from mRNA (Fig. 3.15).

In negative-sense, single-strand RNA viruses (rabies virus) transcription by viral polymerase produces positive sense RNA strands from which new negative-sense RNA is produced (see Fig. 3.15). In the rabies virus this replication occurs in the host cell cytoplasm, but in others (e.g. measles and influenza virus) replication takes place within the nucleus, large numbers of negative-sense RNA molecules being transcribed for new particles.

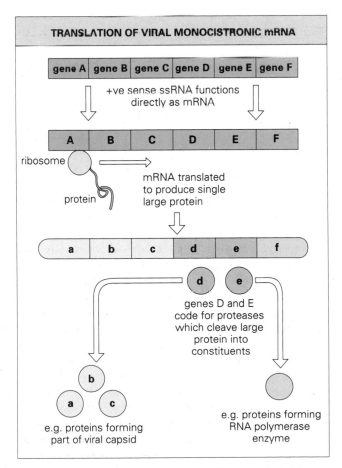

Fig. 3.14 Translation and cleavage of viral proteins from messenger RNA.

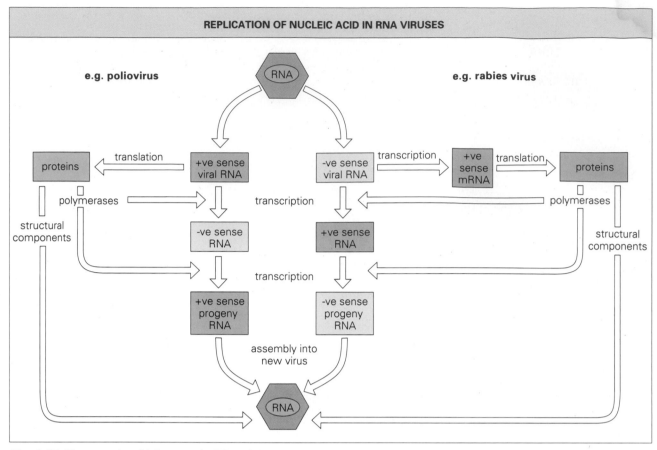

Fig. 3.15 The ways in which genomic RNA of RNA viruses is replicated.

Nucleic acid replication follows a similar pattern in double-stranded RNA viruses (e.g. rotavirus), in that positive sense RNA strands are produced. These then act as templates in a subviral particle, for the synthesis of new negative sense strands to restore the double-stranded condition.

Replication of viral DNA occurs in the host nucleus, except in the case of poxviruses where it takes place in the cytoplasm. Viral DNA may become complexed with host histones to produce stable structures. In herpes viruses, mRNA translated in the cytoplasm produces a DNA polymerase that is necessary for the synthesis of new viral DNA; adenoviruses use both viral and host enzymes for this purpose. In retroviruses, synthesis of new viral RNA occurs in the nucleus, host RNA polymerase transcribing from the viral DNA that has become integrated into the host genome (see Fig. 3.13). Hepatitis B virus, a double-stranded DNA virus, is unique in using a single-strand RNA intermediate, transcribed from its DNA, in order to synthesize new DNA.

Assembly and release of new virus particles
Assembly of virus particles involves the association of replicated nucleic acid with newly synthesized capsomeres to form a new nucleocapsid. This may take place in the cytoplasm or in the nucleus of the host cell. Enveloped viruses go through a further stage before release. Envelope proteins and glycoproteins, translated from viral mRNA, are inserted into areas of the host cell membrane (usually the plasma membrane). The progeny nucleocapsids associ-

ate specifically with the membrane in these areas, via the glycoproteins, and bud through it (Fig. 3.16). As a result the new virus acquires the membrane plus viral molecules as an outer envelope (see also Chapter 22). Viral enzymes (e.g. the neuraminidase of influenza virus) may assist in this process. Host enzymes (e.g. cellular proteases) may also play an important role in cleaving the initial large envelope proteins, a process that is necessary if the progeny viruses are to be fully infectious. In the case of herpes viruses, acquisition of a membrane occurs as the nucleocapsids bud from the inner nuclear membrane. Release of enveloped viruses can occur without causing cell death so that infected cells may continue to shed virus particles for long periods.

Insertion of viral molecules into the host cell membrane results in the host cell becoming antigenically different, in that non-self molecules are presented to the immune system. Expression of viral antigens in this way is a major factor in the development of anti-viral immune responses.

The outcome of infection

Lytic, persistent and latent infections
Although infection by viruses does not always result in the immediate death of the host cell, in 'lytic' infections it does. The virus goes through a cycle of replication, producing many new virus particles. Release of these particles is associated with lysis, i.e. destruction of the cell. This is

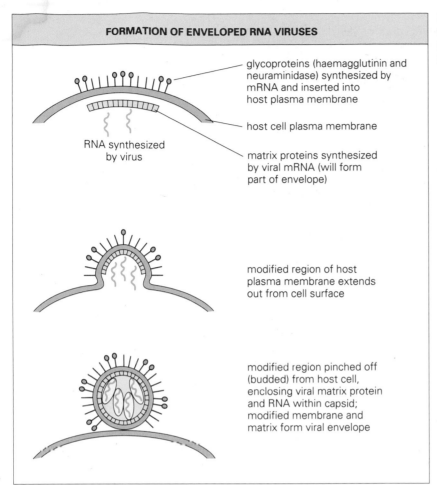

FORMATION OF ENVELOPED RNA VIRUSES

glycoproteins (haemagglutinin and neuraminidase) synthesized by mRNA and inserted into host plasma membrane

host cell plasma membrane

RNA synthesized by virus

matrix proteins synthesized by viral mRNA (will form part of envelope)

modified region of host plasma membrane extends out from cell surface

modified region pinched off (budded) from host cell, enclosing viral matrix protein and RNA within capsid; modified membrane and matrix form viral envelope

Fig. 3.16 Release of enveloped RNA virus by budding through host cell membrane. Influenza A virus is shown in this example.

the typical consequence of infection with polio- or influenza virus. With other infections, such as hepatitis B, the cell may remain alive and continue to release virus particles at a slow rate. These 'persistent' infections are of great epidemiological importance, as the infected person may act as a symptomless carrier of the virus, providing a continuing source of infection (see Chapter 15). In both lytic and persistent infections the virus undergoes replication; in latent infections it remains quiescent. The genetic material of the virus may exist in the host-cell cytoplasm (herpes virus) or be incorporated into the genome (retroviruses), but replication does not take place until some signal triggers a release from latency. When this occurs viral replication begins and may then produce a lytic infection. The stimuli that result in release are not fully understood in all cases. In herpes simplex infection stress can activate the virus, resulting in an active infection seen as cold sores. With HIV, antigenic stimulation of infected cells may provide the signal which leads to activation.

Transformation and oncogenes

Lytic, persistent and latent infections involve essentially normal host cells, although the activity of the virus may severely disrupt cellular metabolic and regulatory processes. Some viruses, however, have the capacity to 'transform' the host cell, malignant transformation being the change of a differentiated host cell into a tumour or cancer cell (see Chapter 16). Characteristic of such transformed cells

are changes in morphology, behaviour and biochemistry, and loss of controlled growth patterns. Transformed cells lose contact inhibition, continue to divide, and form random aggregations. They become invasive and can form tumours if injected into animals. However, not all transformed cells give rise to harmful tumours *in vivo*. Warts, for example, are benign growths caused by one group of papovaviruses.

Cancer-inducing viruses are found in several different groups and include both DNA and RNA viruses (see Chapter 16). Although the end results of transformation may be similar, the mechanisms involved differ between different viruses. However, all involve interference with the normal regulation of division and response to external growth-promoting and growth-inhibiting factors. These changes come about after viral nucleic acid is incorporated into the host genome. In one of the best-analysed cases, that of the Rous sarcoma virus (a retrovirus which causes cancer in chickens), transformation arises from the introduction into the host genome of a viral 'oncogene', the *src* gene. This codes for enzymes (tyrosine-specific protein kinases) involved in phosphorylation of tyrosine residues in target proteins. Several growth-regulating factors act through specific membrane receptors that have tyrosine-specific protein kinase activity i.e. they phosphorylate tyrosine residues in target proteins; one result of up-regulation of this activity, therefore, is that normal host cell growth regulation is lost.

EXAMPLES OF RETROVIRAL ONCOGENES			
class of gene product	oncogene	virus	disease
Tyrosine kinases	*fms* *ros* *src* *yes*	FeLV ALV ALV ALV	⎤ ⎥ sarcoma ⎥ ⎦
Serine/threonine kinases	*mos*	MuLV	sarcoma
Growth factors	*sis*	FeLV	sarcoma (platelet-derived growth factor)
Growth factor receptor	*erb*B	ALV	erythroid leukaemia (epidermal growth factor)
Hormone receptor	*erb*A	ALV	erythroid leukaemia (thyroid hormone)
GTP-binding proteins	Ha-*ras* Ki-*ras*	MuLV MuLV	sarcoma erythroid leukaemia
DNA-binding proteins	*myb* *myc* *fos*	ALV ALV/FeLV MuLV	myeloblast leukaemia carcinoma osteosarcoma

Fig. 3.17 Oncogenes – gene products, viruses known to carry them, and associated animal diseases. ALV/FeLV/MuLV, avian, feline and murine leukaemia viruses.

More than 20 retroviral oncogenes are now known, and these can be grouped into classes based on the nature and function of their gene products (Fig. 3.17). Only one retrovirus (human T cell leukaemia virus, HTLV 1 and 2) is of major importance as a cancer-causing virus in man. Paradoxically this neither possesses a viral oncogene nor directly activates a cellular oncogene (see below). By contrast, several retroviruses are known to cause cancers in animals.

Viral and cellular oncogenes – which came first?

Oncogenes are designated by short acronyms, preceded by 'v' if a viral oncogene is described (e.g. v-*myc*) or by 'c' if a cellular (host) oncogene (e.g. c-*myc*). DNA probes made from copies of the Rous sarcoma virus *src* oncogene have revealed complementary DNA in both infected and normal chicken cells, as well as in cancerous and normal human cells. This striking finding has since been repeated with many other retroviral oncogene sequences. Although this is a surprising finding, it has to be seen in context – retroviral-related gene sequences can make up as much as 0.03–0.3% of the mammalian genome. What is surprising is that oncogene sequences have been identified in a wide variety of animals, from man to fruit-flies, implying that they are conserved because of some valuable function. We are faced then with a chicken-and-egg situation; which came first, host or viral oncogenes? The fact that host oncogenes contain introns, whereas viral oncogenes do not, and that their chromosomal positions are fixed, imply that they, and not the viral forms, are the original genes. Viral oncogenes are therefore considered to have arisen from incorporation of host oncogenes into the viral genome during viral replication.

From what we now know about the gene products of viral oncogenes we can guess that cellular oncogenes (or 'proto-oncogenes') probably play an important role in host cell-growth regulation. They may code for growth factors themselves, for cell-surface receptor molecules which bind specific growth factors, for components of intracellular signalling systems, or for DNA-binding proteins which act as transcription factors.

The Rous sarcoma virus *src* oncogene is incorporated within the viral genome adjacent to the gene coding for viral envelope proteins (Fig. 3.18). Unlike other strongly transforming viruses the Rous virus has all three genes (*gag*, *pol* and *env*) necessary for replication; in the others (termed 'defective' transforming viruses), incorporation of an oncogene results in deletion of genetic material in the regions coding for the *pol* and/or *env* genes, so preventing replication. This becomes possible only with help from genetically complete helper viruses

Oncogenes can be carried from one cell to another within the same host, or from one host to another. This can occur through 'vertical' transmission (from mother to offspring) through passage of viruses in gametes, across the placenta or in milk. It can also occur by 'horizontal' transmission, the virus passing in saliva, urine, etc. (see Chapter 11).

Transformation of a cell occurs when viral oncogenes are incorporated into the host genome (as in Rous sarcoma virus) or when viral DNA is inserted near to a cellular oncogene. The former may be due to mutations in the oncogene sequence while in the viral genome (single base changes in cellular oncogenes being known to confer the ability to transform normal cells). The latter may reflect altered expression of the host oncogene, through disturbance of normal regulatory influences. Altered expression can occur whether the insertion is of a retroviral oncogene or of non-oncogenic viral DNA; it can also occur as a result

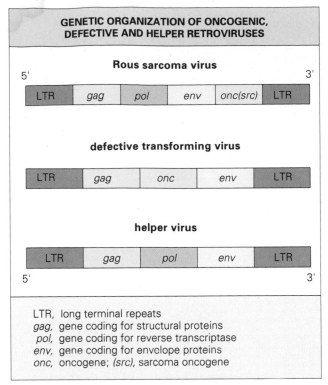

GENETIC ORGANIZATION OF ONCOGENIC, DEFECTIVE AND HELPER RETROVIRUSES

Rous sarcoma virus

5'   3'

| LTR | gag | pol | env | onc(src) | LTR |

defective transforming virus

| LTR | gag | onc | env | LTR |

helper virus

| LTR | gag | pol | env | LTR |

5'   3'

LTR, long terminal repeats
gag, gene coding for structural proteins
pol, gene coding for reverse transcriptase
env, gene coding for envelope proteins
onc, oncogene; (src), sarcoma oncogene

Fig. 3.18 Rous sarcoma virus can transform the host cell and replicate because it has both the oncogene *src* and a complete genome. Some transforming viruses are defective – they carry the oncogene, but lack genes for full replication. Helper virus can supply these genes.

of exposure to a variety of carcinogens. The products of cellular oncogenes are normally used in series to regulate cellular proliferation in a carefully controlled manner. Viral oncogene products, or over-expressed cellular oncogene products, short-circuit and overload this complex control system, with the result that cell division is unregulated.

Major groups of viruses

The classification of viruses into the major groups (families) is based upon a few simple criteria. These include the type of nucleic acid in the genome, the number of nucleic acid strands and their polarity, the mode of replication, and the size, structure and symmetry of the virus particle. Within each family are a number of genera containing the individual species of virus, details of which are given in the Appendix. The characteristics of the major groups and their most important members are summarized in figure 3.19.

THE BACTERIA

Bacteria are ubiquitous. Many are of direct or indirect benefit to man, either because of the uses to which they can be put commercially or because of the roles they play in maintaining the environment in which we live. Compared with the huge numbers of species of free-living bacteria there are relatively few which cause disease, but some of these have had an enormous impact upon human welfare. Their importance has focussed attention accordingly, so that the majority are now well-known and well-studied. Nevertheless, new pathogens continue to emerge and the significance of previously unrecognized infections becomes apparent. A recent and dramatic example of this concerns infection with *Legionella*, the cause of Legionnaires' disease.

Classification of the bacteria is well-established and uses both phenotypic and genotypic data. For the purposes of clinical microbiology the former are of most practical value, and rest on an understanding of bacterial structure and biology.

Structure

Bacteria are 'procaryotes' (see Chapter 2) and have a characteristic cellular organization (Fig. 3.20). Their genetic information is carried in a long, double-stranded, circular molecule of DNA. By analogy with eucaryotes this can be termed a 'chromosome', but the organization of the genome is different in that no introns are present, the DNA comprising a continuous coding sequence of genes. The chromosome is not localized within a distinct nucleus; no nuclear membrane is present and the DNA is tightly coiled into a region known as the 'nucleoid'. In some species extrachromosomal DNA is also present, carried in small, circular plasmids. The cell cytoplasm contains many ribosomes, but no other organelles and many of the metabolic functions performed in eucaryote cells by membrane-bound organelles such as mitochondria are carried out by the cell membrane. In all bacteria except mycoplasmas the cell is surrounded by a complex cell wall, the nature of which forms an important classificatory characteristic (see below). External to this wall may be capsules, flagella and pili. These outer layers and external structures play important roles in the host-parasite relationship.

Cell wall

The nature of the cell wall determines the classification of a bacterium as a Gram-positive or Gram-negative organism. Gram staining is a basic microbiological procedure for detection and identification (see Chapter 18). The main structural component of the cell wall is a 'peptidoglycan' (mucopeptide or murein), a mixed polymer of hexose sugars (*N*-acetylglucosamine and *N*-acetyl muramic acid) and amino acids. In Gram-positive bacteria this forms a thick (20–80nm) layer external to the cell membrane, and may contain other macromolecules. In Gram-negative species the peptidoglycan layer is thin (5–10nm) and is overlaid by an outer membrane, anchored to lipoprotein molecules in the peptidoglycan. The principle molecules of the outer membrane are lipopolysaccharides and lipoprotein (Fig. 3.21).

The polysaccharides and charged amino acids in the peptidoglycan layer make it highly polar, providing the bacterium with a thick hydrophilic surface. It is this property which allows Gram-positive organisms to resist the activity of bile in the intestine. Conversely, the layer is digested by lysozyme, an enzyme present in body secretions, which therefore has bactericidal properties. Synthesis of peptidoglycan is disrupted by penicillin and cephalosporin antibiotics (see Chapter 35).

MAJOR GROUPS OF VIRUSES						
DNA viruses						
virus family	**envelope present**	**capsid symmetry**	**particle size (nm)**	**DNA mol. wt (x10⁻⁶)**	**DNA structure***	**medically important viruses**
Parvoviridae	no	icosahedral	22	2	ss linear	B19 virus
Papovaviridae	no	icosahedral	55	3–5	ds circular, supercoiled	papilloma virus , polyomavirus (JC, BK)
Adenoviridae	no	icosahedral	75	23	ds linear	adenovirus
Hepadnaviridae	yes	icosahedral	42	1.5	ds incomplete circular	hepatitis B virus
Herpesviridae	yes	icosahedral	100**	100–150	ds linear	herpes simplex virus, varicella-zoster virus, cytomegalovirus, Epstein–Barr virus
Poxviridae	yes	complex	250x400	125–185	ds linear	smallpox virus, vaccinia virus
RNA viruses						
virus family	**envelope present**	**capsid symmetry**	**particle size (nm)**	**DNA mol. wt (x10⁻⁶)**	**RNA structure***	**medically important viruses**
Picornaviridae	no	icosahedral	28	2–3	ss linear, non-segmented, +ve sense	poliovirus, rhinovirus, hepatitis A virus, enteroviruses
Reoviridae	no	icosahedral	75	15	ds linear, 10 segments	reovirus, rotavirus, Colorado tick fever
Togaviridae	yes	icosahedral	40–70	4	ss linear, non-segmented, +ve sense	rubella virus, yellow fever virus
Retroviridae	yes	icosahedral	100	7†	ss linear, 2 segments, +ve sense	HIV, HTLV
Coronaviridae	yes	helical	100	5	ss linear, non-segmented, +ve sense	coronavirus
Calciviridae	no	icosahedral	35–40	2.6	ssRNA +ve sense	Norwalk agent
Orthomyxoviridae	yes	helical	80–120	4	ss linear, 8 segments, -ve sense	influenza virus
Paramyxoviridae	yes	helical	150	6	ss linear, non-segmented, -ve sense	measles, mumps, parainfluenza, respiratory syncytial viruses
Rhabdoviridae	yes	helical	75x180	3–4	ss linear, non-segmented, -ve sense	rabies virus
Arenaviridae	yes	helical	80–130	5	ss circular, 2 segments with cohesive ends, -ve sense	lymphocytic choriomeningitis virus
Bunyaviridae	yes	helical	100	5	ss circular, 3 segments with cohesive ends, -ve sense	California encephalitis, sandfly fever viruses
Filoviridae	yes	complex	80x(800–900)	4.2	ss RNA, -ve sense	Marburg, Ebola virus

* ss, single stranded; ds, double stranded
** the herpesvirus nucleocapsid is 100nm, but the envelope varies in size; the entire virus can be as large as 200nm in diameter
† retrovirus RNA contains 2 identical molecules of mol. wt 3.5 x10⁶

Fig. 3.19 Summary of major families of viruses. The scrapie type agents (responsible for Kuru, Creutzfeld-Jacob disease) are not included because they are not viruses and their status remains unclear (see Appendix).

In Gram-negative bacteria the outer membrane is also hydrophilic, but the lipid components of the constituent molecules give hydrophobic properties as well. Entry of hydrophilic molecules such as sugars and amino acids is necessary for nutrition, and this is achieved through special channels or pores, formed by proteins called 'porins'. The lipopolysaccharide (LPS) in the membrane confers both antigenic properties (the 'O antigens' from the carbohydrate chains) and toxic properties (the 'endotoxin' from the lipid A component; see Chapter 16).

In the Gram-positive mycobacteria the peptidoglycan layer has a different chemical basis for cross-linking to the lipoprotein layer and the outer envelope contains a variety of complex lipids (mycolic acids). These create a waxy layer which alters both the staining properties of these organisms (the so-called acid-fast bacteria) and gives considerable resistance to drying and other environmental factors. Mycobacterial cell wall components also have a pronounced adjuvant activity – i.e. they promote immunological responsiveness.

External to the cell wall may be an additional capsule of high molecular weight polysaccharides that give a slimy surface (in the case of the anthrax bacillus the capsule is made of amino acids). This surface provides protection against phagocytosis by host cells and is therefore important in determining virulence, as has been shown with *Streptococcus pneumoniae*, where only a few capsulated organisms cause a fatal infection in mice whereas unencapsulated mutants cause no disease.

Many bacteria possess flagella, long helical filaments extending from the cell surface (Fig. 3.22), which generate propulsive forces and enable bacteria to move in their environment. These may be restricted to the poles of the cell, singly (polar) or in tufts (lopotrichous), or distributed over the general surface of the cell (peritrichous). The structure of bacterial flagella is quite different from that of eucaryote flagella and the forces that result in movement are generated quite differently (being ATP-independent). The ability to move allows positive and negative responses to chemical stimuli (chemotaxis). Flagella

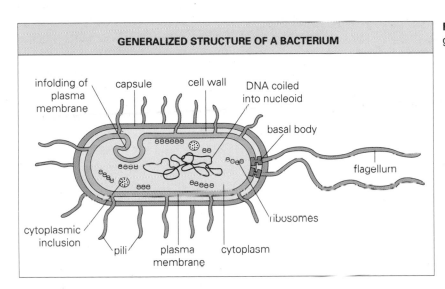

GENERALIZED STRUCTURE OF A BACTERIUM

infolding of plasma membrane

capsule

cell wall

DNA coiled into nucleoid

basal body

flagellum

ribosomes

cytoplasmic inclusion

pili

plasma membrane

cytoplasm

Fig. 3.20 Diagrammatic structure of a generalized bacterium.

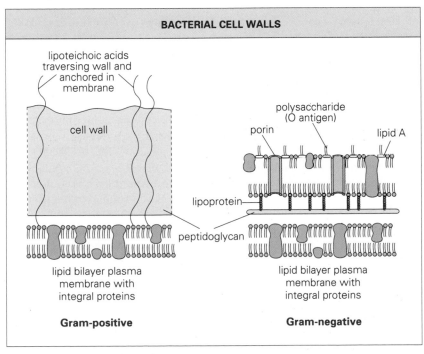

BACTERIAL CELL WALLS

lipoteichoic acids traversing wall and anchored in membrane

cell wall

polysaccharide (O antigen)

porin

lipid A

lipoprotein

peptidoglycan

lipid bilayer plasma membrane with integral proteins

lipid bilayer plasma membrane with integral proteins

Gram-positive

Gram-negative

Fig. 3.21 Construction of the cell walls of Gram-positive and Gram-negative bacteria.

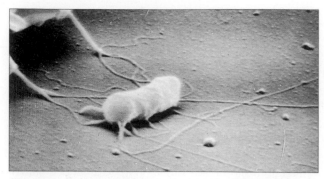

Fig. 3.22 Scanning electron micrograph of *Salmonella* showing peritrichous flagella. Courtesy of DK Banerjee.

are built of protein components (flagellins) which are strongly antigenic. These antigens, the H antigens, are important targets of protective antibody responses.

Pili are another form of bacterial surface projection, somewhat more rigid than flagella and not concerned with movement. Their function is that of attachment, either to other bacteria (the 'sex' pili) or to host cells (the 'common' pili). Adherence to host cells involves specific interactions between component molecules of the pili (adhesins) and molecules present in host cell membranes. For example, the adhesins of *E. coli* interact with fucose/mannose molecules on the surface of intestinal epithelial cells (see Chapter 25). Where there are many pili present they may help to prevent phagocytosis, thus reducing host resistance to bacterial infection. Although immunogenic, their antigens can be changed, allowing the bacteria to avoid recognition by the immune system. The mechanism for this 'antigenic variation' has been elucidated in the gonococci, and is known to involve recombination of genes coding for 'constant' and 'variable' regions of pili molecules.

Metabolism and growth

All pathogenic bacteria are 'heterotrophic', that is they obtain energy by oxidation of preformed organic molecules acquired from their environment. Metabolism of these molecules (carbohydrates, lipids and proteins) yields adenosine triphosphate (ATP) as an energy source. Metabolism may be aerobic, where the final electron acceptor is O_2, or anaerobic, where the final acceptor is an organic molecule. In the first, complete utilization of an energy source such as glucose produces 38 molecules of ATP; in the second, where respiration is incomplete, only 2 molecules of ATP are produced. Anaerobic respiration (fermentation) is therefore less efficient, but can be used where substrates are readily available, as they usually are in the host's body. The requirement for O_2 in respiration may be 'obligate' or it may be 'facultative', some organisms being able to switch between aerobic and anaerobic respiration. Those that use fermentation pathways often use the major product pyruvate in secondary fermentations by which additional energy can be generated.

Bacteria obtain nutrients primarily by taking up small molecules (amino acids, oligosaccharides, small peptides) across the cell wall; in Gram-negative species larger molecules can also be taken up and used, after preliminary digestion in the periplasmic space. Uptake and transport of nutrients into the cytoplasm is achieved by the cell membrane, using a variety of transport mechanisms, including facilitated diffusion and active transport. Oxidative metabolism also takes place at the membrane-cytoplasm interface.

Some species require only minimal nutrients in their environment, having considerable synthetic powers, whereas others have complex nutritional requirements. *Escherichia coli* for example can be grown in media providing only glucose and inorganic salts; streptococci, on the other hand, will grow only in complex media providing them with many organic compounds.

Regulation of enzyme production

Bacteria have a number of processes to regulate the production of enzymes, allowing them to maximize their utilization of nutrients in the environment (Fig. 3.23). One is 'enzyme repression', where the presence in the environment of the end product of a particular metabolic pathway inhibits the production of enzymes involved in that pathway. The end product acts as a 'co-repressor' and turns off mRNA production. This prevents synthetic sources being wasted. Another process is 'enzyme induction', where synthesis of an enzyme is turned on when the appropriate substrate is present. In this case, the substrate (or a similar molecule) acts as the 'inducer', and induces the production of mRNA coding for the enzyme concerned. In both these processes, control of mRNA production is achieved at the level of transcription from DNA, the inducer or co-repressor combining with a repressor protein to alter its activity. Inducers prevent repressor proteins from binding to the operator region of the genes to be transcribed, allowing transcription to take place; co-repressors activate repressor molecules and allow them to bind to the operator and thus prevent transcription. Both affect the transcription of a consecutive group of genes, an 'operon', controlled by a single operator region.

Enzyme induction and repression are examples of negative control; positive control mechanisms also exist, as for example in 'catabolite repression'. Here, when glucose is present there is repression of enzymes necessary for utilization of other substrates. When glucose is exhausted levels of cyclic AMP (cAMP) rise in the cell. cAMP binds to a 'catabolite activator protein' which facilitates binding of RNA polymerase to DNA, permitting transcription of the mRNA necessary for synthesis of the other enzymes. A further form of control is 'attenuation', seen for example in the synthesis of tryptophan. If this is readily available in the cell a leader peptide is translated from the mRNA, as this is transcribed from the operon coding for the proteins needed for tryptophan synthesis. This peptide blocks further transcription. If no tryptophan is available, no leader peptide is translated and transcription continues.

Reproduction

The normal form of reproduction in bacteria is binary fission. During this process the circular DNA is replicated bidirectionally along each strand, each daughter cell receiving one original and one replicated strand.

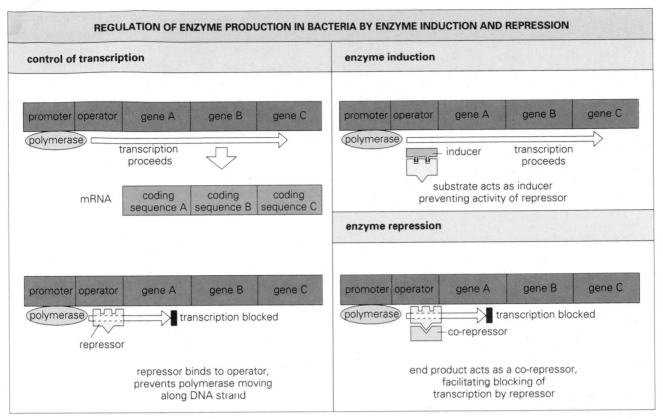

REGULATION OF ENZYME PRODUCTION IN BACTERIA BY ENZYME INDUCTION AND REPRESSION

control of transcription

enzyme induction

enzyme repression

Fig. 3.23 How bacteria regulate the production of enzymes used to metabolize substrates in their environment. On the left is a schematic diagram showing generalized transcription control; on the right how substrate molecules or end product molecules turn on or turn off transcription from DNA.

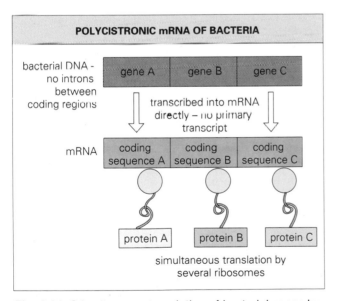

POLYCISTRONIC mRNA OF BACTERIA

Fig. 3.24 Stimultaneous translation of bacterial genes by multiple ribosomes.

Replication of DNA is closely coupled to growth and cell division, the cell membrane participating in this by providing a septum between daughter cells to which newly replicated DNA adheres.

Under optimum conditions bacteria can divide rapidly. *Escherichia coli* can divide every 20 minutes *in vitro* in a nutrient medium and every 1 to 2 hours in a minimal medium. Under *in vitro* conditions growth and division

continue until the population size is such that all available nutrients are exhausted, or toxic metabolic products accumulate to a point at which the bacteria are adversely affected. *In vivo* conditions are different in that nutrient supplies are renewable and harmful metabolites may be removed. On the other hand, growth and division may be inhibited by the immune response (or by antibiotic treatment).

The capacity for rapid growth and division is a major factor in bacterial pathogenesis. Only a few organisms are necessary to initiate a potentially overwhelming infection. However, not all pathogens are capable of rapid division. Mycobacteria, for example, divide only once every 24 hours and infections develop relatively slowly.

Rapid growth and division requires an abundant and efficient machinery by which mRNA can be translated into new proteins. Bacterial cytoplasm is rich in ribosomes, with RNA accounting for 35% of dry weight in rapidly growing cells. This abundance means that the rate of protein synthesis is controlled not by altering the time taken to synthesize the end product but by the frequency with which translation occurs on each mRNA molecule. Bacterial mRNA is polycistronic, and can be translated by several ribosomes simultaneously (Fig. 3.24). Similarly, more mRNA can be produced by multiple transcription occurring simultaneously.

This emphasis on protein synthesis in bacteria makes their synthetic processes an obvious target for chemotherapy. Many antibiotics function by inhibiting transcription (e.g. rifampicin) or translation (e.g. streptomycin, erythromycin).

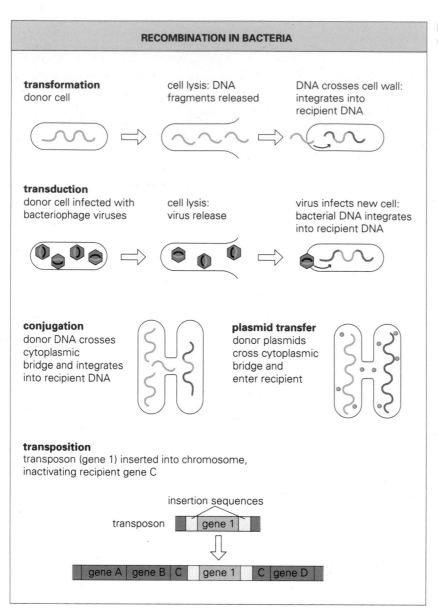

Fig. 3.25 Five ways in which genetic recombination can take pace.

Mutation and recombination

Bacteria are haploid organisms, the chromosome encoding one copy of each gene. Replication of the DNA is a precise process which results in each daughter cell acquiring an exact copy of the parental genome. Changes in the genome can occur by two processes, mutation and recombination, resulting in progeny which may express phenotypic characters that are different from those of the parent. This is of considerable significance in terms of virulence and drug resistance.

Mutation. Changes in the sequence of nucleotides in the DNA molecule can occur spontaneously or under the influence of external agents (mutagens). Point mutations – changes in single nucleotides – alter the triplet code, but may not necessarily result in detectable changes in the proteins eventually transcribed. More comprehensive changes in the DNA involve deletion, replacement, insertion or inversion of several or many bases. The majority of these changes are likely to be harmful to the organism, but a few may be beneficial and confer some selective advantage through production of different proteins.

Recombination. New genotypes can arise in bacteria not only by mutation but also by recombination between the genetic material of one individual and that of another. Recombination brings about larger changes in the genome and, since these normally involve functional genes, are likely to be expressed phenotypically. Recombination occurs in several ways – transformation, transduction, conjugation and plasmid transfer, and transposition (Fig. 3.25).

Transformation. Certain bacteria are able (competent) to take up DNA fragments from related species across the cell wall. Such DNA fragments may be present in the environment of a competent cell as a result of lysis of other organisms, with release of their DNA and its breaking up into smaller lengths. After uptake the double-stranded donor DNA is reduced to a single strand, which can then be integrated into the recipient's chromosome. This process was first discovered in *Streptococcus pneumoniae*, where it was associated with conversion of a non-encapsulated strain of pneumococcus into an encapsulated strain.

Transduction. In this form of recombination DNA is introduced into a recipient cell by a bacteriophage – a bacteria-infecting virus particle. As part of their replication cycle in viruses, bacteriophages may incorporate host-cell DNA into their capsids, either random components of host DNA or specific genes located near to the site of insertion of viral nucleic acid. If these altered particles successfully infect another cell then the bacterial DNA carried can be integrated into the chromosome of the recipient. Such transfer occurs in two forms: 'generalized' transduction, when the virus particle carries only bacterial DNA and 'specialized' transduction, when both viral DNA and bacterial DNA are carried. In the latter case only a specific set of host genes are transduced; in the former almost any host gene may be involved.

Conjugation and plasmid transfer

In addition to the DNA contained within the chromosome, bacteria may have extrachromosomal DNA in the form of plasmids. These are independent, self-replicating units, some of which are relatively large (conjugative plasmids, 60–120 kilobases) and carry several genes, while others are quite small (non-conjugative plasmids, 1.5–15 kilobases). The genes carried control several activities, both of the plasmid itself and of the parent cell. These include plasmid replication, production of sex pili, conjugation, DNA transfer, antibiotic resistance and toxin production. Our knowledge of the detailed behaviour of plasmids and of their molecular biology comes largely from studies with *E. coli.*

Conjugation involves contact between two bacteria and transfer of DNA (plasmid and/or chromosomal) from one to the other. Conjugative plasmids have genes which code for the formation of sex pili, and for changes to the cell surface which allow contact to be made and maintained. Other plasmid genes regulate the transfer of plasmid DNA and of donor chromosomal DNA across a cytoplasmic bridge. In *E. coli* one class of well-studied conjugative plasmids (F factor) becomes stably integrated into the bacterial chromosome, allowing high frequency recombination (Hfr) of quite large regions of bacterial DNA to take place. Such integration characterizes particular strains of bacteria – the Hfr strains. In low frequency recombination, the F factor is not integrated to the same degree, but is cut out of the host chromosome and transferred with only a small part of the genome. The F factor, like other conjugative plasmids, is transferred between cells at high frequency, rapidly spreading throughout a population. Transfer initiated by conjugative plasmids can result in the mobilization and transfer of non-conjugative plasmids as well.

The significance of plasmid transfer. Plasmid transfer is important because it occurs rapidly within populations, so spreading genes controlling new phenotypic characteristics, including the ability to produce new molecules. The most significant of these are concerned with antibiotic resistance and toxin production.

The widespread use of antibiotics against bacteria has applied a strong selection pressure in favour of organisms able to resist antibiotic agents. In the majority of cases resistance is due to the presence of resistance genes in transferable plasmids (R factors; see Chapter 35). These are known to have existed before the era of mass antibiotic treatments, but they have become widespread in many species as a result of selection. R factors are transferred in conjugations involving one of two types of sex pili (F or I pili) and may carry genes for resistance to several drugs. For example common R factors confer resistance to tetracycline, chloramphenicol, streptomycin and sulphonamides; many others exist conferring resistance to a wide spectrum of antibiotics. Recombination can occur between R factors, so that individual plasmids can be responsible for new combinations of multiple drug resistance. In most cases resistance results from the ability of the cell carrying the plasmid to synthesize new enzymes which inactivate the antibiotic.

In addition to drug resistance, plasmids can also confer the properties of toxin production and cellular adhesion upon bacteria. For example, the virulent enterotoxigenic forms of *E. coli* produce a plasmid-coded enterotoxin which alters fluid secretion by intestinal cells. In *Staphylococcus aureus* both an enterotoxin and a number of enzymes involved in bacterial virulence (haemolysin, fibrinolysin) are coded for by plasmid genes. The production of toxins by bacteria and their pathological effects are discussed in detail in Chapter 16.

The ability of plasmids to insert DNA sequences into chromosomal DNA is not only important to the clinical microbiologist because of its effects on resistance and virulence, but also as a means of manipulating organisms experimentally. Plasmids have been exploited by molecular biologists as vectors for DNA in genetic engineering (Fig. 3.26). They can now be constructed artificially and used to transfer genes across species barriers, so that defined gene products can be synthesized in large quantities by suitable recipient organisms.

Transposons

In both procaryotes and eucaryotes it is possible for genes, or groups of genes to move from one site to another in the genome. The ability to make such transpositions reflects the existence of moveable (transposable) elements - 'transposons' or 'jumping genes'. These genetic units have characteristic, specific base sequences (insertion sequences) flanking their genes, which make it possible for the transposon DNA to be inserted at homologous insertion sequences within existing DNA strands (see Fig. 3.25). There are a number of types of transposon known, but for our purposes the most important are those present in plasmids, which allow the integration of plasmids, or plasmid DNA, into the bacterial genome. Drug resistance genes are often components of plasmid transposons. The ease with which transposons can move into or out of DNA sequences means that interchange can occur between plasmids and host, from host into plasmids, and from plasmid to plasmid, thus providing for extensive genetic recombination.

Endospores

Certain bacteria are able to form highly resistant spores – endospores – within their cells, which enable them to survive

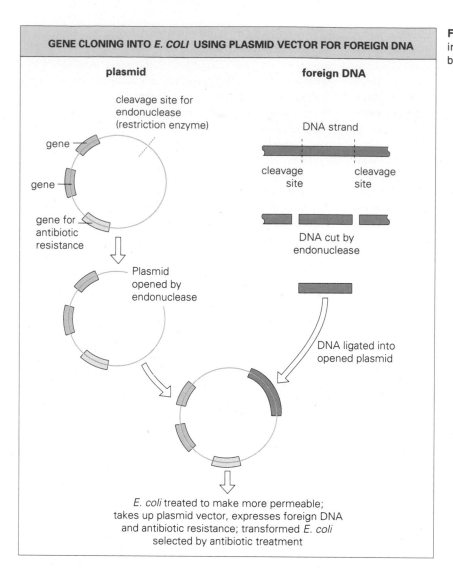

GENE CLONING INTO *E. COLI* USING PLASMID VECTOR FOR FOREIGN DNA

plasmid

foreign DNA

gene

gene

cleavage site for
endonuclease
(restriction enzyme)

DNA strand

cleavage
site

cleavage
site

gene for
antibiotic
resistance

Plasmid
opened by
endonuclease

DNA cut by
endonuclease

DNA ligated into
opened plasmid

E. coli treated to make more permeable;
takes up plasmid vector, expresses foreign DNA
and antibiotic resistance; transformed *E. coli*
selected by antibiotic treatment

Fig. 3.26 The use of plasma vectors to introduce foreign DNA into *E. coli* – a basic step in gene cloning.

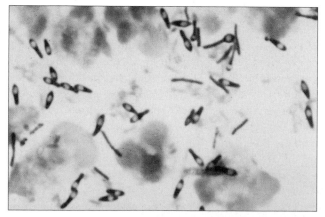

Fig. 3.27 *Clostridium tetani* with terminal spores.

adverse conditions. They are formed when the cells are unable to grow, for example when environmental conditions change or when nutrients are exhausted, but never by actively growing cells. The spore has a complex multi-layered coat surrounding a new bacterial cell, which forms the core of the endospore. There are many differences in composition between endospores and normal cells, notably the presence of dipicolinic acid and a high

calcium content, both of which are thought to confer the endospore's extreme resistance to heat and chemicals.

Because of their resistance, spores can remain viable in a dormant state for many years, reconverting rapidly to normal existence when conditions improve. When this occurs a new bacterial cell grows out from the spore and resumes vegetative life.

Endospores are abundant in soils and those of the pathogenic bacteria *Clostridium* and *Bacillus* are a particular hazard (Fig. 3.27). Tetanus and anthrax, caused by these bacteria are both associated with endospore infection of wounds, the bacteria developing from the spores once in appropriate conditions.

Major groups of bacteria

The major groups of bacteria causing infectious disease in man can be considered either in terms of their classification into families, genera etc., or in terms of their most important diagnostic features. In this book we shall use the second, as this reflects the characteristics most likely to be relevant to clinical practice. These include staining properties, shape and respiratory pathways. More detailed summaries of members of these major groups are shown in figure 18.18, and are included in the Appendix.

THE FUNGI

Although the fungi are eucaryotes, they belong to a king-dom that is distinct from plants and animals. Characteristically they are multinucleate or multicellular organisms, with a thick cell wall, growing as thread-like fila-ments (hyphae), but many other growth forms occur. Of these the mushroom and the single-celled yeasts are most familiar. Fungi are ubiquitous in the environment as decomposers, and are of enormous importance commer-cially in baking, brewing and in pharmaceutics. They are also a world-wide cause of human infections. Free-living fungi digest material externally by release of enzymes; pathogenic species can also do this, but are able to take up nutrients directly from host tissues.

Major groups of fungi

The fungi responsible for human diseases can be divided into two major groups either on the basis of their growth forms, or on the type of infection they cause (Fig. 3.28). Pathogens exist as branched filamentous forms or as yeasts; some show both growth forms in their cycle and are known as 'dimorphic' fungi. In filamentous forms (e.g. *Trichophyton*) the hyphae extend as a result of transverse divisions, the mass of hyphae forming a 'mycelium'. Asexual reproduction results in the formation of sporangia which liberate the spores by which the fungus is dispersed; spores are a common cause of infection after inhalation. In yeast-like forms (e.g. *Cryptococcus*) the characteristic form is the single cell, which reproduces by division. Budding may also occur, with the 'bud' remaining attached, forming pseudohyphae. Dimorphic forms (e.g. *Histoplasma*) form hyphae at environmental temperatures but occur as yeast cells in the body, the switch being tem-perature-induced. *Candida* is an important exception in the dimorphic group, showing the reverse condition and forming hyphae within the body.

Two types of infection (mycoses) are recognized – super-ficial mycoses, where the fungus grows at the body surface in skin, hair and nails, and deep mycoses, with involvement of internal organs. The first are usually mild, but the second can be life threatening. The superficial pathogens are spread by direct contact, whereas the deep mycoses often result from the opportunistic growth of fungi in indi-viduals with impaired immune competence (see Chapter 33). Free-living fungi can also cause disease indirectly as a consequence of toxins released into materials used as food (e.g. the aflatoxins).

Many of the fungi that cause disease are free-living organisms, and are acquired by inhalation or by entry through wounds. Some exist as part of the normal body flora (e.g. *Candida*) and are innocuous unless the body's defences are compromised in some way. The filamentous forms grow extracellularly, but yeasts can survive and mul-tiply within phagocytic cells, both macrophages and neu-trophils. Neutrophils are important defensive cells and play a major role in controlling the establishment of invad-ing fungi. Species that are too large for phagocytosis can still be killed by extracellular factors released from phago-cytes as well as by other components of the immune

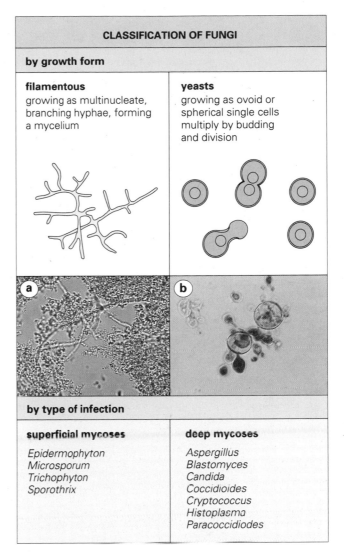

Fig. 3.28 Two ways to classify fungi that causes disease – by growth form, and by type of infection. (a) Hyphae in skin scraping from a ringworm lesion. Courtesy of DK Banerjee. (b) Spherical yeasts of *Histoplasma*. Courtesy of Y Clayton and G Midgley.

response. Some species, notably *Cryptococcus neoformans* prevent phagocytic uptake because they are surrounded by a polysaccharide capsule (see Chapter 27).

The major groups of fungi important in causing human disease are shown in figure 3.29.

THE PROTOZOA

Protozoa are single-celled eucaryotes which occur widely as free-living organisms in the environment, but which are also important parasites of humans. The prevalence of infections is greatest in warmer countries. Malaria for example is very common in tropical and subtropical regions, and is one of the world's major infectious dis-eases. Infections with other species are also common in temperate regions.

Transmission of protozoan parasites occurs in a variety of ways, the two commonest being injection via the bites of blood-sucking insects and accidental ingestion of infective stages. The geographical restriction of some species reflects both the distribution of vector insect species and

IMPORTANT FUNGAL DISEASES				
type	anatomic location	representative disease	genus of causative organism(s)	growth form
Superficial Cutaneous	hair shaft, dead layer of skin	tinea versicolor	*Malassezia*	Y
	epidermis, hair, nails	dermatophytosis (ringworm)	*Microsporum, Trichophyton Epidermophyton*	F
Subcutaneous	subcutis	sporotrichosis mycetoma	*Sporothrix* several genera	Y* F
Deep Systemic	internal organs	coccidioidomycosis histoplasmosis blastomycosis paracoccidioidomycosis	*Coccidioides Histoplasma Blastomyces Paracoccidioides*	** Y Y Y
Opportunistic	internal organs	cryptococcosis candidiasis aspergillosis	*Cryptococcus Candida Aspergillus*	Y Y† F*

Y, yeast; F, filamentous; * growth form in the body; † also forms pseudohyphae

** *Coccidioides* has an unusual growth form with yeast-like endospores within a spherule

Fig. 3.29 Summary of Fungi that cause important diseases.

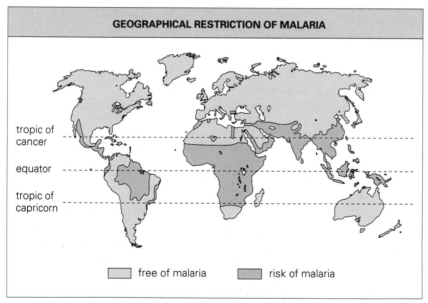

GEOGRAPHICAL RESTRICTION OF MALARIA

tropic of cancer

equator

tropic of capricorn

free of malaria   risk of malaria

Fig. 3.30 Environmental requirements for the development of malaria parasites in their mosquito host limit the distribution of the disease to the tropics.

the climatic conditions (primarily temperature) necessary for the parasites to complete their development in the insect (Fig. 3.30). Orally acquired infections are less dependent on climatic factors, although transmission by the faecal-oral route is obviously favoured by low standards of social and personal hygiene, and by increased survival of infective stages in warm, damp conditions.

Protozoa infect all the major tissues and organs of the body. They live as intracellular parasites in a wide variety of cells or as extracellular parasites in the blood, intestine or urogenital system (Fig. 3.31). Intracellular species obtain nutrients from the host cell, either by direct uptake of small molecules or by ingestion of host cytoplasm.

Extracellular species feed by direct nutrient uptake or by ingestion of host cells. Reproduction in man is usually asexual, by binary or multiple division of growing stages (trophozoites). Sexual reproduction is normally absent or restricted to the insect vector phase; *Cryptosporidium* is exceptional in undergoing sexual reproduction in man. The ability to undergo asexual reproduction gives the organism the potential for a rapid increase in number, particularly where host defence mechanisms are impaired. For this reason some protozoans are most pathogenic in the very young (particularly neonates, e.g. *Toxoplasma*) and in immunocompromised individuals (e.g. *Cryptosporidium* and *Pneumocystis* in AIDS patients).

Transmission between hosts depends on production of resistant stages, which pass out of the body and are subsequently taken up by another host. Insect vectors are also involved in transmission, infective stages developing after the insect has fed on an infected individual; these are then introduced into a new host at the next blood meal. In a few cases infection occurs by sexual contact, by inhalation or by ingestion of infective stages while these are in the body of another host.

The interface between host and parasite in protozoa is the parasite's plasma membrane. Many sophisticated strategies have evolved to avoid the consequences of immune recognition of this surface. For example, trypanosomes undergo repeated antigenic variation of surface antigens, malaria parasites show polymorphisms in dominant surface antigens, and amoebae can consume complement at the cell surface. Although intracellular stages are removed from direct contact with many effectors (notably antibody, complement and phagocytes) their antigens may be expressed at the surface of the host cell, which can then be a target for cytotoxic effectors. Survival within cells, particularly within macrophages (*Leishmania*, *Toxoplasma*) involves a variety of devices to evade or inactivate the harmful effects of intracellular enzymes or reactive oxygen and nitrogen metabolites.

Classification

Protozoa are classified into four main divisions, reflecting their structure, mobility and way of life. One division, the Sporozoa, contains only intracellular parasites. the other three include free-living as well as parasitic species - they are divided primarily on the basis of their means of locomotion (Fig. 3.32). None of the species within the ciliate group cause significant human disease. Protozoa of medical importance are summarized in figure 3.33.

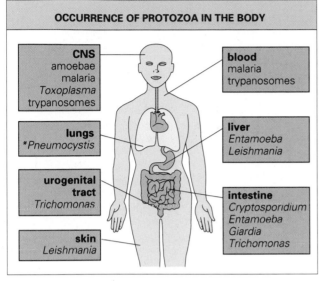

Fig. 3.31 The occurence of protozoan parasites in the body. *Included for convenience. Now believed to be a fungus.

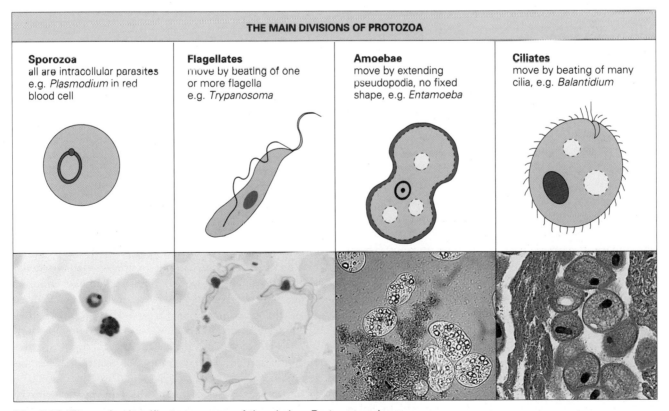

Fig. 3.32 The main classificatory groups of the phylum Protozoa and examples of disease-causing species. Courtesy of R Muller and JR Baker, WE Farrar, and J Newman.

FEATURES OF MEDICALLY IMPORTANT PROTOZOA			
location	species	mode of transmission	disease
Intestinal tract	*Entamoeba histolytica* *Giardia lamblia* *Cryptosporidium* spp.	ingestion of cysts in food	amoebiasis giardiasis cryptosporidiosis
Urogenital tract	*Trichomonas vaginalis*	sexual	trichomoniasis
Blood and tissue	*Trypanosoma* spp. *T. cruzi*	reduviid bug	trypanosomiasis Chagas' disease
	T. gambiense *T. rhodesiense*	tsetse fly	sleeping sickness
	Leishmania spp. *L. donovani*	sand fly	visceral leishmaniasis (kala-azar)
	L. tropica, L. mexicana *L. braziliensis*	sand fly	cutaneous leishmaniasis mucocutaneous leishmaniasis

	Plasmodium spp.
	    P. vivax, P. ovale
	    P. malariae
		Anopheles mosquito	malaria

	P. falciparum	*Anopheles* mosquito	malaria
	Toxoplasma gondii	ingestion of cysts in raw meat; contact with soil contaminated by cat faeces	toxoplasmosis
	Pneumocystis carinii	inhalation	pneumonia

Fig. 3.33 Summary of the location, transmission and diseases caused by protozoan parasites.

THE HELMINTHS

The term 'helminth' is used for all groups of worms that live as parasites. As far as man is concerned, there are three main groups to consider, the tapeworms (Cestoda), flukes (Trematoda or Digenea) and roundworms (Nematoda) (Fig. 3.34). The first two belong to the same phylum, the Platyhelminthes or flatworms, the third are included in separate phylum.

Helminths are generally large organisms with a complex body organization. Although invading larval stages may measure only 100 to 200 microns adult worms may be centimetres or even metres long. As with the protozoa they are commonest in warmer countries, but the intestinal species occur quite frequently in temperate regions.

Transmission occurs in four distinct ways (Fig. 3.35): 1) by the faecal–oral route, when infective eggs or larvae are swallowed; 2) by swallowing an infective larval stage in the tissues of another host; 3) by active penetration of the skin by the larval stage; and 4) in the bite of a blood-sucking insect.

The greater frequency of helminth infections in tropical and sub-tropical regions reflects the climatic conditions that favour survival of infective stages, the socio-economic conditions that facilitate faecal-oral contact, the practices involved in food preparation and consumption, and the availability of suitable vectors. Those species that are more generally distributed are commonest in children, in individuals closely associated with domestic animals and in individuals with particular food preferences.

With the exception of the nematode *Trichinella spiralis*, helminths are extracellular parasites, their size dictating this habit. Many occur in the intestine (adult tapeworms exclusively so), whereas others live in the deeper tissues. Almost all organs of the body can be parasitized. Flukes and nematodes actively feed on host tissues or on the intestinal contents; tapeworms have no digestive system and absorb pre-digested nutrients. Unlike the protozoa, the majority of helminths do not replicate within the host. In its simplest form, as in intestinal worms, sexual reproduction results in production of eggs which are released from the host in faecal material. In others, eggs and larvae may accumulate within the host but do not mature. Certain tapeworm larval stages can reproduce asexually in man. The nematode *Strongyloides* is exceptional in that eggs produced in the intestine can hatch there, releasing infective larvae which reinvade the body – the process of 'autoinfection'. A similar phenomenon occurs with the tapeworm *Taenia solium*.

The outer surfaces of helminths provide the primary host-parasite interface. In tapeworms and flukes the surface is a complex plasma membrane which can present antigens to the host and be damaged by effector mechanisms.

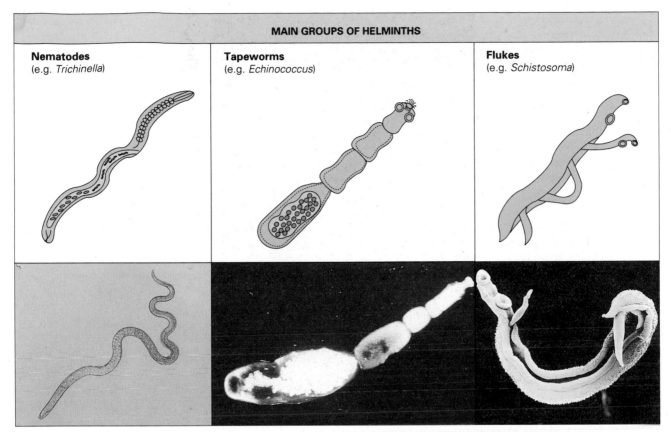

MAIN GROUPS OF HELMINTHS

Nematodes
(e.g. *Trichinella*)

Tapeworms
(e.g. *Echinococcus*)

Flukes
(e.g. *Schistosoma*)

Fig. 3.34 The main classificatory groups of parasitic worms (helminths) and examples of disease-causing species. Courtesy of R Muller and JR Baker, V Southgate and the publishers of *Systemic Parasitology*.

In both groups there are parasite-protective mechanisms which prevent the host damaging the outer surface. Thus, the nematode outer surface is a tough, collagenous cuticle which, although antigenic, is largely resistant to immune attack. However, smaller larval stages may be damaged by host granulocytes and macrophages. Worms also release large amounts of soluble antigenic material in their excretions and secretions, and this plays an important role both in immunity and pathology.

Classification

Platyhelminths, or flatworms, have flattened bodies, covered by a cytoplasmic tegument. Flukes have an anterior mouth, leading into a blindly-ending intestine, whereas tapeworms have no digestive system. Characteristically all flatworms have combinations of muscular suckers and hooks for attachment to the host. The body is muscular and mobile, and filled with reproductive organs. Most flukes are hermaphrodites apart from the schistosomes which have separate sexes. Tapeworms are hermaphrodites, with their reproductive organs replicated along the length of the body (the strobila) in a series of identical segments or 'proglottids'. Proglottids form continuously at a zone behind the head (scolex) of the worm and move along the strobila. They mature sexually, fertilization occurs, and the terminal 'gravid' proglottids become filled with mature eggs. Eventually these proglottids detach and pass out in the faeces. In both flukes and tapeworms, eggs develop into larvae that must pass through one or more

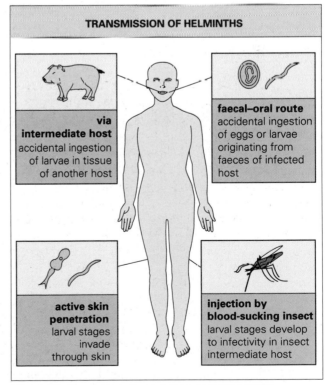

TRANSMISSION OF HELMINTHS

via intermediate host
accidental ingestion of larvae in tissue of another host

faecal–oral route
accidental ingestion of eggs or larvae originating from faeces of infected host

active skin penetration
larval stages invade through skin

injection by blood-sucking insect
larval stages develop to infectivity in insect intermediate host

Fig. 3.35 How helminth parasites enter the body.

intermediate hosts and develop into other larval stages before the parasite is again infective to man. In flukes the first intermediate host is always a snail. The only exception is the tapeworm *Hymenolepis nana*, which can go through a complete cycle from egg to adult in the same host.

The nematodes have long cylindrical bodies covered by a cuticle, with an anterior mouth and a through gut. Roundworms generally lack specialized attachment organs, but some species, notably hookworms, have well developed mouth capsules by which they can clamp onto host tissues whilst feeding (Fig. 3.36). Nematodes have separate sexes, and while most liberate fertilized eggs, *Trichinella spiralis* and the filarial worms release early-stage larvae directly into the host's body. Development from egg or larva to adult can be direct and occur in a single host, or may be indirect, requiring development in the body of an intermediate host. Classification within the nematodes is complex; for practical purposes only two categories need be considered: 1) those which mature within the gastrointestinal tract (some of which may migrate through the body during development) and 2) those which mature in deeper tissues.

Helminths and disease
All the major groups of helminths can cause human disease (Fig 3.37–3.39).

Tapeworms
Adult tapeworms, acquired by eating undercooked or raw meat containing the larval stages, frequently infect humans but are relatively harmless despite their potential for reaching a large size. Humans can also act as the intermediate hosts for certain species, and the development of larval stages in the body can cause severe disease (see Fig. 3.37).

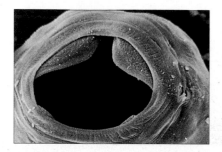 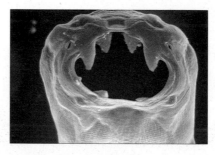

Fig. 3.36 Scanning electron micrographs of the anterior ends of adult *Necator* (a) showing cutting plates in the mouth, and *Ancylostoma* (b) showing teeth for biting into the mucosa. Courtesy of LM Gibbons.

Fig. 3.37 Summary of the location, transmission and other hosts used by tapeworms that infect humans.

HUMAN TAPEWORM INFECTIONS			
species	**acquired from**	**other hosts**	**site in humans**
adult worms			
Taenia saginata	larvae in beef	none	intestine
Taenia solium	larvae in pork	none	intestine
Diphyllobothrium latum	larvae in fish	fish-eating mammals	intestine
Hymenolepis nana	eggs, or larvae in beetles	rodents	intestine
*Hymenolepis diminuta**	larvae in insects	rats, mice	intestine
*Dipylidium caninum**	larvae in fleas	dogs, cats	intestine
larval worms			
Taenia solium (cysticercosis)	eggs in food or water contaminated with human faeces	pigs	brain, eyes
Echinococcus granulosus (hydatid disease)	eggs passed by dogs	sheep	liver, lung, brain
*Echinococcus multilocularis**	eggs passed by carnivores	rodents	liver
Pseudophyllid tapeworms* (sparganosis)	larvae in other hosts	many vertebrates	subcutaneous tissues, eyes
Taenia multiceps	eggs passed by dogs	sheep	brain, eye, subcutaneous tissue
* rare infections			

HUMAN FLUKE INFECTIONS		
species	**acquired from**	**site in humans**
Schistosoma haematobium	penetration of skin by larval stages released from snails	blood vessels of bladder
Schistosoma japonicum		blood vessels of intestine
Schistosoma mansoni		blood vessels of intestine
Clonorchis sinensis	ingesting fish infected with larval stages	liver
Fasciola hepatica	ingesting vegetation (cress) with larval stages	liver
Paragonimus westermani	ingesting crabs infected with larval stages	lungs

Fig. 3.38 Summary of the location and transmission of flukes that infect humans.

HUMAN NEMATODE INFECTIONS		
species	**acquired by**	**site in humans**
transmitted person-to-person		
Ascaris lumbricoides	ingestion of eggs	small intestine
Enterobius vermicularis	ingestion of eggs	large intestine
Hookworms		
Ancylostoma duodenale	skin penetration	small intestine
Necator americanus	by infective larvae	small intestine
Strongyloides stercoralis	skin penetration by infective larvae; autoinfection	small intestine (adults) general tissues (larvae)
Trichuris trichiura	ingestion of eggs	large intestine
transmitted person-to-person via arthropod vector		
Brugia malayi	bite of mosquito carrying infective larvae	lymphatics (adults) blood (larvae)
Onchocerca volvulus	bite of Simulium fly carrying infective larvae	skin (larvae, adults) eye (larvae)
Wuchereria bancrofti	bite of mosquito carrying infective larvae	lymphatics (adults) blood (larvae)
Loa loa	bite of deer fly carring infective larvae	tissues
zoonoses transmitted from animals		
Angiostrongylus cantonensis	ingestion of larvae in snails, crustacea	CNS (larvae)
Anisakis simplex	ingestion of larvae in fish	stomach, small intestine (larvae)
Capillaria phillipinensis	ingestion of larvae in fish	small intestine (adults, larvae)
Toxocara canis*	ingestion of eggs passed by dogs	tissues, CNS (larvae)
Trichinella spiralis*	ingestion of larvae in pork, wild mammals	small intestine (adults) muscles (larvae)

* These species are the commonest in this group

Fig. 3.39 Summary of the location and transmission of nematodes that infect humans.

Flukes

Several species of fluke can mature in humans, developing in the intestine, lungs, liver and blood vessels. The most important, both in terms of prevalence and pathology, are the blood flukes or schistosomes, the cause of schistosomiasis or bilharzia. Three main species – *S. haematobium, S. japonicum* and *S. mansoni* – are responsible for human disease, while two or three are of lesser significance (see Fig. 3.38).

Nematodes

Several of the many species of nematode that infect man are highly specific and can mature in no other host. Others have a much lower host specificity, being acquired accidentally as zoonoses, with humans acting either as the intermediate or the final host after picking up infection from domestic animals or in food (see Fig. 3.39).

THE ARTHROPODS

Human beings are attacked by a wide variety of arthropods, most of which feed briefly on blood. Many species of insects are blood feeders of this type, notably mosquitoes, midges, biting flies, bugs and fleas. Blood meals are also taken by ticks, which feed for prolonged periods after becoming firmly attached by their mouthparts. Ticks are frequently able to feed on several species of host, and many animal ticks will quite happily engorge on man. Species of mites also feed on man, chiggers, the larvae of trombiculid mites, being a familiar example. A few species (Fig. 3.40) have more permanent contact with the human, e.g. the head- and body-forms of the louse *Pediculus humanus,* and the crab louse *Phthirus pubis.* These species reproduce on the body or in clothing and can cause pathological reactions as a consequence of their feeding activity. Only one species of arthropod, the scabies mite *Sarcoptes scabei* lives permanently on man, burrowing into the superficial layers of skin (see Fig. 3.40) to feed and to lay eggs. Because of this constant association, heavy infections can build up, particularly on individuals with reduced immune responsiveness. The burrowing activity eventually leads to severe inflammatory responses and an exudate that forms an encrustation on the skin (see Chapter 28).

In addition to the discomfort and occasionally more serious consequences of arthropod infestation, there is the much greater hazard of disease transmission. Arthropods transmit pathogens of all major groups, from viruses to worms; some, e.g. mosquitoes and ticks transmit a wide variety of organisms while others, e.g. tsetse flies, transmit only one. The ways in which transmission occurs varies from the purely mechanical, where the mouthparts of the vector act as a contaminated syringe, to the biological, where the arthropod is a true host for the pathogen, which needs to undergo developmental or propagative changes before it can once again infect man. The range of pathogens transmitted in these various ways is summarized in figure. 3.41.

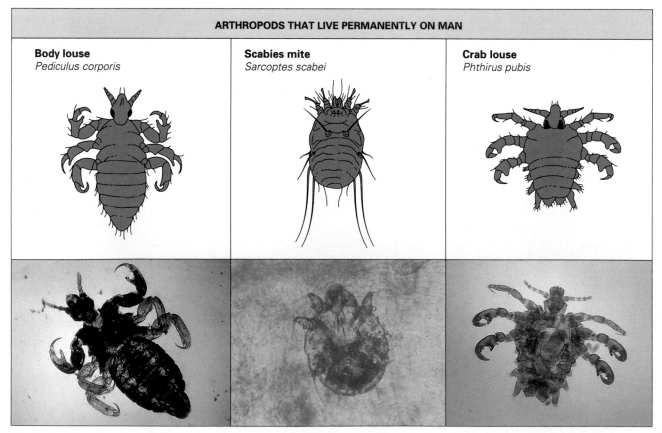

ARTHROPODS THAT LIVE PERMANENTLY ON MAN

Body louse
Pediculus corporis

Scabies mite
Sarcoptes scabei

Crab louse
Phthirus pubis

Fig. 3.40 The most important ectoparasitic arthropods that lived permanently on the human body. Courtesy of CC Kibbler and MJ Wood.

The ability of arthropods to transmit infections poses a constant threat of zoonoses to human beings. Some, such as yellow fever, have been know for many years, whereas others, such as viral encephalitides and Lyme disease, have been recognized only comparatively recently. The organisms transmitted may have evolved as mammalian pathogens that have become secondarily adapted for a phase in arthropods to improve dispersal and transmission, or may have evolved as arthropod pathogens that have become secondarily adapted to mammals.

THE NORMAL FLORA

The preceding sections have focussed primarily on organisms that are quite clearly parasites or pathogens. Their presence in the body is often associated with pathological changes and they are rarely found in healthy individuals. Identification of these organisms is therefore an important indication of actual or potential disease states. Other organisms covered in this chapter may cause disease under certain circumstances – in the newborn, in stressed, traumatized or immunocompromised individuals – but usually co-exist quite peacefully in a balanced relationship with their host. Many of these form what is termed the 'indigenous' or 'normal' flora of the body, a collection of species routinely found in the normal, healthy individual.

Some of these species are positively beneficial to the host, their importance for health sometimes being revealed quite dramatically under stringent antibiotic therapy. Although it is not possible to eliminate the normal flora of the skin or intestine, antibiotics can drastically reduce their numbers to a minimum. The host may then be overrun by introduced pathogens or by overgrowth of organisms normally present in small numbers.

The normal flora is acquired rapidly during and shortly after birth and changes continuously throughout life. The constituent organisms present at any given time reflect the age, nutrition and environment of the individual concerned. It is therefore difficult to define the normal flora very precisely, because it is to a large extent environmentally determined. This can be well illustrated by data from NASA astronauts, who were rendered relatively bacteriologically sterile by antibiotic treatment prior to their space flights. It took only six weeks after the flight for them to repopulate their flora, and the repopulating species were precisely those of their immediate neighbours. Similarly, apparently healthy children in developing countries have a quite different bowel flora from that seen in Western children. Breast-fed infants have lactic acid streptococci and lactobacilli in their gastrointestinal tract, whereas bottle-fed children show a much greater variety of organisms.

Why flora?

The term 'flora' is used because the majority of the organisms are bacteria. It has been estimated that humans have approximately 10^{13} cells in the body and something like

INFECTIOUS DISEASES TRANSMITTED BY ARTHROPODS		
	disease	arthropod vector
Viruses Arboviruses	dengue fever yellow fever encephalitides haemorrhagic fevers	mosquitoes mosquitoes mosquitoes, ticks ticks, mosquitoes
Bacteria Yersinia pestis Borrelia recurrentis Borrelia burgdorferi	plague relapsing fever Lyme disease	fleas soft ticks hard ticks
Rickettsias R. prowazeki R. mooseri R. rickettsiae R. akari	epidemic typhus endemic (murine) typhus spotted fever rickettsial pox	lice, ticks fleas ticks mites
Protozoa Trypanosoma cruzi T.b. rhodesiense T.b. gambiense Plasmodium spp. Leishmania spp.	American trypanosomiasis (Chagas disease) African trypanosomiasis (sleeping sickness) malaria leishmaniasis	reduviid bugs tsetse flies mosquitoes sandflies
Worms Wuchereria and Brugia Onchocerca	lymphatic filariasis onchocerciasis	mosquitoes simulium flies

Fig. 3.41 Summary of infectious diseases transmitted by arthropods.

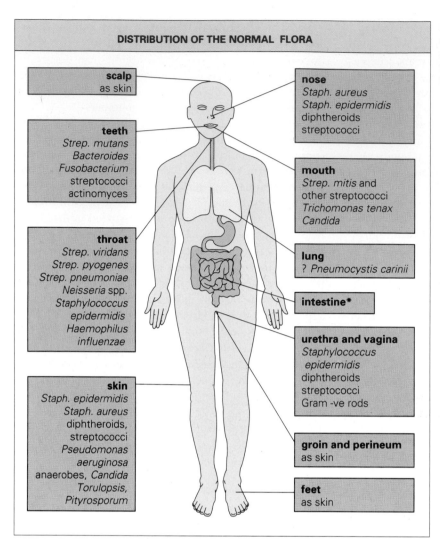

DISTRIBUTION OF THE NORMAL FLORA

scalp
as skin

teeth
Strep. mutans
Bacteroides
Fusobacterium
streptococci
actinomyces

throat
Strep. viridans
Strep. pyogenes
Strep. pneumoniae
Neisseria spp.
Staphylococcus epidermidis
Haemophilus influenzae

skin
Staph. epidermidis
Staph. aureus
diphtheroids,
streptococci
Pseudomonas aeruginosa
anaerobes, Candida
Torulopsis,
Pityrosporum

nose
Staph. aureus
Staph. epidermidis
diphtheroids
streptococci

mouth
Strep. mitis and
other streptococci
Trichomonas tenax
Candida

lung
? Pneumocystis carinii

intestine*

urethra and vagina
Staphylococcus epidermidis
diphtheroids
streptococci
Gram -ve rods

groin and perineum
as skin

feet
as skin

Fig. 3.42 Examples of organisms that occur as members of the normal flora and their location on the body. *Those found in the intestine are detailed in figure 3.43.

10^{14} bacteria associated with them, the majority in the large bowel. Members of groups such as viruses, fungi and protozoa can also be found regularly in healthy individuals, although these form only a minor component of the total population of resident organisms.

Location of the normal flora

Organisms occur in those parts of the body that are exposed to, or communicate with, the external environment, namely the skin, nose and mouth, and intestinal and urogenital tracts. Internal organs and tissues are normally sterile. A list of the main organisms found in these sites is given in figure 3.42.

Skin

Different regions of the skin support different flora, being largely determined by the degree of humidity available. Exposed dry areas have relatively few resident organisms on the surface, whereas moister areas (axillae, perineum, between toes, scalp) support much larger populations. *Staphylococcus epidermidis* is one of the commonest species, making up some 90% of the aerobes and occurring in densities of 10^3-10^4 per cm²; *Staph. aureus* may be present in the moister regions.

Anaerobic diphtheroids occur below the skin surface in hair follicles, sweat and sebaceous glands, *Propionibacterium acnes* being a familiar example. Changes in the skin occurring during puberty often lead to increased numbers of this species, which can be associated with acne. A number of fungi, including *Candida*, occur on the scalp and around the nails. They are infrequent on exposed skin, but can cause infection in moist skin folds (intertrigo).

Nose and mouth

Both of these sites can be heavily colonized by bacteria, streptococci, staphylococci, diphtheroids and Gram-negative cocci being common. Some of the species found as part of the flora in healthy individuals are potentially pathogenic (e.g. *Staph. aureus, Strep. pneumonia. Strep. pyogenes, Neisseria meningitidis, Lactobacillus, Candida*). The mucous membranes of the mouth can have the same microbial density as the large intestine, numbers approaching 10^{11} per gram wet weight of tissue. The surfaces of the teeth and the gingival crevices carry large numbers of anaerobic bacteria. Plaque is a film of bacterial cells anchored in a polysaccharide matrix which the organisms secrete. When teeth are not cleaned regularly plaque may accumulate rapidly and the activities of certain bacteria, notably *Streptococcus mutans*, may lead to dental decay (caries). Acid, fermented by these organisms from carbo-

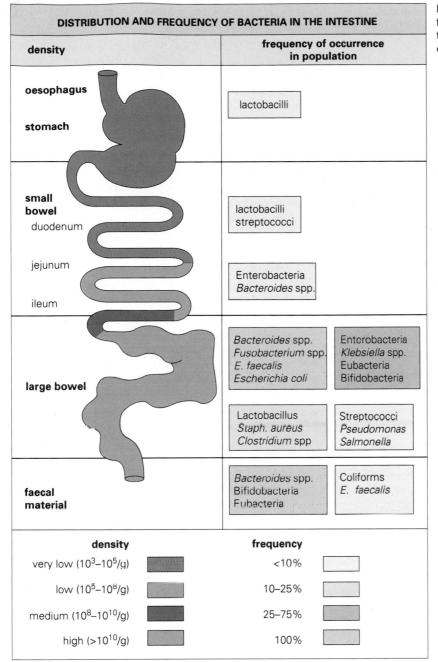

DISTRIBUTION AND FREQUENCY OF BACTERIA IN THE INTESTINE	
density	**frequency of occurrence in population**
oesophagus **stomach**	lactobacilli
small bowel duodenum jejunum ileum	lactobacilli streptococci
	Enterobacteria *Bacteroides* spp.
large bowel	*Bacteroides* spp. *Fusobacterium* spp. *E. faecalis* *Escherichia coli* / Enterobacteria *Klebsiella* spp. Eubacteria Bifidobacteria
	Lactobacillus *Staph. aureus* *Clostridium* spp / Streptococci *Pseudomonas* *Salmonella*
faecal material	*Bacteroides* spp. Bifidobacteria Eubacteria / Coliforms *E. faecalis*

density		frequency	
very low (10^3–10^5/g)		<10%	
low (10^5–10^8/g)		10–25%	
medium (10^8–10^{10}/g)		25–75%	
high (>10^{10}/g)		100%	

Fig. 3.43 The longitudinal distribution, frequency of occurrence and densities of the bacteria making up the normal flora of the human gastrointestinal tract.

hydrates, can attack dental enamel. The prevalence of dental decay is linked with diet, and caries has been one of the commonest infectious diseases in the Western World. Normal individuals may also harbour protozoan species in the mouth.

The pharynx and trachea carry their own normal flora, which may include both α and β haemolytic streptococci as well as a number of anaerobes, staphylococci (including Staph. aureus), neisseriae and diphtheroids. The respiratory tract is normally quite sterile, despite the regular intake of organisms by breathing. However substantial numbers of clinically normal people may carry *Pneumocystis carinii*, which is considered by some to be a component of the normal 'flora'.

Gastrointestinal tract

The density of microorganisms increases as one passes along the gastrointestinal tract from the stomach to the large intestine (Fig. 3.43). Stomach contents harbour only transient organisms, the acidic pH providing an unfavourable environment and forming an effective barrier. However, the gastric mucosa may be colonized by acid-tolerant lactobacilli and streptococci. The upper intestine is only lightly colonized (10^4 organisms per gram) but populations increase markedly in the ileum, where streptococci, lactobacilli, enterobacteria and *Bacteroides* may all be present. In the large bowel bacterial numbers are very high (estimated at 10^{11} per gram) and many different species can be found. The vast majority (95–99%) are anaerobes, *Bacteriodes* being especially common and a major component of faecal material. A number of harmless protozoans occur in the intestine (e.g. *Entamoeba coli*) and these can be considered as part of the normal flora, despite being animals.

Urogenital tract

The urethra in both sexes is relatively lightly colonized, although *Strep. epidermidis*, *E. faecalis* and diphtheroids may be present. In females the vagina supports an extensive flora of bacteria and fungi, the composition of which undergoes age-related changes. Before puberty the predominant organisms are staphylococci, streptococci diphtheroids and *E. coli*. Subsequently *Lactobacillus aerophilus* predominates, its fermentation of glycogen being responsible for the maintenance of an acid pH, which prevents overgrowth by other vaginal organisms. A number of fungi occur, including *Candida*, which can overgrow to cause the pathogenic condition 'thrush' if the vaginal pH rises and competing bacteria diminish. The protozoan *Trichomonas vaginalis* may also be present in healthy individuals.

Advantages and disadvantages of the normal flora

It is quite clear that in many cases members of the normal flora are positively beneficial to the host, although the benefits conferred vary in their importance. An important role is prevention of colonization by potential pathogens. Skin bacteria produce fatty acids which discourage other species from invading; gut bacteria release a number of factors with antibacterial activity (bacteriocins, colicins) and metabolic waste products, which, together with lack of available oxygen, prevent the establishment of other species; vaginal lactobacilli maintain an acid environment that suppresses growth of other organisms. The sheer number of bacteria present in the normal flora of the intestine means that almost all of the available ecological niches become occupied; these species therefore outcompete others for living space. The value of this competition is seen when antibiotic treatment removes a large part of the normal flora, leading to colonization by pathogenic species. A well documented example of this is seen after treatment with clindamycin, when overgrowth by *Clostridium difficile*, which survives treatment, gives rise to pseudomembranous colitis.

Gut bacteria also release a number of organic acids, which might have some metabolic value to the host; they also produce B vitamins and vitamin K in amounts large enough to be valuable should the diet be deficient. In addition, the antigenic stimulation provided by the intestinal flora is thought to be important in ensuring the normal development of the immune system.

What happens when the normal flora is absent? For many years it has been possible to produce germ-free mice, rats pigs, monkeys, even horses. This is technically demanding, and is done by delivering infants via caesarean section into sterile containers (isolators) and providing sterile food, water and air. Germ-free animals tend to live longer, presumably because of the complete absence of pathogens, and develop no caries (see Chapter 20). However, they have a less well developed immune system and are very vulnerable to introduced microbial pathogens. There is no doubt that the germ-free state would be extremely hazardous to human beings. At the time of birth, however, we are germ-free, and acquire our normal flora during and immediately after birth, to the accompaniment of intense immunological activity.

The disadvantages of the normal flora lie primarily in the potential for spread into previously sterile parts of the body. This may happen under a variety of circumstances, for example when the intestine is perforated or the skin is broken, during extraction of teeth (when viridans streptococci may enter the bloodstream), or when organisms such as *E. coli* from the perianal skin ascend the urethra and cause urinary tract infection. Overgrowth by potentially pathogenic members of the normal flora can occur when the composition of the flora changes (e.g. after antibiotics), when the local environment changes (e.g. increases in stomach or vaginal pH) or when the immune system becomes ineffective (e.g. AIDS, clinical immunosuppression). Under these conditions, the potential pathogens take the opportunity to increase their population size or invade tissues, so becoming harmful to the host. An account of diseases associated with such opportunistic infections is given in Chapter 33.

SUMMARY

The wide variety of organisms that cause infectious diseases can be grouped into six main categories – viruses, bacteria, fungi, protozoa, helminths and arthropods. Each has distinctive properties which determine the ways in which the organisms interact with their hosts, and therefore contribute to the characteristics of the diseases they cause. Among these properties are structural and molecular make up, metabolic strategies and reproductive processes. Some species, however, are postively beneficial to the health of the host. The normal flora, the organisms that live on or within the body without causing disease, play an important role in protection against the establishment of pathogenic microbes.

Further Reading

Joklik WK, Willett HP, Amos B, Wilfert CM, eds. *Zinsser Microbiology*. 20th edn. Connecticutt: Appleton and Lange, 1992.

Mandell GL, Douglas RG, Bennett JE. *Principles and practice of infectious diseases*. 3rd edn. London: Churchill-Livingstone, 1990.

Parker MT, Collier, LH, eds. *Topley and Wilson's principles of bacteriology*. 8th edn. London: Edward Arnold, 1990.

section *1*

THE ADVERSARIES

part 2 **Host Defence Mechanisms**

4 THE INNATE DEFENCES OF THE BODY

INTRODUCTION

In the preceding chapters, we have outlined some of the fundamental characteristics of the myriad types of micro- and macroparasites which may infect the body. We now turn to consider the ways in which the body seeks to defend itself against infection from these organisms.

A relatively sharp distinction should be drawn between what are termed the 'innate' and the 'adaptive' immune defences. When an organism infects the body, the defence systems already in place may well be sufficient to prevent replication and spread of the infectious agent, thereby preventing development of disease. These established mechanisms are referred to as constituting the 'innate' immune system. However, should innate immunity be insufficient to parry the invasion by the infectious agent, the 'adaptive' immune system then comes into action, although it takes time to reach its maximum efficiency (Fig. 4.1). When it does take effect, it eliminates the infective organism, allowing recovery from disease.

The main feature distinguishing the adaptive response from the innate mechanism is that specific memory of infection is imprinted on the adaptive immune system, so that should there be a subsequent reinfection by the same agent, a particularly effective response comes into play with remarkable speed. It is worth emphasizing, however, that there is close synergy between the two systems, with the adaptive mechanisms greatly improving the efficiency of the innate response.

The contrasts between these two systems are set out in figure 4.2. On the one hand are the soluble factors such as lysozyme and complement, together with the phagocytic cells which contribute to the innate system, and on the other the lymphocyte-based mechanisms which produce antibody and so-called T lymphocytes, the main elements of the adaptive immune system. Not only do these lymphocytes provide improved resistance by repeated contact with a given infectious agent, but the memory with which they become endowed shows very considerable specificity to

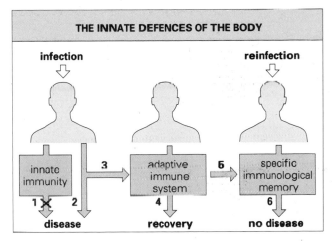

Fig. 4.1 Innate and adaptive immunity. An infectious agent first encounters elements of the innate immune system. These may be sufficient to prevent disease (1) but if not, disease will result (2). The adaptive immune system is then activated (3) to produce recovery (4) and a specific immunological memory (5). Following reinfection with the same agent no disease results (6); the individual has acquired immunity to the infectious agent.

that infection. For instance, infection with measles virus will induce a memory to that microorganism alone and not to another virus, such as rubella.

DEFENCE AGAINST ENTRY INTO THE BODY

Before an infectious agent can penetrate the body, it must overcome the variety of biochemical and physical barriers that operate at the body surfaces. One of the most important of these, of course, is the skin, which is normally impermeable to the majority of infectious agents. Many bacteria fail to survive for long on the skin because of the direct inhibitory affects of lactic acid and fatty acids present in sweat and sebaceous secretions, and the lower pH to which they give rise (Fig. 4.3). However, should there be skin loss, as may occur in burns for example, infection becomes a major problem.

COMPARISON OF INNATE AND ADAPTIVE IMMUNE SYSTEMS		
	innate immune system	adaptive immune system
major elements		
soluble factors	lysozyme, complement, acute phase proteins e.g. C-reactive protein, interferon	antibody
cells	phagocytes natural killer (NK) cells	T lymphocytes
response to microbial infection		
first contact	+	+
second contact	+	++++
	non-specific no memory	specific memory
	resistance not improved by repeated contact	resistance improved by repeated contact

Fig. 4.2 Comparison of innate and adaptive immune systems. Innate immunity is sometimes referred to as 'natural' and adaptive as 'acquired'. There is considerable interaction between the two systems. 'Humoral' immunity due to soluble factors contrasts with immunity mediated by cells. Primary contact with antigen produces weak adaptive and non-adaptive responses, but if the same antigen persists or is encountered a second time there is a much enhanced specific response to that antigen.

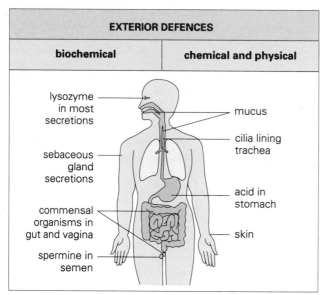

EXTERIOR DEFENCES	
biochemical	chemical and physical

Fig. 4.3 Exterior defences. Most of the infectious agents encountered by an individual are prevented from entering the body by a variety of biochemical and physical barriers. The body tolerates a number of commensal organisms which compete effectively with many potential pathogens.

The membranes lining the inner surfaces of the body secrete mucus, which acts as a protective barrier, inhibiting the adherence of bacteria to the epithelial cells, thereby preventing them from gaining access to the body. Microbial and other foreign particles trapped within this adhesive mucus may be removed by mechanical means, such as ciliary action, coughing and sneezing. The flushing action of tears, saliva and urine, are other mechanical strategies which help to protect the epithelial surfaces. In addition, many of the secreted body fluids contain microbicidal factors, such as the acid in gastric juice, spermine

and zinc in semen, lactoperoxidase in milk and lysozyme in tears, nasal secretions and saliva.

The phenomenon of microbial antagonism associated with the normal bacterial flora of the body, often referred to as 'commensal' organisms, is explained in Chapter 3. These organisms suppress the growth of many potentially pathogenic bacteria and fungi at superficial sites by virtue of the physical advantage of previous occupancy, especially on epithelial surfaces, by competing for essential nutrients, or by producing inhibitory substances such as acid or colicins. The latter are a class of bactericidins which bind to the negatively charged surface of susceptible bacteria and form a voltage-dependent channel in the membrane which kills by destroying the cell's energy potential.

Not withstanding the general effectiveness of these various barriers, microorganisms successfully penetrate the body on many occasions. When this occurs essentially two main defensive strategies come into play, based on 1) the destructive effect of soluble chemical factors, such as bactericidal enzymes, and 2) the mechanism of phagocytosis, which involves the engulfment and killing of microorganisms by specialized cells.

INTRACELLULAR KILLING OF MICROBES BY PHAGOCYTES

Professional phagocytes

Perhaps because of the belief that professionals do a better job than amateurs, the cells which shoulder the main burden of our phagocytic defences have been labelled 'professional phagocytes'. These consist of two major cell families, as originally defined by Elie Metchnikoff, the Russian zoologist (see panel) – the large macrophages and the smaller polymorphonuclear granulocytes which are generally referred to as polymorphs or neutrophils on the basis of the lack of staining of their cytoplasmic granules by haematoxylin/eosin.

Elie Metchnikoff (1845-1916)

This perceptive Russian zoologist can legitimately be regarded as the father of the concept of cellular immunity, in which it is recognized that certain specialized cells mediate the defence against microbial infections. He was intrigued by the motile cells of transparent starfish larvae and made the critical observation that a few hours after the introduction of a rose thorn into these larvae, it became surrounded by these motile cells. A year later, in 1883, he observed that fungal spores can be attacked by the blood cells of daphnia, a tiny metozoan which, also being transparent, can be studied directly under the microscope. He went on to extend his investigations to mammalian leucocytes, showing their ability to engulf microorganisms, a process which he termed 'phagocytosis' (literally, eating by cells,).

Because he found this process to be even more effective in animals recovering from an infection, he came to the conclusion that phagocytosis provided the main defence against infection. He defined the existence of two types of circulating phagocytes: the

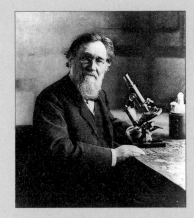

Fig. 4.4 Elie Metchnikoff (1845-1916).

polymorphonuclear leucocyte, which he termed a 'microphage', and the larger 'macrophages'.

Although Metchnikoff held the somewhat polarized view that cellular immunity based upon phagocytosis provided the main if not the only defence mechanism against infectious microorganisms, we now know that through co-operation with humoral factors, in particular antibody and complement, the efficiency of the phagocytic system is enormously enhanced.

Macrophages

These cells originate as bone marrow promonocytes which develop into circulating blood monocytes (Fig. 4.5) and finally become the mature macrophages, widespread throughout the tissues, collectively termed the 'mononuclear phagocyte system' (Fig. 4.6). These macrophages are present throughout the connective tissue and are associated with the basement membrane of small blood vessels. They are particularly concentrated in the lung (alveolar macrophages), liver (Kupffer cells), and the lining of lymph node medullary sinuses and spleen sinusoids (Fig. 4.7) where they are well placed to filter off foreign material (Fig. 4.8). Other examples are the brain microglia, kidney mesangial cells, synovial A cells and osteoclasts in bone. In general, these are long-lived cells which depend upon mitochondria for their metabolic energy and show significant rough-surfaced endoplasmic reticular profiles (Fig. 4.9) related to the formidable array of different secretory proteins which these cells generate.

Polymorphonuclear neutrophils

The polymorph is the dominant white cell in the bloodstream and, like the macrophage, shares a common haemopoietic stem cell precursor with the other formed elements of the blood. It has no mitochondria but utilizes its abundant cytoplasmic glycogen stores for its energy requirements; thus, glycolysis enables these cells

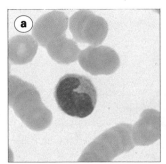
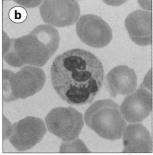

Fig. 4.5 Phagocytic cells. (a) Blood monocytes and (b) polymorphonuclear neutrophils, both derived from bone marrow stem cells. Courtesy of P M Lydyard.

PHAGOCYTES OF THE MONOCYTE/MACROPHAGE SERIES

- brain microglial cells
- alveolar macrophages
- splenic macrophages
- blood monocytes
- lymph node resident and recirculating macrophages
- precursors in bone marrow
- liver Kupffer cells
- kidney mesangial phagocytes
- connective tissue histiocytes
- synovial A cells
- osteoclasts

Fig. 4.6 The mononuclear phagocyte system. Tissue macrophages are derived from blood monocytes which are manufactured in the bone marrow.

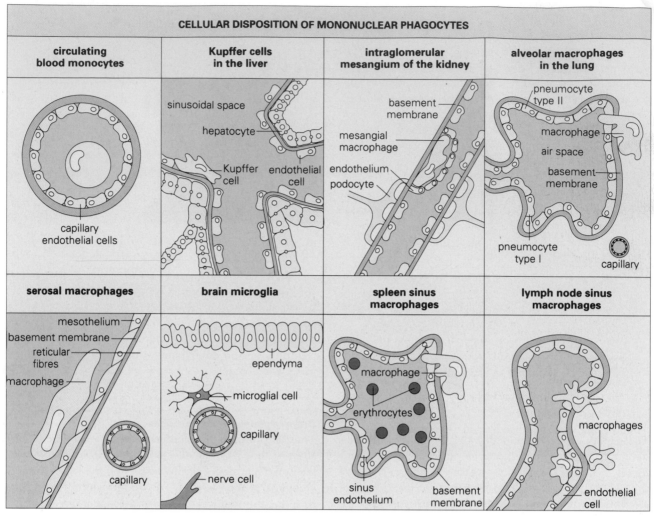

Fig. 4.7 Cellular disposition of mononuclear phagocytes.

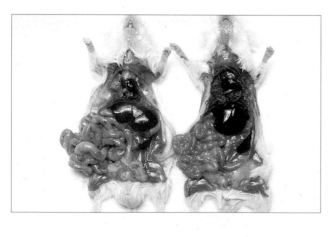

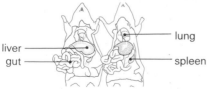

Fig. 4.8 Localization of intravenously injected particles in the mononuclear phagocyte system. A mouse was injected with fine carbon particles and killed five minutes later. Carbon accumulates in organs rich in mononuclear phagocytes – lungs, liver, spleen and areas of the gut wall. The normal organ colour is shown in the control mouse on the left. Courtesy of P Lydyard.

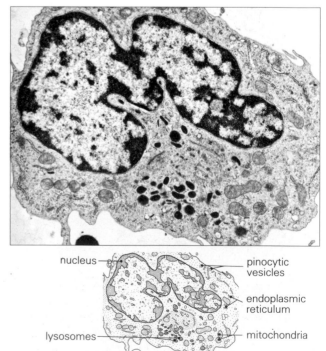

Fig. 4.9 Monocyte (x8 000), with 'horseshoe' nucleus. Phagocytic and pinocytic vesicles, lysosomal granules, mitochondria and isolated profiles of rough-surfaced endoplasmic reticulum are evident. Courtesy of B Nichols. Copyright Rockfeller University Press.

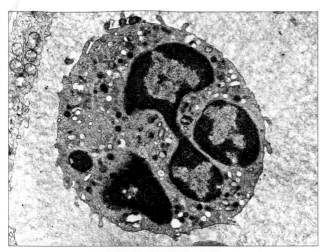

Fig. 4.10 Neutrophil. The multi-lobed nucleus and cytoplasmic granules are well displayed. Courtesy of D McLaren.

to function under anaerobic conditions, such as those in an inflammatory focus. It is a non-dividing, short-lived cell with a segmented nucleus; the cytoplasm is characterized by an array of granules, including the primary azurophilic granule which contains myeloperoxidase, some lysozyme and families of cationic proteins, the secondary 'specific' granules associated with lactoferrin and lysozyme, and the tertiary granules typical of the conventional lysosome with acid hydrolases (see Figs 4.5 and 4.10). As a very crude generalization, it may be said that the polymorphs provide the major defence against pyogenic (pus-forming) bacteria, while the macrophages are thought to be at their best in combatting those organisms that are capable of living within the cells of the host.

PHAGOCYTOSIS

The first event in the uptake and digestion of a microorganism by the professional phagocyte involves the attachment of the microbe to the surface of the cell (Fig. 4.11). The attachment itself usually represents a somewhat primitive recognition mechanism, probably involving carbohydrate elements on the infectious agent. The attached particle may now initiate the ingestion phase by activating an actin–myosin contractile system which sends arms of cytoplasm around the particle until it is completely enclosed within a vacuole (phagosome; Figs 4.11 and 4.12). Shortly afterwards, the cytoplasmic granules fuse with a phagosome and discharge their contents around the incarcerated microorganism which is then the target of a dastardly array of killing mechanisms.

THE KILLING PROCESS

As phagocytosis is initiated, there is a vigorous burst of oxygen consumption resulting from a dramatic increase in activity of the hexose monophosphate shunt. This generates NADPH and reduces molecular oxygen through a unique plasma membrane cytochrome system to a series of powerful microbicidal agents, namely superoxide anion, hydrogen peroxide, singlet oxygen and hydroxyl radicals

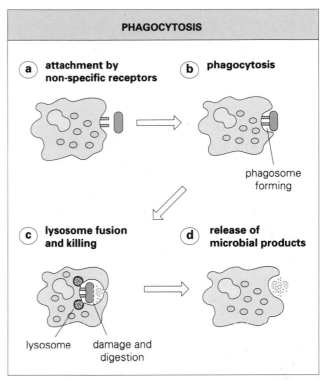

PHAGOCYTOSIS

a attachment by non-specific receptors

b phagocytosis

phagosome forming

c lysosome fusion and killing

d release of microbial products

lysosome   damage and digestion

Fig. 4.11 Phagocytosis. Phagocytes attach to microorganisms via their non-specific cell surface receptors (a). If the membrane now becomes activated by the attached infectious agent, it is taken into a phagosome by pseudopodia which extend around it (b). Once inside, lysosomes fuse with the phagosome to form a phagolysosome (c). The infectious agent is killed by a battery of microbicidal mechanisms, and the microbial products released (d).

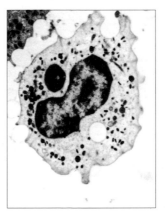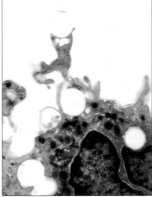

Fig. 4.12 Electron micrographic study of phagocytosis. These two micrographs show human phagocytes engulfing latex particles. x3000 (left); x4500 (right). Courtesy of CHW Horne.

(Fig. 4.13; see also Chapter 12). Subsequently, the peroxide, in association with myeloperoxidase, generates a potent halogenating system from halide ions which is capable of killing both bacteria and viruses.

As superoxide anion is formed, the enzyme superoxide dismutase acts to convert it to molecular oxygen and hydrogen peroxide, but in the process consumes hydrogen ions. Thus initially there is a small increase in pH which facilitates the anti-bacterial function of the families of cationic proteins derived from the phagocytic granules.

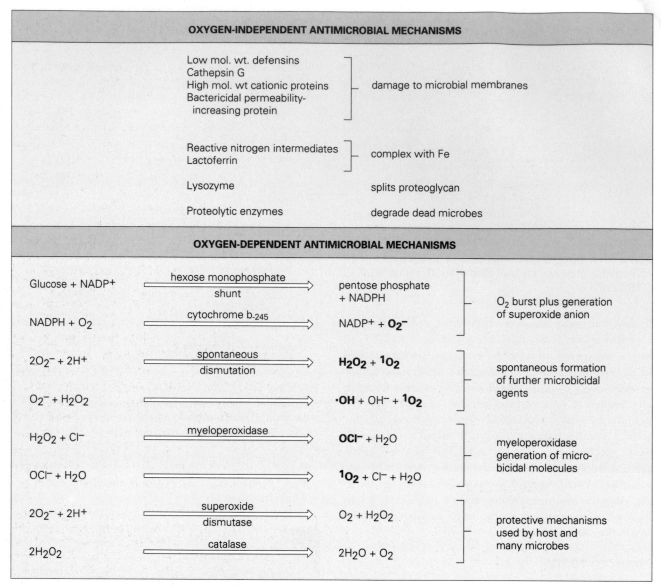

Fig. 4.13 Anti-microbial mechanisms in phagocytic vacuoles. Microbicidal species in bold letters. O_2^-, superoxide anion; $^1O_2$, singlet (activated) oxygen; $\cdot OH$, hydroxyl free radical. Reactive nitrogen intermediates such as nitric oxide (NO) are derived from asparagine.

These molecules damage microbial membranes both by the action of cathepsin G and by direct adherence to the microbial surface. Other granule-derived factors are lactoferrin and reactive nitrogen intermediates like nitric oxide, which through their ability to complex iron, deprive bacteria of an essential growth element, and lysozyme which splits the proteoglycan cell wall of bacteria. The pH now falls, so that the dead or dying microorganism is extensively degraded by acid hydrolytic enzymes and the degradation products are released to the exterior.

RECRUITMENT OF DEFENSIVE PHAGOCYTES

The need for chemotaxis

Phagocytosis cannot occur unless the bacterium first attaches to the surface of the phagocyte, and clearly this cannot happen unless both have become physically close to each other. There is therefore a need for a mechanism that mobilizes phagocytes from afar and targets them onto the bacterium. Many bacteria produce chemical substances such as formyl methionyl peptides which directionally attract leucocytes, a process known as 'chemotaxis'. However, this is a relatively weak signalling system and evolution has provided the body with a far more effective magnet which utilizes a complex series of proteins collectively termed 'complement'.

Activation of the complement system

Complement resembles blood clotting, fibrinolysis and kinin formation in being a major triggered enzyme plasma system. Such systems are characterized by their ability to produce a rapid, highly amplified response to a trigger stimulus, mediated by a cascade phenomenon in which the product of one reaction is the enzymic catalyst of the next. The most abundant and most central component is C3 (complement components are designated by the letter 'C' followed by a number) and the cleavage of this molecule is at the heart of all complement-mediated phenomena.

In normal plasma, C3 undergoes spontaneous activation at a very slow rate, to generate the split product C3b. This is able to complex with another complement component, factor B, which is then acted upon by a normal plasma enzyme, factor D, to produce the C3 splitting enzyme C3bBb. This C3 convertase can then split new molecules of C3 to give C3a (a small fragment), and further C3b. This represents a positive feedback circuit with potential for runaway amplification; however, the overall process is restricted to a tick-over level by powerful regulatory mechanisms which break the unstable soluble-phase C3 convertase into inactive cleavage products (Fig. 4.14).

In the presence of certain molecules, such as the carbohydrates on the surface of many bacteria, the C3 convertase can become attached and stabilized against breakdown. Under these circumstances, there is active generation of new C3 convertase molecules and what is known as the 'alternative' complement pathway can swing into full tempo (see also Chapter 5).

Complement synergizes with phagocytic cells to produce an acute inflammatory response

Activation of the alternative complement pathway with a consequent splitting of very large numbers of C3 molecules has important consequences for the orchestration of an integrated anti-microbial defence strategy (Fig. 4.15). Large numbers of C3b produced in the immediate vicinity of the microbial membrane, bind covalently to that surface and act as opsonins – molecules which make the particle they coat more susceptible to engulfment by

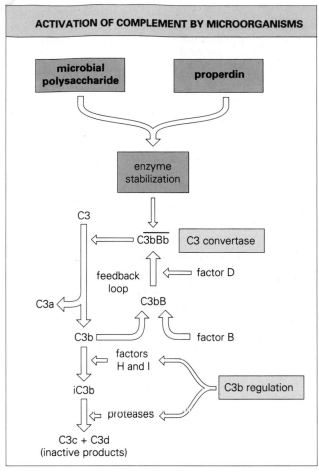

Fig. 4.14 Activation of complement by microorganisms.

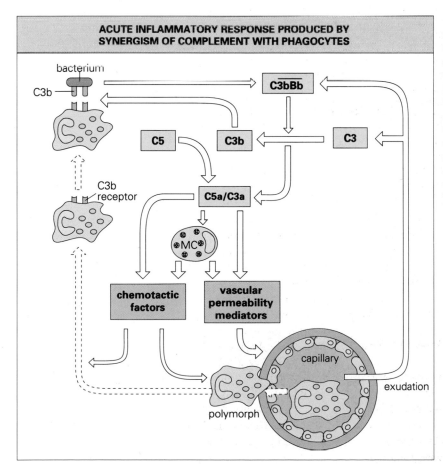

Fig. 4.15 The defensive strategy of the acute inflammatory reaction initiated by bacterial activation of the alternative complement pathway. Activation of the C3bBb C3-convertase by the bacterium, leads to the generation of C3b (which binds to the bacterium), C3a and C5a, and recruitment of mast cell (MC) mediators. These in turn cause capillary dilatation and exudation of plasma proteins, and chemotactic attraction and adherence of polymorphs to the C3b-coated bacterium. The polymorphs are then activated for the final kill.

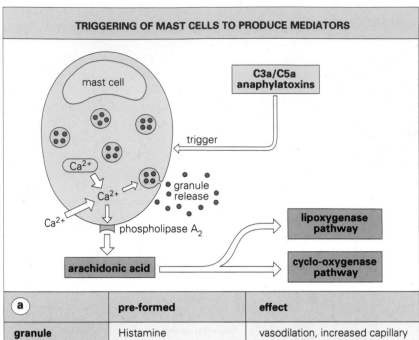

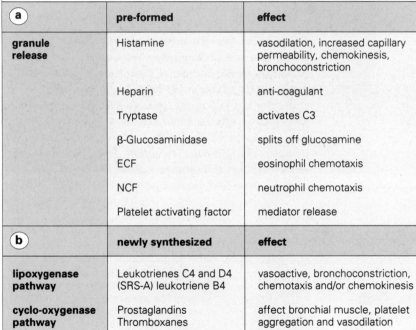

TRIGGERING OF MAST CELLS TO PRODUCE MEDIATORS

(a)	pre-formed	effect
granule release	Histamine	vasodilation, increased capillary permeability, chemokinesis, bronchoconstriction
	Heparin	anti-coagulant
	Tryptase	activates C3
	β-Glucosaminidase	splits off glucosamine
	ECF	eosinophil chemotaxis
	NCF	neutrophil chemotaxis
	Platelet activating factor	mediator release
(b)	**newly synthesized**	**effect**
lipoxygenase pathway	Leukotrienes C4 and D4 (SRS-A) leukotriene B4	vasoactive, bronchoconstriction, chemotaxis and/or chemokinesis
cyclo-oxygenase pathway	Prostaglandins Thromboxanes	affect bronchial muscle, platelet aggregation and vasodilation

Fig. 4.16 Mast cell triggering leading to release of mediators by two major pathways: (a) release of pre-formed mediators present in the granules, and (b) the metabolism of arachidonic acid produced through activation of a phospholipase. Intracellular Ca^{2+} and cAMP are central to the initiation of these events but details are still unclear. ECF, eosinophil chemotactic factor; NCF, neutrophil chemotactic factor. Chemotaxis refers to directed migration of granulocytes up the concentration gradient of the mediator, whereas chemokinesis describes randomly increased motility of these cells.

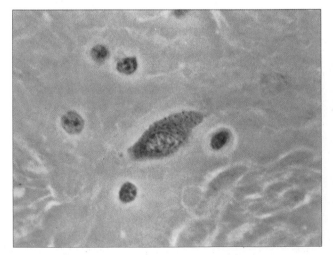

Fig. 4.17 Histological appearance of human (gut) connective tissue mast cells. This micrograph shows the dark blue cytoplasm with brownish granules. Alcian blue and Safranin, x600. Courtesy of TSC Orr.

phagocytic cells (see below). This C3b, together with the C3 convertase, acts on the next component in the sequence, C5, to produce a small fragment C5a, which together with C3a, has a direct effect on mast cells to cause their degranulation. Consequently mediators of vascular permeability and factors chemotactic for polymorphs are released. The nature of this degranulation process and of the products to which it gives rise are shown in figures 4.16–4.18, while the circulating equivalent of the tissue mast cell, the basophil, is shown in figure 4.19.

The vascular-permeability mediators increase the permeability of capillaries by modifying the intercellular forces between the endothelial cells of the vessel wall. This allows the exudation not only of fluid, but of plasma components including more complement, to the site of the infection. These mediators (Fig. 4.20) also up-regulate molecules such as intercellular adhesion molecule-1 (ICAM-1) and endothelial cell-leucocyte adhesion molecule-1 (ELAM-1; Fig. 4.20) which bind to specific complementary molecules

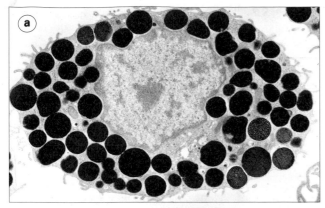

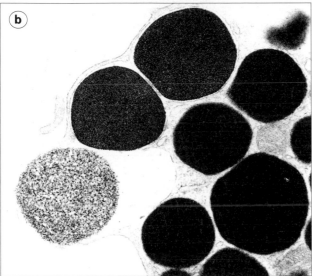

Fig. 4.18 Electron micrographs of rat peritoneal mast cells. These show the undegranulated cell with its electron-dense granules (upper, x6000) and a granule in the process of exocytosis (lower, x30 000). Courtesy of TSC Orr.

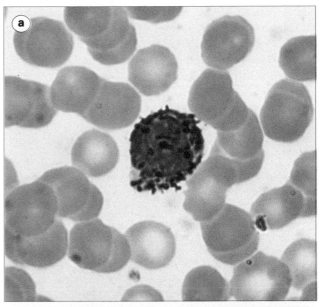

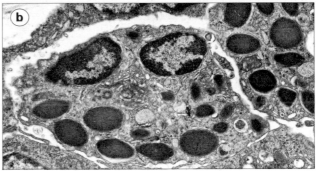

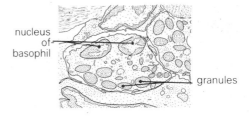

Fig. 4.19 Morphology of the basophil. (a) This blood smear shows a typical basophil with its deep violet-blue granules. Wright's stain, x1500. (b) Electron micrograph showing the ultrastructure of the basophil. Basophils in guinea pig skin showing the characteristic randomly distributed granules. x6000. Courtesy of D McLaren.

on the polymorphs and encourage them to stick to the walls of the capillaries, a process termed 'margination'.

The chemotactic factors, on the other hand, provide a chemical gradient which attracts marginated polymorphonuclear leucocytes from their intravascular location, through the walls of the blood vessels, and eventually leads them to the site of the C3b coated bacteria which initiated the whole activation process. Polymorphs have a well-defined receptor for C3b on their surface, and as a result, the opsonized bacteria adhere very firmly to the surface of these newly arrived cells.

The processes of capillary dilatation (erythema), exudation of plasma proteins and also of fluid (oedema) due to hydrostatic and osmotic pressure changes, and the accumulation of neutrophils are collectively termed the 'acute inflammatory response', and represent a highly effective way of focusing the phagocytic cells onto complement-coated microbial targets.

It also seems clear that the macrophage can be stimulated by certain bacterial toxins such as the lipopolysaccharides (LPS), by the action of C5a and by the phagocytosis of C3b-coated bacteria, to secrete other potent mediators of acute inflammation which reinforce the mast-cell directed pathway (see Fig. 4.20).

FURTHER HUMORAL INNATE DEFENCE MECHANISMS

The cytolytic effect of complement

We have already introduced the idea that following the activation of C3, the next component to be cleaved is C5; the larger C5b fragment which results becomes membrane bound. This subsequently binds components C6, C7 and C8 which form a complex capable of inducing a critical conformational change in the terminal component C9. The unfolded C9 molecules become inserted into the lipid bilayer and polymerize to form an annular 'membrane attack complex' (MAC; Figs 4.21 and 4.22). This behaves as a transmembrane channel which is fully permeable to electrolytes and water. Because of the high internal colloid osmotic pressure of cells, there is a net influx of sodium ions frequently leading to lysis.

Acute phase proteins

Certain proteins in the plasma, collectively termed 'acute phase proteins' increase in concentration in response to early 'alarm' mediators such as interleukin-1 (IL-1), IL-6 and tumour necrosis factor (TNF), released as a result of infection or tissue injury. While many acute phase reactants such as C-reactive protein increase dramatically (Fig. 4.23), others show more moderate rises, usually less than five-fold (Fig. 4.24). In general, these proteins are thought to subserve defensive roles.

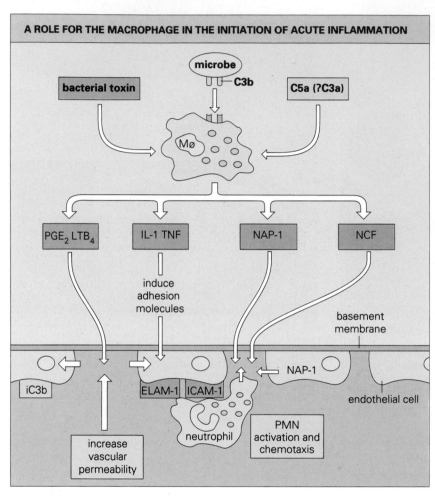

Fig. 4.20 A role for the macrophage (Mø) in the initiation of acute inflammation. Stimulation induces macrophage secretion of mediators. Blood neutrophils stick to the adhesion molecules on the endothelial cell and use this to provide traction as they force their way between the cells, through the basement membrane (with the help of secreted elastase) and up the chemotactic gradient. During this process they become progressively activated by NAP-1 (neutrophil activating peptide-1). NCF, neutrophil chemotactic factor; PGE_2, prostaglandin E_2; LTB_4, leukotriene B_4; IL-1, interleukin-1; TNF, tumour necrosis factor; ELAM-1, endothelial cell leucocyte adhesion molecule-1; ICAM-1, intercellular adhesion molecule-1.

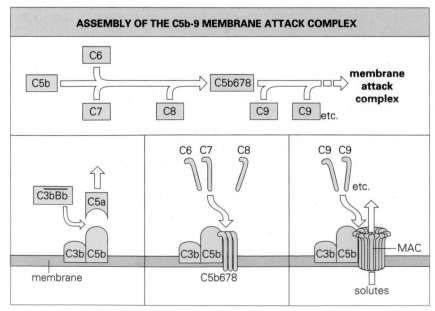

Fig. 4.21 Assembly of the C5b-9 membrane attack complex. Once C5b is membrane bound, C6 and C7 attach themselves to form the stable complex, C5b67, which interacts with C8 to yield C5b678. This unit has some effect in disrupting the membrane, and also causes the polymerization of C9 to form tubules traversing the membrane. The tube is referred to as a membrane attack complex (MAC). Disruption of the membrane by this structure permits the free exchange of solutes, which is primarily responsible for cell lysis.

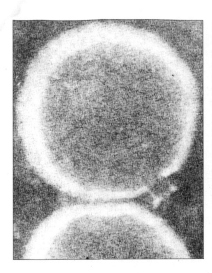

Fig. 4.22 Electron micrograph of the membrane attack complex. The funnel-shaped lesion is due to a human C5b-9 complex that has been reincorporated into lecithin liposomal membranes. x234 000. Courtesy of J Tranum-Jensen and S Bhakdi.

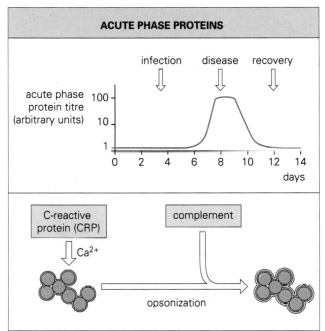

Fig. 4.23 Acute phase proteins, here exemplified by C-reactive protein, are serum proteins which increase rapidly in concentration (sometimes up to 100–fold) following infection (graph). They are important in innate immunity to infection. C-reactive protein (CRP) recognizes and binds, in a Ca^{2+} dependent fashion, to molecular groups found on a wide variety of bacteria and fungi. In particular it binds the phosphocholine moiety of pneumococci. The CRP acts as an opsonin and activates complement with all the associated sequelae.

Other extracellular anti-microbial factors

There are many microbicidal agents that operate at short range within phagocytic cells, but which also appear in a number of body fluids in concentrations adequate to have inhibitory effects on infectious agents directly. For example, lysozyme is present in fluids such as tears and saliva, in amounts that are capable of acting against the proteoglycan wall of susceptible bacteria. Similarly, lactoferrin may appear in the circulation at levels which complex iron and deprive bacteria of this important growth factor. Whether normally short-range acting agents such as reactive oxygen metabolites or tumour necrosis factor (a cytotoxic molecule produced by macrophages and other cell types)

ACUTE PHASE PROTEINS PRODUCED IN RESPONSE TO INFECTION IN THE HUMAN	
acute phase reactant	**role**
dramatic increases in concentration:	
C-reactive protein	fixes complement, opsonizes
mannose binding protein	fixes complement, opsonizes
α_1 acid glycoprotein	transport protein
serum amyloid A protein	?
moderate increases in concentration:	
α_1 proteinase inhibitors	inhibit bacterial proteases
α_1 anti-chymotrypsin	inhibit bacterial proteases
C3, C9, factor B	increase complement function
caeruloplasmin	O_2^- scavenger
fibrinogen	coagulation
angiotensin	blood pressure
haptoglobin	bind haemoglobin
fibronectin	cell attachment

Fig. 4.24 Acute phase proteins produced in response to infection in the human. Adapted from Stadnyk and Gauldie, 1991.

can reach concentrations in the body fluids that are adequate to allow them to act at a distance from the cell producing them will be discussed in later chapters particularly when considering the mechanisms by which the blood-borne forms of parasites such as malaria are attacked.

Interferons

These represent a family of broad spectrum anti-viral molecules that are widely present in the animal kingdom (discussed further in Chapter 12). They were first recognized by the phenomenon of viral interference, in which a cell infected with one virus is found to be resistant to super-infection by a second unrelated virus. Leucocytes produce many different α-interferons (IFN-α), while fibroblasts and probably all cell types synthesize IFN-β. A third type (IFN-γ) is not a component of the innate immune system and will be discussed in the next chapter as a member of the important cytokine family.

When cells are infected by a virus, they synthesize and secrete interferon, which binds to specific receptors on nearby uninfected cells. The bound interferon exerts its antiviral effect by facilitating the synthesis of two new enzymes which interfere with the machinery used by the virus for its own replication. The mechanism of action of interferon is discussed more fully in Chapter 12; the net result is to set up a cordon of infection-resistant cells around the site of virus infection, so restraining its spread (Fig. 4.25). That interferon is highly effective *in vivo* is supported by experiments in which mice injected with an antiserum to murine interferon were found to be killed by several hundred times less virus than was needed to kill the controls. It should be emphasized, however, that interferon seems to play a significant role in recovery from, as distinct from prevention of, viral infections.

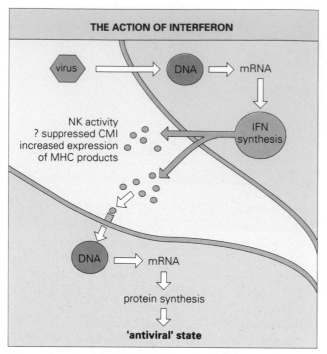

THE ACTION OF INTERFERON

virus → DNA → mRNA

NK activity
? suppressed CMI
increased expression
of MHC products

IFN synthesis

DNA → mRNA

↓

protein synthesis

↓

'antiviral' state

Fig. 4.25 The action of interferon. Virus infecting a cell induces the production of interferon. This is released and binds to interferon receptors on other cells. The interferon induces production of anti-viral proteins which are activated if virus enters the second cell.

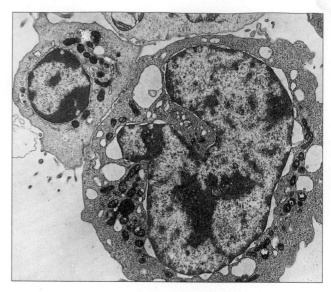

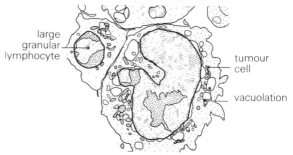

large granular lymphocyte

tumour cell

vacuolation

Fig. 4.26 Electron micrograph of a large granular lymphocyte (LGL) killing a tumour cell. LGLs bind to and kill IgG antibody-coated (see Fig. 5.10), and even non-coated, tumour cells. It is essential for the membranes of the two cells to be closely apposed in order for LGL to deliver the 'kiss of death'. x4500. Courtesy of P Lydyard.

EXTRACELLULAR KILLING

Natural killer cells

There is a widely held view that viruses represent fragments of the genome of multicellular organisms that have achieved the ability to exist in an extracellular state. The small number of genes present in the viral genome, however, do not include those required for viral replication. Accordingly, it is essential for viruses to penetrate the cells of an infected host in order to subvert the cells' replicative machinery towards viral replication. Clearly, it is in the interests of the host to try to kill such infected cells before the virus has had a chance to reproduce. Natural killer (NK) cells are cytotoxic cells which appear to have evolved to carry out just such a task. These are large granular lymphocytes (Fig. 4.26) which attach themselves to structures, presumably glycoproteins, which appear on the surface of virally infected cells and which allow them to be differentiated from normal cells; activation of the NK cell results in extracellular release of its granule contents into the space between the target and effector cells. Perhaps the most important of the cytotoxic agents released are the perforin molecules, which resemble C9 in many respects, expecially in their ability to insert into the membrane of the target cell and polymerize to form annular transmembrane pores, like the membrane attack complex. Such a structure leads to death of the target cell (Fig. 4.27).

Subsidiary cytotoxic mechanisms may involve molecules which resemble tumour necrosis factor (TNF). TNF was first recognized as a product of activated macrophages. These cells are known to be capable of killing certain other cells, particularly some tumour cells, presumably by the production of a cell poison. Yet a further mode of cytotoxicity can be turned on by the activated macrophage, involving the direct 'burning' of the surface of another cell by means of a stream of reactive oxygen intermediates, produced at the macrophage membrane by the respiratory oxygen burst, as discussed previously.

Eosinophils

It takes little imagination to realise that professional phagocytes are far too small to be capable of physically engulfing large parasites such as helminths. An alternative strategy, such as killing by an extracellular broadside of the type discussed above, would seem to be a more appropriate form of defence. Eosinophils appear to have evolved to fulfil just this role. These polymorphonuclear relatives of the neutrophil have distinctive cytoplasmic granules which stain strongly with acidic dyes (Fig. 4.28) and have a characteristic appearance at the ultrastructural level. A major basic protein (MBP) has been identified in the core of the granule, while the matrix has been shown to contain an eosinophilic cationic protein, a peroxidase and a perforin-like molecule. The cells have surface receptors for C3b and when activated, generate copious amounts of active oxygen metabolites.

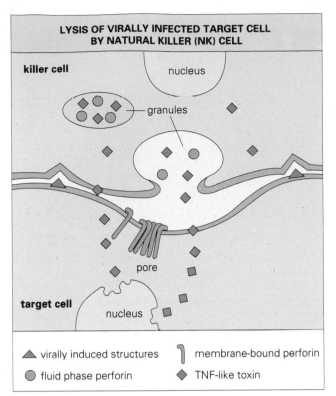

Fig. 4.27 Schematic model of lysis of virally infected target cell by natural killer (NK) cell. As the NK receptors bind to the surface of the virally infected cell, there is exocytosis of granules and release of cytolytic mediators into the intercellular cleft. A calcium dependent conformational change in the perforin enables it to insert and polymerize within the membrane of the target cell to form a transmembrane pore which leads to cell lysis. The granules and the cytosol itself contain a toxin resembling tumour necrosis factor (TNF) which mediates a calcium-independent fragmentation of nuclear DNA.

Many helminths can activate the alternative complement pathway, but although resistant to C9 attack, their coating with C3b allows adherence to the eosinophils through their C3b surface receptors. Once activated, the eosinophil launches its extracellular ammunition, which includes the release of MBP and the cationic protein to damage the parasite membrane, with a possibility of a further 'chemical burn' from the oxygen metabolites and 'leaky porous plug' formation by the perforins.

SUMMARY

The vital importance of the innate system of immune defence, consisting of a formidable barrier to entry and second line phagocytes and circulating soluble factors, is underlined by the colonization of the body by normally non-pathogenic ('opportunistic') microorganisms which occurs whenever there is a hereditary or acquired deficiency in any of these functions.

The main phagocytic cells are polymorphonuclear neutrophils and macrophages. Organisms adhere to their surface, activate the engulfment process and are taken inside the cell where they fuse with cytoplasmic granules. A formidable array of oxygen-dependent and oxygen-independent microbicidal mechanisms then come into play.

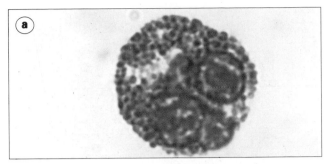

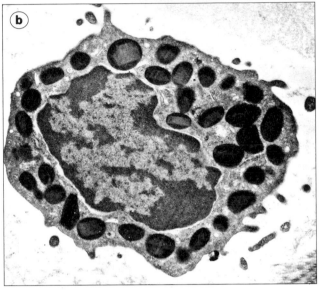

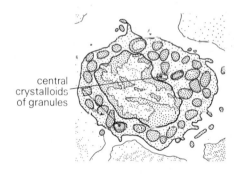

Fig. 4.28 The eosinophil granulocyte, is capable of extracellular killing of parasites (e.g. worms) by release of its granule contents. (a) Morphology of the eosinophil. This blood smear enriched for granulocytes shows an eosinophil with its multilobed nucleus and heavilystained cytoplasmic granules. Leishman stain. x1800. Courtesy of P Lydyard. (b) Electron micrograph showing the ultrastructure of a guinea pig eosinophil. The mature eosinophil contains granules with central crystalloids. x8000. Courtesy of D McLaren.

The complement system, a multicomponent triggered enzyme cascade, is used to attract phagocytic cells to the microbes and engulf them. The most abundant component, C3, is split by a convertase enzyme formed from its own cleavage product C3b and factor B and stabilized against breakdown caused by factors H and I, through association with the microbial surface. As it is formed, C3b becomes linked covalently to the microorganism. The next component C5, is activated to yield a small peptide, C5a, while residual C5b binds to the surface and assembles the terminal components C6–9 into a membrane attack complex which is freely permeable to solutes and can lead to

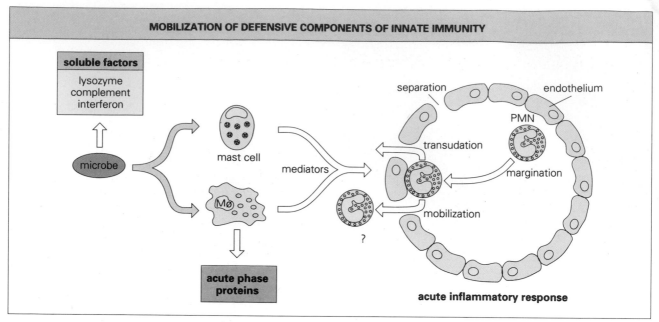

Fig. 4.29 Mobilization of defensive components of innate immunity. C', complement; Mø, macrophage.

osmotic lysis. In addition, C5a is a potent chemotactic agent for polymorphs and greatly increases capillary permeability. C3a and C5a act on mast cells causing the release of further mediators such as histamine, leukotriene B4 and tumour necrosis factor with effects on capillary permeability and adhesiveness, and neutrophil chemotaxis. They also activate neutrophils, which bind to the C3b-coated microbes by their surface C3b receptors and then ingest them. The influx of polymorphs and the increase in vascular permeability constitute the potent anti-microbial acute inflammatory response. Inflammation can also be initiated by tissue macrophages which subserve a similar role to the mast cell, since signalling by bacterial toxins, C5a or by iC3b-coated bacteria adhering to surface complement receptors causes release of TNF, LTB$_4$, PGE$_2$, neutrophil chemotactic factor and a neutrophil activating peptide.

Other humoral defences involve the acute phase proteins such as C-reactive protein. Viral replication can be blocked by interferons and virally infected cells can be killed by large granular lymphocytes with natural killer (NK) activity. Extracellular killing can also be effected by C3b-bound eosinophils. which may be responsible for the failure of many large parasites to establish a foothold in potential hosts

It is probably true to say that engulfment and killing by phagocytic cells is the mechanism used to dispose of the majority of microbes, and the mobilization and activation of these cells by orchestrated responses such as the acute inflammatory reaction (Fig. 4.29) is a key feature of innate immunity. However, by no means every organism is readily susceptible to phagocytosis or even to killing by complement or lysozyme and this brings us to the role of the adaptive immune response, as explored in the following chapter.

Further Reading

Alt F, Marrack P, Roitt IM, eds. *Curr Opinions in Immunol.* Journal series. London: Current Science. 1988 onwards.

Nichols B, Bainton DF, Farquhar MG. Differentiation of monocytes: origin, nature and fate of their azurophil granules. *J Cell Biol* 1971; **50:** 498–515.

Roitt IM. *Essential Immunology*, 7th edn. Oxford: Blackwell Scientific Publications, 1991.

Roitt IM, Brostoff J, Male D. *Immunology*, 2nd edn. London: Gower Medical Publishing, 1987.

Stadnyk AW, Gauldie J. The acute phase protein response during parasitic infection. *Immunol Today* 1991; **7:** A7–A12.

Wilson GS, Miles AA, Parker MT, eds. *Topley and Wilson's principles of bacteriology, virology and immunity*, 7th edn. Baltimore: Williams and Wilkins, 1983.

Zychlinsky A *et al.* Cytolytic mechanisms of the immune system. *Curr Opinions in Immunol* 1988; **1:** 63–69.

5 ADAPTIVE RESPONSES PROVIDE A QUANTUM LEAP IN EFFECTIVE DEFENCE

INTRODUCTION: THE NEED FOR 'TAILOR-MADE' IMMUNE DEFENCES

In the last chapter, we discussed the many ways in which the primary or innate defences of the body may counteract microbial infection. However, the extraordinary number of different microorganisms that surround us and their powerful ability to mutate, frequently result in infectious agents that can find ways around these innate defences. For example, the surface of some microbes fail to activate the alternative complement pathway, while others that can activate this pathway, do so at the end of flagelli, so that the membrane activation complex is planted at a site distant from the body of the organism and hence causes no damage. In other cases, microorganisms that are taken into the body of the macrophage, develop subterfuges that prevent the development of the awesome battery of microbicidal mechanisms which this cell normally expresses (see Chapter 12). Cells infected with certain viruses may prove to be insusceptible to the cytotoxic action of NK cells, or the viruses may be only weak stimulators of interferon so that cell-to-cell transmission of the virus proceeds unchecked. Yet another microbial subterfuge would be the production of bacterial toxins that can kill the phagocyte if not neutralized.

It is clear then that the body needs to provide immune defences that can be 'tailor-made' to each individual variant of the different species of microorganism. Ideally, these should link the organism directly into the various killing mechanisms of the innate system. In this chapter, we shall see how evolution has achieved just this by inserting specific recognition sites on antibody molecules and on certain lymphocytes. When an infectious agent enters the body, the white cells respond to it and produce a reaction that is specific for that particular microorganism. Furthermore, the magnitude of this response increases with time, often to quite high levels, so that we speak of this as an 'adaptive' or 'acquired' response.

ANTIBODY ACTS AS AN ADAPTOR TO FOCUS THE ACUTE INFLAMMATORY REACTION

Antibodies are synthesized by host B lymphocytes (so called because they mature in the bone marrow) when they make contact with an infectious microbe which acts as a foreign antigen, i.e. it generates antibodies. Each antibody has a recognition site, complementary in shape to the surface of the foreign antigen, which enables it to bind with varying degrees of strength to that antigen.

Other sites on the antibody molecule are specialized for such functions as activating the complement system and inducing phagocytosis by macrophages and polymorphs (Fig. 5.1). Thus, when a microbial antigen is coated with several of these adaptor antibody molecules, it can induce

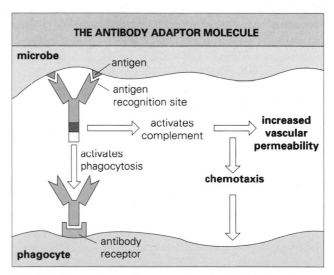

Fig. 5.1 The antigen adaptor molecule. Antibodies (anti-foreign bodies) are produced by host lymphocytes on contact with invading microbes which act as antigen (i.e. generate antibodies). Each antibody has a recognition site enabling it to bind antigen, and a backbone structure capable of some secondary biological action, e.g. activating complement and phagocytosis.

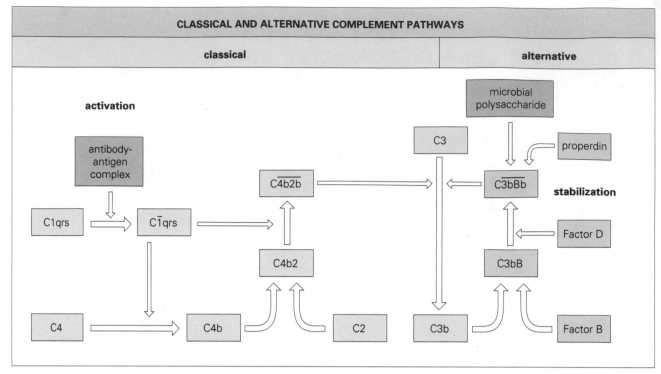

Fig. 5.2 The complex of antibody with microbial antigen activates the first component of the 'classical' pathway leading to cleavage of C3 through the C4b2b C3 convertase. This contrasts with the activation of the 'alternative' pathway which depends upon stabilization of the C3 convertase (C3bBb) on the microbial surface. The classical pathway in general is antibody dependent, the alternative pathway is not.

complement fixation and phagocytosis, processes which the microbe may well have evolved to avoid otherwise. In this way, the reluctant microorganism becomes drawn into the innate defence mechanism of the acute inflammatory response. We will now examine the ways in which antibody can mediate these different phenomena.

Antibody complexed with antigen activates complement through the 'classical' pathway

When antibody molecules bind an antigen, the resulting complex activates the first component of complement, C1, converting it into an esterase. This initiates a second route of complement activation (Fig. 5.2) termed the 'classical' pathway mainly because scientists discovered it before the 'alternative' pathway, although the evidence indicates that the latter is of greater antiquity in evolutionary terms. The activated first component splits off a small peptide from each of the succeeding components C4 and C2, the residual fragments forming a composite, the C4b2b complex, which has the enzymatic ability or property of a C3 convertase. It has a similar function to the alternative pathway C3 convertase C3bBb, and the sequence of events following the splitting of C3 is now indistinguishable from that occurring in the alternative pathway. C3a and C5a anaphylatoxins are formed and C3b binds to the surface of the microbe–antibody complex (Fig. 5.3). Subsequently, the later components are assembled into a membrane attack complex which may help to kill the microorganism if it has been focused by antibody onto a vulnerable site.

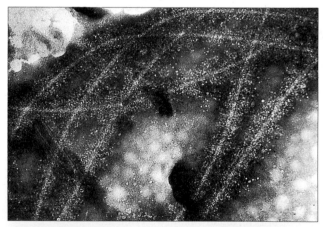

Fig. 5.3 Electron microscopy of C3-coated salmonella flagellae. The flagellae have been incubated with anti-flagella antibody and complement. The electron-dense material extending 30nm on either side of each flagellum , is believed to be C3b. The intepretation of this is that complement fixation by antibody results in a heavy macromolecular coating of C3b on biological membranes to which complement has been fixed. x900 000. Courtesy of A Feinstein and E Munn.

The acute inflammatory reaction can also be initiated by antibody bound to mast cells

A specialized antibody, immunoglobulin E (IgE), has a backbone site with high affinity for specific receptors on the surface of mast cells. When microbial antigen attaches to these cell-bound antibodies, the surface receptors are cross-linked and transduce a signal to the interior of the cell which leads to the release of mediators capable of effecting increases in vascular permeability and chemotaxis of polymorphs (Fig. 5.4). Thus, we see that antibody, either by activating complement or by directly causing mast cell degranulation, can bring about an acute inflammatory reaction at the site of the infectious agent.

Antigen–antibody complexes activate phagocytic cells

Other sites on the backbone of certain types of antibody molecule bind to specialized receptors on the surface of phagocytic cells. If there is more than one antibody in the antigen–antibody complex, these receptors are cross-linked and induce the cell to put out arms of cytoplasm which enclose the complex in a phagocytic vacuole (Fig. 5.5). Note also that there is a 'bonus effect' of multivalent binding of reversible ligand–receptor links; for example, the association constant for a complex binding through two antibody molecules to the phagocyte is the product rather than the sum of the individual association constants.

ANTIBODY CAN BLOCK IMPORTANT MICROBIAL REACTIONS

Because of its size, the antibody molecule can block interactions by combining with one of the two reacting molecules. For example, an antibody directed against the influenza haemagglutinin will prevent the virus from attaching to its specific receptor on a cell, making it unable to infect that cell (Fig. 5.6). Likewise, antibodies to an essential transport molecule on a bacterial surface can prevent the uptake of that nutrient and cause a metabolic block. As a last example, an antibody to a bacterial toxin prevents damage to cells with which it would otherwise react.

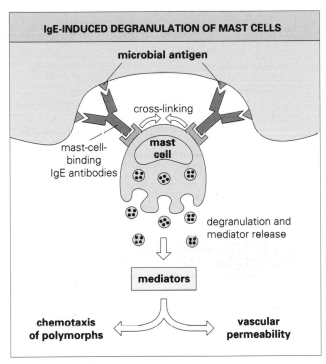

Fig. 5.4 Degranulation of mast cells by interaction of microbial antigen with specific antibodies of the IgE class which bind to special receptors on the mast cell surface. The cross-linking of receptors caused by this interaction leads to the release of mediators which induce an increase in vascular permeability and attract polymorphs, i.e. provoke an acute inflammatory reaction at the site of the microbial antigen.

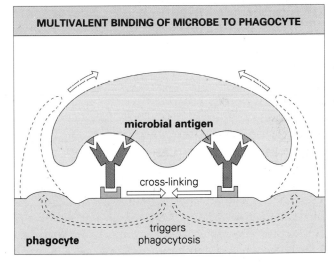

Fig. 5.5 The binding of a microbe to a phagocyte by more than one antibody cross-links the antibody receptors on the phagocyte surface and triggers phagocytosis of the microorganism.

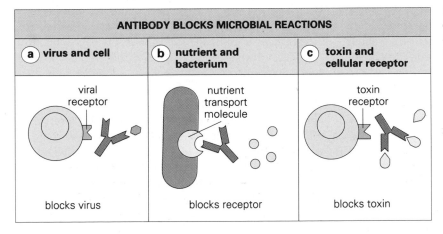

Fig. 5.6 Antibody, because of its size, can block interactions between (a) virus and cell, (b) nutrient and bacterium and (c) toxin and cellular receptor.

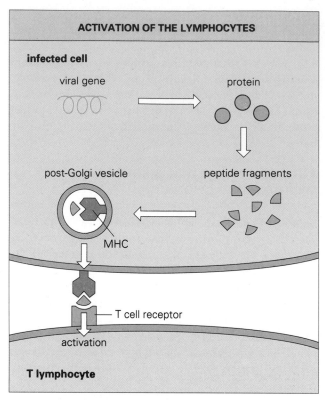

ACTIVATION OF THE LYMPHOCYTES

Fig. 5.7 T lymphocytes are activated when their specific cell surface receptors recognize an infected cell by binding to a surface MHC molecule that is associated with a peptide fragment of a degraded intracellular microorganism.

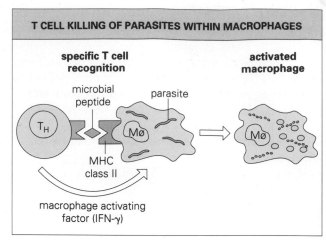

T CELL KILLING OF PARASITES WITHIN MACROPHAGES

Fig. 5.8 T$_H$ cells trigger the killing of parasites within macrophages. Recognition of the infected macrophage by the T$_H$ cell receptor result in lymphocyte activation with release of interferon-γ (IFN-γ). This then activates the macrophage, which turns on its microbicidal mechanisms to kill the intracellular parasite.

T LYMPHOCYTES IMPROVE DEFENCE AGAINST INTRACELLULAR ORGANISMS

Viruses and a number of different species of microorganisms can live within cells, where they are shielded from attack by antibody. The body has evolved a defence system against such organisms based upon the T lymphocyte, so called because it matures in the thymus gland. The system works in the following way. As microorganisms go through their various life cycles they sometimes die within the cells they infect. The proteins derived from these dead organisms are fragmented by intracellular enzymes ('processing'), and the peptides incorporated into cytoplasmic vacuoles where they associate with a molecule of the major histocompatibility complex (MHC). MHC molecules were originally discovered because of their ability to bring about the most violent rejection of grafts interchanged between members of the same species. We now know that one of their important functions is to act as surface markers. Class I MHC molecules are present on virtually every cell in the body, and therefore can be used as a marker for a 'cell'. Class II MHC appear mainly on macrophages and B cells. The specialized receptor on the T lymphocyte, which is analogous to an antibody molecule in its ability to recognize foreign antigen, is specialized for binding to the complex of MHC molecule and peptide derived from the intracellular organism. Thus, when it recognizes these two moi-

eties together, the T lymphocyte binds to an infected cell of a type indicated by the class of the MHC. The T lymphocyte then becomes activated (Fig. 5.7) and, depending upon its particular characteristics, sets in train an effector mechanism that deals with the intracellular microorganisms, as explained below.

T lymphocytes help macrophages to kill intracellular parasites

The task of recognizing macrophages that have unwelcome guests such as listeria or tubercle bacilli living within them, falls to a subset of lymphocytes called the T helper (T$_H$) cells. When a specific T$_H$ cell combines with a complex of MHC class II and microbial peptide on the surface of an infected macrophage, it is triggered to release macrophage activating factors, notably interferon-γ (IFN-γ; see Chapter 12). This unleashes previously suppressed microbicidal mechanisms within the macrophage, so leading to death of the intracellular parasites (Fig. 5.8).

T lymphocytes inhibit intracellular replication of viruses

Cells infected with virus express a complex consisting of class I MHC and a virally derived peptide on their surface. This is recognized by the specific receptor on cytotoxic T (T$_C$) cells which are thus led into close proximity to their virally infected target; the target cell is then killed by similar extracellular mechanisms to those described in the last chapter under 'natural killer cells'. Since the virally derived peptides appear on the cell surface at a very early stage of infection, the T$_C$ cells kill the cell before the virus has had an opportunity to replicate significantly and the host has won an important battle. The natural killer (NK) cell fulfils a similar function, but because it lacks the specialized receptor for recognizing the particular viral peptide in association with class I MHC, its chances of binding

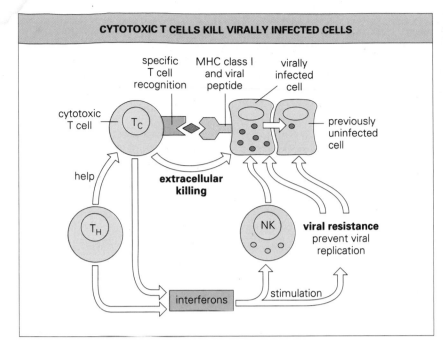

CYTOTOXIC T CELLS KILL VIRALLY INFECTED CELLS

Fig. 5.9 Cytoxic T cells (T$_C$) specifically recognize and kill virally infected cells before the virus replicates. Natural killer (NK) cells can do the same, though far less effectively; however their activity is enhanced by interferons produced by T$_C$ and T$_H$ cells. Local production of interferons also prevents adjacent cells from becoming infected by intercellular viral transport.

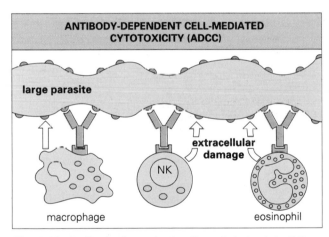

ANTIBODY-DEPENDENT CELL-MEDIATED CYTOTOXICITY (ADCC)

Fig. 5.10 Antibody-dependent cell-mediated cytotoxicity (ADCC). Different effector cells bind to the parasite surface through their receptor for antibody and damage the parasite target. The antibodies essentially belong to the IgG class (see Chapter 6).

strongly to the surface of the infected target cell are very much less than those of the T$_C$ cell. However, it is of interest that both the cytotoxic T cell and the T helper cell are capable of releasing interferons that markedly improve the performance of the NK cell, so making a useful integrated system. Nonetheless, the main responsibility of these interferons is to render adjacent cells resistant to replication of viral particles which gain entrance through intercellular transport mechanisms (Fig. 5.9).

EXTRACELLULAR ATTACK ON LARGE INFECTIOUS AGENTS IS AIDED BY ANTIBODY

Where a parasite is demonstrably larger than a phagocytic cell, it is physically impossible for phagocytosis to occur.

However, it is still possible for the defensive cells to deliver an extracellular attack on the surface of the parasite. This can occur through the phenomenon of 'antibody-dependent cell-mediated cytotoxicity' (ADCC) in which effector cells bind through their surface receptors to antibody molecules coating the target cell (Fig. 5.10). The result of this interaction is to induced activation of the effector cell and the release of materials which damage the parasite target. Major cell types that indulge in this type of activity are the macrophage, the eosinophil and the natural killer cell, which in this context of antibody-mediated killing, is often referred to as a K cell.

LOCAL DEFENCE AT MUCOSAL SURFACES

The immune mechanisms involving the acute inflammatory response and T cell mediated systems, operate well within the milieu of the body. It is worth examining the special nature of the defences required to protect the body at the mucosal surfaces which face the exterior such as the lung and the gastrointestinal tract (Fig. 5.11). The first line of defence is aimed at preventing the microbe from adhering to the mucosal surface, which is a prerequisite for penetration of the body. Aside from the innate mechanism of mucus production, a special antibody, immuno-globulin A (IgA), is actively secreted into the lumen and is present at a high concentration associated with the mucosal surface. When coated with such antibodies, the adherence of infectious agents is very greatly diminished. Mast cells tend to cluster in the submucosal region and should a microorganism break through the mucosal barrier, it could encounter a mast cell which has bound the specialized IgE antibody to its surface; on reaction with this surface antibody, the mast cell is triggered to

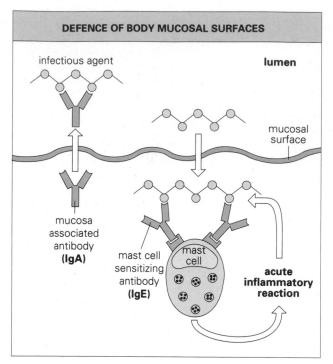

Fig. 5.11 Defence of body mucosal surfaces. A specialized antibody associated with the mucosal surface (secretory immunoglobulin A) blocks adherence of the microbe to the mucosa and hence entry into the body. An infectious agent gaining entrance to the body will fire IgE-sensitized mast cells which cluster beneath the surface and generate a protective acute inflammatory response.

release mediators of the acute inflammatory reaction. By increasing vascular permeability, these mediators will bring about the flooding of the site with plasma proteins, including other classes of antibody and complement, while chemotactic agents will attract polymorphonuclear leucocytes.

The presence of larger parasites such as nematodes within the lumen of the gut poses special problems. It is thought that antigens derived from the nematode may penetrate into the submucosal space and activate T and B cells and degranulate sensitized mast cells. The latter will produce an acute inflammation at the mucosal surface and almost certainly leads to an outflow of antibody, complement and probably effectors of ADCC into the lumen, where they can interact with the parasite and inflict metabolic damage. In the meantime, the interaction with sensitized T helper cells will lead to the release of soluble factors, termed lymphokines, among which will be a mediator that is capable of stimulating the goblet cells lining the intestinal villi. These release their mucins into the lumen where they coat the damaged parasite and facilitate expulsion from the body (Fig. 5.12) .

SUMMARY

The evolution of the adaptive response has provided the body with a very powerful series of mechanisms which extend and exploit the innate mechanisms of defence. As

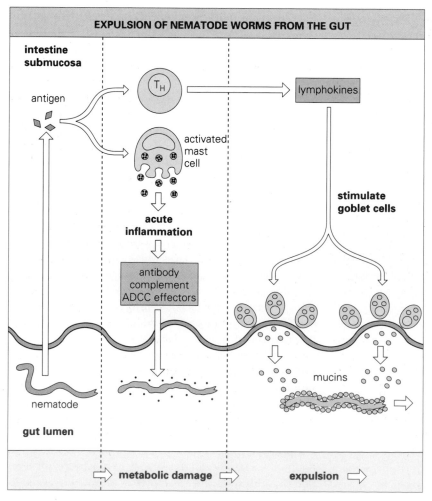

Fig. 5.12 Expulsion of nematode worms from the gut. Worm antigen is thought to trigger an acute inflammatory reaction in the submucosa which facilities, complement and possibly ADCC effectors which damage the parasite. Soluble factors (lymphokines), released by antigen-specific trigger of T helper cells, stimulate the secretion by goblet cells of mucins which coat the worm and aid its expulsion.

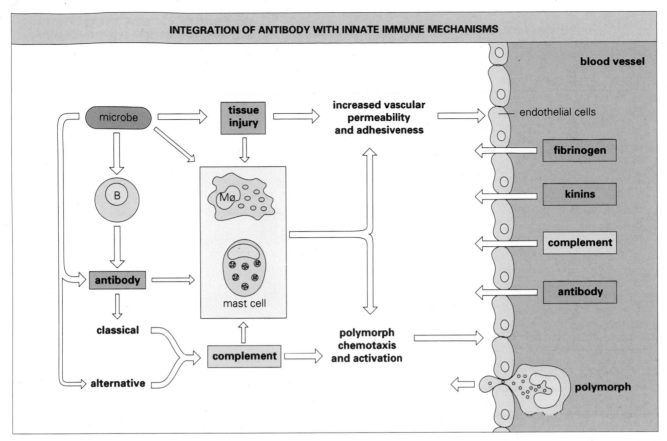

Fig. 5.13 Integration of antibody with the innate immune mechanisms leading to the production of a protective acute inflammatory reaction. The activated endothelial cells allow exudation of soluble proteins from the circulation and express accessory molecules which aid the binding of the polymorphs to the capillary wall and their subsequent escape into the infected site.

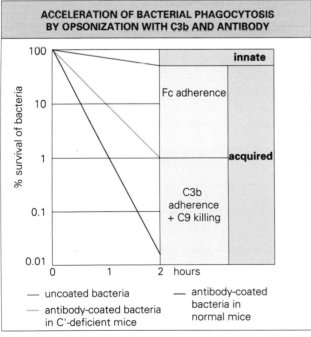

Fig. 5.14 The slow rate of phagocytosis of uncoated bacterial (innate immunity) is increased many-fold by acquired immunity through coating with antibody and then C3b (opsonization). Killing may also take place through the C5-9 terminal complement components. This is a hypothetical but realistic situation; the natural proliferation of the bacteria has been ignored.

we have seen, the characteristic of this lymphocyte-mediated action is to build up the defence against each particular infecting organism into a major response. In the majority of cases, the effector mechanisms lead the organism back into the innate systems of defence, such as phagocytosis, complement activation, macrophage intracellular killing, and so forth.

Taking a brief bird's eye view of the adaptive responses, humoral immunity, mediated by antibody produced by B lymphocytes, is effective in neutralizing bacterial toxins and by interacting with complement, mast cells and poly-morphs, produces the acute inflammatory reaction (Fig. 5.13). This response is especially effective against extracel-lular microbes and the quantum leap provided by antibody in the clearance of extracellular bacteria from the blood is clearly shown in the example in figure 5.14. By contrast, the T cell mediated response is directed to intracellular organisms. The T helper cells interact with macrophages by producing lymphokines, firstly chemotactic factors, and secondly interferon-γ which activates phagocytic cells to switch on their intracellular anti-microbial mechanisms. Cytotoxic T cells are effective against viruses, killing virally infected targets and preventing the spread of virus through the local production of interferons.

Figure 5.15 emphasizes the close interactions between innate and acquired mechanisms leading to defence against extracellular microorganisms on the one hand,

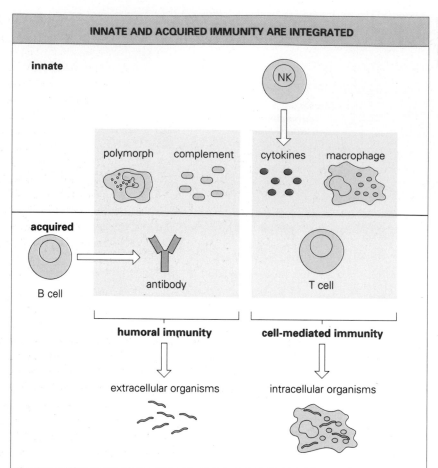

INNATE AND ACQUIRED IMMUNITY ARE INTEGRATED

innate

NK

polymorph   complement   cytokines   macrophage

acquired

B cell

antibody   T cell

humoral immunity   **cell-mediated immunity**

extracellular organisms   intracellular organisms

Fig. 5.15 The mechanisms of innate and acquired immunity are integrated to provide the basis for humoral and cell-mediated immunity respectively

and intracellular infections on the other. In keeping with these concepts, deficiencies in humoral immunity from whatever cause, predispose the individual to infection by extracellular organisms, whereas defects in T cell mediated responses are primarily associated with intracellular infections.

The first contact with antigen evokes a response that leaves behind a memory of the encounter, so that the subsequent response to second contact with antigen is more powerful and more rapid in its evolution than on the first occasion. The cellular bases for these phenomena are explained in a later chapter, but it will be clear that the production of memory by primary interaction with antigen provides the basis for vaccination, where the first contract is with an avirulent form of the microorganism or its component antigens. The other point to stress at this stage is the specificity of memory, so that infection with measles for example, produces a subsequent immunity to that virus, but does not afford protection against an unrelated virus such as mumps.

Further Reading

Roitt IM. *Essential Immunology*, 7th edn. Oxford: Blackwell Scientific Publications, 1990.

Roitt IM, Brostoff J, Male DK, eds. *Immunology*, 2nd edn. London: Gower Medical Publishing, 1987.

Klein J, ed. *Immunology*. Oxford: Blackwell Scientific Publications, 1990.

Law SKA, Reid KBM. *Complement*. In Focus series. Male DK, ed. Oxford: IRL Press, 1988.

Goldschmeider I, Gotschlich EC, Artenstein MS. Human immunity to the meningococcus. I. The role of humoral antibodies. *J Exp Med* 1969;**129**:1307.

6 THE BASIS OF ANTIGEN RECOGNITION

INTRODUCTION: WHAT ARE ANTIGENS?

In the last chapter we became familiar with the idea that an infectious agent can generate antibodies within the host. Each different type of microbial molecule to which antibodies bind, is called an 'antigen'. Different antibodies bind to different antigens, providing each antibody with its own particular specificity. To be more precise, each antibody binds to an individual part of the antigen termed an 'antigenic determinant' or, preferably, an 'epitope'. A given antigen can display several different epitopes, or sometimes several identical epitopes, on its surface depending on the degree of symmetry of the molecule (Fig. 6.1). Since each individual antibody is complemen-

tary in shape to a given epitope, its specificity resides in its binding to that epitope rather than to the antigen molecule as a whole. Furthermore, each antigen has its own particular set of epitopes not usually shared with other antigens, so that the collection of antibodies in an antiserum is effectively specific for that antigen.

It is broadly true to say that the more distant a molecule is in evolutionary terms, the more antigenic it is for a given host. The less foreign a molecule is phylogenetically, the more it resembles the components of the host itself. Thus, the immune response is correspondingly weaker since the mechanisms of so-called immunological tolerance set up in early life act to inhibit the response of the lymphoid system to self (i.e. auto-) antigens.

Antigens are usually large molecules and are very frequently proteins. Examples include the envelope and nucleoproteins from viruses, the membrane proteins and exotoxins of bacteria, and many of the surface components of different parasitic organisms. The complex array of bacterial cell-wall carbohydrates provide a rich variety of different antigens, most of them characteristic of the particular organisms with which they are associated. Glycolipids can also be antigenic, but uncomplicated lipids and nucleic acids tend to be non-antigenic partly because of their close structural resemblance to self and partly due to the inability of T helper cells to recognize them.

MOLECULES INVOLVED IN ANTIGEN RECOGNITION

Immunoglobulins

Structure
The immunoglobulins are based on a unit structure consisting of four polypeptide chains, two heavy and two light, as shown in figure 6.2. Each chain is composed of individual globular domains (Fig. 6.3), and whereas the N-terminal domains in a given antibody population show very high variability in amino acid structure, the remaining domains are relatively constant (see Fig. 6.2).

ANTIGENS AND THEIR CORRESPONDING ANTIBODIES

antigen   antibody

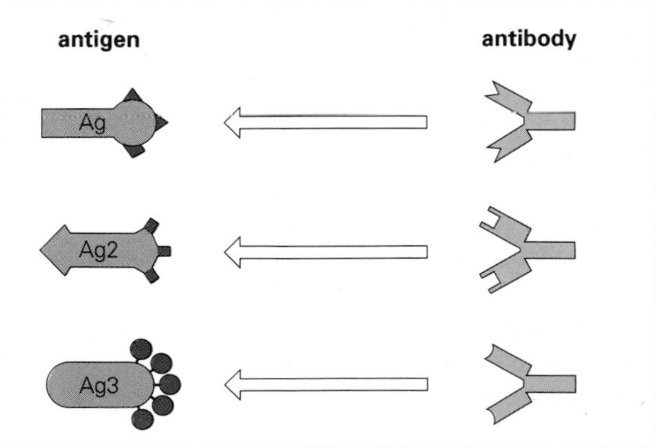

Fig. 6.1 Antigens and their corresponding antibodies. Antibodies recognize and combine with a number of different sites on the surface of the antigen molecule termed 'epitopes' or sometimes 'antigen determinants'. The epitopes on a given antigen are often different from one another (Ag1) and usually different from those on another antigen (Ag2). Some antigens have repeated epitopes (Ag3). Even simple microorganisms are composed of several different antigens.

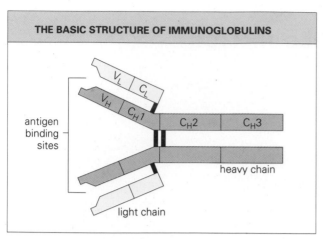

THE BASIC STRUCTURE OF IMMUNOGLOBULINS

Fig. 6.2 The basic structure of immunoglobulin. The unit consists of two identical light polypeptide chains and two identical heavy polypeptide chains linked together by disulphide bonds. Each chain is made up of individual globular domains. Different antibodies have different V_L and V_H domains which are therefore highly variable whereas the remaining domains (C_L and C_H1 etc.) are relatively constant in amino acid structure.

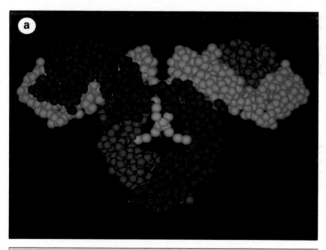

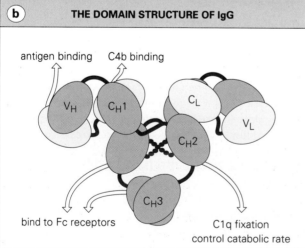

THE DOMAIN STRUCTURE OF IgG

Fig. 6.3 The structure of IgG. (a) Computer generated model of IgG. Heavy chains are shown in blue and red with the two light chains in green. Carbohydrate bound to the Fc portion is shown in turquoise. The structure was determined by EW Silverton *et al.* (1977). The figure was generated by computer graphics using the system developed by RJ Feldmann at the NIH. (b) The domain structure of IgG showing its relationship to function.

designation	IgG	IgA	IgM	IgD	IgE
PHYSICAL PROPERTIES OF MAJOR HUMAN IMMUNOGLOBULINS					
sedimentation coefficient	7S	7S, 9S, 11S*	19S	7S	8S
molecular weight	150 000	160 000 & dimer	900 000	185 000	200 000
number of basic four-peptide units	1	1,2*	5	1	1
heavy chains	γ	α	μ	δ	ε
light chains κ+λ	κ+λ	κ+λ	κ+λ	κ+λ	κ+λ
valency for antigen binding	2	2,4	5(10)	2	2
concentration range in normal serum (mg/ml)	8–16	1.4–4	0.5–2	0–0.4	(2–50) x10⁻⁵
% total immunoglobulin	80	13	6	0–1	0.002

* dimer in external secretion caries secretory component IgA dimer and IgM contain J-chain

Fig. 6.4 Physical properties of the major human immunoglobulins.

In humans, immunoglobulins can be grouped into five major classes on the basis of these constant region domains: immunoglobulin G (IgG), IgA, IgM, IgD and IgE. The major physical characteristics of these immunoglobulins are set out in figure 6.4. Whereas IgG, serum IgA, IgD and IgE exist in the form of the basic four peptide unit, IgM and secretory IgA appear largely as polymeric molecules, IgM being a pentamer and IgA a dimer, the structures of which are based on inter-unit disulphide links (Fig. 6.5).

To complicate the picture further, there are minor variations in the structure of the IgG constant regions which give rise to four subclasses, namely IgG1, IgG2, IgG3 and IgG4. Likewise IgA is subdivided into two subclasses. These classes and subclasses are all present in the blood of normal individuals and are therefore termed 'isotypes'. (The term 'idiotype' refers to the set of epitopes in the variable region of a given immunoglobulin which react with an antiserum raised against it.)

The structural basis of function

The elucidation of the relationship between structure and function was greatly facilitated by studies in which IgG molecules were cleaved by proteolytic enzymes. Papain generates two Fab fragments each of which contains a single binding site for antigen (Fig. 6.6): in addition an Fc portion containing the remaining heavy chain domains is split off and has been shown to mediate a number of immunoglobulin functions, such as classical complement

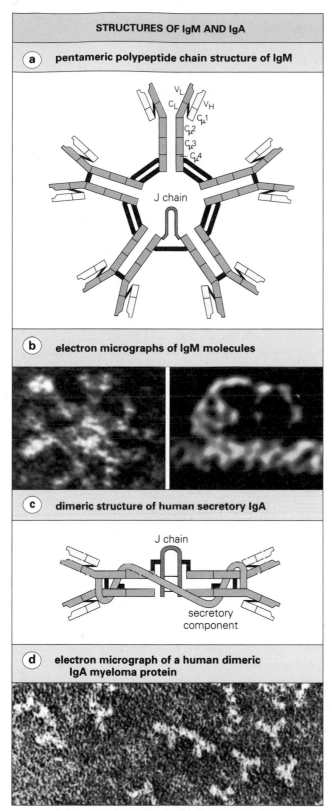

STRUCTURES OF IgM AND IgA

(a) pentameric polypeptide chain structure of IgM

(b) electron micrographs of IgM molecules

(c) dimeric structure of human secretory IgA

(d) electron micrograph of a human dimeric IgA myeloma protein

Fig. 6.5 The structures of IgM and IgA.
(a) Pentameric polypeptide chain structure of IgM. (b) Electron micrographs of IgM molecules in free solution adopting (left) the characteristic star-shaped configuration (x520 000. Courtesy of R Dourmashkin) and (right) a crab-like configuration due to cross-linkage with a single flagellum (x520 000. Courtesy of A Feinstein). (c) Dimeric structure of human secretory IgA. (d) Electron micrograph of a human dimeric IgA myeloma protein. The double Y-shaped appearance indicates that the monomeric subunits are linked end to end through the C-terminal Cα3 domain. x160 000. Courtesy of R Dourmashkin.

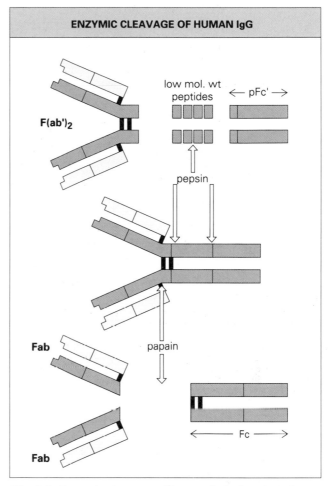

ENZYMIC CLEAVAGE OF HUMAN IgG

Fig. 6.6 Enzymic cleavage of human IgG. Pepsin induces a divalent antigen binding fragment, F(ab')$_2$ and a pFc' fragment composed of 2 terminal C$_H$3 domains. Papain produces two univalent antigen binding fragments, Fab, and an Fc portion containing the C$_H$2 and C$_H$3 heavy chain domains.

fixation and attachment to the Fc receptor sites on accessory cells such as polymorphs and macrophages. Pepsin on the other hand cleaves an F(ab')$_2$ fragment which contains both antigen binding sites. It therefore acts like the full IgG molecule in terms of its ability to link different antigenic molecules together to cause such phenomena as agglutination. With this enzyme, however, the Fc region is partially degraded and secondary biological functions such as complement fixation are lost. The Fab fragments contain the very highly variable domains and it is now clear that the individual binding specificity of each antibody is intimately linked to the hypervariability in amino acid sequence in certain sectors of these variable domains. These 'complementarity determining regions' are arranged together on the surface of the molecule to form the antigen binding site. A basic summary of the biological properties of the major human immunoglobulin classes is given in figure 6.7.

BIOLOGICAL PROPERTIES OF MAJOR IMMUNOGLOBULIN CLASSES IN THE HUMAN					
	IgG	IgA	IgM	IgD	IgE
major characteristics	most abundant internal Ig	protects external surfaces	very efficient against bacteraemia	mainly lymphocyte receptor	initiates inflammation, raised in parasitic infections, causes allergy symptoms
antigen binding	++	++	++	++	++
complement fixation (classical)	++	–	+++	–	–
cross placenta	++	–	–	–	–
fix to homologous mast cells and basophils	–	–	–	–	++
binding to macrophages and polymorphs	++	±	–	–	±

Fig. 6.7 Biological properties of major immunoglobulin classes in the human.

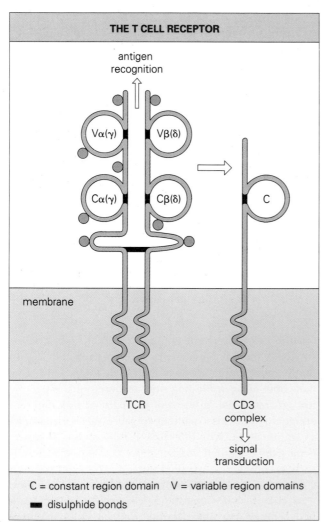

THE T CELL RECEPTOR

antigen recognition

Vα(γ)   Vβ(δ)

Cα(γ)   Cβ(δ)   C

membrane

TCR   CD3 complex

signal transduction

C = constant region domain   V = variable region domains
■ disulphide bonds

Fig. 6.8 The structure of the T cell receptor (TCR). Antigen plus MHC is recognized by the VαCα/VβCβ disulphide-linked transmembrane heterodimer TCR2, or the alternative VγCγ/VδCδ TCR1. The receptor is associated with the CD3 complex which transduces the signal produced by antigen recognition to the cell interior. Based on Clevers H *et al.* (1988).

The T cell receptor

Antigens are recognized not only by antibodies but also by receptors on the surface of the T lymphocyte. These receptors consist of a heterodimer of two transmembrane peptide chains, each of which is folded to form two domains with the characteristic overall structure of those seen in the immunoglobulins (Fig. 6.8). Rather like an Fab fragment from an immunoglobulin molecule, each peptide consists of a variable and a constant domain with hypervariable regions on the variable domain that are presumed to be responsible for individual antigen binding specificity. The majority of T cells have heterodimers composed of α and β chains but a minority, which appear first in foetal development, have γ and δ chains. Whenever the T cell receptor is expressed on the T cell surface, it is always associated with the CD3 transmembrane molecular complex, which transduces the signal induced when the receptor is triggered by contact with antigen, to the interior of the cell.

The major histocompatibility complex

The molecules making up the major histocompatibility complex (MHC) were first discovered through their ability to provoke a dominant rejection response when tissues from one individual were transplanted to another individual of the same species. Quite apart from its contribution to the difficulties of transplant surgery, in recent years it has become abundantly clear that the MHC plays a major role in the operation of T cell immunity, particularly in its function to present antigen to the T cell receptor (see Chapter 5).

The structure of the MHC

In the context of antigen recognition by T cells we are primarily concerned with class I and class II MHC molecules and have no need to discuss class III which are essentially part of the complement system. Class I molecules are made up of a transmembrane heavy chain peptide which is

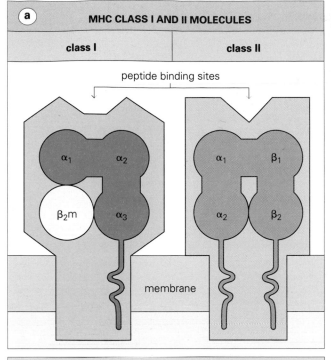

a MHC CLASS I AND II MOLECULES

| class I | class II |

peptide binding sites

α_1 α_2

$\beta_2 m$ α_3

α_1 β_1

α_2 β_2

membrane

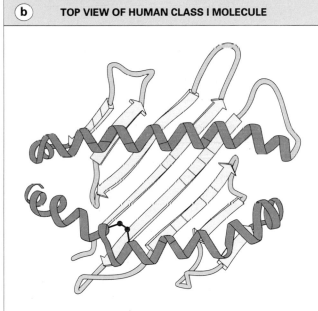

b TOP VIEW OF HUMAN CLASS I MOLECULE

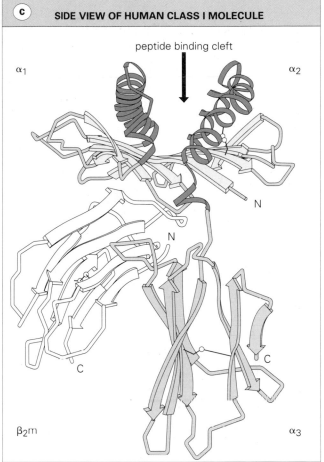

c SIDE VIEW OF HUMAN CLASS I MOLECULE

peptide binding cleft

α_1 α_2

N

N

C C

$\beta_2 m$ α_3

Fig. 6.9 Class I and class II major histocompatibility complex molecules. (a) Diagram showing domains and transmembrane segments; the α-helices and β-sheets are viewed end on. (b) Top surface of human class I molecule (HLA-A2) based on X-ray crystallographic structure. The strands making the β-pleated sheet are shown as thick grey arrows in the amino to carboxy direction, α-helices are represented as helical ribbons. The inside facing surfaces of the two helices and the upper surface of the β-sheet form a cleft. The two black spheres represent an intrachain disulphide bond. (c) Side view showing the cleft and the typical Ig folding of the α3 and β2-microglobulin domains (4 anti-parallel β-strands on one face and 3 on the other). Reproduced from Bjorkman P.I. *et al.* (1987) with permission.

noncovalently associated with the small β2-microglobulin (β2m) molecule (Fig. 6.9). Class II molecules, on the other hand, are composed of two smaller transmembrane peptide chains, α and β. The peptides are arranged in domains that are of comparable size to those of immunoglobulin molecules, and almost certainly share ancestral genes with the latter. However, only the extracellular domains immediately adjacent to the cell membrane and the β2-microglobulin peptide have clear homology with the immunoglobulin domains. The α1 and α2 segments of class I and the α1 and β1 domains of class II have quite an unusual structure which has recently been revealed through x-ray analytical studies. As shown in

figure 6.9, these external domains form a striking cavity, bounded on two sides by α-helical structures, with a floor composed of β-sheet peptide strands. It is as though the groove had been formed from two curved sausages (the α-helices) facing each other on a plate (the β-pleated sheet).

Class I molecules are present on virtually every cell in the body, the most notable exception being the syncytial trophoblast of the placenta. Class II expression is far more restricted; B cells, dendritic cells which present antigen to T cells, and activated macrophages express abundant class II molecules on their surface. However, most other tissues can be induced to express class II molecules under the influence of soluble mediators such as interferon-γ.

GENES IN THE HUMAN MHC (HLA)																
complex	HLA															
MHC class	II			III										I		
genes (chromosome 6)	DP_β DP_α	DQ_β DQ_α	DR_β DR_α	210HB	C4B	210HA	C4A	FB	C2	HSP1	HSP2	TNFα	TNFβ	B	C	A
gene products	HLA-DP	HLA-DQ	HLA-DR	210HB	C4B	210HA	C4A	FB	C2	HSP1	HSP2	TNFα	TNFβ	HLA-B	HLA-C	HLA-A

Fig. 6.10 Genes in the major histocompatibility complex in the human, the HLA system. Class III MHC encodes complement components and other proteins as shown. 210HB, 21-hydroxylase; FB, complement factor B; HSP, 70 kDa heat shock protein; TNF, tumour necrosis factor.

GENES IN THE MOUSE MHC												
complex	H2										Tla	
MHC class	I	II	III						I		I	I
genetic region	K	I	S						D		Qa	Tla
genes (chromosome 17)	K	$A_\beta A_\alpha E_\beta E_\alpha$	C4	Slp	FB	C2	TNFα	TNFβ	D	L	Qa(17)	Tla Qa(12)
gene products	H-2K	I-A I-E	C4	C4'	FB	C2	TNFα	TNFβ	H-2D	H-2L	Qa(2–5)	Tla Qa1,6

Fig. 6.11 Genes in the MHC complex of the mouse.

Gene map of the MHC

A map of the human major histocompatibility gene complex is given in figure 6.10. There are three major class I loci and three class II making a total of six different proteins forming the MHC, known in the human as the 'HLA' system. Each locus is highly polymorphic, i.e. there are a large number of different allelic forms of each protein, so that individuals are genetically highly diverse with respect to HLA tissue types. A comparable map for the mouse MHC, the H-2 system, is given in figure 6.11.

THE GENERATION OF DIVERSITY

We know that the body produces millions of different antibodies capable as a population of recognizing virtually any pathogen that has arisen or might arise. Since this is probably more than the total number of genes in the body, there must be some clever way in which all this diversity is generated. Before examining these mechanisms, we must first look at the genetic building blocks from which the final genes encoding antibody molecules and the T cell receptor are constructed.

Multiple gene segments code for antibody and T cell receptor

The gene segments that code for antibody are grouped into three major clusters on three different chromosomes, coding for κ, λ and heavy chains. In the human, the V_κ, V_λ and V_H regions each consist of 100 or so different gene segments. The other genes involved in forming the variable region of the immunoglobulin peptides are a small series of J minigenes, which contribute to the light chains (Fig. 6.12), and both J and D segments which contribute to the heavy chain (Fig. 6.13). Single genes code for each of the immunoglobulin constant regions. The αβ and γδ T cell receptor peptide chains are coded for by rather similar clusters of gene families. The sequence of events which lead to the final synthesis of κ light chain peptides is shown in figure 6.12 as model for the recombinations which generate the final immunoglobulin gene.

Mechanisms for the generation of diversity

Intra-chain recombination

During the DNA translocation event in, for instance, the H chain variable region, a single V_H gene becomes linked to one D and one J region gene in the pre-B cell. Since there is a random selection and recombination of these genes, the 100 V_H, 12 D and 6 J region genes can give rise to a total of over 7×10^3 (100 x 12 x 6) combinations and therefore antibody specificities. Further variation is produced by variable recombinations at the VD and DJ boundaries giving different junctional sequences, and by the insertion of nucleotides at the N region of the D and J segments. By combining with only one of the constant

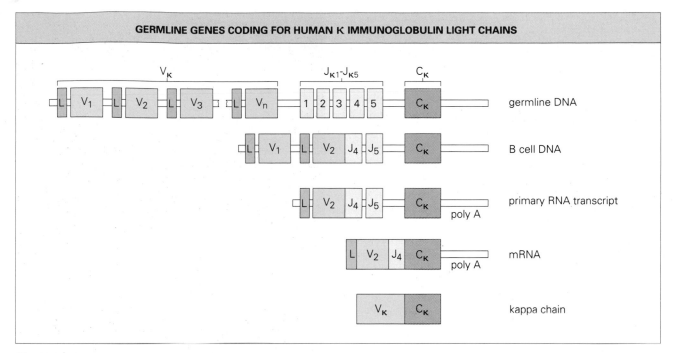

Fig. 6.12 Germline genes encoding human κ immunoglobulin light chains. During differentiation of the pre-B cell, one of the 100 or so V_K genes on the germline DNA is recombined and apposed to one of five J_K minigenes. Each V_K gene is preceded by a leader sequence (L). The B cell transcribes a segment of DNA into a primary RNA transcript which is processed into mRNA by splicing out the intervening nucleotides between the L, VJ and constant region C_K exons. The mRNA becomes associated with the endoplasmic reticulum where it is translated on the ribosomes into κ-light chains.

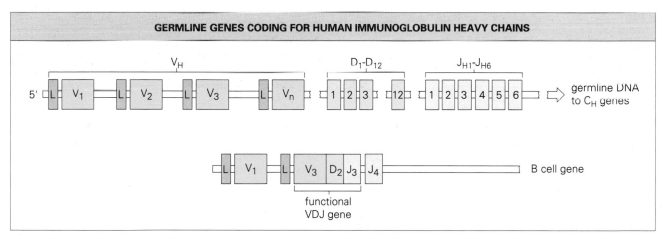

Fig. 6.13 Germline genes coding for human immunoglobulin heavy chains. The heavy chain gene loci combine three segments to produce the exon (VDJ gene) which will code for the V_H domain. One of several hundred V genes recombines with one of twelve D segments, and one of six J segments, to produce a functional VDJ gene, in the B cell. The rearrangement illustrated is only one of the many thousand possible.

region genes at a time, the same antibody specificity can be stitched into any of the different immunoglobulin classes.

Similar considerations show that there could be some 500 different κ chains (100 V_K x 5 J_K) and 600 λ chains, a total of some 1100 light chains, again without considering any of the further recombination strategies which have evolved to squeeze even more variety out of a limited number of gene segments.

Inter-chain amplification

Because any one heavy chain can combine with any one light chain, the total number of different specificities that could be generated is now the product of the number of each type. Thus, using the above figures, random combinations of heavy and light chains would yield at the very least 8×10^6 (7×10^3 multiplied by 1100) different possible combinations. All this from around 600 different gene segments!

The T cell receptor diversity arises by comparable mechanisms and the αβ receptor, for example, may exist in at least 8×10^6 and probably many more different combinatorial associations. The process can be likened in some ways to a child's building set, where a relatively small number of different building blocks can be put together in many thousands of different ways to create a multiplicity of objects.

Somatic mutation

Unlike the T cell receptor the genes coding for the variable region of antibody peptide chains undergo a high rate of somatic mutation, through random replacement of nucleotides during cell division, fairly early in the immune response and almost certainly under the influence of T cell help. As we shall see later, this mechanism provides a means whereby high affinity antibodies can be selected during the adaptive immune response.

THE RECOGNITION OF ANTIGEN BY ANTIBODIES AND T CELLS

Antibody recognizes native antigen

If the native three-dimensional confirmation of a protein antigen is destroyed by denaturation, its ability to combine with its antibody is largely, or more often completely, lost. In other words antibodies formed to the native protein antigen recognize the conformation of the native but not the denatured molecule. Thus, the three-dimensional configuration rather than the linear sequence of amino acids making up the protein is usually of primary consideration, at least in the case of globular proteins. Of course this is helpful to the host as antibodies must react with the components of the infectious organism that are encountered within the body after infection, when they are normally in their native state.

The necessity for intimate complementarity of shape between antigen and antibody (i.e. a lock and key type fit), is evident from the x-ray crystallographic analysis of the complex formed between the Fab fragment of an antibody and its antigen (hen egg white lysozyme in figure 6.14). Amino acids, largely within the special hypervariable regions of the antibody, provide a surface which complements that of the antigen epitope. This allows the two molecules to dock together so that the atomic radii of antigen and antibody are closely opposed over a large area, enabling the relatively weak non-covalent intermolecular forces to operate with high efficiency. These include coulombic, hydrogen bond, hydrophobic and van der Waals' forces which increase greatly in magnitude with a diminution in the distance between the attracting moieties, and if the intermolecular distance is so small that water molecules are excluded, these forces achieve very high levels. Changes in the amino acid sequence in the hypervariable region, by providing different side chains, can destroy the antibody's ability to combine with a particular antigen but may confer the ability to combine with another antigen with a different complementary shape; it is in this way that the specificity of the antibody is mediated.

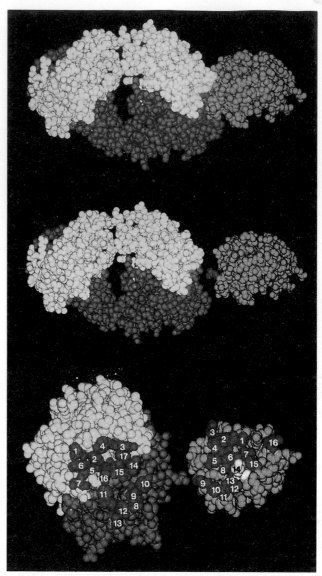

Fig. 6.14 The Fab-lysozyme complex. The upper panel shows lysozyme (green) binding to the hypervariable regions of the heavy (blue) and light (yellow) chains of the Fab fragment of antibody Dl.3. The centre panel shows the complex separated with Glu 121 (red) visible. This residue fits into the centre of the cleft between the heavy and light chains. The lower panel shows the molecules rotated forward 90° to show the contact residues which contribute to the antigen–antibody bond. Courtesy of RJ Poljak; permission from *Science* 1986; **233**: 747-753. Copyright 1986 by the AAAS.

How T cells recognize infected cells

Extracellular microbial antigens are dealt with effectively by circulating antibodies. As discussed earlier T cells, which mediate cellular immunity, have to recognize infected cells as their targets. This involves seeing antigen in the context of an infected cell. The molecular marker used by the body to represent a cell is one or more components of the major histocompatibility complex. For example, cytotoxic T cells must be able to recognize almost any cell type infected with a virus, and since class I MHC molecules are expressed by virtually every cell in the body, they can be employed by the immune system to target the killer T lymphocyte onto the infected cell. In much the same way, class II MHC molecules on the surface of activated

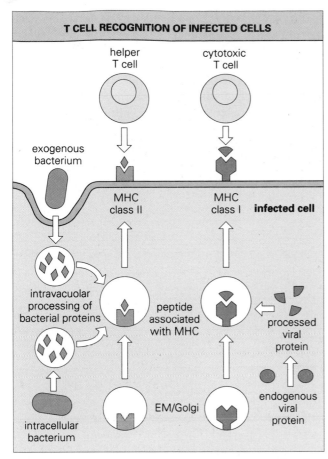

T CELL RECOGNITION OF INFECTED CELLS

Fig. 6.15 T cell recognition of infected cells. The T cell receptor binds to MHC molecule combined with peptide derived from processed antigen, which together act as markers for the cell and the infecting antigen.

macrophages are used to direct the lymphokine-producing T cells onto an infected macrophage, and hence to trigger the release of interferon-γ and other appropriate lymphokines.

Thus, the MHC provides part of the homing signal for the T cell receptor. However, we must still consider how evolution has handled the problem of presenting antigen to the T cell receptor without confusion with extracellular native antigen which might block or divert the T cell from its cellular target. The problem was solved ingeniously (if one may use such a word): the intracellular components of the microbe are degraded and the resulting peptide fragments transported to the surface of the cell to be presented in association with the MHC molecule. As discussed in Chapter 5, such peptides bind firmly into the cleft in the MHC molecule, and the T cell receptor, by binding to this complex of degraded antigen plus MHC, is targetted onto the two components, which thus provide markers of the infecting antigen and the cell which is infected (Fig. 6.15).

T cell subpopulations are assisted in binding firmly to their correct target cell by accessory molecules; thus, the CD4 molecule on T helper cells binds to the non-polymorphic part of MHC class II molecules, whereas the CD8 molecule on cytotoxic T cells binds to the MHC class I molecules on the infected target cell. Other accessory molecules such as LFA-1 (leucocyte function antigen-1) and ICAM-1 (intercellular adhesion molecule-1), and CD2 and LFA-3 (Fig. 6.16) have also been recognized as subserving similar roles with respect to increasing the strength of intercellular reactions. There is evidence that the CD4, CD8 and CD2 molecules may also be involved in processing the signal received by the T cell receptor.

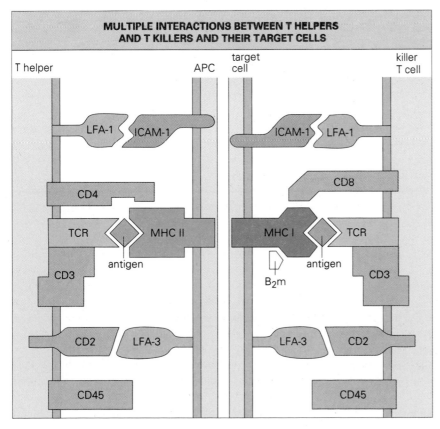

MULTIPLE INTERACTIONS BETWEEN T HELPERS AND T KILLERS AND THEIR TARGET CELLS

Fig. 6.16 Multiple interactions between T helper and T killer cells and their antigen-presenting and target cells, which present antigen in association with MHC class I and II. TCR, T cell antigen-specific receptor; CD45, leucocyte common antigen; LFA-1, lymphocyte function antigen; ICAM-1, intercellular adhesion molecule; CD2, receptor for LFA-3-like molecule on sheep erythrocytes.

SUMMARY

The complex series of individual surface regions (epitopes) on each foreign antigen are recognized by a tremendous variety (millions) of antibodies and T cell receptors. This amazing diversity is generated from pools of minigenes which are randomly combined to produce the peptide chains that form these recognition molecules.

Antibodies are fashioned to be complementary in shape to native antigens so that they can react with and destroy or neutralize extracellular infectious agents or their secreted toxins. T cells, on the other hand, have to recognize infected cells and do so by using a dual code: the intracellular microbe is coded for by its processed protein components, which appear as peptides on the surface of the cell in close association with major histocompatibility complex (MHC) molecules which themselves act as a code for 'cells'.

It should always be borne in mind, however, that although many antigens in a given microorganism may induce an immune response, only a select few are 'protective' in the sense that they generate antibodies or T cell responses which successfully defend the host against the infection.

Further Reading

Roitt IM *Essential Immunology*, 7th edn. Oxford: Blackwell Scientific Publications, 1991.

Roitt IM, Brostoff J, Male DK, eds. *Immunology*, 2nd edn. London: Gower Medical Publishing, 1989.

Sela M. Antigenicity: some molecular aspects. *Science* 1989; **166**: 1365.

Abbas AK, Litchtman AH, Pober JS, eds. *Cellular and molecular immunology*. Philadelphia: W.B. Saunders Company, 1991.

Silverton EW *et al*. Three-dimensional structure of an intact human immunoglobulin. *Proc Natl Acad Sci USA* 1977; **74**: 5240–5144.

Clevers H *et al*. The T-cell receptor/CD3 complex: a dynamic protein ensemble. *Ann Rev Immunol* 1988; **6**: 629–662.

Bjorkman P *et al*. Structure of the human class I histocompatibility antigen, HLA-A2. *Nature* 1987; **329**: 506–512.

7 THE CELLULAR BASIS OF ADAPTIVE IMMUNE RESPONSES

Contents

INTRODUCTION: THE NATURE OF LYMPHOCYTES

The relationship to primary and secondary lymphoid tissues

Lymphocytes are derived from stem cells which differentiate within the primary lymphoid organs (bone marrow and thymus), where they mediate the immune responses to antigens. From here they colonize the secondary lymphoid tissues (Fig. 7.1). The lymph nodes are concerned with the generation of immune responses to antigens which drain into them from the tissues, while the spleen is concerned primarily with antigens which reach it from the bloodstream. In addition, unencapsulated aggregates of lymphoid tissue lie in the mucosal surface where they have the job of responding to antigens from the environment by producing antibodies for mucosal secretions. These defenders of the mucosal surfaces are collectively grouped under the heading of 'mucosa-associated lymphoid tissue' or MALT (see Fig. 7.1).

Resting and activated lymphocytes have totally different morphologies

The resting lymphocyte is a small cell with a large nucleus and relatively scant cytoplasm. Its functions are to recirculate and to recognize antigen but most of its other potential functions are suppressed so that the chromatin in the nucleus is condensed and tends to stain rather heavily. Most resting lymphocytes have an agranular appearance with a high nuclear to cytoplasmic ratio (Fig. 7.2). However, a small proportion of T cells have a slightly lower nuclear to cytoplasmic ratio and possess granules in the

ORGANIZED LYMPHOID TISSUE			
primary lymphoid organ	thymus	bone marrow	
	(T) ⇐ (S) ⇒ (B)		
	encapsulated		unencapsulated
secondary lymphoid organ	lymph node	spleen	MALT
immune response	to antigens in tissues	to antigens in blood	to antigens at mucosal surfaces

Fig. 7.1 Organized lymphoid tissue. Stem cells (S) arising in the bone marrow differentiate into immunocompetent T and B cells in the primary lymphoid organs. These cells then colonize the secondary lymphoid tissues where immune responses are organized. MALT, mucosa-associated lymphoid tissue.

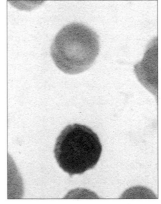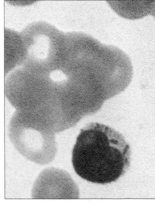

Fig. 7.2 Morphological heterogeneity of lymphocytes. The small agranular lymphocyte (left) has a high nuclear:cytoplasmic ratio. The large granular lymphocyte (right) has azurophilic granules in the cytoplasm and a lower nuclear:cytoplasmic ratio. The dark nuclear staining is produced by condensed chromatin. Geimsa stain, x 1000. Courtesy of P Lydyard.

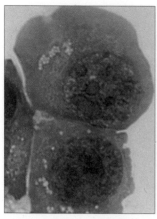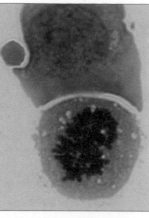

Fig. 7.3 Mitogen/antigen-induced lymphocyte activation. On stimulation by pokeweed mitogen, these T and B cells show increased basophilia in the cytoplasm and an increase in the cell volume (left). The chromosomes condense and can be clearly seen during metaphase (right). Giemsa stain, x 2000. Courtesy of P Lydyard.

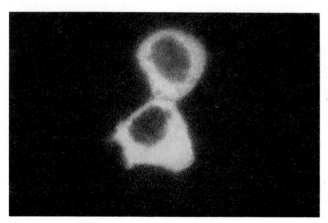

Fig. 7.4 The immunofluorescent staining of intracytoplasmic immunoglobulin in plasma cells. Human plasma cells treated with fluoresceinated anti-human IgM (green) and rhodaminated anti-IgG (red) show distinct intracytoplasmic staining, indicating that plasma cells normally manufacture only one class of antibody. x 3000. Courtesy of P Lydyard.

SURFACE MARKERS ON T AND B CELLS			
function/identity	CD designation	T cells	B cells
antigen receptors			
Surface immunoglobulin	—	–	++
T cell αβ, γδ	—	++	–
TCR signal transducer	CD3	++	–
receptors for			
Sheep red cells (rosettes: antigen non-specific)	CD2	++	–
MHC class II (mainly T helpers)	CD4	++	–
MHC class I (cytotoxic/suppressors)	CD8	++	–
Complement (CR2)	CD21	–	++
Complement (CR1)	CD35	+	++
FcγII	CDw32	–	++
Fcε	CD23	–	+
IL–2 (α-chain)	CD25	act*	act*
MHC			
Class I	—	++	++
Class II	—	act*	++
other markers			
Differentiation marker	CD5	++	subset
Restricted leucocyte common antigen	CD45R	memory	+
* activated cells only			

Fig. 7.5 Surface markers on T and B cells.

cytoplasm, so that they often referred to as 'large granular lymphocytes', or LGLs. Upon activation by contact with antigen, the lymphocytes becomes derepressed, the nucleus stains less densely, and the cytoplasm enlarges. Many of the cells also undergo mitotic division (Fig. 7.3). B cells will ultimately synthesize and secrete antibody and they acquire the morphology of plasma cells (Fig. 7.4).

B and T cells can be distinguished by their surface markers

As they differentiate into populations with differing functions, B and T cells acquire molecules on their surface which reflect these specializations. It is possible to produce homogeneous antibodies of a single specificity, termed 'monoclonal antibodies', which can recognize such surface markers. When laboratories from all over the world compared the monoclonal antibodies they had raised, it was found that groups or clusters of monoclonal antibodies were recognizing the same molecule on the surface of

the lymphocyte. Each surface molecule so defined, was referred to as a 'CD' molecule (Fig. 7.5), where CD refers to a 'cluster determinant'.

EACH LYMPHOCYTE EXPRESSES A RECEPTOR OF UNIQUE SPECIFICITY ON ITS SURFACE

Among the surface markers on the B and T cells referred to above are the antigen receptors, present on the plasma membrane. B cells possess surface immunoglobulin whereas the T cell receptor on the surface of the T lymphocyte acts as an antigen recognition unit (see Fig. 7.5). We now know that despite the very large number of different components that could be combined together in multiple ways to give a diversity of surface receptors, each B lymphocyte rearranges its germ-line genes coding for these receptors

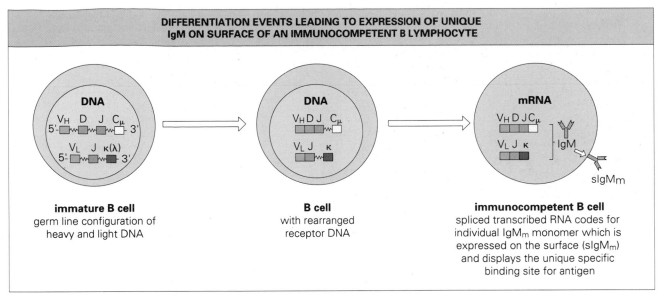

DIFFERENTIATION EVENTS LEADING TO EXPRESSION OF UNIQUE IgM ON SURFACE OF AN IMMUNOCOMPETENT B LYMPHOCYTE

DNA

V_H D   J C_μ
5'—☐—ⱳ—☐—ⱳ—☐—☐— 3'

V_L J $\kappa(\lambda)$
5'—☐—ⱳ—☐—ⱳ—■— 3'

immature B cell
germ line configuration of
heavy and light DNA

DNA

V_H D J C_μ
☐☐☐—ⱳ—☐

V_L J κ
☐☐—ⱳ—■

B cell
with rearranged
receptor DNA

mRNA

V_H D JC$_\mu$
☐☐☐☐

V_L J κ
☐☐☐ $\Big\}$ IgM

sIgM$_m$

immunocompetent B cell
spliced transcribed RNA codes for
individual IgM$_m$ monomer which is
expressed on the surface (sIgM$_m$)
and displays the unique specific
binding site for antigen

Fig. 7.6 Differentiation events leading to the expression of unique IgM on the surface of an immunocompetent B lymphocyte. Leader sequences have been omitted for simplicity.

so that it selects one and only one of the specificities for each receptor polypeptide chain. It then expresses that receptor molecule on its surface (Fig. 7.6). Once this occurs, the other genes coding for these antigen receptors in the lymphocyte are no longer utilized. In other words, following this genetic rearrangement process, the lympho-cyte becomes committed to the synthesis and expression of a single receptor type. An analogous process occurs in the rearrangement of the αβ and γδ genes coding for the T cell receptor. Just as for B cells, each T cell expresses one and only one specific combination of receptor pep-tides, and therefore shows a single specificity to which it is committed for the whole of its lifespan.

ANTIGEN SELECTS AND CLONALLY EXPANDS LYMPHOCYTES BEARING COMPLEMENTARY RECEPTORS

Because lymphocytes can express such a large number of different possible specificities, perhaps of the order of mil-lions, there must of necessity only be a relatively small number that have a particular specificity. Thus, when a microbe invades the body, the total number of lympho-cytes initially committed to recognizing the antigens which go to make up the microbial constitution, are relatively small and must be expanded to obtain a sufficient number to protect the host. Evolution has provided a masterful solution to this problem. When a microbe enters the body, its component antigens combine with only those lympho-cytes whose surface receptor is complementary to the shape of those antigens. The cells which bind antigen become activated and proliferate clonally to form a large population of cells derived from the original. In the case of B cells, a large proportion of these clonally expanded lymphocytes become dedicated to the synthesis and secre-tion of antibodies. Since these plasma cells are derived from a parent cell that is already committed to the produc-tion of only one specific antibody, the final product is identical to the molecule that was posted on the surface of the original antigen-recognizing cell. We therefore have the production of large amounts of antibody, which like that on the surface of the parent cell, must combine with invading antigen (Figs 7.7 and 7.8).

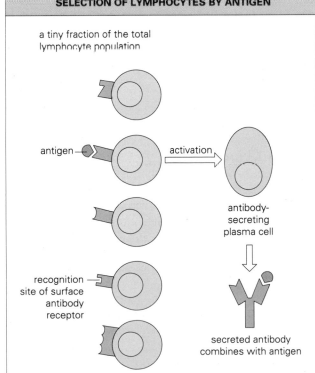

SELECTION OF LYMPHOCYTES BY ANTIGEN

a tiny fraction of the total lymphocyte population

antigen

activation

antibody-secreting plasma cell

recognition site of surface antibody receptor

secreted antibody combines with antigen

Fig. 7.7 Activation of B cells by combination of antigen with specific surface antibody receptors. Only those B cells whose surface receptor is complementary in shape to the antigen are activated. For simplicity, only the combining site of the surface antibody is shown.

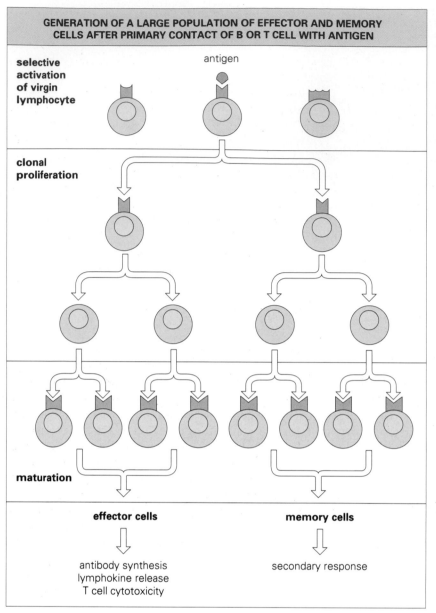

GENERATION OF A LARGE POPULATION OF EFFECTOR AND MEMORY CELLS AFTER PRIMARY CONTACT OF B OR T CELL WITH ANTIGEN

selective activation of virgin lymphocyte

antigen

clonal proliferation

maturation

effector cells

memory cells

antibody synthesis
lymphokine release
T cell cytotoxicity

secondary response

Fig. 7.8 Generation of a large population of effector and memory cells after primary contact of B or T cell with antigen. A fraction of the progeny of the original antigen-reactive lymphocytes become non-dividing memory cells, whereas the others become the effector cells of humoral or cell-mediated immunity. Memory cells require fewer cycles before they develop into effectors, thus shortening the reaction time for the secondary response.

A similar process of T cell clonal selection and expansion occurs with T cells, producing a large number of effectors with the same specificity as the original parent cell; some of these cells release lymphokines, whereas others have cytotoxic functions so that they act as effectors of T cell mediated immunity. In the case of both B and T cells, a fraction of the clonally expanded population become resting memory cells (see Fig. 7.8). Thus a larger number of cells in the population are capable of recognizing the microbial antigen in any subsequent infection than were present in the initial virgin population that existed before the primary infection occurred.

SECONDARY IMMUNE RESPONSES ARE BIGGER AND BRISKER THAN PRIMARY RESPONSES

The increased number of lymphocytes specific for a given antigen present in the memory pool produced by the primary response, give rise to a much stronger antibody response on the second contact with antigen. This provides the principle for vaccination (Fig. 7.9). The microbe or antigen to be used for vaccination, is modified in such a way that it no longer produces disease or damage, but still retains the majority of its antigenic shapes. The primary response produced by the vaccination will give rise to a pool of memory cells which can generate an abundant secondary response when subsequent contact with the antigen is made during a natural infection.

ANTIBODY PRODUCTION FREQUENTLY REQUIRES T CELL HELP

T-independent antigens

Some antigens stimulate B cells without the need for intervention by T lymphocytes. These so-called T-independent antigens are of two main types. The first type contain molecular features which enable them to stimulate a wide variety of B cells independently of their specific antigen

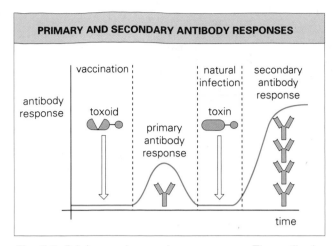

Fig. 7.9 Primary and secondary responses. The antibody response on the second contact with antigen is more rapid and more intense. Thus, following vaccination with a benign form of the antigen (a chemically modified form of tetanus toxin in the example shown) to produce a primary response, subsequent contact with antigen in the form of a natural infection evokes the more efficient secondary response.

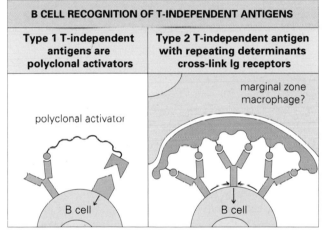

Fig. 7.10 B cell activation by T-independent antigens. The requirements for an antigen-presenting cell for type 2 antigens is still uncertain.

receptors; they are thus referred to as 'polyclonal activators'. Those B cells carrying a surface receptor which recognizes epitopes on the polyclonal activator, focuses the molecule on their surfaces and are preferentially stimulated relative to the remainder of the B cell population (Fig. 7.10). The second type of T-independent antigen involves repeating determinants which can cross-link immunoglobulin receptors on the B cell and apparently stimulate the lymphocyte directly (see Fig. 7.10). One feature of both these types of T-independent antigen is that they give rise mainly to low affinity IgM rather than IgG antibody responses, and rarely induce a memory response.

T-dependent antigens

The majority of antigens will stimulate B cells only if they have the assistance of T helper cells (Fig. 7.11). The sequence of events is as follows. In stage 1 the antigen is processed by an antigen-presenting cell which degrades it and places a peptide derived from it on its surface in association with MHC class II, as discussed in the last chapter. This complex is recognized by and primes a T helper cell with a complementary receptor on its surface. In stage 2 a B cell with surface receptors complementary to an epitope on the original antigen, captures the antigen on its receptor, internalizes it and after processing, also presents a derived peptide on its surface in association with endogenous MHC class II molecules. This is the complex against which the T helper cell was originally primed, and recognition of processed antigen by the primed T helper causes stimulation of the B cell with subsequent activation, proliferation and maturation.

It should be noted that although the T helper cell recognizes a processed determinant of the antigen, the B cell is programmed to make only antibody with the same specificity as its surface receptor, and therefore the antibodies which finally result will be those directed against the epitope on the antigen recognized by the B cell surface receptor.

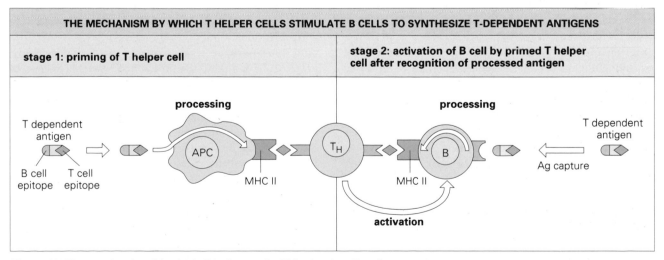

Fig. 7.11 The mechanism by which T helper cells (T$_H$) stimulate B cells to synthesize antibody to T-dependent antigens. See text for a detailed description of the sequence of events.

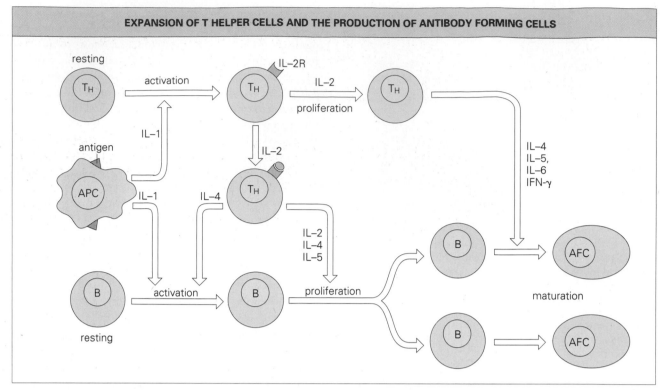

Fig. 7.12 Expansion of T helper cells and the production of antibody forming cells (AFC) from resting B cells involves the action of cytokines.

CYTOKINES ARE SOLUBLE FACTORS INVOLVED IN INTERCELLULAR COMMUNICATION DURING THE IMMUNE RESPONSE

Interactions between the antigen presenting cell (APC), the T helper cell and the B cell are effected by the recognition of processed antigen in association with MHC class II by the T cell receptor, as indicated in figure 7.11. Following this recognition process, the cells act on each other by releasing soluble factors which react with the appropriate complementary surface receptors on the target cell. As may be seen from figure 7.12, the APC provides an important triggering factor for the T helper cell – interleukin-1 (IL-1). In the activated T cell, the gene encoding the interleukin-2 receptor (IL-2R) is derepressed and the IL-2R molecule is expressed on the surface of the lymphocytes. A subpopulation of T helper cells is also induced to synthesize IL-2 , which acts as a growth factor for T cells by combining with the IL-2 receptor and causing proliferation. Other cytokines, as these soluble factors are termed, are produced (Fig. 7.13) which among other things play a role in the activation, proliferation and maturation of B cells, in the switch of B cells from IgM production, and perhaps in the generation of mutations in the variable region of the immunoglobulin gene, leading to the possibility of the selection of high affinity antibody molecules during the immune response. The formation of memory B cells is also almost certainly under the influence of T lymphocyte control.

UNLIMITED EXPANSION OF CLONES MUST BE CHECKED BY REGULATORY MECHANISMS

Once lymphocyte clones are activated by antigen, they clearly cannot be allowed to go on dividing indefinitely, otherwise they would completely fill the body of the host. Fortunately, there are several mechanisms which regulate the irresponsible expansion of these dividing lymphocytes.

One of the most important factors controlling the immune response is the concentration of antigen. There would of course be a distinct evolutionary advantage in a system where the immune response is switched on by antigen and switched off when the antigen is no longer present. It is perhaps not surprising then that selective processes have guided the production of such a system, in which the immune response is antigen-driven through the direct effect of antigen on the lymphocyte receptors. As the antigen is eliminated by metabolic catabolism and by clearance through the operation of the immune response, the drive to the immune system disappears.

Antibody itself also has feedback potential. IgM produced early in the response has a positive feedback which stimulates the response in its fledgling stages. By contrast, IgG in sufficient concentrations produces negative feedback and acts to down-regulate the immune response. There is also considered to be a population of T-suppressor cells which act to down-regulate both T helper cells and B cells, whether through antigen-specific or idiotype-specific mechanisms. The epitopes on one lymphocyte receptor

(a) CYTOKINES: HORMONES OF THE IMMUNE SYSTEM

factor	source	actions
IL-1 α/β	macrophages	inflammatory
IL-2	T cells	T and B cell proliferation
IL-3	T cells	pluripotent growth
IL-4	T cells	T and B proliferation, activation of macrophages
IL-5	T cells	eosinophil differentiation, B cell growth
IL-6	T cells	B cell differentiation
IL-7	T cells	B and T cell proliferation
IL-8	T cells	PMN activation
IL-9	T cells	mast cell growth
IL-10	T cell/B cell, macrophages	cytokine inhibition
IFN-α	multiple	anti viral
IFN-β	multiple	anti viral
IFN-γ	T cells, NK cells	anti viral, activation of macrophages, MHC induction
TNF-α	monocytes	cytotoxicity, cachexia, fever
TNF-β	T cells	cytotoxicity, cachexia, fever
TGF-β	T cell/macrophages	inhibits activation of NK and T cells, macrophages; inhibits proliferation of B and T cells
GM-CSF	T cells	growth of granulocytes and monocytes
G-CSF	macrophages	growth of granulocytes
M-CSF	macrophages	growth of monocytes

Fig. 7.13 The cytokines. (a) Known cytokines and their actions. (b) Cellular interactions mediated by cytokines. S, stem cells; MS, myeloid stem cell; LS, lymphoid stem cell; PC, plasma cell; PMN, polymorphonucleocyte; T$_H$, helper cell; T$_C$, cytotoxic T cell; IFN, interferon; TNF, tumour necrosis factor; TGF, transforming growth factor; GM-CSF, granulocyte-macrophage colony stimulating factor. Adapted from Playfair JHL, 1987.

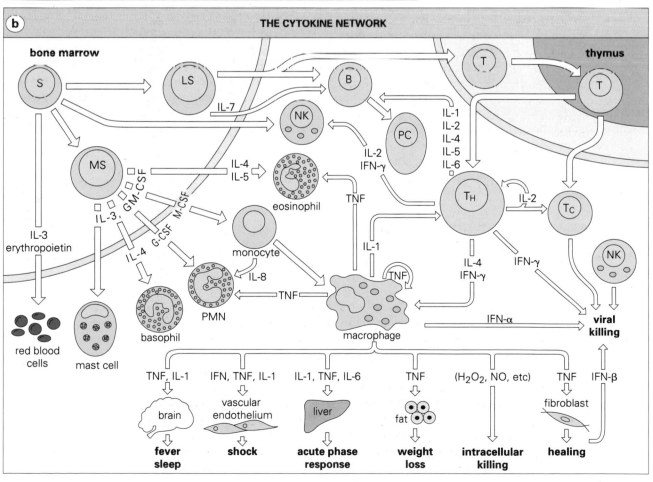

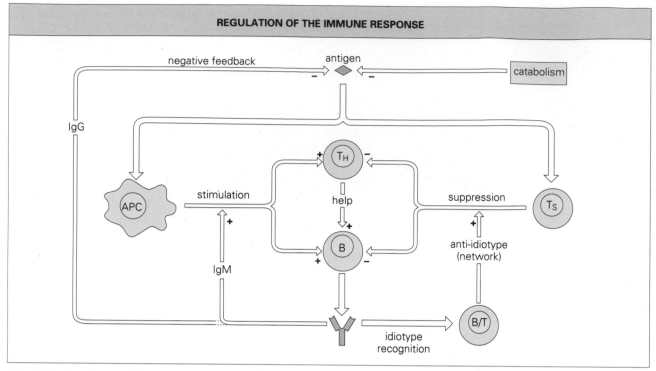

Fig. 7.14 Regulation of the immune response. T help for cell-mediated immunity is subject to similar regulation. The recruitment of B cells by anti-idiotypic T helper cells and direct activation of anti-idiotype T suppressors by idiotype-positive T helpers have been omitted for the sake of clarity. APC, antigen presenting cell; T_H, T helper cell; T_S, T suppressor cell.

(idiotype) recognized by the receptor on another lymphocyte (the anti-idiotype) can form a network of interactions through which suppression may be mediated (Fig. 7.14)

TOLERANCE MECHANISMS PREVENT IMMUNOLOGICAL SELF-REACTIVITY

To avoid reaction against the body's own components, it is essential for the immune system to develop non-reactivity or 'tolerance' to self-molecules. In essence, it is thought that cells which are auto-reactive are either eliminated by some form of clonal deletion or made anergic early in the life of the cell, or sometimes silenced through T suppressor systems later in life (Fig. 7.15).

T cells are more readily tolerized than B cells at a given antigen concentration and there is extremely good evidence that self-molecules present in the thymus can lead to the deletion or 'anergy' of the specific T cell clone. B cells in contact with relatively high concentrations of self proteins are also subject to clonal deletion or anergy but there is less need to tolerize other B cells in the sense that autoreactive B cells directed to thymus-dependent antigens will be unable to respond (helpless) if the corresponding T helpers to that molecule have been tolerized, be it through clonal deletion or T suppression (see Fig. 7.15).

Unresponsiveness will also result if self-components cannot be seen or recognized by the immune system. This may occur because, over a long period of time, the repertoire has lost the genes giving rise to autoreactive receptors. However, even if autoreactive T cells are present, they will not be activated if the self-antigen is not presented in processed form, in combination with MHC class II in adequate concentrations. Thus, they will also be unable to react with the whole molecules that constitute the surface array on cells which do not express class II. Since most cells express class I, it seems reasonable to assume that the cytotoxic T cells capable of reacting against cells expressing processed intracellular components have been deleted, are helpless or are suppressed.

SUMMARY

Each lymphocyte expresses either antibody or a T cell receptor with a single specificity for antigen. A lymphocyte bearing a complementary antibody or T cell receptor on its surface, will bind antigen, be activated, profilerate to form a clone, and differentiate into antibody forming cells or effectors of cell-mediated immunity, and also form a large pool of memory cells. Second contact with antigen stimulates this pool of memory cells to produce a larger and faster response than the primary reaction. Thus, vaccination with a benign form of the antigen prepares the individual for an effective response when second contact with antigen occurs during a natural infection.

Many antigens require T cell help before they can activate B cells and the interactions are mediated by a variety of soluble cytokines. The unlimited expansion of clones is restricted by antigen concentration, antibody feedback and T suppression. Reactivity to self is prevented by a variety of tolerance mechanisms.

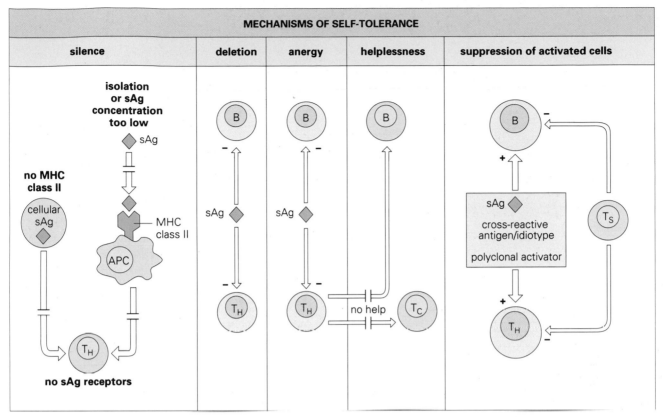

Fig. 7.15 Mechanisms of self-tolerance. Self antigens (sAg) will not provoke a response if there is insufficient processed peptide–class II complex or if there are no auto-reactive T cells. Both B and T cells can be silenced by clonal deletion or made anergic (still living but unresponsive) by contact with self-antigen. B cells and cytotoxic T cells cannot function without T cell help.

Inadvertent stimulation of available autoreactive cells may be checked by T suppressors. Cells that are dead, unreactive or suppressed are shown in grey. sAg, self antigen; APC, antigen presenting cell; T_H, T helper; T_S, T suppressor; T_C, cytotoxic-T cell precursor. Modified from Roitt IM, 1991.

Further Reading —————————————————————————————

Roitt IM. *Essential Immunology* 7th edn. Oxford: Blackwell Scientific Publications, 1991.

Roitt IM, Brostoff J, Male DK, eds. *Immunology* 2nd edn. London: Gower Medical Publishing, 1989.

Raff M. The immune system. In: Alberts, B *et al.* eds. *The Molecular Biology of the Cell*. 2nd edn, New York: Garland Publishing, 1989.

Playfair JHL. Immunology at a glance. 4th edn. Oxford: Blackwell Scientific Publications, 1987.

Contents

INTRODUCTION

The individual components and the overall functional activity of the innate and adaptive defence systems can be assessed both qualitatively and quantitatively by a wide variety of techniques, as outlined in this chapter. Furthermore, just as antigen preparations are used to measure antibodies, so antibodies themselves can be used to identify their corresponding antigens. For more detailed examples of the application of these techniques, please refer to Chapter 18.

INNATE IMMUNITY

Complement

The overall biological activity of complement in serum can be assayed by its ability to effect the lysis of antibody-sensitized red cells through activation of the classical pathway and insertion of the terminal cytolytic complement components (Fig. 8.1). The relative haemolytic activity of a number of different serum samples can be assessed simultaneously by placing the sample in a well punched into agar gel that contains a suspension of antibody-coated red cells; the size of the clear plaque in the agar surrounding the well is a reflection of the overall lytic complement activity in that sample.

Additionally, it is sometimes of value to assess the opsonic activity of complement in the serum sample, by looking at its ability to facilitate the uptake of a microbial particle by a phagocytic cell (Fig. 8.2).

The activities of individual components of the complement system can be evaluated either by their ability to be titrated into a complement-dependent lytic system in which the component to be tested is lacking, or by direct immunochemical measurement often using gel precipitation reactions (see below).

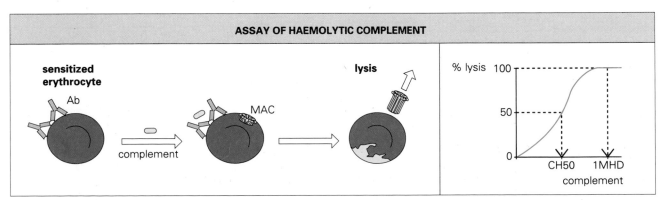

ASSAY OF HAEMOLYTIC COMPLEMENT

Fig. 8.1 The lysis of red cells sensitized by antibody (left) is used to assay the haemolytic complement activity of a serum sample (MAC, membrane attack complex). The curve (right) shows lysis of antibody-sensitized red cells with increasing amounts of complement. Because of the sigmoid shape of the curve, the minimum haemolytic dose (MHD) cannot be measured as accurately as the amount giving 50% haemolysis (CH50) so the latter is preferred as a unit.

Phagocytosis

The ability of neutrophils to become phagocytic and concurrently to bring about the reduction of molecular oxygen, can be assayed by the nitroblue tetrazolium (NBT) test. When yellow NBT dye is added to blood, it forms complexes with the heparin or fibrinogen present in the sample. These complexes are then phagocytosed by neutrophils that have been activated by the addition of exogenous endotoxin. The dye complex is taken into the stimulated neutrophils and substitutes for oxygen by acting as a substrate for the reduction process, forming as a result a blue insoluble formazan (Fig. 8.3).

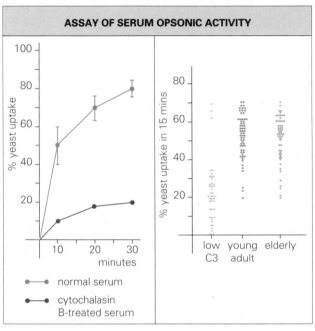

Fig. 8.2 Opsonic activity of serum. (a) Time course for the uptake of PMN from 12 healthy donors of yeast opsonized with the same normal serum, and uptake of yeast by PMN from one donor after treatment with cytochalasin B (40μg/ml) which inhibits phagocytosis. (b) The distribution of opsonic activity for 150 sera from young healthy, elderly and pathological sera. Redrawn from Kerr *et al.*, 1983.

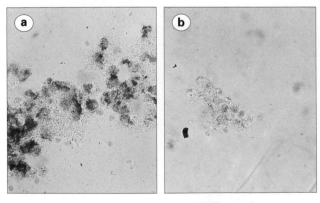

Fig. 8.3. The nitroblue tetrazolium (NBT) test for phagocytosis by neutrophils. (a) Endotoxin-stimulated polymorphs take up the dye and reduce it to a blue formazan. (b) The patient with chronic granulomatous disease lacks the cytochrome system required to reduce oxygen and the dye remains in its oxidized form.

ASSAYS FOR ANTIGENS AND ANTIBODIES

Gel precipitation reactions

When antigen and antibody meet in solution at sufficiently high concentrations, their mulivalency results in the formation of aggregates which usually precipitate. These precipitation reactions can be visualized more usefully and sensitively by allowing the antigen and antibody to diffuse towards each other through agar gels (Fig. 8.4). Each antigen reacts with a corresponding set of antibodies present within the serum; the resulting individual antigen–antibody systems form separate lines of precipitation in the gel, provided there is no immunochemical relationship (i.e. cross-reaction between the antigens). The gel precipitation system can also be used to identify the relationship between two different antigen systems and it is possible to establish whether two antigens are immunologically identical, non-identical or partially identical (i.e. cross-reactive; Fig. 8.5).

The concentration of antigen in a given fluid can be ascertained by placing it in a well punched into an agar gel containing antibody and then allowing the antigen to diffuse into the gel to form a precipitin ring. The diameter of the ring increases with increasing concentration of antigen (Fig. 8.6). A more sensitive assay can be obtained by electrophoresing the antigen into the antibody-containing gel to form 'rockets' whose length is related to the antigen concentration (Fig. 8.7).

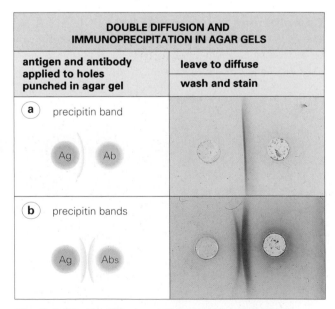

Fig. 8.4 Double diffusion and immunoprecipitation in agar gels. The opaque lines formed can be better visualized by staining. (a) Precipitin band formed with a single antigen. The two independent antigens in (b) give separate precipitation bands with their corresponding antibody sets (Abs), coexisting within the complex

Agglutination reactions

Antibodies directed against antigens present on the surface of red cells cause cross-linking in such a way that when the cells are allowed to sediment in a microtitre agglutination tray, they form a mat on the bottom of the well rather than a tight button (Fig. 8.8). This system can be used to detect antibodies against any antigen that can be linked, whether covalently or non-covalently, to the surface of the red cell or even to other particles such as latex (see Chapter 18). It can also be used to detect antigens, e.g. hepatitis B surface antigens, if specific antibody has been linked to the particle surface.

The complement fixation test

The consumption of complement can form the basis of a test for either antigen or antibody, provided the immune complex is capable of activating the complement system. The complement fixation test (CFT) is carried out as follows (Fig. 8.9). Serum to be tested for antibody is mixed

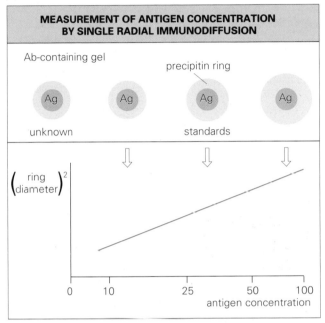

MEASUREMENT OF ANTIGEN CONCENTRATION BY SINGLE RADIAL IMMUNODIFFUSION

Fig. 8.6 Measurement of antigen concentration by single radial immunodiffusion. Antigen diffuses into the gel and forms a precipitate at equivalence such that the square of the diameter of the ring is linearly related to antigen concentration. Unknowns can be read off a standard curve by interpolation. A reversal of the system gives a measure of antibody concentration.

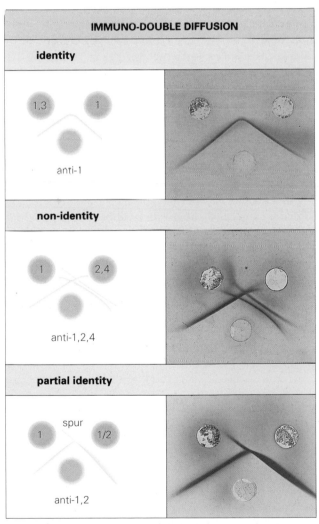

IMMUNO-DOUBLE DIFFUSION

Fig. 8.5 The relationship between two antigens can be investigated by placing them in adjacent wells in agar and allowing them to react with antiserum from a third well. Reactions of (a) identity, (b) non-identity and (c) partial identity can be defined but only with respect to the antibodies present in a given antiserum. The greater the number of epitopes recognized by an antiserum, the more likely it is that these relationships will emerge. The converse also holds; for example, if anti-1 only was added to (c) it would have indicated identity.

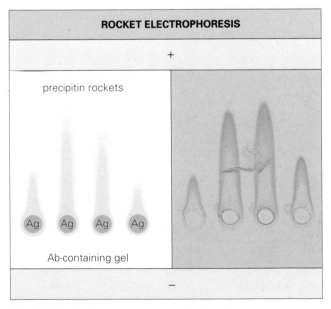

ROCKET ELECTROPHORESIS

Fig. 8.7 Rocket electrophoresis. Antigen is electrophoresed into agar containing antibody and standard samples used to obtain a calibration curve of 'rocket' height versus antigen concentration.

with the known antigen. If antibodies are present, complexes will be formed (Fig. 8.9a) which will consume some or all of the complement subsequently added (b). The consumption of complement is measured by adding indicator red cells coated with a subagglutinating amount of erythrocyte antibody (c); any residual complement will lyse these indicator cells. Clearly, the system can be turned around so that a standard antiserum can be used to look for antigen in a given sample.

Immunoassays for antigen and antibody

Radioimmunoassay of antigen

The binding of radioactively labelled antigen to a limited but standard amount of antibody can be partially inhibited by addition of unlabelled antigen. The extent of this inhibition can be used as a measure of the unlabelled material that has been added. The principle of this form of saturation analysis is outlined in figure 8.10. In essence this method measures the ratio of free antigen to that bound to antibody. In practice, this is usually achieved by binding the antibody to a plastic surface, to facilitate the separation of bound from free antigen. In another variation, unlabelled test antigen is added to solid-phase antibody, and the percentage occupancy of antibody sites, which is proportional to antigen concentration, is determined by adding a labelled second antibody.

There is a tendency now to replace the radioisotope with enzymatic, chemiluminescent or time-resolved fluorescent labels, the latter two giving assays of very high sensitivity.

Solid phase assay of antibody

Solid phase antigen can be used to assay antibody in a given sample. The amount of antibody binding to the solid phase antigen is a measure of the antibody content of the original sample, and can be detected by adding a second antibody conjugated either with a radioactive label, or with an enzyme that produces a colour reaction with a given substrate. Such enzymes include phosphatase or peroxidase and the method is termed the 'enzyme-linked immunosorbent assay' (ELISA; Fig. 8.11). Another valuable test for the qualitative analysis of antigen–antibody

---

THE HAEMAGGLUTINATION TEST FOR ANTIBODIES USING RED CELLS SENSITIZED BY ANTIGEN

red cell antigen	antigen-sensitized red cell

red cell antigen

sensitizing antigen

reciprocal serum dilution

2 4 8 16 32 64 128 256 512 1024 pos. neg.

test sera

Fig. 8.8 The haemagglutination test for antibodies using red cells sensitized by antigen. Doubling dilutions of sera are made (horizontal row), with positive and negative controls in vertical rows 11 and 12 respectively. A tight button of cells indicates a negative reaction.

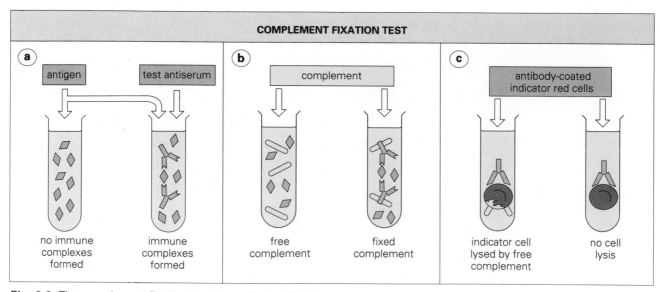

COMPLEMENT FIXATION TEST

a antigen test antiserum

no immune complexes formed

immune complexes formed

b complement

free complement

fixed complement

c antibody-coated indicator red cells

indicator cell lysed by free complement

no cell lysis

Fig. 8.9 The complement fixation test for antibody. With the same system, a known antiserum can be used to assay antigen.

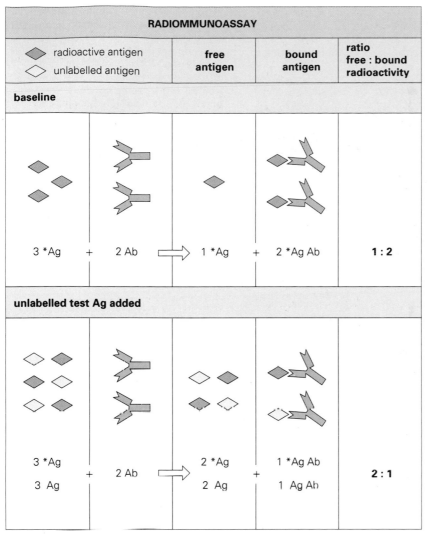

RADIOMMUNOASSAY			
◆ radioactive antigen ◇ unlabelled antigen	**free antigen**	**bound antigen**	**ratio free : bound radioactivity**
baseline			
3 *Ag + 2 Ab ⟹	1 *Ag +	2 *Ag Ab	**1 : 2**
unlabelled test Ag added			
3 *Ag 3 Ag + 2 Ab ⟹	2 *Ag 2 Ag +	1 *Ag Ab 1 Ag Ab	**2 : 1**

Fig. 8.10 The principle of radiommunoassay, simplified by assuming a very highly avid antibody and one combining site per antibody molecule. (a) If 3 mol of radiolabelled antigen (Ag) are added to 2 mol of antibody (Ab), 1 mol of Ag will be free and 2 bound to Ab. The ratio of the counts of free to bound will be 1:2. (b) If 3 mol of unlabelled Ag plus 3 mol radiolabelled Ag are added to the Ab, again only 2 mol of total Ag will be bound, but since the Ab cannot distinguish labelled from unlabelled Ag, half will be radioactive. The remaining antigen will be free and the ratio of free to bound radioactivity changes to 2:1. This ratio will vary with the amount of unlabelled Ag added, enabling the construction of a calibration curve (below).

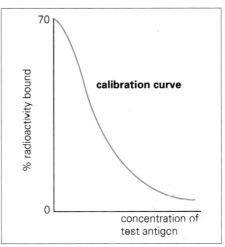

interactions is 'immunoblotting', the principle of which is set out in figure 8.12. The initial electrophoretic step is carried out in the denaturing detergent sodium dodecyl sulphate (SDS), and the success of the technique depends to a considerable extent on the degree to which the antigen regains a confirmation that is capable of binding antibody after subsequent transfer to a nitrocellulose membrane.

Immunohistological reactions

Antibodies coupled to fluorescent dyes or to enzymes with chromogenic substrates (as in the ELISA test) can be used to visualize a microbial antigen either in the free state or within tissues (Fig. 8.13). The method can be made more sensitive or can be adapted to the detection of antibody, by labelling a second antibody in an indirect test. An example showing the application of this technique to demonstrate antibodies to *Treponema pallidum* is given in Chapter 18.

Effects of antibodies on microbial activity

A number of tests focus on the ability of antibodies to inhibit some biological faculty of the microorganisms in question. The anti-streptolysin O test is one such assay, in which the streptolysin O toxin is neutralized by antibody. The extent to which the test serum can be diluted before it fails to prevent the toxin from lysing red cells, provides a convenient titre (Fig. 8.14). The ability of antibody to block the metabolic activity of microbes in culture or to immobilize flagellated bacteria are other examples. In the case of

SOLID PHASE ASSAY FOR ANTIBODY	
1 sensitize plate with antigen	
2 wash	antigen
3 add test antibody	antibody
4 wash	
5 add radiolabelled ligand	radiolabelled ligand
6 wash	
7 count	

Fig. 8.11 Solid phase assay for antibody. The binding of antibody in the test serum to solid phase antigen is measured by the binding of a labelled second reagent, usually an antibody labelled with radioactivity or an enzyme which can be detected by a colour reaction (ELISA).

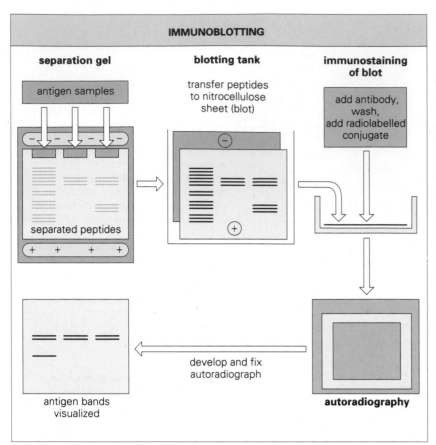

Fig. 8.12 Immunoblotting. Antigen samples are electrophoresed in an SDS polyacrylamide gel or an isoelectric focusing gel and the resolved molecules transferred electrophoretically to a nitrocellulose membrane. The blot is treated with specific antibody, washed, and then a radiolabelled conjugate to detect antibodies bound to the blot. The antigen bands that have bound the antibody are visualized by autoradiography. This technique can be modified for use with an enzyme-coupled conjugate.

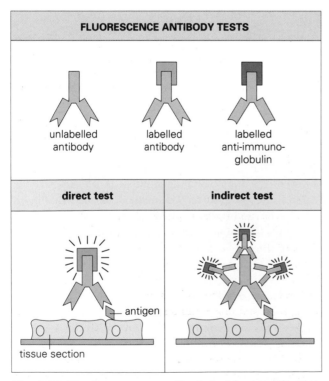

Fig. 8.13 The fluorescence antibody test for identification of tissue antigens or their antibodies. The fluorescent label can be replaced by an enzyme and the distribution of the product of a chromogenic substrate viewed in a normal light microscope.

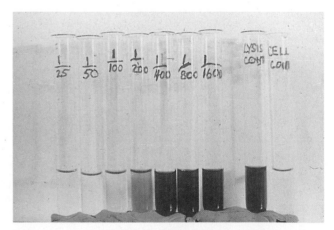

Fig. 8.14 Anti-streptolysin O (ASO) test. The O-toxin lyses red cells and test serum is diluted out until it no longer inhibits lysis by a standard level of toxin. Positive and negative controls are included in the test (right).

cytopathic viruses, antibodies which block viral infectivity can be assayed by their ability to reduce the number of plaques formed when the viruses are innoculated into a tissue or a cell culture. Antibodies can also mask viral molecules such as the influenza haemagglutinin which are involved in specific adherence to cells (see Chapter 18).

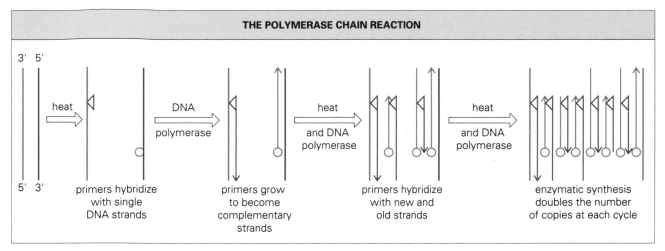

THE POLYMERASE CHAIN REACTION

Fig. 8.15 The polymerase chain reaction. The short oligonucleotide primers hybridize with the nucleotide sequences on complementary strands at each end of the DNA fragment to be expanded. These, together with a heat-stable polymerase, produce millions of copies of the fragment after several cycles.

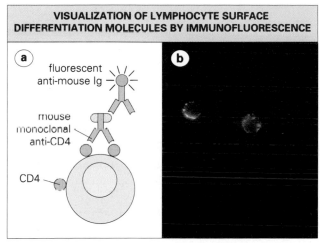

VISUALIZATION OF LYMPHOCYTE SURFACE DIFFERENTIATION MOLECULES BY IMMUNOFLUORESCENCE

Fig. 8.16 Visualization of lymphocyte surface differentiation molecules by immunofluorescence. (a) The double antibody test utilizing mouse monoclonal antibodies to the required surface molecule. (b) Direct demonstration of antibody receptors on the surface of two B lymphocytes by a fluorescent anti-immunoglobulin. Aggregation and capping of the surface receptors by the anti-Ig reagent is evident.

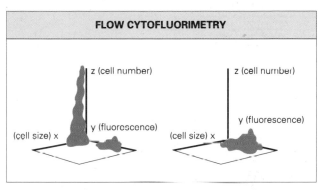

FLOW CYTOFLUORIMETRY

Fig. 8.17 Flow cytofluorimetry. Cells in the sample are stained with specific fluorescent reagents to detect surface molecules and then stream one at a time past a laser. Each cell is measured for size (forward light scatter) and granularity (90° light scatter), as well as for red and green fluorescence, to detect two different surface markers. The 3-dimensional plots show a whole lymphocyte population (left) and a CD8+ population obtained by cell sorting (right), stained with anti-CD8.

Non-immunological tests for microbes

Microorganisms within a sample can be expanded by natural growth under appropriate culture conditions and then examined morphologically under the light and electron microscopes; the individual protein, carbohydrate and lipid components can be analysed biochemically (see Chapter 18), in addition to their identification as antigens by the immunological methods discussed above.

It is now possible to identify the genome of a given microorganism using the polymerase chain reaction (PCR), even if very few organisms are present in the sample. Where the nucleotide sequence of the gene being sought is known, appropriate primers can be added to the sample which allow a DNA polymerase to generate very high numbers of gene copies (Fig. 8.15). These can easily be identified with a gene probe.

LYMPHOCYTES

Enumeration

Lymphocyte differentiation is accompanied by the expression of related molecules on the cell surface. Detection of these molecules by immunofluorescent techniques allows their enumeration and, in addition, their classification into different subpopulations (Fig. 8.16). Monoclonal antibodies are widely used to define these differentiation molecules and increasing use is being made of the technique of flow cytofluorimetry (Fig. 8.17), a more rapid and less laborious means of analysing lymphocyte subpopulations than conventional fluorescent microscopy.

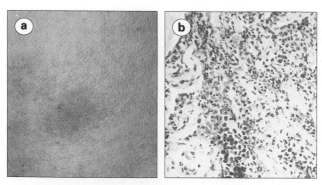

Fig. 8.18 Tuberculin-type delayed sensitivity. The dermal response to antigens of leprosy bacillus in a sensitive subject (the Fernandez reaction) is characterized (a) by red induration maximal at 48–72 hours, and (b) by dense infiltration of the injection site with lymphocytes and macrophages. H & E stain, x80.

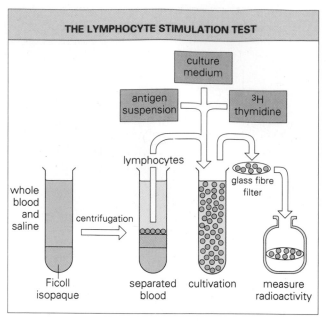

Fig. 8.20 Lymphocyte stimulation assessed by incorporation of radioactive thymidine. A high count indicates that lymphocytes have proliferated and confirms their sensitivity to the antigen.

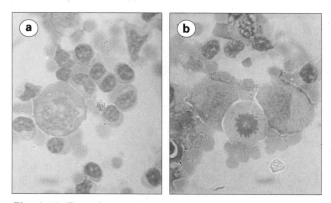

Fig. 8.19 Transformed lymphocytes (lymphoblasts). (a) Lymphocytes from a normal subject cultured for 7 days with purified protein derivative (PPD) from tuberculosis bacilli. (b) Similar culture from a patient with primary tuberculosis showing large numbers of blast cells and mitotic figures.

T cell sensitization

The development of T effector cells dedicated to a particular antigen can frequently be revealed by intradermal challenge with that antigen, which usually gives rise to erythema and induration, peaking at around 48 hours (Fig. 8.18). This time course has led to the reaction being described as 'delayed-type hypersensitivity' (see Chapter 9).

Overall responsiveness of the T cell population can be probed by using a material such as phytohaemagglutinin or Concanavalin A, which are polyclonal stimulators in the sense that they activate T cell populations independently of their precise antigen specificity. However, when peripheral blood cells are incubated with antigen *in vitro*, the specifically sensitized T cells, which represent only a very small fraction of the total, become activated and divide. Examination of the cultures will reveal blast cells and mitotic divisions (Fig. 8.19), but the most convenient way of assessing the response is by the incorporation of radiolabelled thymidine which provides a measure of cell proliferation (Fig. 8.20).

Stimulated T cells also release cytokines, which can now be studied in great detail. Originally, cytokines were recognized by their activity within a biological assay, with specificity being confirmed by abrogation of activity with a specific antibody. However, with the advent of cloned cytokines, and monoclonal antibodies directed against them, there is a strong move towards immunoassay of the individual cytokines.

Cytotoxic T cells

The ability of cytotoxic T cells to attack targets such as virally infected cells, is conventionally assayed by prelabelling the target with a radioisotope such as ^{51}Cr, and then looking for the release of isotopes into the supernatant from damaged cells (Fig. 8.21).

Antibody-forming cells

It is possible to enumerate the number of cells synthesizing antibody within a given lymphocyte population by the 'sandwich immunofluorescent technique', in which the fixed antibody-forming cell is treated first with antigen and then with a fluorescent second layer of antibody directed to that antigen. It is generally thought to be more convenient, however, to detect cells secreting antibody by plaque techniques, in which each individual cell gives rise to a number of events which can very readily be ascertained by eye, with minimal magnification. In the original 'Jerne' technique, the antibody-forming cell population was mixed with erythrocytes that had been sensitized with the

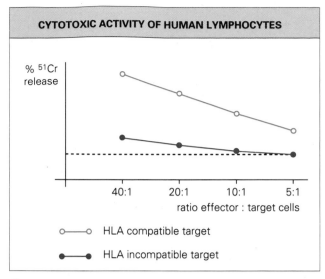

Fig. 8.21 Measurement of cytotoxic activity of human lymphocytes against influenza-infected target cells. Only those targets, that share HLA haplotype with the cytotoxic cell donor are attacked (haplotype restriction) with consequent release of ^{51}Cr. The dotted line indicates background release of isotype from target cells incubated in the absence of effector cells.

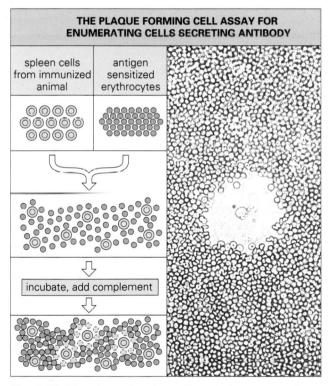

Fig. 8.22 The plaque forming cell assay for enumerating cells secreting antibody. Following incubation with antibody-forming cells, the surrounding red cells become coated with antibodies and can subsequently be lysed by complement.

appropriate antigen on their surface. The secreted antibody coats the antigen-sensitized erythrocytes and these are revealed by addition of complement which causes lysis and a clear plaque within the cell mixture (Fig. 8.22).

A more recent method is the so-called 'Elispot' technique, which can be adapted for identifying cells secreting any molecule against which antibodies can be derived (Fig 8.23). The example in the figure shows the application of

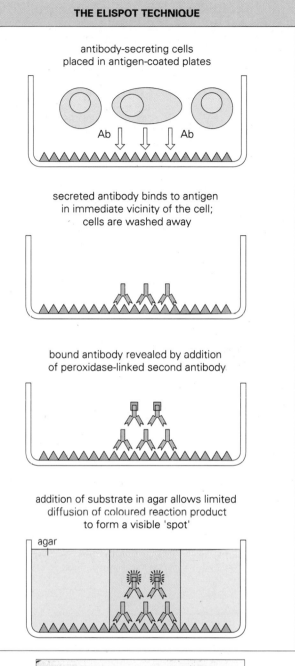

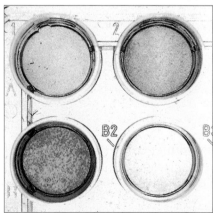

Fig. 8.23 Elispot system for enumerating antibody-forming cells. The lower picture shows spots formed by cells making autoantibodies to thyroglobulin revealed by alkaline phosphatase-linked anti-immunoglobulin. The bottom right-hand well is a control using cells of irrelevant specificity. Courtesy of P Hutchings.

ASSAYS FOR ANTIGENS AND ANTIBODIES	
test	**principles**
Gel precipitation	antigen/antibody precipitates are visualized in gels
Complement fixation	consumption of complement by an antigen/antibody mixture is measured
Agglutination	antigens on the surface of particles are cross-linked by antibody and agglutinate
Immunoassay for antigen	unlabelled test antigen inhibits binding of labelled antigen to fixed amount of antibody
Immunoassay for antibody	antibody binding to solid-phase antigen is visualized by labelled anti-immunoglobulin
Immunohistology	antibody binding to antigen in a tissue can be visualized by labelled reagents
Effects on microbial activity	antibody can block specific microbial functions e.g. metabolism, motility, toxicity
Non-immunological tests for microbes	expand by culture and identify morphologically; expand genes by polymerase chain reaction

Fig. 8.24 Assays for antigens and antibodies.

this method to demonstrate cells secreting autoantibody to thyroglobulin, but clearly this technique could also be applied to the measurement of T cells secreting individual lymphokines.

SUMMARY

The most important components of the innate immune mechanisms that can be studied in the diagnostic laboratory are 1) complement, as evidenced by the ability of serum to be cytocidal for antibody-coated cells and to opsonize microbes for adherence to phagocytes; and 2) phagocytosis, usually evaluated by the respiratory burst induced by agents such as endotoxin.

The many different types of assay for antigens and antibodies are summarized in figure 8.24.

Lymphocytes and their subsets are enumerated by flow cytofluorimetry, utilizing fluorescent monoclonal antibodies directed against discriminating differentiation molecules. Helper T cells sensitized to specific antigens can be revealed by the ability of antigen to induce proliferation and cytokine release *in vitro* and delayed-type hypersensitivity dermal responses *in vivo*. Cytotoxic T cells, such as those directed against virally infected cells, cause the release of radioactive chromium (^{51}Cr) from prelabelled target cells in culture. Antibody-forming cells can be enumerated by the plaque or Elispot techniques.

Further Reading

Hudson L, Hay FC. *Practical immunology*. 3rd edn. Oxford: Blackwell Scientific Publications, 1989.

Johnstone A, Thorpe R. *Immunochemistry in practice*. 2nd edn. Oxford: Blackwell Scientific Publications, 1987.

Kerr MA *et al*. The effect of C3 levels on yeast opsonization by normal and pathological sera: identification of a complement-independant opsonin. *Clin Exp Immunol* 1983; **54**: 793–800.

Sheehan C. *Clinical immunology: principles and laboratory diagnosis*. Philadelphia: JB Lippincott, 1990.

9 IMMUNOLOGICAL REACTIONS PRODUCING TISSUE DAMAGE

Contents

INTRODUCTION: AN INAPPROPRIATE IMMUNE RESPONSE CAN CAUSE TROUBLE FOR THE HOST

Just as mercenaries may turn capriciously upon their paymasters, the immune defence systems of the body may become disloyal and give rise to damage within the tissues of the host. This may happen if the invading microbe or antigen is present in relatively large amounts, or if the humoral and cellular immune state is at heightened level. We speak of a state of 'hypersensitivity', and Coombs and Gell have clarified our thinking to a considerable extent by defining four types of hypersensitivity reactions (see Fig. 9.17) which may be provoked by inappropriate action of the adaptive immune systems. However, before we consider these it would be logical to look at the way in which the innate immune mechanisms themselves can cause hypersensitivity.

INNATE IMMUNE MECHANISMS CAN SOMETIMES LEAD TO DISEASE

These are largely related to inappropriate complement activation. For example, the endotoxins released in Gram-negative septicaemia activate the alternative pathway and lead to platelet destruction through immune adherence of C3b-coated endotoxin to platelets, followed by destruction and release of clotting factors.

The spontaneous activation of the complement system in normal life is controlled by a series of regulatory proteins. Should any of these be deficient, this control is lost. Thus, the gross lack of active C1 inhibitor in hereditary angioedema, for example, leads to recurring episodes of acute circumscribed non-inflammatory oedema mediated by a vasoactive C2 fragment (Fig. 9.1).

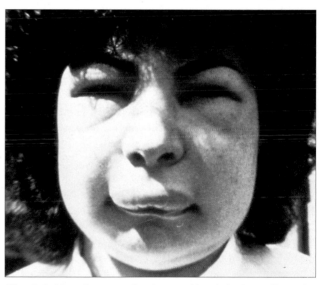

Fig. 9.1 Hereditary angioedema with marked swelling of the upper lip. Courtesy of RP Warin.

IgE–MAST CELL INTERACTIONS MAY CAUSE ANAPHYLAXIS (TYPE I HYPERSENSITIVITY)

The activation of mast cells by antigen cross-linking surface IgE receptors through attachment to bound IgE antibodies, was discussed earlier in the context of the initiation of an acute inflammatory reaction (see Chapter 4). This occurs through the release of mediators that bring about an increase in vascular permeability and chemotaxis of polymorphs and other cell types. Excessive release of mediators causes anaphylaxis through the constriction of smooth muscle and the lowering of blood pressure through capillary dilatation. Anaphylaxis can be local if

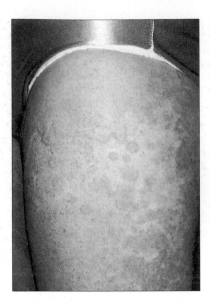

Fig. 9.2 Urticarial weals on the thigh due to a type I anaphylactic reaction. Courtesy of R StC Barnetson and D Gawkrodger.

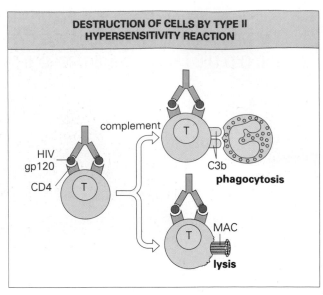

DESTRUCTION OF CELLS BY TYPE II HYPERSENSITIVITY REACTION

Fig. 9.3 Destruction of cells by type II hypersensitivity reaction. In the example shown, CD4+ T cells have bound the gp120 envelope protein of the AIDS virus HIV. Coating of the cell with antibodies to gp120 leads to complement activation and deposition of C3b molecules on the cell surface, which mediate destruction of the T cell by a C3b receptor-bearing phagocyte. Cells may also be killed by lysis through insertion of the post C3 membrane attack complex (MAC) formed by the terminal complement components.

these reactions occur in a site such as the eye or lung, causing hay fever and asthma respectively, or in the skin causing urticaria (Fig. 9.2). Systemic release of these mediators can cause death through generalized anaphylaxis.

ANTIBODY ON THE SURFACE OF HOST CELLS CAN RESULT IN CYTOTOXICITY (TYPE II HYPERSENSITIVITY)

An antigen adhering to, or that is an endogenous component of, the surface of a host cell which then becomes coated with antibody, may be eliminated by phagocytic cells. This process is enhanced by activation of C3. Killing of the cell may also occur if the terminal components of the complement system become activated and the membrane attack complex (MAC) is inserted into the plasma membrane (Fig. 9.3).

The antibody-coated cell itself can also become the target for extracellular cytotoxic attack by natural killer (NK) cells with Fc receptors or myeloid cells which become closely apposed to the membrane of the target and deliver lethal 'hits'. This process is referred to as 'antibody-dependent cell-mediated cytotoxicity' or ADCC (see Chapter 5).

DEPOSITION OF IMMUNE COMPLEXES MAY MEDIATE TISSUE DAMAGE (TYPE III HYPERSENSITIVITY)

Mechanisms leading to tissue damage
Excessive formation of antigen and antibody complexes can lead to tissue damage through platelet aggregation, complement activation and the stimulation of macrophages, as outlined in figure 9.17 and illustrated in Chapter 16.

Locally formed complexes can induce inflammatory lesions

Reactions to inhaled antigens
Repeated exposure to inhaled dusts containing antigens such as microbial spores, may eventually produce a high

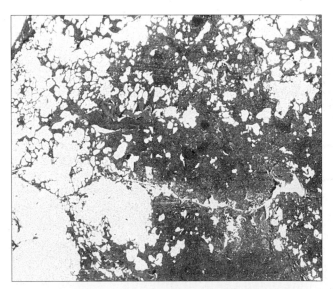

Fig. 9.4 Changes in the lung in human extrinsic allergic alveolitis resulting from a type III hypersensitivity reaction to inhaled foreign antigen. The section shows considerable destruction of the alveoli with regions of heavily stained inflammation and fibrosis. H & E stain, x150. Courtesy of G Boyd.

level of circulating precipitating antibody. When this occurs, inhaled antigen can react with antibody in the lung and become deposited locally as an immune complex, which can give rise to type III hypersensitivity reactions. This will lead to replacement of normal alveolar tissue with fibrous material and consequently to respiratory disorders (Fig. 9.4).

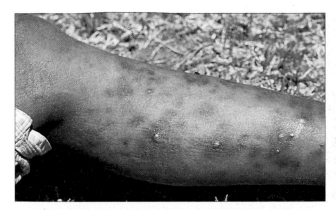

Fig. 9.5 Erythema nodosum leprosum characterized by red indurated areas with pustule formation on the leg of a leprosy patient. Courtesy of R StC Barnetson and D Gawkrodger.

Reactions to internal antigens

Type III reactions are often provoked by the local release of antigen from infectious organisms within an individual with high antibody levels. Thus, chemotherapy may cause an abrupt release of microbial antigens, which in such individuals will produce quite dramatic immune complex mediated reactions, such as erythema nodosa leprosum in the skin of dapsone treated lepromatous leprosy patients (Fig. 9.5).

Circulating immune complexes are often associated with disease

Soluble immune complexes in the circulation are normally cleared by phagocytic mechanisms but when the antigen is persistent as in chronic infections and autoimmune disease, circumstance can arise in which the complexes become deposited in different sites within the vascular bed. A probable mechanism by which small and large complexes may be deposited at different anatomical sites in relationship to be basement membrane in the kidney glomerulus is outlined in Chapter 16. Actual examples of immune complex deposition in kidney glomeruli and in artery walls are illustrated in figures 9.6 and 9.7.

EFFECTOR T CELLS CAN PROVOKE TYPE IV HYPERSENSITIVITY REACTIONS

Unlike the other three forms of hypersensitivity which are mediated by antibody, type IV hypersensitivity is based essentially on the action of the CD4+ helper T cells (see Fig. 9.17). Contact with antigen causes the release of soluble factors from the sensitized T helpers which have amongst their many actions a chemotactic effect on macrophages and an ability to activate these cells once they arrive on the scene. Should the antigen, perhaps in the form of a chronic microbial infection within the macrophage, be one which is difficult to eliminate and therefore is persistent, the T cell stimulation will continue and the activated macrophages, under the prolonged influence of lymphokines, may turn into so-called 'epithelioid' cells and many will fuse to form giant cells, both of which contribute to the characteristic structure known as a 'chronic granuloma' (Fig. 9.8). This may be looked upon

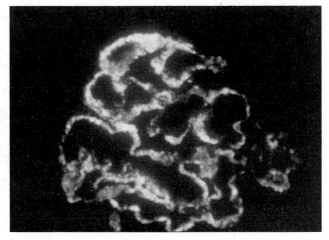

Fig. 9.6 Type III hypersensitivity membranous glomerulonephritis showing the granular peripheral capillary loop deposits of immune complexes which may form after infection with viruses such as hepatitis B or Epstein-Barr. Courtesy of P Sweny.

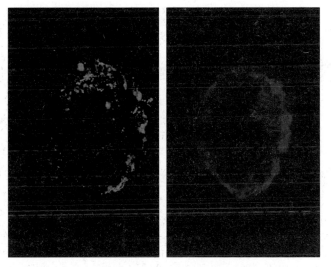

Fig. 9.7 Immune complexes in renal artery following infection with hepatitis B virus. These two serial sections are stained with fluoresceinated anti-hepatitis B antigen (left) and rhodaminated anti-IgM (right). Courtesy of A Nowoslawski.

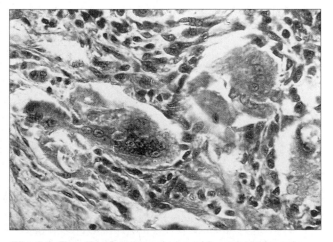

Fig. 9.8 Type IV granuloma induced by streptococcal cells walls. Note the epithelioid and giant cells.

as a strategy by which the body tries to wall off a site in which non-eradicable microbial organisms are located. The CD4+ T cells may also enable cytotoxic T cell precursors to mature and cause damage to tissues containing virally infected cells against which they are specifically directed. The killing of virally infected cells before the virus has had the opportunity to replicate is an important normal defense mechanism; it is only when this occurs on an excessively large scale, as in viral hepatitis, that damage to host tissue becomes a serious issue. It is also likely that cytotoxic T cells recognizing processed antigen on the surface of macrophages could bring about their destruction and this may contribute to some of the tissue damage seen within the centre of a chronic granuloma (Fig. 9.9).

The type IV hypersensitivity state can often be revealed by intradermal injection of antigen to produce the so-called 'delayed-type hypersensitivity' (DTH) response. Following the injection, appropriately sensitized T-cells trafficking through the region of antigen deposition are activated and draw into the site mononuclear cells of the lymphocyte and macrophage families, as shown in figure 8.18. The skin becomes reddened and indurated due to the cellular infiltration, with the reaction being maximal at around 48 hours as in the well-known Mantoux test for hypersensitivity to tuberculin (Fig. 9.10).

HYPERSENSITIVITY DAMAGE CAN ARISE THROUGH AUTOIMMUNE RESPONSES

The phenomenon of autoimmune disease

Not all B and T lymphocytes capable of reacting with self antigens are tolerized, and it is possible to immunize normal animals with certain autoantigens in adjuvants such as 'Complete Freund's (a water in oil emulsion of the antigen mixed with killed tubercle bacilli; see Chapter 36) and evoke autoimmune responses. Antibodies reacting with self, termed 'autoantibodies', and T cell responses, may arise spontaneously in a number of animal models.

Autoimmune responses appear to arise spontaneously in human beings and are very frequently associated with certain diseases. To a first approximation, these disorders can be divided into two main groups. The first, termed 'organ-specific diseases', are so-called because the immune response is targetted to a particular organ and the damage seen as a result of the hypersensitivity reaction is localized to that given organ. For example, in Hashimoto's disease of the thyroid, the gland is damaged by infiltrating mononuclear inflammatory cells associated with the appearance of thyroid-specific autoantibodies in the circulation (Fig. 9.11) The other group, the 'non-organ specific

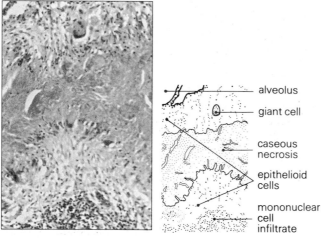

alveolus
giant cell
caseous necrosis
epithelioid cells
mononuclear cell infiltrate

Fig. 9.9 A tuberculous section of lung showing epithelioid and giant cells characteristic of a granulomatous reaction. There is marked caseation and necrosis within the granuloma. H&E stain, x75. Courtsy of R StC Barnetson and D Gawkrodger.

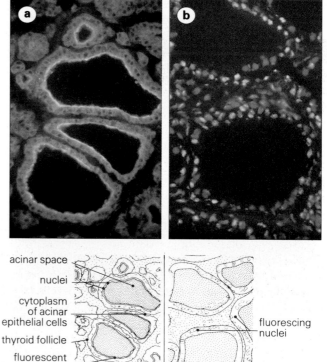

acinar space
nuclei
cytoplasm of acinar epithelial cells
thyroid follicle
fluorescent apical margin
fluorescing nuclei

Fig. 9.11 Autoantibodies demonstrated by double layer immunofluorescence. Unfixed thyroid sections are treated with patient's serum and the fluoresceinated rabbit anti-human immunoglobulin. (a) Serum from a patient with Hashimoto's disease, with thyroid-specific antibodies reacting with the cytoplasm and apical cell surface. (b) Serum from a patient with systemic lupus erythematosus (SLE) with non-organ specific antibodies to nuclear DNA.

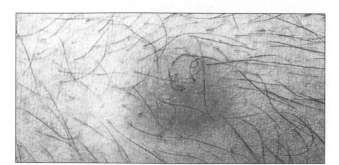

Fig. 9.10 The Mantoux test showing a type IV hypersensitivity cell-mediated reaction with characteristic induration and erythema, in response to intradermal injection of purified protein derivative from *Mycobacterium tuberculosis*.

diseases', are essentially those disorders grouped under the heading of 'rheumatological'. In general, they are associated with the appearance of antibodies lacking specificity for any given organ, such as antibodies to DNA (see Fig. 9.11) and to IgG (rheumatoid factor; Fig. 9.12). It may also be said that the tissue damage in this group is largely mediated by immune complexes. Some representatives of human autoimmune disease are listed in figure 9.13.

The potential for induction of autoimmunity by microbial infection

Induction through antigenic cross-reaction

A non-tolerized autoreactive B cell capable of recognizing a given epitope on a self-antigen will not be triggered if the T cells reacting with the self-molecule have been tolerized. However, a microbial antigen bearing an epitope which cross-reacts with the self-antigen, will stimulate the autoreactive B cell because of the presence of new T helper epitopes on the microbial antigen to which the host has not been tolerized. The resulting antibody synthesized by the triggered B-cell will then be an autoantibody in that it will react with the epitope on the self-antigen (Fig. 9.14).

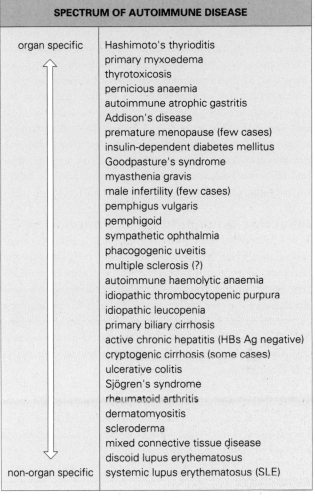

SPECTRUM OF AUTOIMMUNE DISEASE	
organ specific	Hashimoto's thyrioditis
	primary myxoedema
	thyrotoxicosis
	pernicious anaemia
	autoimmune atrophic gastritis
	Addison's disease
	premature menopause (few cases)
	insulin-dependent diabetes mellitus
	Goodpasture's syndrome
	myasthenia gravis
	male infertility (few cases)
	pemphigus vulgaris
	pemphigoid
	sympathetic ophthalmia
	phacogogenic uveitis
	multiple sclerosis (?)
	autoimmune haemolytic anaemia
	idiopathic thrombocytopenic purpura
	idiopathic leucopenia
	primary biliary cirrhosis
	active chronic hepatitis (HBs Ag negative)
	cryptogenic cirrhosis (some cases)
	ulcerative colitis
	Sjögren's syndrome
	rheumatoid arthritis
	dermatomyositis
	scleroderma
	mixed connective tissue disease
	discoid lupus erythematosus
non-organ specific	systemic lupus erythematosus (SLE)

Fig. 9.13 Autoimmune diseases cover a spectrum from organ specific to non-organ specific or systemic. This depends on whether the reponse is primarily against antigens localized to particular organs or against widespread antigens.

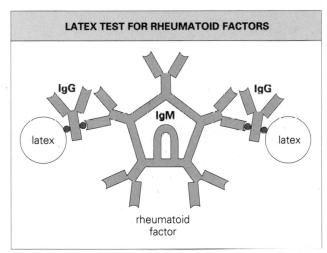

LATEX TEST FOR RHEUMATOID FACTORS

IgG   IgG

IgM

latex   latex

rheumatoid factor

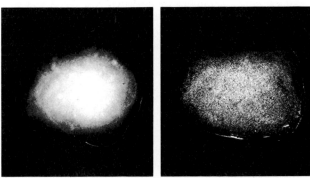

Fig. 9.12 Demonstration of rheumatoid factors, autoantibodies (IgM) to IgG Fc region, present in the serum of patients with rheumatoid arthritis (RA) and certain other systemic autoimmune disorders. Latex particles coated with human IgG are agglutinated by serum from an RA patient (left) but not from a normal individual (right).

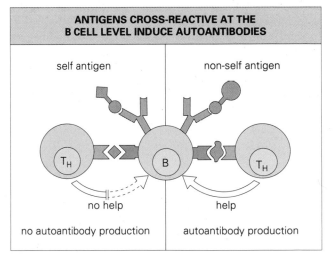

ANTIGENS CROSS-REACTIVE AT THE B CELL LEVEL INDUCE AUTOANTIBODIES

self antigen   non-self antigen

T_H   B   T_H

no help   help

no autoantibody production   autoantibody production

Fig. 9.14 A B cell recognizing an epitope present on self-antigen cross reacts with a similar self epitope coincidentally present on a microbial antigen. B cells do not normally respond to self-antigen because the self reactive Th cells are functionally deleted (tolerized), but if the B cell encounters the cross-reactive microbial antigen, it can present peptides of the antigen to non-self reactive T_H cells, and become activated.

However, when the microbial antigen is cleared, the stimulus for autoantibody production will cease since there will be no T helper epitopes available. The situation may be quite different with epitopes which cross-react at the T cell level because of their similarity in primary amino acid sequence. There is evidence that a peptide from a microbe which includes a similar sequence to that present in the self-protein may be capable of priming an autoreactive T cell which the self protein had previously been unable to stimulate. However, once primed it appears that the self-peptide sequence can boost the primed cell and therefore maintain the autoimmune reaction in the absence of the inciting microbial T cell epitope (Fig. 9.15).

Induction through idiotype interactions

It will be recollected that an idiotype is a collection of epitopes on a given lymphocyte receptor recognized by the receptor on another lymphocyte which acts as an anti-idiotype. A relatively common (public) idiotype on an anti-microbial T or B cell may provoke an anti-idiotype response, which is then capable of stimulating autoreactive T or B cells whose receptors bear an idiotype in common with that of the original anti-microbial lymphocyte receptors (Fig. 9.16).

Yet another possibility is that a virus will stimulate an anti-viral response that may generate an anti-idiotype capable of behaving as an autoantibody to the viral receptor because it acts in certain ways as a structural image of the original virus (see Fig. 9.16)

SUMMARY

The normal defence mechanisms, when excessively heightened or inappropriate, can give rise to host damage. Sometimes, elements of the innate immune response may be unacceptably activated, as when the complement system is driven inexorably by bacterial endotoxins or by constitutional lack of a regulatory control factor. Inappropriate expression of adaptive immune responses can also lead to hypersensitivity reactions, conveniently classified by Coombs and Gell under four main headings, as summarized in figure 9.17. The uneasy truce between self-reactive lymphocytes and body autoantigens can be broken by cross-reactions resulting from microbial infections and this can evoke an autoimmune response leading to autoaggressive disease.

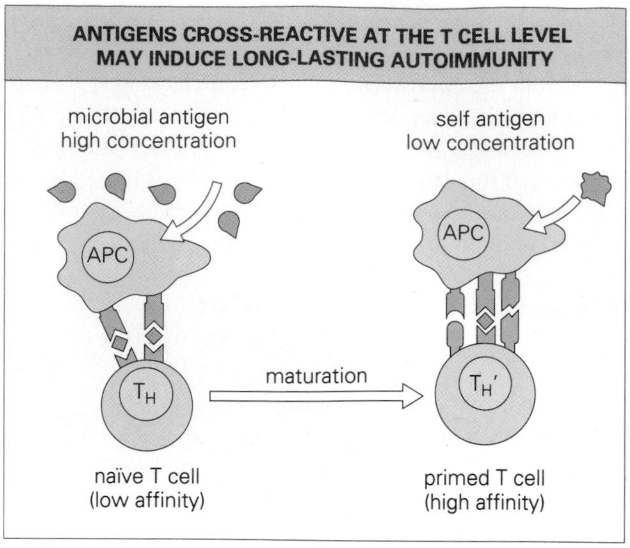

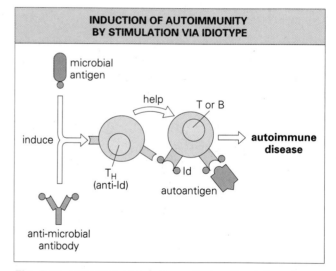

Fig. 9.15 Naïve T_H cells usually cannot be primed by processed self antigen either because of low concentration or low affinity. They can be stimulated by cross-reacting microbial antigens at higher concentration or with higher affinity. Because of increased expression of accessory molecules such as LFA-1 and CD2, the primed cell now has a higher affinity for self peptides and can react with them.

Fig. 9.16 Induction of autoimmunity by stimulation via idiotype. Autoimmunity could arise if self-reactive T or B cells carry a public idiotype (Id) which cross-reacts with the idiotype on antibody stimulated by a microbial agent or even with a structure on the microbe itself.

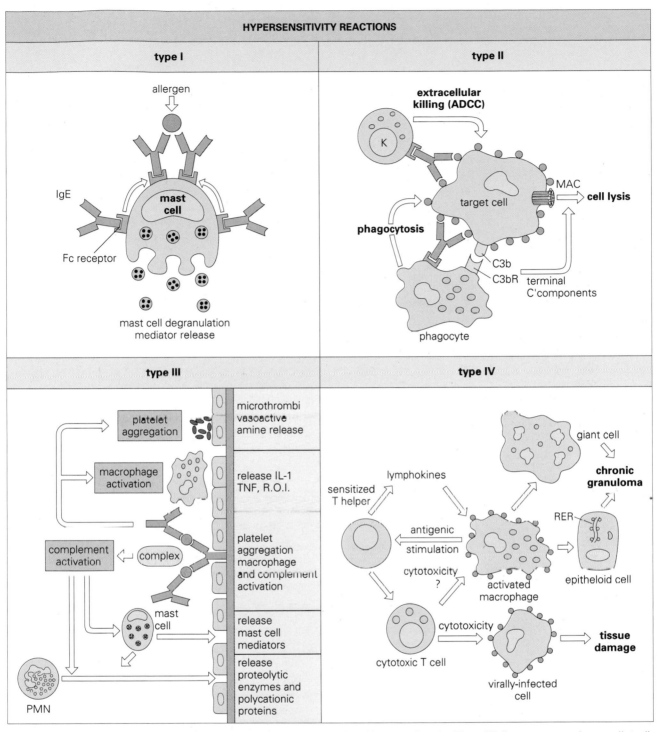

Fig. 9.17 Four types of hypersensitivity reactions based on adaptive immunological responses: **Type I** (immediate) hypersensitivity. Cross-linking of IgE receptors through interaction of bound IgE with allergen leads to degranulation of the mast cell and synthesis of new mediators. This causes smooth muscle constriction and lowering of blood pressure through capillary dilatation. **Type II** (antibody-mediated) hypersensitivity. Antibodies bound to antigens on the host cell surface adhere to Fcγ receptors on effector cells. Associated C3b molecules deposited on the target cell surface then bind to C3b receptors on the effector cells. These events lead to phagocytosis, and to extracellular killing by myeloid cells and large granular lymphocytes with Fcγ receptors (K cells), the phenomenon of 'antibody dependent cell mediated cytotoxicity' (ADCC). Any further reaction with the terminal components of the complement system results in insertion of the membrane attack complex (MAC) and cell lysis. **Type III** (immune complex-mediated) hypersensitivity. Immune complexes deposited in the tissues or blood vessels activate complement, triggering release of mast cell mediators and attracting polymorphs whose granules release molecules that cause tissue damage. Further damage results from platelet microthrombus induced anoxia, and from cytokines and reactive oxygen intermediates secreted by activated macrophages. **Type IV** (delayed) hypersensitivity. Persistent stimulation of antigen-sensitized CD4+ T helper cells by chronically infected macrophages leads to excessive macrophage activation, with transformation to epithelioid cells and fusion to giant cells which make up the typical granuloma. Tissue damage also results from cytotoxic T cell killing of virally infected cells, which can become excessive if viral spread outstrips the rate at which immune defences can be mobilized.

Further Reading —————————————————————————————————————

Brostoff J, Scadding BK, Male DL, Roitt IM. *Clinical immunology.* London: Gower Medical Publishing, 1991.

Roitt IM, Brostoff J, Male DL. *Immunology.* 3rd edn. London: Gower Medical Publishing, 1993.

section 2

CONFLICTS

10 CONFLICTS: THE BACKGROUND TO INFECTIOUS DISEASE

Contents

INTRODUCTION

Vertebrates have been continuously exposed to microbial infections throughout their hundreds of millions of years of evolution. As a result of this constant conflict, with disease or death as the penalty for inadequate defences, they have developed highly efficient recognition (early warning) systems for foreign invaders, and effective inflammatory and immune responses to restrain their growth and spread, and to eliminate them from the body. The fundamental basis for these defences has been described earlier (see Chapters 4–9). If these responses were completely effective, however, microbial infections would be few in number and would be terminated rapidly; microorganisms would not be allowed to persist in the body for long periods. But microorganisms, faced with the anti-microbial defences of the host species, have evolved and developed a variety of characteristics which enable them to bypass or overcome these defences. They must undergo certain steps if they are to successfully infect the host and maintain themselves in nature and at each step the requirement is clear (Fig. 10.1). Furthermore microorganisms multiply exceedingly rapidly compared with their vertebrate hosts, the generation time of an average bacterium being an hour or less, as compared with about 20 years for the human host. Consequently microorganisms evolve with extraordinary speed in comparison with their hosts. This rapid rate of evolution ensures that they are always many steps ahead of the host's antimicrobial defences. Indeed if there are possible ways around the established defences, microorganisms are likely to have discovered and taken advantage of them. Infectious micro-organisms, therefore, owe their success to this ability to adapt and evolve, exploiting weak points in the host defences. The ways in which the phagocytic and immune defences may be overcome are shown in figure 10.2 and are described in Chapters 12 and 15.

OBLIGATORY STEPS FOR INFECTIOUS MICROORGANISMS		
step	**requirement**	**phenomenon**
Attachment ± entry into body	evade natural protective and cleansing mechanisms	entry (infection)
Local or general spread in the body	evade immediate local defences	spread
Multiplication	increase numbers (many will die in the host, or en route to new hosts)	multiplication
Evasion of host defences	evade immune and other defences long enough for the full cycle in the host to be completed	microbial answer to host defences
Shedding from body (exit)	leave body at a site and on a scale that ensures spread to fresh hosts	transmission
Cause damage in host	not strictly necessary but often occurs*	pathology, disease

Fig. 10.1 Obligatory steps for infectious microorganisms. *A certain amount of damage may be inevitable if shedding is to occur, as in the case of the common cold, diarrhoea or the shedding of vesicle fluid or pus.

HOST DEFENCES AND MICROBIAL EVASION STRATEGIES

defence	microbial evasion strategy	mechanism	example
Microbe rinsed away from epithelial surface by host secretions (plus ciliary activity in respiratory tract)	Bind firmly to epithelial surface	Surface molecule on microbe attaches to 'receptor' molecule on host epithelial cell	Influenza, Rhinovirus Chlamydia, Gonococcus
	Interfere with ciliary activity	Produce ciliotoxic/ciliostatic molecule	*Bordetella pertussis* Pneumococci, *Pseudomonas*
Microbe ingested and killed by phagocyte	Interfere with function (e.g. chemotaxis) of phagocyte or kill it (before or after phagocytosis)	Release leucocidins, antiphagocytic haemolysins etc.	Staphylococci, Streptococci *Shigella, E. coli, Pseudomonas*
	Inhibit phagocytosis	Microbial outer wall or capsule impedes phagocytosis	Pneumococci, *Treponema pallidum, H. influenzae*
	Inhibit lysosomal fusion	Microbe liberates molecule from phagosome	*M. tuberculosis, Toxoplasma gondii*
	Resist killing and multiply in phagocyte	Unknown; may involve exit from phagosome (*Listeria*)	*Brucella* sp., *Listeria monocytogenes* Measles, Dengue viruses
Host molecules (lactoferrin, transferrin etc.) restrict availability of free iron needed by microbe	Microbe competes with host for iron	Microbe possesses avidly iron-binding molecules (siderophores)	Pathogenic *Neisseria E. coli, Pseudomonas*
Complement activated with anti-microbial effects	Interfere with alternative pathway complement activation	Fully sialylated bacterial surface	K antigen of *E. coli*, Group B meningococcus
	Inactivate complement components	Production of an elastase	*Pseudomonas aeruginosa*
	Microbial antigen (polysaccharides) project beyond microbial surface	C activation occurs away from microbial surface and damage thus avoided	Gram-negative bacteria
	Interfere with complement-mediated phagocytosis	C3b receptor on microbe competes with that on phagocyte. Complement access blocked	*Candida albicans, Toxoplasma gondii* M protein of *Strep. pyogenes*
Host cell membrane as barrier to intracellular microbe	Traverse host cell membrane	Fusion protein in viral envelope	Influenza, HIV
	Suffer uptake by phagocyte and resist killing	See above	See above
	Enter cell by active penetration	Microbial enzymes mediate cell penetration	Trypanosomes, *Toxoplasma gondii*

Host defence	Microbial evasion strategy	Mechanism	Examples
Infected host produces interferons to inhibit virus replication	Induce a poor interferon response	HBc of hepatitis B suppresses IFN-β production	Hepatitis B, Rotaviruses
	Enjoy insensitivity to interferons	Prevent activation of interferon-induced enzymes	Adenovirus
Infected host produces antimicrobial antibody	Destroy antibody	Bacterium liberates IgA protease	Gonococcus, *H. influenzae* Streptococci
	Fail to induce protective antibody	Infect lymphoid cells?	Scrapie agents
	Display Fc receptor on microbial surface	Antibody bound to microbe in upside-down position	Staphylococci (Protein A), Trypanosomes Certain streptococci, Herpes simplex virus Cytomegalovirus
	Avoid immune recognition	Acquire coating of host molecules	Hydatid disease, Schistosomiasis
Infected host produces antimicrobial cell-mediated immune response	Invade T cells and interfere with their function or kill them	Virus envelope molecule binds to CD4 on helper T cell surface	HIV
	Switch on T cells or B cells non-specifically, non-productively	Polyclonal activation of B cells Polyclonal activation of T cells by release of T cell mitogens	EB virus, *Mycoplasma pneumoniae* Staphylococcal toxins
Antimicrobial immune response recognizes infected cells and destroys them, or liberates cytokines with antimicrobial effects	Microbe in cell fails to display microbial antigens on cell surface	Antiviral antibody modulates and removes viral antigens	Measles
		Viral antigens not synthesized or not transported to surface membranes	Herpes simplex virus in sensory neurones
Antimicrobial immune response	Infect glands or epithelial surfaces relatively inaccessible to circulating antibody or immune cells	Virus has tropism for cells in glands or on surfaces	Cytomegalovirus, Rabies virus (salivary glands)
	Suppress immune responses	Invade immune tissues	HIV, Measles
	Vary microbial antigens either in individually infected host, or during spread in host community	Switch on different surface antigens	*Trypanosoma* sp., *Borrelia recurrentis*
		Mutation, genetic recombination	Influenza virus, streptococci, gonococci

Fig. 10.2 Host defences and microbial evasion strategies. Microbes evolve fast and are generally one step ahead in this ancient conflict, but it must be remembered that the antimicrobial defences themselves represent the host's answer to invading microbes.

10.3

EVERY INFECTION IS A RACE

The speed with which host adaptive responses can be mobilized is crucial. *Every infection is a race* – between the capacity of the microorganism to multiply, spread and cause disease and the ability of the host to control and finally terminate the infection (Fig. 10.3). For instance, if there is a 24 hour delay before an important host response comes into operation, this can give a decisive advantage to a rapidly growing microorganism. From the host's point of view, it may allow enough damage to be done to cause disease. More importantly from the microbe's point of view, it may give the microbe the opportunity to be shed from the body in larger amounts or for an extra day or two. A microbe that achieves this will be rapidly selected for in evolution.

The picture of conflict between host and parasite, usually and appropriately described in military terms, is central to an understanding of the biology of infectious disease. As with military conflicts, adaptation on both sides (see panel) has tended to lessen the amount of damage and death in the host population, leading to a more stable and balanced relationship. The successful parasite gets what it can from the host without causing too much damage, and in general the more ancient the relationship the less damage is done. Many microbial parasites, not only the normal flora (see Chapter 3) but also polioviruses, meningococci and pneumococci etc., live for the most part in peaceful co-existence with their human host.

Some microorganisms remain at body surfaces, perhaps spreading locally but failing to invade deeper tissues. These include the common cold viruses, wart viruses, mycoplasmas and skin fungi. Often the disease is mild, but when powerful toxins are produced and act either locally (cholera) or at distant sites (diphtheria) severe illness may occur.

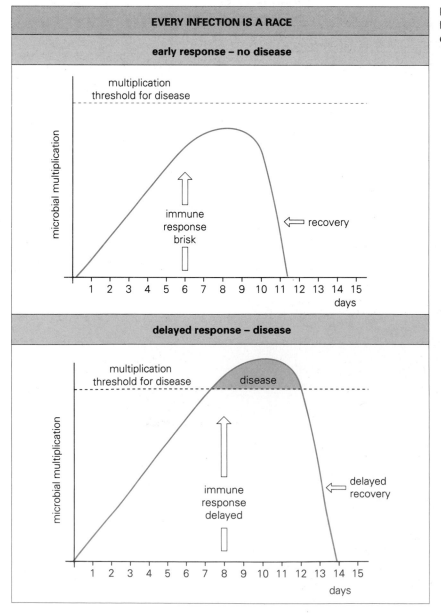

Fig. 10.3 Every infection is a race. Delays in mobilizing host adaptive defences can lead to disease or death.

Myxomatosis

Myxomatosis provides a well-studied, classic example of the evolution of an infectious disease in a highly susceptible population. Myxomavirus, which is spread mechanically by mosquitoes, normally infects South American rabbits (*Sylvilagus brasiliensis*), but they remain perfectly well, developing only a virus-rich skin swelling at the site of the mosquito bite. The same virus in the European rabbit (*Oryctolagus cuniculus)* causes a rapidly fatal disease.

Myxomavirus was successfully introduced into Australia in 1950 as an attempt to control the rapidly increasing rabbit population. Initially, more than 99% of infected rabbits died (Fig. 10.4), but then two fundamental changes occurred. First, new, less lethal strains of virus appeared and replaced the original strain. This occurred because rabbits infected with these strains survived for longer and their virus was therefore more likely to be transmitted. Second, the rabbit population changed its character, as those that were genetically more susceptible to the infection were eliminated. In other words, the virus selected out the more resistant host, and the less lethal virus strain proved to be a more successful parasite. If the rabbit population had been eliminated the virus would also have died out, but the host–parasite relationship quite rapidly settled down to

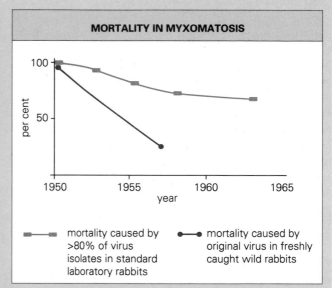

Fig. 10.4 Myxomatosis is the best-studied example of the appearance in a host population of a devastating, lethal microbe, which gradually settles down to a state of more balanced pathogenicity. *V. cholerae* has progressed in this direction, and perhaps HIV is destined to tread the same path.

reach a state of better balanced pathogenicity. And, of course, Australia's rabbit problem remained unsolved.

Four types of infection can be distinguished (Fig. 10.5), where:

1) The microorganism has specific mechanisms for attaching to or penetrating the body surfaces of the normal healthy host (e.g. most viruses and certain bacteria);

2) The microorganism is introduced into normal healthy host by a biting arthropod (malaria, plague, typhus, yellow fever);

3) The microorganism is introduced into an otherwise normal, healthy host via skin wound or animal bite (clostridia, rabies, *Pasteurella multocida*);

4) The microorganism is unable to infect a normal, healthy host unless there is impairment of surface or systemic defences (Chapter 33); e.g. burns, insertion of foreign bodies (cannulae and catheters), urinary tract infections in male (stones, enlarged prostate, see Chapter 23), bacterial pneumonia following initial viral damage (e.g. post-influenza), or depressed immune responses (immunosuppressive drugs or diseases such as HIV).

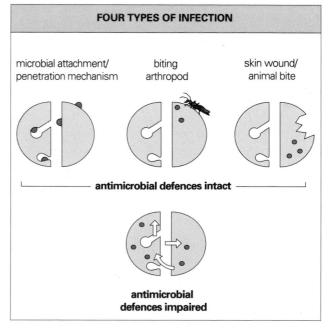

Fig. 10.5 Four types of microbial infection can be distinguished. Surface or systemic defences of the host can be impaired in a variety of ways (see text).

CAUSATION IN INFECTIOUS DISEASES

Humans are host to a large number of different microorganisms. In addition to the scores of microbes that form the normal flora there are more than one hundred that quite commonly cause infection (some of them remaining in the body for many years afterwards), and several hundred others that are responsible for less common infections. Against this rich background of parasitic activity, how do we prove that a certain microorganism is the culprit in a given disease? In some instances (anthrax, cholera, tetanus) the causative microorganism was identified and incriminated at an early stage, but in the case of glandular fever and viral hepatitis it was not so easy. In 1890 Robert Koch (see panel) set out as 'postulates' the criteria he felt to be necessary for a microorganism to be accepted as the cause of a given disease. These were:

1) The microbe must be present in every case of the disease;

2) The microbe must be isolated from the diseased host and grown in pure culture;

3) The disease must be reproduced when a pure culture is introduced into a non-diseased susceptible host;

4) The microbe must be recoverable from an experimentally infected host.

However, certain modifications were needed in order to include certain bacterial diseases and the new world of virological diseases. The microbe could not always be grown in the laboratory (*Treponema pallidum*, wart viruses), and for certain microbes there was (initially) no susceptible animal species (hepatitis B, EB virus). The criteria were modified, therefore, on several occasions to accomodate these problems and finally reformulated and brought up to date by A S Evans in 1976.

In the early days of microbiology Koch's postulates brought a welcome clarity. The germ theory of disease causation had only recently been set out, following Koch's classic studies on anthrax (1876) and tuberculosis (1882), and methods for isolating microbes in pure culture and identifying them were only just being developed. Nowadays, with our vastly increased technology and understanding of infection, those attempts to make lists and apply rigid criteria may seem old fashioned. Perhaps we can now reach conclusions about causation using enlightened common sense. For instance, we recognize that diseases sometimes do not appear until many years after a specific infection (SSPE, Creutzfeld-Jakob disease; see Chapter 27). Nevertheless, grey areas remain, especially in

Robert Koch (1843–1910)
In 1876, while in general practice in Berlin, Robert Koch (Fig. 10.6) isolated the anthrax bacillus, and became the first to show a specific organism as the cause of a disease. In 1882 he discovered *Mycobacterium tuberculosis* as the cause of tuberculosis. He then went on to lead the 1883 expedition to Egypt and India, and discovered the cause of cholera – *Vibrio cholerae.*

Koch was the founder of the 'germ theory' of disease, which maintained that certain diseases were caused by a single species of microbe. In 1890, he set out his 'postulates' as ground-rules (see text).

New techniques were necessary to meet the exacting requirements of the postulates, and Koch became the first to grow bacteria in 'colonies', initially on potato slices and later, with his pupil Petri, on solid gelatin media.

Koch himself could not reproduce cholera in animals, however, and not all microbes could be cultivated. His neat rules therefore had to be modified. Nevertheless, he brought order and clarity to medicine - until then diseases were attributed to miasmas or mists, to punishments from the Gods or devils, or to unfortunate conjunctions of the stars and planets. However, there was resistance to his ideas - a distinguished Munich physician Max Von Petternkofer, felt that he had put paid to the new theory when he drank a pure culture of *V. cholerae* and suffered no more than mild diarrhoea!

During the next 20 years much was achieved by Koch's disciples, who included Albert Neisser (1879, the gonococcus), F. Escherich (1885, *E. coli*) and K. Shiga (1898, *Shigella*). Koch himself became a professor at Berlin University and was awarded the Nobel prize in 1905.

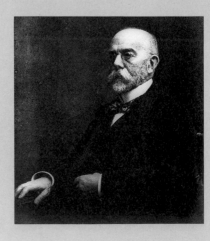

Fig. 10.6
Robert Koch
(1843–1910).

diseases of possible/probable microbial aetiology where the microbe does not act alone. Cofactors or genetic and immunological factors in the host may play a vital part. Examples include:

- The cancers associated with viruses (hepatitis B, genital wart viruses, EB virus);

- Diseases of possible microbial origin, but where a number of different microbes may be involved (post-viral fatigue syndrome, exacerbations of multiple sclerosis);

- Diseases that might be infectious but occur only in the very small proportion of genetically predisposed individuals (rheumatoid athritis, juvenile diabetes);

Finally, there are two interesting possibilities which could give problems in assigning disease aetiology, although neither have yet been shown to apply to human disease: 1) in some infections the DNA of the causative virus is integrated into the genome of the host, and is transmitted vertically. It thus behaves as a genetic attribute. This is known to occur, for instance, with mammary tumour virus in mice; 2) the causative microbe, having triggered off the disease process, disappears completely from the body and is no longer detectable. This is known to be the case in the cerebellar hypoplasia occurring in hamsters and cats after intrauterine infection with parvoviruses. There are no known examples in humans.

FREQUENCY OF CLINICALLY APPARENT DISEASE	
infection	approximate % with clinically apparent disease*
Pneumocystis carinii	0
Poliomyelitis (child)	0.1–1.0
EB virus (1-5 yr old child)	1.0**
Rubella	50
Influenza (young adult)	60
Whooping cough Typhoid Malaria Anthrax	>90
Gonorrhoea (adult male) Measles	99
Rabies HIV (?)	100
* on primary infection ** 30–75% in young adults	

Fig. 10.7 The likelihood of developing clinical disease often depends on age and sex, as shown. When there is a lengthy incubation period the proportion with clinical disease may increase with time, from a few per cent to (probably) 100% in the case of HIV.

THE BIOLOGICAL RESPONSE GRADIENT

It is uncommon for a microbe to cause exactly the same disease in all infected individuals. Hence a physician must be able to make a diagnosis when only some of the possible signs and symptoms are present. The exact clinical picture depends on many variables, such as infecting dose and route, age, sex, presence of other microbes, nutritional status, genetic background, and so on. Infections such as measles or cholera give a fairly regular disease picture but others such as syphilis cause such a wide spectrum of pathology that Sir William Osler (1849–1919) stated that "He who knows syphilis, knows medicine".

There is great variation not only in the nature but also in the severity of clinical disease. Many infections are asymptomatic in more than 90% of individuals, the clinically characterized illness applying to only an occasional unfortunate host (Fig. 10.7). This illness can be very mild or severe. Asymptomatically infected individuals are important because although they develop immunity and resistance to reinfection, they are not identified, move normally in the community, and can infect others. Clearly there is little point in isolating a clinically infected patient when there is a high frequency of asymptomatically infected individuals in the community. This phenomenon can be represented as an 'iceberg' (Fig. 10.8).

SUMMARY

This book is based on the concept of a conflict between microbe and host. Faced with host defences (Part 2), the microbes (Part 1) have developed answers, and in turn the host defences have had to be modified although slowly, in response. Every infectious disease is the result of this ancient conflict. Details of the host–microbe conflict will now be given (Chapter 11–16), followed by an outline of diagnostic methods (Chapters 17, 18), and then a central account of infectious diseases according to the bodily systems involved (Chapters 19–31).

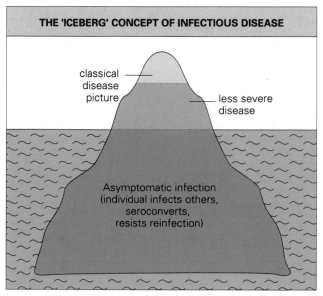

Fig. 10.8 The 'iceberg' concept of infectious disease.

Further Reading

Burnet FM, White DO. *The natural history of infectious disease* 4th edn. Cambridge: Cambridge University Press, 1972.

Mims CA. *The pathogenesis of infectious disease* 3rd edn. London: Academic Press, 1987.

Falkow W. Koch's postulates applied to microbial pathogenicity. *Rev Inf Dis* 1988; **10**: S 274.

11 ENTRY, EXIT AND TRANSMISSION

Contents

INTRODUCTION

The mammalian host can be considered as a series of body surfaces (Fig. 11.1). To establish themselves on or in the host, microorganisms must either attach to or penetrate one of these body surfaces. The outer surface, covered by skin, and usually fur, protects and isolates the body from the outside world, forming a dry, horny, relatively impermeable outer layer. Elsewhere, however, there has to be more intimate contact and exchange with the outside world. Hence in the alimentary, respiratory and urinogenital tracts, where food is absorbed, gases exchanged, and urine and sexual products released, the lining consists of one or more layers of living cells. In the eye the skin is replaced by a transparent layer of living cells, the conjunctiva. All these body surfaces have well developed cleansing and defence mechanisms and entry of microorganisms always has to occur in the face of these natural mechanisms (see Chapter 4). Successful microorganisms therefore possess efficient mechanisms for attaching to and often traversing these body surfaces.

BODY SURFACES AS SITES OF MICROBIAL INFECTION AND SHEDDING

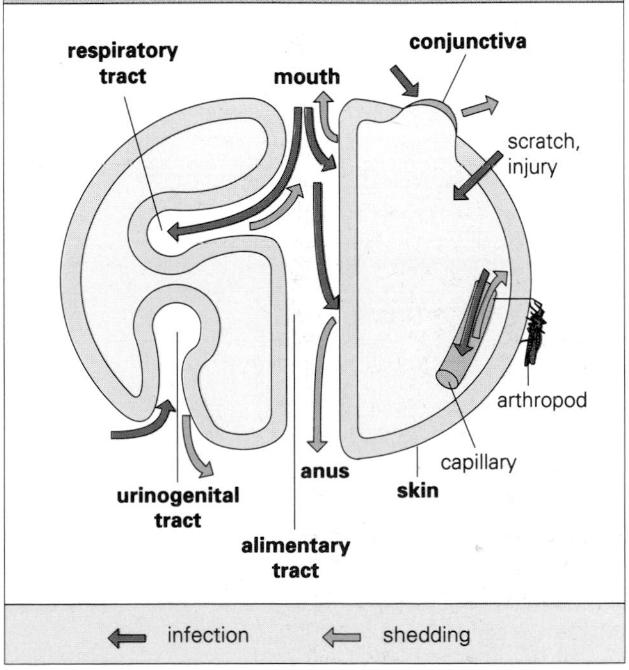

Fig. 11.1 Body surfaces as sites of microbial infection and shedding.

There are often specific molecules on the microbe that bind to receptor molecules on host cells, either at the body surface (viruses, bacteria etc.) or in tissues (viruses). These receptor molecules, which are not, of course, present for the benefit of the virus or other infectious agent, have specific functions in the life of the cell. Very occasionally the receptor molecule is present only in certain cells, which are then uniquely susceptible to infection. Examples include the CD4 receptor for HIV and the C3d receptor for EB virus. In these cases the presence of the receptor molecule determines virus tropism and accounts for the distinctive pattern of infection. Receptors are thus critical determinants of cell susceptibility not only at the body surface but in all tissues. After binding to the susceptible cell, the microorganism can multiply at the surface (mycoplasma, *Bordetella pertussis*) or enter the cell (viruses, chlamydia) and infect it (see Chapter 13).

If they are to be transmitted to a fresh host, microorganisms must also exit from the body. They are either shed in large numbers in secretions and excretions, or are available in blood for uptake by blood-sucking arthropods, needles and so on.

SKIN AS A SITE OF ENTRY

Microorganisms infecting or entering the body via the skin are listed in figure 11.2. On the skin microorganisms other than residents of the normal flora (see Chapter 3) are soon inactivated, especially by fatty acids (skin pH is about 5.5), and probably by substances in sebaceous or other glands, and materials produced by the normal flora of the skin. Skin bacteria may enter hair follicles or sebaceous glands (styes, boils) or teat canal (staphylococcal mastitis).

Several types of fungi (the dermatophytes) infect the non-living keratinous structures (stratum corneum, hair, nails) produced by the skin. Infection is established as long as the parasites rate of downward growth into the keratin exceeds the rate of shedding of the keratinous product. When the latter is very slow, as in the case of nails, the infection is more likely to become chronic.

More commonly infection takes place at the site of wounds, abrasions or burns. Even a small break in the skin can be a portal of entry if virulent microorganisms such as streptococci, leptospira or hepatitis B virus are present at the site.

Biting arthropods such as mosquitoes, ticks, fleas and sandflies (see Chapter 31) penetrate the skin during feeding and can thus introduce infectious agents or parasites into the body. The arthropod transmits the infection and is an essential part of the life cycle of the microorganism. Sometimes the transmission is mechanical, the microorganism contaminating the mouth parts without multiplying in the arthropod. In most cases, however, the infectious agent multiplies in the arthropod and as a result of millions of years of adaptation causes little or no damage to that host. After an incubation period it appears in the saliva or feces and is transmitted during a blood feed. The mosquito for instance, injects saliva directly into host tissues as an anticoagulent, whereas the human body louse defecates as it feeds, and *Typhus rickettsiae* present in the feces are introduced into the bite wound when the host scratches the affected area.

The conjunctiva can be regarded as a specialized area of skin. It is kept clean by the continuous flushing action of tears, aided every few seconds by the windscreen wiper action of the eyelids. Hence the microorganisms that infect the normal conjunctiva (chlamydia, gonococci) must have

MICROORGANISMS THAT INFECT VIA THE SKIN		
microorganism	disease	comments
Arthropod-borne viruses	various fevers	150 distinct viruses, transmitted by infected arthropod bite
Rabies virus	rabies	bite from infected animals
Vaccinia virus	skin lesion	vaccination against smallpox
Wart viruses	warts	infection restricted to epidermis
Staphylococci	boils etc.	commonest skin invaders
Rickettsia	typhus, spotted fevers	infestation with infected arthropod
Leptospira	leptospirosis	contact with water containing infected animals urine
Streptococci	impetigo, erysipelas	concurrent pharyngeal infection in one-third of cases
Bacillus anthracis	cutaneous anthrax	systemic disease following local lesion at inoculation site
Treponema pallidum and *pertenue*	syphilis, yaws	warm, moist skin is more susceptible
Yersinia pestis	plague	bite from infected rodent flea
Plasmodia	malaria	bite from infected mosquito
Trichophyton sp. and other fungi	ringworm, athletes foot	infection restricted to skin, nails, hairs
Anklostoma duodenale (or *Necator americanus*)	hookworm	silent entry of larvae through skin of e.g. foot
Filarial nematodes	filariasis	bite from infected mosquito, midge, blood-sucking fly
Schistosoma sp.	schistosomiasis	larvae (cercariae) from infected snail penetrate skin during wading or bathing

Fig. 11.2 Microorganisms that infect via the skin. Some remain restricted to the skin (wart viruses, ringworm), while others enter the body after growth in the skin (syphilis) or after mechanical transfer across the skin (arthropod-borne infections, schistosomiasis).

efficient attachment mechanisms (see Chapter 21). Interference with local defences, due to decreased lachrymal gland secretion, conjunctival or lid damage, allows even non-specialist microorganisms to establish themselves.

RESPIRATORY TRACT AS A SITE OF ENTRY

Air normally contains suspended particles, including smoke, dust and microorganisms. Efficient cleansing mechanisms (see Chapter 20 and 22) deal with these constantly inhaled particles. With about 500–1000 microorganisms per m³ inside buildings, and a ventilation rate of 6 litres per minute at rest, as many as 10 000 microorganisms per day are introduced into the lungs. In the upper or lower respiratory tract inhaled microorganisms like other particles, will be entrapped in mucus, carried to the back of the throat by ciliary action and swallowed. Those that invade the normal healthy respiratory tract avoid this fate because they have developed specific mechanisms for doing so.

The ideal strategy is to attach firmly to the surfaces of cells forming the mucociliary sheet. Specific molecules on the organism (often called adhesins) bind to receptor molecules on the susceptible cell (Fig. 11.3). Examples of such respiratory infections are given in figure 11.4.

Another way of interfering with cleaning mechanisms is by inhibiting ciliary activity; this helps invading microorganisms to establish themselves in the respiratory tract. *B. pertussis* for instance not only attaches to respiratory epithelial cells, but also interferes with ciliary activity, and other bacteria (Fig. 11.5) produce various ciliostatic substances, whose nature is generally unknown.

Inhaled microorganisms reaching the alveoli encounter alveolar macrophages, whose function is to remove foreign particles and keep these air spaces clean. Most microorganisms are destroyed by these macrophages, but one or two pathogens have learnt either to avoid phagocytosis or to avoid destruction after phagocytosis. Tubercle bacilli, for instance, survive in these cells and respiratory tuberculosis is thought to be initiated in this way. The vital role of macrophages in anti-microbial defences is dealt with more thoroughly in Chapters 12 and 14. Alveolar macrophages are damaged following inhalation of toxic asbestos particles and certain dusts, and this leads to increased susceptibility to respiratory tuberculosis.

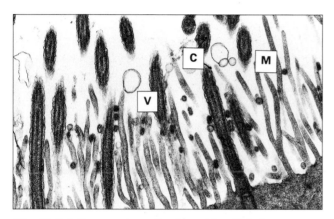

Fig. 11.3 Influenza virus attachment to ciliated epithelium. Influenza virus particles (V) attached to cilia (C) and microvilli (M). Electron micrograph of thin section from organ culture of guinea-pig trachea 1 hour after addition of virus. Courtesy of R E Dourmashkin.

Fig. 11.4 Microbial attachment in the respiratory tract.

MICROBIAL ATTACHMENT IN THE RESPIRATORY TRACT			
microorganism	disease	microbial adhesin	receptor on host cell
Influenza virus	influenza	haemagglutinin	neuraminic acid-containing glycoprotein
Rhinovirus, Coxsackie A viruses	common cold	capsid protein	ICAM1-type molecule
Parainfluenza virus type 1 Respiratory syncytial virus	respiratory illness	envelope protein	glycoside
Adenoviruses	respiratory illness	capsid protein (penton fibre)	?
Mycoplasma pneumoniae	atypical pneumonia	mycoplasmal molecule on 'foot'	neuraminic acid
Neisseria meningitidis	carrier state	molecule on pili	?
Haemophilus influenzae *Strep. pneumoniae* *Klebsiella pneumoniae*	respiratory disease	surface molecule	carbohydrate sequence in glycolipid

INTERFERENCE WITH CILIARY ACTIVITY IN RESPIRATORY INFECTIONS		
MEDIATED BY INFECTING MICROORGANISMS		
microorganisms	**action**	**mechanisms**
Bordetella pertussis	interference with ciliary activity	unknown
Haemophilus influenzae	interference with ciliary activity	unknown
Pseudomonas aeruginosa	interference with ciliary activity	at least 7 ciliostatic substances produced by bacteria
Mycoplasma pneumoniae	interference with ciliary activity	ciliostatic substance produced
OTHER CAUSES		
cause	**mechanisms**	**importance**
Viral infection	ciliated cell dysfunction or destruction by influenza, measles	+++
Atmospheric pollution (automobiles, cigarette smoking etc.)	acutely impaired mucociliary function	?+
Inhalation of unhumidified air (indwelling tracheal tubes, general anaesthesia)	acutely impaired mucociliary function	+
Chronic bronchitis Cystic fibrosis	chronically impaired mucociliary function	+++

Fig. 11.5 Interference with ciliary activity in respiratory infections. Although microbes can actively interfere with ciliary activity (top), a more general impairment of mucociliary function (bottom) acts as a predisposing cause of respiratory infection.

INTESTINAL TRACT AS A SITE OF ENTRY

Apart from the general flow of intestinal contents, there are no particular cleansing mechanisms in the intestinal tract, except in so far as diarrhoea and vomiting can be included in this category. Under normal circumstances multiplication of resident bacteria is counterbalanced by their continuous passage to the exterior with the rest of the intestinal contents. Ingestion of a small number of non-pathogenic bacteria followed by growth in the lumen of the alimentary canal, produces only relatively small numbers within 12–18 hours, the normal intestinal transit time. Thus if they are to establish themselves and multiply in large numbers, infecting bacteria must attach themselves to the intestinal epithelium (Fig. 11.6), and thereby avoid being carried straight down the alimentary canal to be excreted with the rest of the intestinal contents. The concentration of microorganisms in feces depends on the balance between the production and removal of bacteria in the intestine. Thus *Vibrio cholerae* (Figs 11.7 and 11.8) and the rotaviruses both establish specific binding to receptors on the surface of intestinal epithelial cells. For *V. cholerae*, establishment in surface mucus may be sufficient for infection and pathogenicity. The fact that certain bacteria infect mainly the large bowel (*Shigella* sp.) or

small intestine (most salmonella) indicates the presence of specific receptor molecules on epithelial cells in those sections of the alimentary canal.

Crude mechanical devices rather than specific molecular adhesion, are used for the attachment and for entry of certain parasitic protozoans and worms. *Giardia lamblia* for example, adheres closely to the microvilli of the epithelial cells by its own microvillar sucking disc. Hookworms attach to the intestinal mucosa by means of a large mouth capsule, containing hooked teeth or cutting plates. Other worms, e.g. *Ascaris*, maintain their position by 'bracing' themselves against peristalsis; tapeworms adhere closely to the mucus covering the intestinal wall, the anterior hooks and sucker playing a relatively minor role in the largest worms. A number of worms actively penetrate into the mucosa as adults (Trichinella, Trichuris) or traverse the gut wall in order to enter deeper tissues (e.g. the embryos of *Trichinella*, released from the female worm, and the larvae of *Echinococcus* hatched from ingested eggs).

The likelihood of infection in the intestinal tract is certainly affected by the presence of mucus, acids, enzymes and bile. Mucus protects epithelial cells, perhaps acting as a mechanical barrier to infection. It may contain molecules that bind to microbial adhesins, thus blocking attachment to host cells. It also contains secretory IgA antibodies which

MICROBIAL ATTATCHMENT IN THE INTESTINAL TRACT			
microorganism	**disease**	**attachment site**	**mechanism**
Poliovirus	poliomyelitis	intestinal epithelium	viral capsid protein reacts with specific receptor on cell (perhaps ICAM*)
Vibrio cholerae	cholera	intestinal epithelial cell	specific bacterial molecule (adhesin)** binds to fucose/ mannose receptor on cell
E. coli (certain strains)	diarrhoea	intestinal epithelial cell	specific bacterial molecule (adhesin)** binds to fucose/ mannose receptor on cell
S.typhi	enteric fever	intestinal epithelial cell	specific bacterial molecule (adhesin)** binds to fucose/ mannose receptor on cell
Shigella sp.,	dysentery	colonic epithelium	unknown
Giardia lamblia	diarrhoea	duodenal, jejunal epithelium	protozoa bind to mannose-D phosphate on host cell; also have mechanical sucker
Entamoeba histolytica	dysentry	colonic epithelium	amoebae bind to asialofetuin on host cell
Ankylostoma duodonalo	hookworm	intestinal epithelium	four hooked teeth

* intracellular adhesion molecule; has important functions in inflammatory and 'social' life of cells. Acts as receptor molecule for poliovirus on cells *in vitro*
** often on pili or fimbriae (e.g. up to 200 pili, each bearing adhesions, on *E. coli*)

Fig. 11.6 Microbial attachment in the intestinal tract.

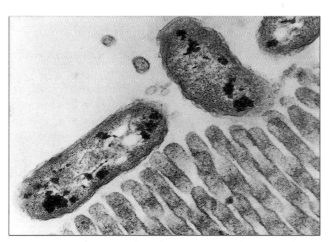

Fig. 11.7 Attachment of *Vibrio cholerae* to brush border of rabbit villus. Thin section electron micrograph, x10 000. Courtesy of E T Nelson.

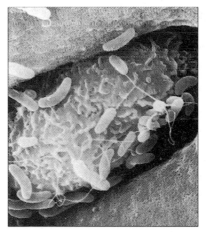

Fig. 11.8 Adherence of *Vibrio cholera* to M cells in human ileal mucosa. Courtesy of T Yamamoto.

protect the immune individual against infection. Motile microorganisms (*V. cholerae*, salmonellae and certain strains of *E. coli*) can propel themselves through the mucus layer and are thus more likely to reach epithelial cells to make specific attachments; *V. cholerae* also produces a mucinase that probably helps its passage through the mucus. Non-motile microorganisms, in contrast, rely on random and passive transport in the mucus layer.

As might be expected, microorganisms infecting by the intestinal route are often capable of surviving in the presence of acid, proteolytic enzymes and bile. This also applies to microorganisms shed from the body by this route (Fig. 11.9).

All organisms infecting by this route must run the gauntlet of acid in the stomach. The fact that tubercle bacilli resist acid conditions favours the establishment of intestinal tuberculosis, but most bacteria are acid sensitive and prefer slightly alkaline conditions. For instance, volunteers who drank different doses of *V. cholerae* contained in 60 ml saline showed a 10 000-fold increase in

MICROBIAL SUCCESS IN THE GASTROINTESTINAL TRACT		
property	**examples**	**consequence**
specific attachment to intestinal epithelium	poliovirus, rotavirus, *V. cholerae*	microorganism avoids expulsion with other gut contents and can establish infection
motility	*V. cholerae*, certain *E. coli* strains	bacteria travel through mucus and more likely to reach susceptible cell
Production of mucinase (neuraminidase)	*V. cholerae*	may assist transit through mucus
Acid resistance	*M. tuberculosis*	encourages intestinal tuberculosis (acid labile microorganisms depend on protection in food bolus or in diluting fluid) increased susceptibility in individuals with achlorhydria
	enteroviruses (hepatitis A, poliovirus, coxsackieviruses, echoviruses)	infection and shedding from gastrointestinal tract
Bile resistance	salmonella, shigella, enteroviruses	intestinal pathogens
	Enterococcus faecalis, *E. coli*, proteus, pseudomonas	establish residence
Resistance to proteolytic enzymes	reoviruses in mice	permits oral infection other examples?
Anaerobic growth	*Bacteroides fragilis*	most common resident bacteria in anaerobic environment of colon

Fig. 11.9 Microbial properties that aid success in the gastrointestinal tract.

susceptibility to cholera when 2g of sodium bicarbonate was given with the bacteria. The minimum disease-producing dose without bicarbonate was 10^8 bacteria and 10^4 bacteria with bicarbonate. Similar experiments have been done in volunteers with *Salmonella typhi* where the minimal infectious dose of 100–10 000 bacteria was again significantly reduced by the ingestion of sodium bicarbonate.

When the infecting microorganism penetrates the intestinal epithelium (shigella, *Salmonella typhi*, hepatitis A and other enteroviruses) final pathogenicity depends on subsequent multiplication and spread, on toxin production, cell damage, and inflammatory and immune responses.

Microbial exotoxins, endotoxins and proteins can be absorbed from the intestine on a small scale. Diarrhoea generally promotes the uptake of protein, and absorption of protein also takes place more readily in the infant, which in some species needs to absorb antibodies from milk. As well as large molecules, particles the size of viruses can also be taken up from the intestinal lumen. This occurs particularly in certain sites, such as those where Peyer's patches occur. These are isolated collections of lymphoid tissue lying immediately below the intestinal epithelium, which in this region is highly specialized, consisting of so called M cells. M cells take up particles and foreign proteins, delivering them to underlying immune cells with which they are intimately associated by means of cytoplasmic processes.

URINOGENITAL TRACT AS A SITE OF ENTRY

The urinogenital tract is a continuum, so that microorganisms can spread easily from one part to another, and the distinction between vaginitis and urethritis, or between urethritis and cystitis is not always easy or necessary (see Chapters 23 and 24). The urinary tract is nearly always invaded from the exterior, via the urethra. Urine in the bladder is normally sterile, and since the urethra is flushed with urine every few hours, an invading microorganism must first and foremost avoid being washed out during urination.

Successful invaders (e.g. gonococci) have therefore developed specialized attachment mechanisms (Fig. 11.10), enabling them to establish themselves in the urethra. A defined peptide on the bacterial pili binds to a carbohydrate polymer on the urethral cell, and the cell is then induced to engulf the bacterium. This is referred to as parasite-directed endocytosis and also occurs with chlamydia. Spread to the bladder is no easy task especially in the male, where the (flaccid) urethra is 20cm long (Fig. 11.11). Hence urinary infections in males are rare, unless organisms are introduced by catheters or when the flushing activity of urine is impaired (see Chapter 23). Things are different in the female. Not only is the urethra much shorter (5cm) but it also suffers from a perilous proximity to the anus (see Fig. 11.11), which is a constant source of

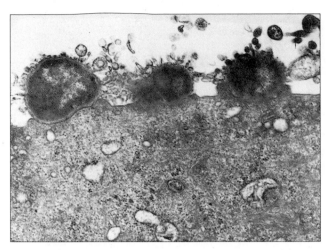

Fig. 11.10 Adherence of gonococci to surface of human urethral epithelial cell. Courtesy of P J Watt.

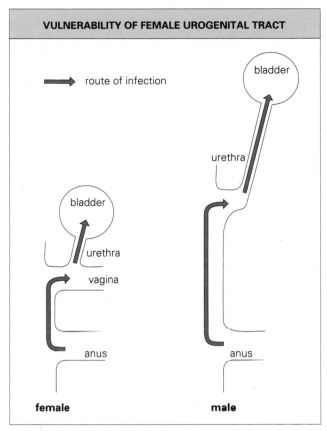

Fig. 11.11 The female urinogenital tract is particularly vulnerable to infection, due mainly to topographical considerations.

intestinal bacteria. Urinary infections are about 14-times more common in women and at least 20% women have a symptomatic urinary tract infection at some time during their life. The invading bacteria often begin by colonizing the mucosa around the urethra and probably have special attachment mechanisms to cells in this area. Bacterial invasion is favoured by the mechanical deformation of the urethra and surrounding region that occurs during sexual intercourse, which can lead to urethritis and cystitis. Bacteruria is about 10-times more common in sexually active women than in nuns.

The bladder is more than an inert receptacle and in its wall there are intrinsic, but poorly understood, defence mechanisms. These include a protective layer of mucus, and the ability to generate inflammatory responses, produce secretory antibodies and immune cells.

The vagina has no particular cleansing mechanisms, and repeated introductions of a contaminated, sometimes pathogen-bearing foreign object (the penis) makes the vagina particularly vulnerable to infection, forming the basis for sexually-transmitted diseases (see Chapter 24). Nature has responded by providing additional defences. During reproductive life the vaginal epithelium contains glycogen because of the action of circulating oestrogens, and certain lactobacilli colonize the vagina, metabolizing the glycogen to produce lactic acid. As a result the normal vaginal pH is about 5.0, which inhibits colonization by all except the lactobacilli and certain other streptococci and diphtheroids. Normal vaginal secretions contain up to 10^8 per ml of these commensal bacteria. If other microorganisms are to colonize and invade they must either have specific mechanisms for attaching to vaginal/cervical mucosa, or take advantage of impaired defences (presence of tampons, oestrogen imbalance). These are the microorganisms responsible for sexually transmitted infections.

OROPHARYNX AS A SITE OF ENTRY

Commensal microorganisms in the oropharynx are described in Chapter 20. A natural cleansing mechanism is provided by the flushing action of saliva (about a litre a day, needing 400 swallows), aided by masticatory and other movements of the tongue, cheek and lips. Additional defences include secretory IgA antibodies, antimicrobial substances such as lysozyme, the normal flora, and the antimicrobial activities of leucocytes present on mucosal surfaces and in saliva. Material borne backwards from the nasopharynx is firmly wiped against the pharynx by the tongue during swallowing and microbes therefore have an opportunity to enter the body at this site. Factors that reduce mucosal resistance allow commensal and other bacteria to invade, as in the case of gum infections due to vitamin C deficiency, or *Candida* invasion (thrush) due to changed resident flora after broad spectrum antibiotics. When salivary flow is decreased for 3–4 hours, as between meals, there is a four-fold increase in the number of bacteria in saliva (see Chapter 20). In dehydrated patients salivary flow is greatly reduced and the mouth soon becomes overgrown with bacteria. As at all body surfaces, there is a shifting boundary between good behaviour by residents and tissue invasion, according to changes in host defences.

TYPES OF INFECTION AND THEIR ROLE IN TRANSMISSION				
type of infection	host defences	microbial evasion mechanism	examples	value of infection in transmission
Respiratory tract	mucociliary clearance	adhere to epithelial cells interfere with ciliary action	influenza virus pertussis	essential
	alveolar macrophage	replicate in alveolar macrophage	legionella, tuberculosis	essential
Intestinal tract	mucus, peristalsis	adhere to epithelial cells	rotavirus, salmonella	essential
	acid, bile	resist acid, bile	poliovirus	essential
Liver	Kupffer cells and endothelial cells	localize in sinusoid, bypass Kupffer cells and endothelial cells	hepatitis viruses	essential: microbe from liver → bile → gut (HepA); microbe from liver → blood (HepB, yellow fever)
Reproductive tract	flushing action of urine and sexual secretions, mucosal defences	adhere to urethral/vaginal epithelial cells	gonococcus, chlamydia	essential
Urinary tract	flushing action of urine	adhere to urethral/epithelial cells	E. coli	no value
		reach urine from tubular epithelium	polyoma virus	valuable
Central nervous system	enclosed in bony 'box' of skull and vertebral canal	reach CNS via nerves or blood vessels that enter skull or vertebral canal	bacterial meningitis, viral encephalitis (e.g. rabies)	no value (except rabies)
Skin, mucosa	layers of constantly shed cells (mucosa) dead keratinized cell layers (skin)	invade skin/mucosa from below	varicella, measles	essential
		infect basal epidermal layer	papillomaviruses	essential
		infect via minor abrasions	staphylococci, streptococci	valuable
		penetrate intact skin	schistomiasis, ankylostomiasis, anthrax	essential
Vascular system	skin	injection of microbe by biting vector	malaria, yellow fever	essential

Fig. 11.12 Types of infection. For each type of host defence the successful microbe has an answer, which may or may not be important for transmission.

Invading microorganisms must, like the residents, be capable of attaching to mucosal or tooth surfaces. For instance, different types of streptococci make specific attachments, via lipoteichoic acid molecules on their pili, to the buccal epithelium and tongue (resident *Streptococcus salivarius*), to teeth (resident *Streptococcus mutans*), or to pharyngeal epithelium (invading *Streptococcus pyogenes*).

EXIT AND TRANSMISSION

Nearly all microorganisms are shed from body surfaces, this being the route of exit to the outside world and to the next host. Some, however, are extracted from inside the body by vectors – the blood-sucking arthropods that trans-

mit yellow fever, malaria and filarial worms, etc. Figure 11.12 shows types of infection and their value in transmission of the microbe, with a summary of host defences and the ways in which they are evaded. Transfer from one host to another forms the basis for the *epidemiology* of infectious disease. Transmission depends in the first place on three factors:

1) Number of microorganisms shed. Obviously the more virus particles, bacteria, protozoa, eggs etc. that are shed, the greater the chance of reaching a fresh host. There are many hazards. Most of the shed microorganisms die, and only a very occasional one survives to perpetuate the species.

11.8

MICROBIAL RESISTANCE TO DRYING AS A FACTOR IN TRANSMISSION		
stability on drying	examples	consequence
stable	tubercle bacilli staphylococci	spread more readily in air (dust, dried droplets)
	clostridial spores anthrax spores	spread readily from soil
unstable	*Neisseria meningitidis* streptococci *Bordetella pertussis* common cold viruses influenza virus measles	require close (respiratory) contact
	gonococci HIV *Treponema pallidum*	require close (sexual) contact
	polioviruses hepatitis A *Vibrio cholerae* leptospira	spread via water, food
	yellow fever virus malaria trypanosomes	spread via vectors (i.e. remain in a host)
	larvae/eggs of worms	need moist soil (except pinworms)

Fig. 11.13 Microbial resistance to drying as a factor in transmission. Microbes that are already dehydrated (spores, artificially freeze-dried viruses etc.) are also less susceptible to thermal inactivation. Spores can survive for years in soil.

2) Stability in the environment. As one might expect, microorganisms that resist drying spread more rapidly in the environment than those that are sensitive to drying (Fig. 11.13). The latter depend for spread on close contact, on vectors, or on contamination of food and water.

Microorganisms also remain infectious for longer periods in the external environment when they are resistant to thermal inactivation. Certain microorganisms have developed special forms (e.g. clostridial spores, amoebic cysts), that enable them to resist drying, heat inactivation and chemical insults and this testifies to the importance of stability in the environment. Once dried, and if still alive, microorganisms are more thermostable. Drying directly from the frozen state (freeze-drying) can make them very resistant to environmental temperatures. The fact that spores and cysts are dehydrated accounts for much of their stability.

3) The number of microorganisms required to infect a fresh host. That is, the efficiency of infection. This varies greatly between microorganisms, and helps us to understand many aspects of transmission. For instance, volunteers ingesting ten *Shigella dysenteriae* bacteria (from other humans) will become infected, whereas as many as 10^6 *Salmonella* sp. (from animals) are needed to cause food poisoning. The route of infection also matters. A single tissue culture infectious dose of a human rhinovirus instilled into the nasal cavity causes a common cold; although this dose contains many virus particles, about 200 such doses are needed when applied to the pharynx. As few as ten gonococci can establish infection in the urethra, but many thousand times this number are needed to infect the mucosa of the oropharynx or rectum.

Transmission also depends on genetic factors in the microorganisms, so that some strains of a given microorganism are more readily transmitted than others. This property may vary independently of the ability to do damage and cause disease (pathogenicity or virulence).

Activities of the infected host may increase the efficiency of shedding and transmission. Coughing and sneezing are reflex activities that benefit the host by clearing foreign material from the upper and lower respiratory tract. But they also benefit the microorganism. Strains that are better at increasing fluid secretions or irritating respiratory epithelium will induce more coughing and sneezing, will be transmitted more effectively and will therefore be positively selected for. Similar arguments can be applied to the equivalent intestinal activity – diarrhoea. Diarrhoea eliminates the infection more rapidly (prevention of diarrhoea often prolongs intestinal infection), while from the microbes point of view it is a magnificent material for contamination of the environment and spread of the microorganism to fresh hosts.

TYPES OF TRANSMISSION

Transmission is at its most effective when it takes place directly from human to human. The commonest, worldwide infections are spread by the respiratory, fecal-oral or venereal routes. A separate set of infections are acquired from animals, either directly from vertebrates (the zoonoses) or from biting arthropods. It is a striking feature of these infections that they are not transmitted, or transmitted very poorly, from human to human. Types of transmission are illustrated in figure 11.14.

TRANSMISSION FROM THE RESPIRATORY TRACT

Effective shedding from the nasal cavity depends on an increase in nasal secretions, and is helped by sneezing and coughing. In a sneeze (Fig. 11.15) up to 20 000 droplets are produced, and during a common cold, for instance, many of them will contain virus particles.

A smaller number of microorganisms (hundreds) are expelled from the mouth, throat, larynx and lungs during coughing (whooping cough, tuberculosis). Talking is a less important source of airborne particles, but produces them especially when the consonants f, p, t and s are used. It is surely no accident that the many of most abusive works in the English language begin with these letters, so that a spray of droplets (possibly infectious) is delivered with the abuse!

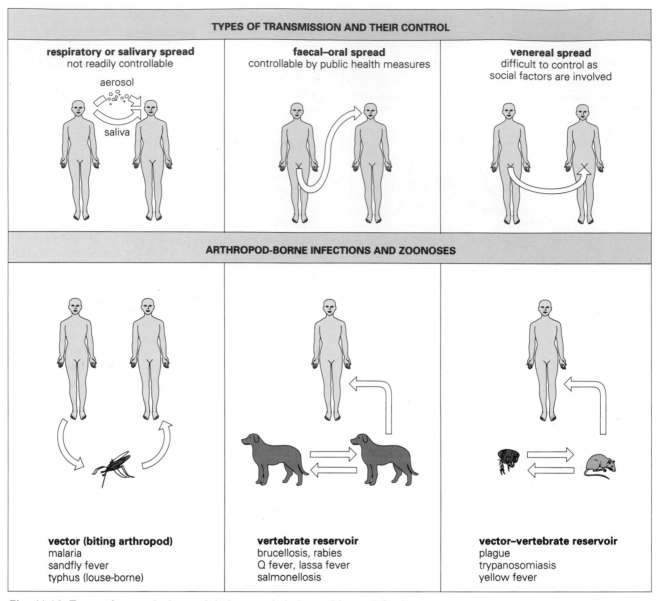

TYPES OF TRANSMISSION AND THEIR CONTROL

respiratory or salivary spread
not readily controllable

aerosol

saliva

faecal–oral spread
controllable by public health measures

venereal spread
difficult to control as
social factors are involved

ARTHROPOD-BORNE INFECTIONS AND ZOONOSES

vector (biting arthropod)
malaria
sandfly fever
typhus (louse-borne)

vertebrate reservoir
brucellosis, rabies
Q fever, lassa fever
salmonellosis

vector–vertebrate reservoir
plague
trypanosomiasis
yellow fever

Fig. 11.14 Types of transmission and their control. Arthropod-borne infections and zoonoses cell be controlled by controlling vectors, or by controlling animal infection. There is virtually no person-to-person transmission of these infections.

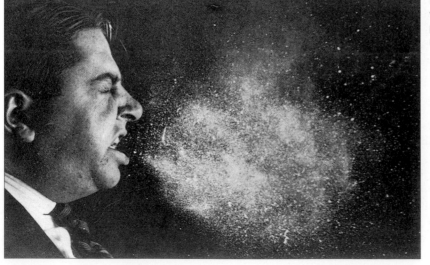

Fig. 11.15 Droplet dispersal following a violent sneeze. Most of the 20 000 particles seen are coming from the mouth. Courtesy of the AAAS.

The largest droplets fall to the ground after travelling 4m or so and the rest settle according to size. Those up to $10\mu M$ in diameter can be trapped on the nasal mucosa. The smallest ($1–4\mu M$ diameter) are kept suspended for an indefinite period by normal air movements and it is particles of this size that are likely to pass the turbinate baffles in the nose and reach the lower respiratory tract. Respiratory infections spread rapidly when people are crowded together indoors – for instance the common cold in schools or offices, and meningococcal infections in military recruits. This is perhaps why respiratory infections are common in winter. The air in ill-ventilated rooms is also more humid; favouring survival of suspended microorganisms such as streptococci and enveloped viruses. As another factor air conditioning can give dry air, and mucociliary activity is impaired under these circumstances.

Respiratory spread is in one sense, unique. Material from a person's respiratory tract can be taken up, unchanged and straight away into the respiratory tract of another individual. This is in striking contrast to the material expelled from the gastrointestinal tract, and helps explain why such infections spread so rapidly when people are indoors.

Although coughs and sneezes give a dramatic picture of the spread of respiratory infections, there is clear evidence that in addition handkerchiefs, hands and other objects can carry infection (e.g. common cold viruses) from one individual to another. Transmission from the infected conjunctiva is referred to in Chapter 21.

It is not only initial localization or the presence of receptors that determine which part of the respiratory tract is infected. There are other factors. For instance, it can assumed that rhinoviruses arrive in the lower respiratory tract on a large scale, but they fail to grow there because, like leprosy bacilli, they prefer the cooler temperature of the nasal mucosa.

TRANSMISSION FROM THE INTESTINAL TRACT

If there are enough susceptible individuals in the vicinity, the spread of an intestinal microorganism seems assured, as long as it appears in the feces in large enough numbers and hygiene is poor. Diarrhoea gives it an additional advantage, and the key role of diarrhoea in transmission has been referred to in the last section. During most of human history, there has been a large scale recycling of fecal material back into the mouth and this continues in developing countries. The attractiveness of the fecal-oral route for microorganisms and parasites is reflected in the great variety that are transmitted in this way. Intestinal infections have been to some extent controlled in developed countries. The great public health reforms of the 19th Century were responsible for the introduction of adequate sewage disposal and a supply of purified water. For instance, in England 200 years ago there were no flushing toilets, no sewage disposal and much of the drinking water was contaminated. Cholera and typhoid could spread easily, and in London the Thames became an open sewer. Nowadays, as in other cities, a complex underground disposal system separates sewage from drinking water.

HUMAN INFECTIONS TRANSMITTED VIA URINE		
infection	details	value in transmission
Schistosomiasis	parasite eggs excreted in bladder	+++
Typhoid	bacterial persistence in bladder scarred by schistosomiasis	+
Polyoma virus infection	commonly excreted in urine in normal pregnancy	?
Cytomegalovirus infection	commonly excreted in infected children	?
Leptospirosis	infected rats, dogs excrete bacteria in urine	++
Lassa fever (and South American hemorrhagic fevers)	persistently infected rodent excretes virus in urine	+++

Fig. 11.16 Human infections transmitted via urine. Schistosomiasis is the major infection transmitted in this way, the eggs undergoing development in snails before reinfecting humans. Viruses are shed in urine after infecting tubular epithelial cells in the kidney.

Intestinal infections are still spread in developed countries but via food and fingers, rather than water and flies. Hence, although each year in the UK there are dozens of cases of typhoid acquired on visits to foreign lands, the infection is not transmitted to others.

The microorganisms that appear in feces have generally multiplied in the lumen or wall of the intestinal tract, but there are a few that are shed into bile. For instance, hepatitis A (enterovirus 72) enters bile after replication in liver cells.

TRANSMISSION FROM THE URINOGENITAL TRACT

Urine can contaminate food, drink and living space, but although urinary tract infections are common, most are not spread via urine. Those that are, are listed in figure 11.16. Microorganisms shed from the urinogenital tract are generally transmitted as a result of mucosal contact with susceptible individuals. In other words, they are transmitted as a result of sexual activity and cause sexually transmitted diseases (STD). If there is a discharge, organisms are carried over epithelial surfaces and transmission is more likely to take place. Hence, some of the most successful sexually transmitted microorganisms (gonococci, chlamydia) induce a discharge. Other are transmitted effectively from mucosal sores (ulcers) as in the case of *Treponema pallidum* or herpes simplex. The human papilloma viruses are transmitted from genital warts or from foci of infection in the cervix where the epithelium, although apparently normal, shows dysplasia and contain infected cells (see Chapter 24).

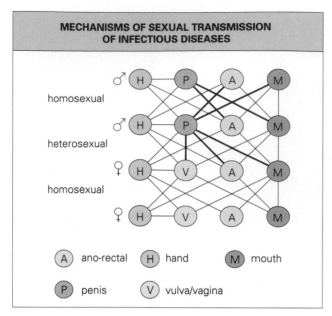

MECHANISMS OF SEXUAL TRANSMISSION OF INFECTIOUS DISEASES

homosexual

heterosexual

homosexual

| A | ano-rectal | H | hand | M | mouth |
| P | penis | V | vulva/vagina |

Fig. 11.17 The mechanisms of sexual transmission of infection. Redrawn from Wilcox, 1981.

HUMAN INFECTIONS TRANSMITTED BY SALIVA	
microorganisms	comments
Herpes simplex Mumps	infection generally during childhood
Cytomegalovirus EB virus	adolescent/adult infection is common
Rabies virus	shed in saliva of infected dogs, wolves, jackals, vampire bats etc.
Pasteurella multocida	bacteria in upper respiratory tract of dogs, cats etc. appears in saliva and transmitted via bites, scratches
Streptobacillus moniliformis	present in rat saliva and infects man (rat bite fever)

Fig. 11.18 Human infections transmitted via saliva.

The transmission of these infections is determined by social and sexual activity. Recent changes in human numbers and way of life have had a dramatic influence on STDs. Among other things, increasing population density, increased movement of people, the decline of the idea that sexual activity was sinful and the knowledge that (until AIDS) STDs were treatable, have led to increased numbers of sexual partners. Pregnancy is avoidable and the contraceptive pill, by discouraging the use of mechanical barriers to conception, has favoured the spread of such infections. Condoms have been shown to reliably retain herpes simplex virus, HIV, chlamydia and gonococci in simulated coital test of the syringe and plunger type (see Chapter 24).

STDs, however, are transmitted with far less speed and efficiency than respiratory or intestinal infections. Influenza can be transmitted to a multitude of others in the course of an innocent hour in a crowded room, or a rotavirus to a score of children during a morning at preschool. STDs however, must spread to each person by a separate sexual act, and even the most energetic lover could not transmit on this scale. Promiscuity is essential. Frequent sexual activity is not enough without promiscuity, because stable partners can do no more than infect each other. Nevertheless, the increased general level of promiscuity in society, together with extraordinary activity by certain individuals (e.g. prostitutes) has permitted a dramatic rise in incidence of STDs.

Because almost all mucosal surfaces of the body can be involved in sexual activity, microorganisms have had increasing opportunity to infect new bodily sites. Thus, the meningococcus, a nasopharyngeal resident, is sometimes recovered from the cervix, the male urethra, or the anal canal. The gonococcus and occasionally chlamydia infect the throat and anal canal. Possibilities are illustrated in all their complexity in figure 11.17, limited only, it seems, by anatomical considerations. It is no surprise that genito-oro-anal contacts have sometimes allowed intestinal infections

such as salmonella, giardia, hepatitis A, shigella, and pathogenic amoebae to spread directly between individuals, in spite of good sanitation and sewage disposal.

It might be expected that semen is involved in the transmission of infection, and this is the case in virus infections of animals such as blue-tongue and foot-and-mouth disease. In humans cytomegalovirus is often present in large amounts in semen, and the fact that it is also recoverable from the cervix suggests that sexual transmission occurs. Hepatitis B and HIV are also present in semen, and although the amounts are probably small, it plays a part in both homosexual and heterosexual transmission.

The female genital tract can also be a source of infection for the newborn child (see Chapter 26). During passage down an infected birth canal microorganisms can be wiped onto the conjunctiva of the infant or inhaled, leading to conjunctivitis, pneumonia, bacterial meningitis and so on.

TRANSMISSION FROM THE OROPHARYNX

Saliva is often the vehicle of transmission. Microorganisms (e.g. streptococci, tubercle bacilli) reach saliva during upper and lower respiratory tract infections, but certain viruses infect salivary glands and are transmitted in this way. Mumps, herpes simplex, cytomegalovirus and human herpes virus type 6 are shed into saliva. In young children fingers and other objects are regularly contaminated by saliva and each of these infections is acquired via this route. Epstein–Barr virus is also shed into saliva, but perhaps because it is present only in cells or in small amounts, it appears to be transmitted less effectively. In developed countries, people often escape infection during childhood, and become infected as adolescents or adults during the extensive salivary exchanges (mean 4.2ml per hour) that accompany deep kissing. Other infections are transmitted in the saliva of animals, and are included in Fig. 11.18.

INFECTIONS TRANSMITTED FROM THE SKIN		
microorganism	disease	comments
Staphylococci	boils, carbuncles etc., neonatal skin sepsis	pathogenicity varies, skin lesions or nose picking are common sources of infection
Treponema pallidum	syphilis	mucosal surfaces more infectious than skin
Treponema pertenue	yaws	regular transmission from skin lesions
Streptococcus pyogenes	impetigo	vesicular (epidermal) lesions crusting over, common in children in hot, humid climates
Staphylococcus aureus	impetigo	less common; bullous lesions, especially in newborn
Dermatophytes	skin ringworm	different species infect skin, hair, nails
Herpes simplex virus	herpes simplex, cold sore	up to 10^6 infectious units per ml of vesicle fluid
Varicella-zoster virus	varicella, zoster	vesicular skin lesions occur but transmission is usually respiratory*
Coxsackie virus A16	hand, foot and mouth disease	vesicular skin lesions but transmission fecal and respiratory
Papilloma-viruses	warts	many types
Leishmania tropica	cutaneous leishmaniasis	skin sores are infectious
Sarcoptes scabei	scabies	eggs from burrows transmitted by hand (also sexually)

Fig. 11.19 Human infections transmitted from the skin. *Except in zoster, where a localized skin eruption occurs and respiratory tract is generally unaffected.

INFECTIONS TRANSMITTED VIA MILK		
microorganism	type of milk	importance in transmission
Mumps virus	human	–
Cytomegalovirus	human	–
HIV	human	–
HTLV1	human	+
Brucella	cow, goat, sheep	++
Mycobacterium bovis	cow	++
Coxiella burnetii (Q fever rickettsia)	cow	+
Campylobacter jejuni	cow	++
Salmonella sp.	cow	+
Listeria monocytogenes	cow	+
Staphylococcus sp.	cow	+
Streptococcus pyogenes	cow	+
Yersinia enterocolitica	cow	+

Fig. 11.20 Human infections transmitted via milk. Human milk is rarely a significant source of infection. All microbes listed are destroyed by pasteurization.

TRANSMISSION FROM THE SKIN AND SKIN GLANDS

The normal individual sheds desquamated skin scales into the environment at the rate of about 5×10^8 per day, the rate depending on physical activities such as exercise, dressing and undressing. The fine white dust that collects on indoor surfaces, especially in hospital wards, consists largely of skin scales. However, microorganisms from the skin are generally transmitted by direct contact rather than following release into the environment. Microorganisms that are transmitted in this way include potentially pathogenic staphylococci and human papilloma viruses. Different individuals show great variation in staphylococcal shedding, but the reasons are unknown. Dermatophytes (ringworm fungi) are shed from skin and also from hair and nails, the exact source depending on the type of fungus (see Chapter 28). Skin is also an important source of certain other bacteria and viruses, as outlined in figure 11.19.

Milk is from a skin gland, and is therefore considered under this heading. Microorganisms are rarely shed into human milk (mumps, cytomegalovirus, HTLV1), but milk from cows, goats and sheep can be important sources of infection (Fig. 11.20). Other bacteria can be introduced into milk after collection.

TRANSMISSION FROM BLOOD

Blood is often the vehicle of transmission. Microrganism and parasites spread by blood-sucking athropods (see below) can be said to have been shed into the blood. Infectious agents present in blood (hepatitus viruses, HIV) are transmissible also by needles, either in transfused blood or when contaminated needles are used (injections, intravenous drug abuse). The blood is also the source of infection in transplacental transmission and this generally involves initial infection of the placenta (see Chapter 26).

VERTICAL AND HORIZONTAL TRANSMISSION

When transmission is direct from parents to offspring via sperm, ovum, placenta (Fig. 11.21), milk, blood etc. it is referred to as *vertical*. This is because it can be represented as a vertical flow down a page (Fig. 11.22) just like a family pedigree. Other infections, in contrast, are said to be *horizontally* transmitted, an individual infecting unrelated individuals by contact, respiratory, or faecal-oral spread. Vertically transmitted infections can be subdivided as in figure 11.23. Strictly speaking, they are able to maintain themselves in the species without spreading horizontally, as long as they do not affect the viability of the host. Various retroviruses are known to maintain themselves vertically in animals (e.g. mammary tumour virus in milk, sperm, ovum of mice) but this does not appear to be important in humans, except possibly for HTLV1, where milk transfer may be important. There are, however, hordes of retrovirus sequences present in the normal human genome. These DNA sequences are too incomplete to produce infectious virus particles but can be regarded as amazingly successful parasites. They presumably do no harm, and survive in the innermost sanctum of the human species, watched over, conserved and replicated as part of our genetic constitution.

TRANSMISSION FROM ANIMALS

Humans live in a complex ecological system, in daily contact, directly or indirectly, with a wide variety of other animal species, both vertebrate and invertebrate. We not only share our environment with them, we may also share

TRANSPLACENTAL TRANSMISSION OF INFECTION	
microorganism	**effect**
Rubella virus, Cytomegalovirus	placental lesion, abortion, stillbirth, malformation
HIV	childhood AIDS
Hepatitis B virus	antigen carriage in infant, most of these infections perinatal or postnatal
Treponema pallidum	stillbirth, congenital syphilis with malformation
Listeria monocytogenes	meningoencephalitis
Toxoplasma gondii	stillbirth, CNS disease

Fig. 11.21 Human infections transmitted via the placenta.

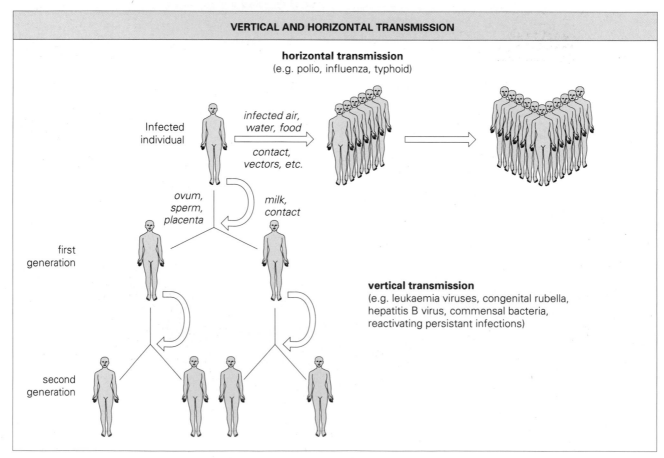

Fig. 11.22 Vertical and horizontal transmission by infection. Most infections are transmitted horizontally, as might be expected in crowded human populations. Vertical transmission becomes more important in small, isolated communities (see Chapter 15).

a common susceptibility to particular pathogens. The degree to which animal contacts transmit infection depends on the type of environment (urban/rural, tropical/temperate, hygienic/insanitary) and on the nature of the contact. Close contact is made with vertebrate animals used for food or as pets, and with invertebrate animals adapted to live or feed on the human body. Less intimate contact is made with many other species, which nevertheless may equally well transmit pathogens. For convenience, animal-transmitted infections can be divided into two categories those involving arthropod and other invertebrate vectors, and those transmitted directly from vertebrates (zoonoses). More detailed accounts of these infections are given in Chapters 30 and 31.

TYPES OF VERTICAL TRANSMISSION		
type	**route**	**examples**
Prenatal	placenta	rubella cytomegalovirus syphilis toxoplasmosis
Perinatal	infected birth canal	gonococcal/chlamydial conjunctivitis
Postnatal	milk or direct contact	cytomegalovirus hepatitis B
Germline	viral DNA sequences in human gonome	many retroviruses

Fig. 11.23 Types of vertical transmission.

Insects, ticks and mites – the bloodsuckers

By far the most important vectors of disease belong to these three groups of arthropods. The number of species capable of transmitting infection, and the range of organisms transmitted, is truly remarkable (Fig. 11.24). In the past, insects have been responsible for some of the most devastating epidemic diseases (fleas for plague, lice for typhus), and even today transmit one of the world's most important infectious diseases – malaria, carried by the *Anopheles* mosquito. The distribution and epidemiology of these infections is determined by the climatic conditions that allow the vectors to breed and the organism to complete its development in their bodies. Some diseases are therefore purely tropical and subtropical, like malaria, sleeping sickness, yellow fever while others are much more widespread, plague and typhus being excellent examples.

Insects may carry pathogens passively on their bodies, or within their intestines. Transfer onto food, or onto the body, occurs directly as a result of the insect regurgitating or defecating. A number of important diseases, such as trachoma, can be transmitted in this way by common species such as houseflies and cockroaches.

More important is transmission by blood-feeding species, all of which have mouth parts adapted for penetrating skin in order to reach blood vessels or to create small pools of blood (Fig. 11.25). The ability to feed in this way provides access to organisms present in the skin or bloodstream. Transmission of pathogens by such species may be purely mechanical, the mouth parts acting as a contaminated hypodermic needle, carrying infection between individuals. More often transmission is biological, the vector acting as a necessary host for the multiplication and development of

ARTHROPOD-BORNE PATHOGENS			
arthropods	**pathogens**	**types**	**disease**
insects houseflies sandflies mosquitoes blackflies	Viruses	Togaviruses Bunyaviruses	yellow fever, dengue febrile diseases, encephalitides haemorrhagic fevers
lice fleas hemipteran bugs	Bacteria	Yersinia Rickettsias Spirochaetes	plague, tularaemia Q fever, spotted fevers, typhus, rickettsialpox relapsing fever, Lyme disease
midges tabanids **acarids** ticks	Protozoa	Trypanosomes Leishmania Plasmodium	sleeping sickness, Chagas' disease leishmaniases malaria
mites	Helminths	Filarial nematodes	lymphatic filariases, loiasis, onchocerciasis

Fig. 11.24 Arthropod-borne pathogens. mosquitoes are a major source of infection. Note that, with the exception of pneumonic plague, none are transmitted from human to human.

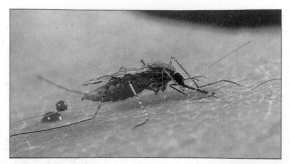

Fig. 11.25 Female *Anopheles* mosquito feeding
Courtesy of C J Webb.

the pathogen. The most important diseases are almost all transmitted biologically, the pathogen being reintroduced into the human host, after a period of time, at the next blood meal. Transmission can be by direct injection, often in the vectors' saliva, or by contamination from feces deposited at the time of feeding.

Other invertebrate vectors

Many invertebrates used for food convey pathogens (Fig. 11.26). Perhaps the most familiar are those shellfish (molluscs and crustacea) associated with food poisoning and acute gastroenteritis. These aquatic animals accumulate viruses and bacteria in their bodies, taking them in from contaminated waste, and transferring them passively. In other cases the relationship between the pathogen and the invertebrate is much closer. Many parasites, especially worms, must undergo part of their development in the invertebrate before becoming human-infective. Humans are infected when they eat the invertebrate (intermediate) host. Dietary habits are therefore an important factor in infection. Aquatic molluscs are also necessary intermediate hosts for schistosomes - the blood flukes. They become infected by larval stages which hatch from eggs passed into water via the urine or faeces of infected people. After a period of development and multiplication large numbers of infective stages (cercariae) escape from the snails. These have the ability to penetrate rapidly through human skin, initiating the infection that will result in adult flukes occupying visceral blood vessels (see Chapter 3).

Zoonoses

Strictly, the term zoonoses can apply to any infection transmitted to humans from infected animals, whether this is direct (by contact or by eating) or indirect (via an invertebrate vector). For our purposes we will restrict zoonoses to infections of vertebrate animals that can be transmitted directly. A very large number of pathogens are transmitted in this way (Fig. 11.27) by a variety of different routes: contact, inhalation, bites, scratches, contamination of food or water, or ingestion as food. The epidemiology of zoonoses depends upon the frequency and the nature of contact between the vertebrate and the human hosts. Some are localized geographically, being dependent for example on restricted food preferences. Where these involve eating uncooked animal products, such as fish or amphibia, a variety of parasites (especially tapeworms and nematodes)

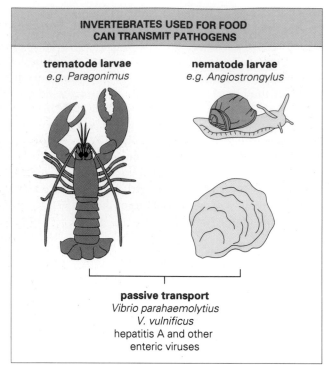

Fig. 11.26 Microorganisms transmitted via invertebrates used for food. Filter-feeding molluscs living in estuaries, near sewage outlets, are common sources of infection.

can be acquired. Others are associated with occupation, for example where this involves contact with raw animal products (butchers in the case of toxoplasmosis, Q fever), or frequent contact with domestic stock (farm workers in the case of brucellosis, dermatophyte fungi). In urban areas, zoonoses are most likely to be acquired by eating or drinking infected animal products or by contact with dogs, cats and other domestic pets.

Domestic pets or pests?

Dogs and cats are the commonest domestic pets, and both are reservoirs of infection for their owners (Fig. 11.28). The pathogens concerned are spread by contact, bites and scratches, vectors and contamination with fecal material. Major infections transmitted in these ways include toxocariasis, primarily from dogs, and toxplasmosis from cats. Both are almost universal in their distribution. Where dogs are used for herding domestic animals, and have access to infected carcasses, humans may acquire hydatid disease from tapeworm eggs passed in dog feces. In many countries this has been, or remains, a most important infection in rural areas.

Many species of birds are kept as pets and some may pass on serious infections to those in contact with them. Contact is most often through inhalation of particulate material contaminated by pathogens. Perhaps the most important of these is psittacosis (caused by *Chlamydia psittaci*) which, despite the common name 'parrot fever', can be acquired from many avian species.

The recent trend in western countries towards keeping unusual or exotic pets (especially reptiles, exotic birds and

HUMAN INFECTIONS TRANSMITTED FROM VERTEBRATES		
pathogens	vertebrate vector	diseases
Viruses		
Arenaviruses	mammal	Lassa fever, lymphocytic choriomeningitis, Bolivian haemorrhagic fever
Pox viruses	mammal	cowpox, orf
Rhabdoviruses	mammal	rabies
Bacteria		
Bacillus anthracis	mammal	anthrax
Brucella	mammal	brucella
Chlamydia	birds	psittacosis
Leptospira	mammal	leptospirosis (Weil's disease)
Listeria	mammal	listeriosis
Salmonella	birds, mammals	salmonellosis
Mycobacterium tuberculosis	mammals	tuberculosis
Fungi		
Cryptococcus	birds	meningitis
Dermatophytes	mammals	ringworm
Protozoa		
Cryptosporidium	mammals	cryptosporidiosis
Entamoeba	mammals	amoebic dysentery
Giardia	mammals	giardiasis
Toxoplasma	mammals	toxoplasmosis
Helminths		
Ancylostoma	mammals	creeping eruption
Echinococcus	mammals	hydatid disease
Taenia	mammals	tapeworms
Toxocara	mammals	toxocariasis (visceral larval migrans)
Trichinella	mammals	trichinellosis

Fig. 11.27 Human infections transmitted directly from vertebrates (birds and mammals).

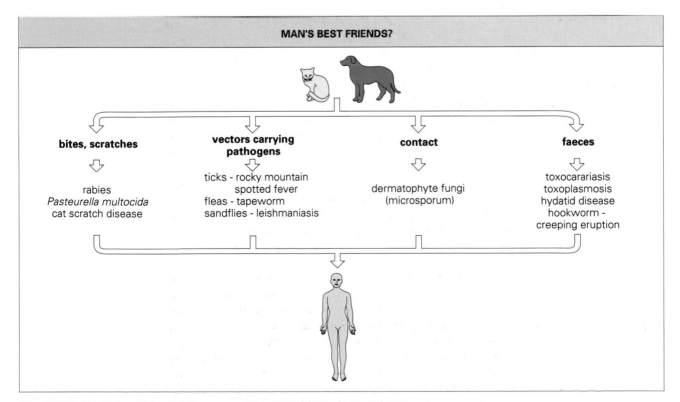

Fig. 11.28 Man's best friends? Zoonoses transmitted from dogs and cats.

mammals) raises new risks of zoonotic infection. Many reptiles, for example, pass human-infective *Salmonella* sp. in their droppings. Exotic birds and mammals may carry a range of potentially infective viruses, that could be transmitted under the correct conditions. Diagnosis of infections under these circumstances may be difficult if the physician does not know of the existence of such pets.

SUMMARY

To establish infection in the host, microbes must attach to or pass across body surfaces. Thus, many microbes have developed attachment mechanisms, either chemical or mechanical in nature, in the respiratory, urinogenital and alimentary tracts. In the skin they generally depend on introduction via small wounds or by arthropod bites. Once they have replicated, microbes must exit from the body in order to be transmitted to fresh hosts. This also takes place across body surfaces. Efficient shedding of microbes from the skin, or respiratory, urinogenital or alimentary tracts, or delivery into the blood or dermal tissues for uptake during arthropod feeding, is therefore a vital stage in their lifecycle. Since many human infections come from animals, either directly (zoonoses) or indirectly (via blood sucking arthropods), their incidence depends on exposure to infected animals or arthropods.

Further Reading

Beachley E.H. Bacterial adherence; adhesion-receptor interactions mediating the attachment of bacteria to mucosal surfaces. *J Inf Dis* 1981;**143**: 325.

Falkow S. Bacterial entry into eukaryotic cells. *Cell* 1991; **65**: 1099–1102

Falkow S. Small P, Isberg R *et al*. A molecular strategy for the study of bacterial invasion. *Rev Inf Dis* 1987; **9**: 450–455.

Green, GM. Defense of the lung. *Am Rev Resp Dis* 1970; **102**: 691.

Marsh M, Helenius A. Virus entry into animal cells. *Adv Virus Res* 1989; **36**: 107–151.

Mims CA. *The pathogenesis of infectious disease*, 3rd edn. London: Academic Press, 1987.

Pearce WA, Buchanan TM. Attachment role of gonococcal pili. *J Clin Invest* 1978; **61**: 931–43.

Rammelkamp CH, Mortimer EA, Wolinsky E. Transmission of streptococcal and staphylococcal infections. *Ann Intern Med* 1964; **60**: 753.

Warren KS. The control of helminths; non-replicating infectious agents of man. *Am Rev Publ Health* 1981; **2**: 101–116.

Wilcox RR. The rectum as viewed by the venereologist. *Br J Ven Dis* 1981; **57**:1–6.

12 NATURAL DEFENCE IN ACTION

Contents

INTRODUCTION

The barrier effect of the skin and mucous membranes, and their adjuncts such as cilia, have already been referred to (see Chapter 11). We now turn to the back-up mechanisms called rapidly into play when an organism has penetrated these barriers – namely complement, the phagocytic and cytotoxic cells, and a variety of cytotoxic molecules, the most important of which are listed in figure 12.1.

COMPLEMENT

The basic biology of the complement system, and its role in inducing the inflammatory response and promoting chemotaxis, phagocytosis and vascular permeability, have been described in Chapter 4. Here we are concerned with its ability to directly damage microorganisms as part of the early response to infection. Contrary to what might be expected from the dramatic lysis of many kinds of bacteria in the test tube, the action of complement *in vivo* is restricted mainly to the *Neisseria*. This is evidenced by the inability of patients deficient in C5, 6, 7, 8 or 9 to eliminate gonococci and meningococci, with the increased risk of developing septicaemia or becoming a carrier.

The lack of effect of complement in other infections may be due to escape strategies by the microorganism. For example, the insertion of the C567 complex is prevented by the long side chains of the cell-wall polysaccharides of smooth strains of salmonellae and by the capsules of staphylococci which, unlike the cell wall, do not activate complement (Fig. 12.2). Mammalian cells (e.g. the neutrophil) can avoid lysis by isolating bound complement molecules to a small portion of membrane and budding this off, and some microorganisms can do the same. Certain bacteria (e.g. streptococci, campylobacter) actively inhibit complement activation, while a covering of non-complement fixing antibody (e.g. IgA) is yet another way of avoiding lysis. Anti-complement activity is also a feature of several protozoal and helminthic infections, an example being leishmania and the hydatid worm *Echinococcus granulosus*.

It should be emphasized that only the alternative pathway of complement activation forms part of this natural 'early defence' system. Activation through the classical pathway occurs only after an antibody response has been made. It

CYTOTOXIC MOLECULES		
host component		
major cell source	molecule	effective against
Liver cells Macrophage	complement C1–3 complement C5–9 C-reactive protein	bacteria, fungi *Neisseria* streptococci
Macrophage Neutrophil	reactive oxygen intermediates (plus peroxidase)	bacteria, fungi malaria
Macrophage	lysozyme interferon (α,β) TNF arginase reactive nitrogen intermediates	Gram-positive bacteria viruses viruses, bacteria, malaria schistosome worms leishmania, malaria
Neutrophil	defensins cathepsins lactoferrin	bacteria, fungi bacteria, fungi bacteria, yeasts
Eosinophil	cationic proteins	schistosome
T lymphocyte	cytokines	viruses some bacteria, fungi, protozoa
Natural killer cell	perforins	viruses
Liver, fat	high density lipoprotein low density lipoprotein (oxidized)	trypanosomes malaria
Kidney	urea	bacteria

Fig. 12.1 Some important cytotoxic molecules that operate against infectious organisms.

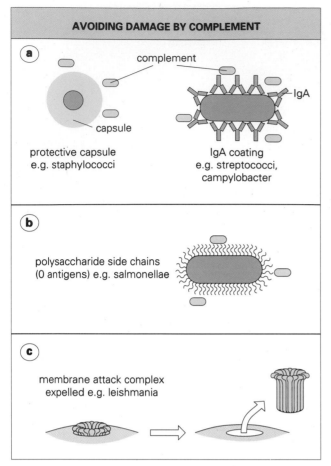

AVOIDING DAMAGE BY COMPLEMENT

(a) complement

capsule

protective capsule
e.g. staphylococci

IgA

IgA coating
e.g. streptococci,
campylobacter

(b) polysaccharide side chains
(0 antigens) e.g. salmonellae

(c) membrane attack complex
expelled e.g. leishmania

Fig. 12.2 Three ways by which microorganisms can avoid damage by complement. (a) Failure to trigger complement. (b) Protection of membrane from attack. (c) Expulsion of the membrane attack complex C5-9.

is not surprising to learn, therefore, that the alternative pathway appears to have evolved first.

C-REACTIVE PROTEIN

Among the acute-phase proteins produced in the course of most inflammatory reactions, C-reactive protein (CRP) is particularly interesting in being an anti-bacterial agent, albeit of very restricted range. CRP is a pentameric β-globulin, somewhat resembling a miniature version of IgM (mol. wt 130 000 as compared to 900 000). It reacts with phosphorylcholine in the wall of some streptococci and subsequently activates both complement and phagocytosis. CRP is produced by liver cells in response to cytokines, particularly IL-6 (see Chapter 7), and levels can rise as much as 1000-fold in 24 hours, a much more rapid response than that of antibody. Thus, CRP levels are often used to monitor inflammation, e.g. in rheumatic diseases. Most of the other acute-phase proteins are produced in increased amounts early in infection, but an anti-microbial role for these has not been proved. Indeed it has been suggested that they may be taken up by certain parasites and used to protect them from immune attack, or to help the parasite gain access to cells (see Chapter 14). However, some acute-phase proteins may be responsible for reducing pathology by binding toxic bacterial products such as lipopolysaccharide.

PHAGOCYTOSIS

Perhaps the greatest danger to the would-be parasite is to be recognized by a phagocytic cell, engulfed, killed and digested. For a description of the various stages of phagocytosis, see Chapter 4. Phagocytes (principally macrophages) are normally found in the tissues, where invading microorganisms are more likely to be encountered. In addition, phagocytes present in the blood (principally the polymorphonuclear leucocytes – PMNs) can be rapidly recruited into the tissues when and where required. Only about 1% of the normal adult bone marrow reserve of 3×10^{12} PMNs are present in the blood at any one time, representing a turnover of about 10^{11} PMNs per day. Most macrophages remain within the tissues and well under 1% are present in the blood as monocytes. PMN's are short-lived, but macrophages can live for many years (see below).

Not surprisingly, successful parasites have evolved numerous ingenious anti-phagocytic devices (Fig. 12.3). These range from killing or inhibiting the phagocyte itself, via more subtle ways of eluding contact, to protection against intracellular death, which allows the microorganism to survive within the phagocyte – a very serious challenge to the host. The ways in which some of these parasite strategies can be countered by the development of adaptive immune responses (antibody and T cells) are described in Chapter 14.

INTRACELLULAR KILLING

The mechanisms by which phagocytes kill the organisms they ingest are traditionally divided into oxidative and non-oxidative, depending on whether the cell consumes oxygen in the process. Respiration in PMNs is non-mitochondrial and anaerobic, and the burst of oxygen consumption, the so called 'respiratory burst' (Fig. 12.4), which accompanies phagocytosis represents the generation of microbicidal reactive oxygen intermediates (ROI).

Oxidative killing

It was the discovery that PMNs from patients with chronic granulomatous disease (CGD) do not consume oxygen after phagocytosing staphylococci that revealed the importance of ROI in bacterial killing. These patients suffer from one of three kinds of genetic defect in a PMN membrane enzyme system involving NADPH oxidase. The normal activity of this system is to progressively reduce atmospheric oxygen to water, with the production of ROI such as the superoxide ion, hydrogen peroxide, and free hydroxyl radicals, all of which can be extremely toxic to microorganisms.

CGD patients are unable to kill staphylococci and certain other bacteria and fungi, which consequently cause deep chronic abscesses. They can, however, deal with catalase-negative bacteria such as pneumococci because these produce, and do not destroy, their own hydrogen peroxide in sufficient amounts to interact with the cell myeloperoxidase, producing the highly toxic hypochlorous acid (HOCl; see Fig. 12.4). The defective PMN from CGD

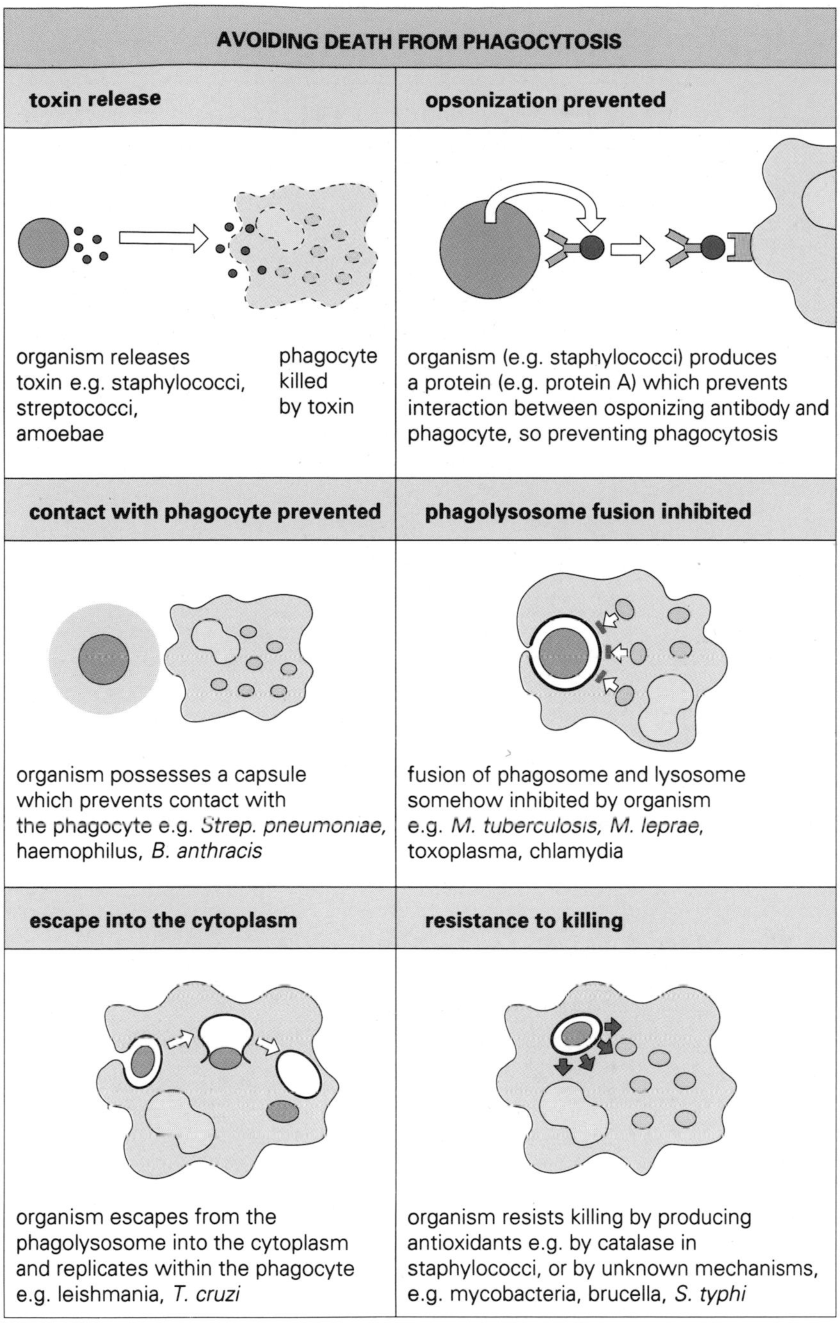

AVOIDING DEATH FROM PHAGOCYTOSIS	
toxin release	**opsonization prevented**
organism releases toxin e.g. staphylococci, streptococci, amoebae — phagocyte killed by toxin	organism (e.g. staphylococci) produces a protein (e.g. protein A) which prevents interaction between osponizing antibody and phagocyte, so preventing phagocytosis
contact with phagocyte prevented	**phagolysosome fusion inhibited**
organism possesses a capsule which prevents contact with the phagocyte e.g. *Strep. pneumoniae*, haemophilus, *B. anthracis*	fusion of phagosome and lysosome somehow inhibited by organism e.g. *M. tuberculosis, M. leprae*, toxoplasma, chlamydia
escape into the cytoplasm	**resistance to killing**
organism escapes from the phagolysosome into the cytoplasm and replicates within the phagocyte e.g. leishmania, *T. cruzi*	organism resists killing by producing antioxidants e.g. by catalase in staphylococci, or by unknown mechanisms, e.g. mycobacteria, brucella, *S. typhi*

Fig. 12.3 Various mechanisms adopted by microorganisms to avoid phagocytosis.

patients can be readily identified *in vitro* by their failure to reduce the yellow dye nitroblue tetrazolium to a blue compound (the 'NBT test'; see Chapter 8).

The way in which ROIs actually kill microorganisms is still somewhat controversial. ROIs can damage cell membranes (lipid peroxidation), DNA, and proteins (including vital enzymes), but in some cases it may be the altered pH that accompanies the generation of ROIs that does the damage. Killing of some bacteria and fungi occurs only at acid pH (e.g. *Candida, E. coli*) and of others at alkaline pH (e.g. staphylococci).

It is hardly surprising that bacteria produce molecules that inactivate ROIs, of which catalase and superoxide dismutase are the best documented (Fig. 12.5).

Non-oxidative killing by phagocytes

Oxygen is not always available for killing microorganisms; indeed some bacteria grow best in anaerobic conditions (e.g. the clostridia of gas gangrene), and oxygen would in any case be in short supply in a deep tissue abscess. It is no surprise, then, that phagocytic cells contain a number of other cytotoxic molecules. The best studied are the proteins in the various PMN granules (Fig. 12.6), which are brought to bear on the contents of the phagosome as the granules fuse with it.

Another phagocytic cell, the eosinophil, is particularly rich in cytotoxic granules (see Fig. 12.6), whose highly cationic (i.e. basic) contents give them their characteristic acidophilic staining pattern. Five distinct eosinophil

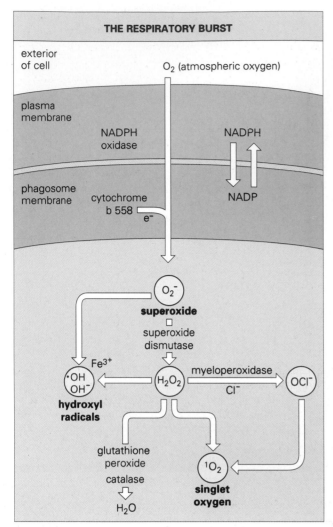

THE RESPIRATORY BURST

exterior of cell

O_2 (atmospheric oxygen)

plasma membrane

NADPH oxidase

NADPH

phagosome membrane

cytochrome b 558

e^-

NADP

O_2^-

superoxide

superoxide dismutase

Fe^{3+}

$\cdot OH$ OH^-

H_2O_2

myeloperoxidase Cl^-

OCl^-

hydroxyl radicals

glutathione peroxide

catalase

H_2O

$^1O_2$

singlet oxygen

Fig.12.4 The principal molecules involved in the respiratory burst. Oxygen is progressively reduced by the addition of electrons (e^-).

SOME ORGANISMS KILLED BY REACTIVE OXYGEN AND NITROGEN SPECIES

Bacteria	Fungi	Protozoa
Staphylococcus aureus	Candida albicans	Plasmodium
E. coli	Aspergillus	Leishmania
Serratia marcescens		(nitric oxide)

Fig. 12.5 Organisms killed by reactive oxygen species.

PMN AND EOSINOPHIL GRANULE CONTENTS

PMN		eosinophil
primary (azurophil)	**specific (heterophil)**	
myeloperoxidase	lysozyme	eosinophil peroxidase
acid hydrolases	lactoferrin	
cathepsins G, B, D	alkaline phosphatase	cationic proteins
defensins	NADPH oxidase	ECP
BPI		MBP
	collagenase	
cationic proteins	histaminase	neurotoxin
lysozyme		lysophospholipase

Fig. 12.6 Contents of polymorphonucleocyte and eosinophil granules. BPI, bactericidal permeability increasing protein; ECP, eosinophil cationic protein; MBP. major basic protein.

cationic proteins are known, and they seem to be particularly toxic to parasitic worms, at least *in vitro*. Because of the enormous difference in size, this type of damage is limited to the outer surfaces of the parasite. The eosinophilia typical of worm infections is presumably an attempt to cope with these large and almost indestructible parasites. It has recently been shown that both the production and the level of activity of eosinophils is under regulatory control by T cells and macrophages, mediated by cytokines such as IL-5 and TNF.

Monocytes and macrophages also contain cytotoxic granules, but their contents are less well characterized. As compared to PMN (Fig. 12.7), macrophages contain little or no myeloperoxidase, but secrete large amounts of lysozyme, an anti-bacterial molecule maintained at a level of about 30 mg per ml in serum, which can rise as high as 800 mg per ml in rare cases of monocytic leukaemia. Macrophages also differ from PMN in being extremely sensitive to activation by bacterial products (e.g. LPS) and T cell products (e.g. IFN-γ). Activated macrophages have a greatly enhanced ability to kill both intracellular and extracellular targets.

A major secreted product of the activated macrophage is nitric oxide (NO), one of the reactive nitrogen intermediates (RNI) generated during the conversion of arginine to citrulline by arginase. NO is strongly cytotoxic to a variety of cell types, and RNI are generated in large amounts during infections (e.g. leishmaniasis, malaria). Arginase can also cause damage by a separate mechanism, deprivation of arginine, which is an essential amino acid for some viruses (e.g. herpes simplex) and parasites (e.g. the liver fluke *Schistosoma*).

CYTOTOXICITY BY LYMPHOCYTES AND NATURAL KILLER CELLS

The well-known cytotoxic or 'killer' T lymphocyte (CTL) is unusual in that both antigen-specific recognition and killing of the target are carried out by the same cell. The recognition step, involving an antigenic fragment which becomes associated with a class I MHC molecule, is discussed in Chapter 6, and displays the high degree of specificity characteristic of adaptive responses (see Chapter 14). The killing mechanism, however, is relatively non-specific. It appears to involve the induction of 'leaks' in the target cell by the insertion of perforin, a 66kDa molecule struc-

PMN AND MACROPHAGES COMPARED		
	PMN	**macrophage**
Site of production	bone marrow	bone marrow, tissues
Duration in marrow	14 days	54 hours
Duration in blood	7–10 hours	20–40 hours (monocyte)
Average lifespan	4 days	months–years
Numbers in blood	$(2.5–7.5)\times10^9/l$	$(0.2–0.8)\times10^9/l$
Marrow reserve	10 x blood	–
Numbers in tissues	(transient)	100 x blood
Principal killing mechanisms	oxidative non-oxidative	oxidative nitric oxide cytokines
Activated by	TNF	TNF, IFN-γ, IL-4 GM-CSF microbial products (e.g. LPS)
Important deficiencies	CGD myeloperoxidase chemotactic Chediak–Higashi	lipid storage diseases
Major secretory products	lysozyme	over 80, including: lysozyme cytokines (TNF, IL-1) complement factors

Fig. 12.7 The major phagocytic cells, PMN and macrophages, differ in a number of important respects.

turally and functionally similar to the terminal complement component C9 (77kDa; Fig. 12.8). Other molecules, including cytokines such as TNF and lymphotoxin may also be involved, and their effects may be either direct or indirect. Target cell death may be due to leakage, to fragmentation of DNA, or to induction of apoptosis, a 'suicide' programme built into all cells.

These mechanisms are thought to operate principally against virus-infected cells, but some cells infected with other intracellular parasites may also be susceptible, including mycobacteria (e.g. *M. leprae* in Schwann cells) and even protozoa (e.g. *Theileria parva* in lymphocytes). Both CD8+ and CD4+ T cells have been implicated. Recent experiments with genetically engineered virus–cytokine constructs in T cell depleted mice indicate that in some cases cytokine release alone may be sufficient for virus killing, in the absence of T cells.

As far as their mechanism of killing is concerned, the large granular lymphocytes (LGL) usually referred to as natural killer (NK) cells appear to resemble CTL fairly closely. The vital difference is their lack of an antigen-specific receptor and therefore the absence of specificity, memory and MHC-restriction in their response. Indeed, it seems that NK cells may be best at recognizing cells that do not express MHC antigens. NK cells are thought of as a more rapid but less specific means of controlling viral and other intracellular infections. Their importance is highlighted by the ability of mice lacking both T and B cells (severe combined immunodeficiency or 'SCID') to control some virus infections, and the same is probably true for SCID in man. Recently, it has been shown that NK cells can secrete interferon and other cytokines (see below), just as T cells can. This further increases the resemblance between these two types of cell.

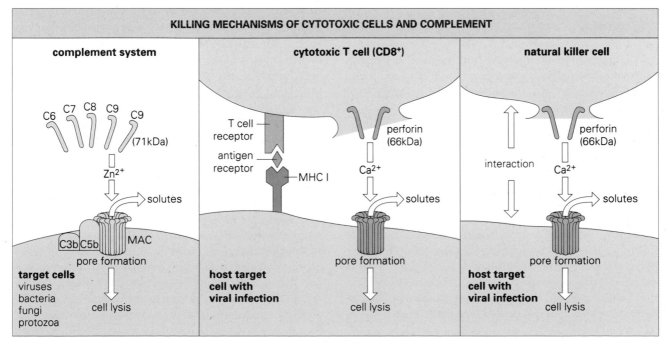

Fig.12.8 Comparison of cytotoxic cells and the lytic mechanisms of the complement system.

HUMAN INTERFERONS			
	IFN-α	IFN-β	IFN-γ
Alternative name	'leucocyte' IFN	'fibroblast' IFN	'immune' IFN
Principal source	all cells	all cells	T lymphocytes
Inducing agent	viral infection (or dsRNA)	viral infection (or dsRNA)	antigen (or mitogen)
Number of species	22*	1	1
Chromosomal location of gene(s)	9	9	12
Antiviral activity	+++	+++	+
Immunoregulatory activity: Macrophage action MHC I upregulation MHC II upregulation	– + –	– + –	++ + +
* each species coded by a different gene			

Fig. 12.9 Human interferons.

CYTOTOXIC LIPIDS

As already mentioned, one of the targets of the toxic oxygen metabolites (ROI) is the lipids of cell membranes. ROI are normally extremely short-lived (fractions of a second) but their toxicity can be greatly prolonged by interaction with serum lipoproteins to form lipid peroxides, which are stable for hours and can pass on the oxidative damage to cell membranes, both of the parasite (e.g. malaria infected red cell) and of the host (e.g. vascular endothelium). The cytotoxic activity of normal serum to some blood trypanosomes has been traced to the high-density lipoproteins, and in cotton rats to a macroglobulin.

CYTOKINES

Early studies with supernatants from cultures of lymphocytes and macrophages revealed a family of non-antigen-specific molecules with diverse activities, including both cell–cell communication and cytotoxicity. These are now collectively known as 'cytokines', and their role in infectious disease is under very active study. The way in which these molecules acquired their sometimes rather misleading names, and the bewildering overlap of function between molecules of quite different structure, are described in detail in Chapter 7.

Cytokines are of importance in infectious disease for two contrasting reasons: they may contribute to the control of infection or to the development of pathology. The latter harmful aspect (of which TNF in septic shock is a good example) is discussed in Chapter 16. The beneficial effects may be direct or, more often, indirect via the induction of some other antimicrobial process (see Chapter 14).

Interferons

The best-established anti-microbial cytokines are the inter-

ferons (Fig. 12.9), whose name is derived from the demonstration in 1957 that virus-infected cells secrete a molecule which interferes with viral replication in bystander cells. Interferons of all three types (α,β and γ) interact with specific receptors on most cells, one for α and β and another for γ, following which they induce an anti-viral state via the generation of at least two types of enzyme, a protein kinase and a 2',5'-oligoadenylate synthetase. Both of these enzymes result in the inhibition of viral RNA translation and thus of protein synthesis (Fig. 12.10). Interferons α and β are produced rapidly within 24 hours of infection, and constitute a major part of the early response to viruses. Interferon-γ (IFN-γ), being mainly a T cell product, is produced later, although in some cases an early IFN-γ response may be mounted by NK cells. Interferons can also inhibit virus assembly at a later stage (e.g. retroviruses), while many of the other effects of IFN also contribute to the anti-viral state, for example the enhancement of cellular MHC expression and the activation of NK cells and macrophages (Fig. 12.11). Unlike cytotoxic T cells, IFN normally inhibits viruses without damaging the host cell. Some intracellular organisms (e.g. leishmania) can counteract the effect of IFN-γ on MHC expression, thus facilitating their own survival.

Though best known for their antiviral activity, interferons have recently been shown to be induced by and active against a wider range of organisms, including rickettsia, mycobacteria, and several protozoa. The lack of any clearcut IFN deficiency syndromes makes it hard to assess their importance in isolation, but may in fact be an indication that IFN deficiency is incompatible with survival. In animal experiments, treatment with antibodies to IFN greatly increases susceptibility to virus infection and, conversely, treatment with IFN has proved useful in some human virus infections, notably chronic hepatitis B (see Chapter 35).

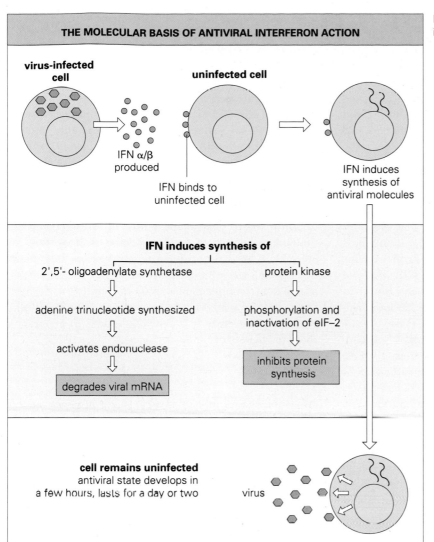

Fig. 12.10 The molecular basis of interferon action.

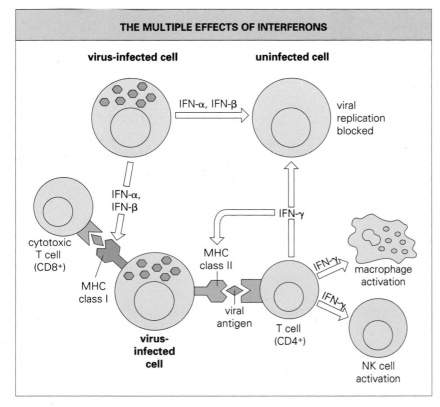

Fig. 12.11 The multiple activities of interferons in virus immunity.

Other cytokines

Tumour necrosis factor (TNF) has been shown to kill cells infected with a number of viruses, though in some cases this may be secondary to the induction of IFN. A striking example of a potentially useful role for TNF in infection is the inhibition of the proliferation of B lymphocytes caused by Epstein–Barr virus (EBV). EBV infection in malaria patients can lead to Burkitt's lymphoma, a monoclonal tumour of B cells, and TNF levels have been shown to be raised in malaria; conceivably, this is part of an attempt to prevent the development of the lymphoma. However, TNF is also thought to contribute to the pathology of malaria as well as that due to bacterial endotoxins (see Chapter 16), which illustrates the often confusing role that cytokines play in infectious diseases of all kinds – 'enough is enough', 'too much is dangerous' seems to be the rule for these powerful molecules. Paradoxically TNF, levels of which are raised in HIV infection, has been found to enhance the replication of HIV in T cells, a 'positive feedback' with worrying potential.

Most of the interleukins have also been shown to contribute to protection in one or more infectious diseases, but in all cases this effect is derived from the activation of macrophages, B cells, eosinophils, etc. Needless to say, parasites have found ways to avoid such activation. For example the South American trypanosome *T. cruzi* can down-regulate receptors for IL-2, while in malaria, circulating soluble IL-2 receptors can block the normal T cell activation by IL-2. Pseudomonas bacteria secrete proteolytic enzymes that cleave IL-2 and IFN-γ , and it seems likely that many similar evasion mechanisms will come to light as systems for the detection of cytokines, their receptors, and their natural inhibitors become more sophisticated.

FEVER: GOOD OR BAD?

A raised temperature almost invariably accompanies infection (see Chapter 32). In many cases the cause can be traced to the release of cytokines such as IL-1 or TNF, which play important roles in both immunity and pathology (see Chapter 15). But the interesting question remains whether the raised temperature itself is of benefit to the host.

Several microorganisms have been shown to be susceptible to high temperature. This was the basis for the 'fever therapy' of syphilis by deliberate infection with blood-stage malaria, and the malaria parasite itself may also be damaged (though it is obviously not totally eliminated) by high temperatures. But in general one would predict that successful parasites were those which were adapted to survive episodes of fever; indeed the 'stress' or 'heat-shock' proteins produced by both mammalian and microbial cells in response to stress of many kinds, including heat, are thought to be part of their protective strategy. On the other hand, several host immune mechanisms might also be expected to be more active at higher temperatures; examples are complement activation, lymphocyte proliferation, and the synthesis of proteins such as antibody and cytokines. Therefore it is probably unwise to generalize about the benefit or otherwise of fever.

SUMMARY

Protection against infectious organisms that penetrate the outer barriers of the skin and mucous membranes is mediated by a number of early defence mechanisms, more rapid though less specific than the adaptive mechanisms based on lymphocyte responses. Important early defence mechanisms include the acute phase response, the complement system, the interferons, the phagocytic cells, and the natural killer cells. Together these act as a first line of defence during the initial hours/days of infection.

Further Reading

Baron S, Tyring SK, Fleischmann WR *et al*. The interferons. Mechanisms of action and clinical applications. *J Am Med Assoc* 1991; **266(10):** 1375–1383.

Clas F, Loos M. Complement and bacteria. In: Whaley K, ed. *Complement in health and disease*. Lancaster: MTP Press, 1987.

Cooper NR. Complement evasion mechanisms of microorganisms. *Immunol Today* 1991; **12:** 327–331.

Liew FY, Cox FEG. Non-specific defence mechanism: the role of nitric oxide. *Immunol Today* 1991; **12 (3):** A17–21.

Morgan BP. Complement membrane attack on nucleated cells: resistance, recovery and non-lethal effects. *Biochem J* 1989; **264:** 1–14.

Pepys MB. Aspects of the acute phase response: the C-reactive protein system. In: *Clinical aspects of immunology*. 4th edn. Oxford: Blackwell Scientific Publications, 1982.

13 SPREAD AND REPLICATION

Contents

INTRODUCTION: SURFACE AND SYSTEMIC INFECTIONS

Many successful microorganisms multiply in epithelial cells at the site of entry on the body surface, but fail to spread to deeper structures or through the body. Local spread takes place readily on a fluid-covered mucosal surface, often aided by ciliary action, and large-scale movements of fluid spread the infection to more distant areas on the surface. This is obvious in the gastrointestinal tract. In the upper respiratory tract high winds (coughing, sneezing) can splatter infectious agents onto new areas of mucosa, or into the openings of sinuses or the middle ear, while the gentler downward trickle of mucus during sleep may seed an infectious agent into the lower respiratory tract. As a result, large areas of the body surface can be involved within a few days, with shedding to the exterior. There is not enough time for a primary immune response to be generated, and therefore non-adaptive responses (interferon, NK cells) are more important in controlling the infection. These surface infections are thus showing a 'hit-and-run' pattern.

In contrast, other microorganisms spread systemically through the body via lymph or blood. They often undergo a complex or stepwise invasion of various tissues before reaching the final site of replication and shedding to the exterior (e.g. measles, typhoid). Surface and systemic infections and their consequences are compared in figure 13.1.

What prevents surface infections from spreading more deeply? Why do the microbes that cause systemic infections leave the relatively safe haven of the body surface to spread through the body, where they will bear the full onslaught of host defences? These are important questions. For instance, what are the factors that persuade meningococci residing harmlessly on the nasal mucosa to invade deeper tissues, reach the blood and meninges, and cause meningitis (see Chapter 27)? The answer is not known.

Temperature, however, is a factor that is known to restrict microbes to body surfaces. Rhinovirus infections, for instance, are restricted to the upper respiratory tract because they are temperature-sensitive, replicating efficiently at 33°C but not at the temperatures encountered in

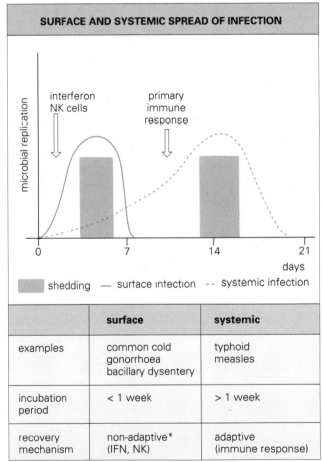

SURFACE AND SYSTEMIC SPREAD OF INFECTION

	surface	systemic
examples	common cold gonorrhoea bacillary dysentery	typhoid measles
incubation period	< 1 week	> 1 week
recovery mechanism	non-adaptive* (IFN, NK)	adaptive (immune response)

Fig. 13.1 Surface and systemic infections.*If there is pre-existing immunity (memory), a secondary immune response comes into operation within 1–2 days.

the lower respiratory tract (37°C). *Mycobacterium leprae* is also temperature-sensitive, which accounts for its replication being more or less limited to nasal mucosa, skin and superficial nerves. Influenza and parainfluenza viruses, however, invade the lung but are restricted to the epithelial surface, partly because these viruses are liberated by budding from the free (external) surface of the epithelial cell, not from the basal layer from where they could spread to deeper tissues (Fig. 13.2).

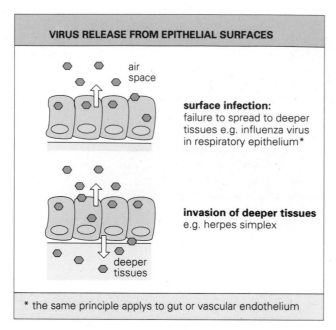

Fig. 13.2 Topography of virus release from epithelial surfaces can determine the pattern of infection.

On the other hand, many microorganisms *need* to spread systemically because they fail to spread and multiply at the site of initial infection, the body surface. In the case of measles or typhoid, there is, for unknown reasons, next to no replication at the site of initial respiratory or intestinal infection. Only after spreading through the body systemically are large numbers of microorganisms delivered back to the same surfaces, where they multiply and are shed to the exterior. Other microorganisms have committed themselves to infection by one route but the major replication occurs at a different site. The microbe must reach the replication site, and there is then no need for extensive replication at the site of initial infection. For instance, mumps and hepatitis A viruses infect via the respiratory and alimentary routes respectively, but multiply in salivary glands (mumps) and liver (hepatitis A).

In systemic infections, therefore, there is a stepwise invasion of different tissues of the body (Fig. 13.3), as in measles and typhoid (Figs 13.4 and 13.5). Although the final sites of multiplication may be essential for microbial shedding and transmission (e.g. measles), they are sometimes completely

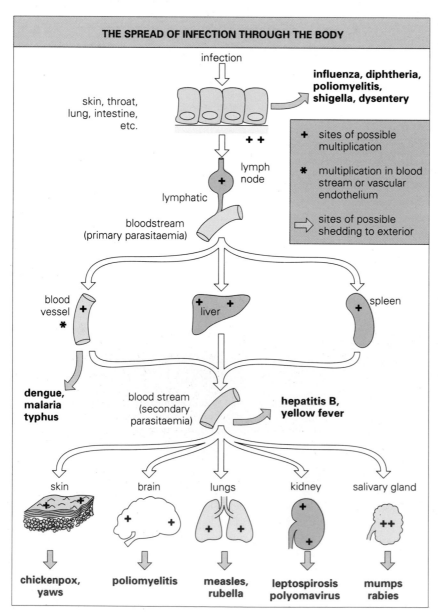

Fig. 13.3 The spread of infection throughout the body. Bone marrow muscle are possible sources for secondary parasitaemia in addition to blood vessels, liver, spleen.

unecessary from this point of view (e.g. meningococcal meningitis, paralytic poliomyelitis). These microbes are not shed to the exterior after multiplying in the meninges or spinal cord.

For the microbe, systemic spread is fraught with obstacles and a major encounter with immune and other defences is inevitable. Microorganisms have therefore been forced to develop strategies for bypassing or countering these defences (see Chapter 15).

MICROBIAL REPLICATION

The rate of replication of the infecting microorganism is of central importance, and doubling times vary from 20 minutes to several days (Fig. 13.6). Rapid replication is essential for hit-and-run (surface) infections, whereas a microorganism that divides every few days (e.g. *M. tuberculosis*) is likely to cause a slowly evolving disease, with a long incubation period. Microorganisms nearly always multiply faster *in vitro* than they do in the intact host, as might be expected if host defences are performing a useful function. In the host, microorganisms are phagocytosed, and killed, and the supply of nutrients may be limited. The net increase in numbers is slower than in laboratory cultures where microbes are not only free from attack by host defences but also every effort has been made to supply them with optimal nutrients, susceptible cells, and so on.

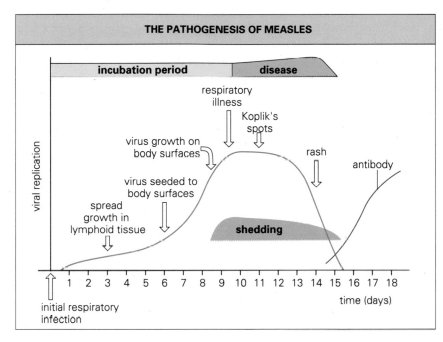

Fig. 13.4 The pathogenesis of measles. Virus invades body surfaces via blood vessels, and reaches surface epithelium first in the respiratory tract where there are only 1-2 layers of epithelial cells, then in mucosae (Koplik's spots) and finally in the skin (rash).

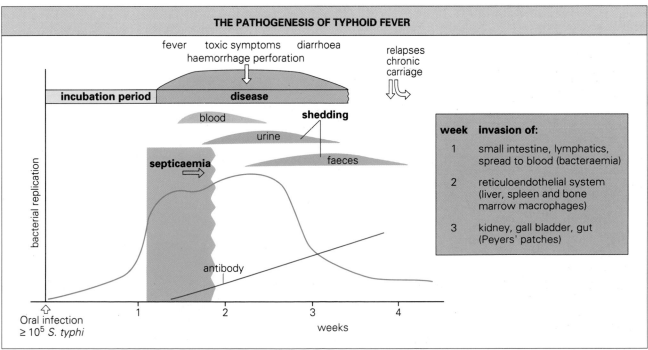

Fig. 13.5 The pathogenesis of typhoid fever.

REPLICATION RATES OF MICROORGANISMS		
microorganism	situation	mean doubling time
Most viruses	in cell*	< 1 hour
Many bacteria e.g. *E.coli* staphylococci	*in vitro*	20–30 minutes
Salmonella typhimurium	*in vitro* *in vivo*	30 minutes 5–12 hours
Mycobacterium tuberculosis	*in vitro* *in vivo*	24 hours many days
Mycobacterium leprae[†]	*in vivo*	2 weeks
Treponema pallidum[†]	*in vivo*	30 hours
Plasmodium falciparum	*in vitro/in vivo* (erythrocyte or hepatic cell)	8 hours

* but some viruses show greatly delayed replication or delayed spread from cell to cell

[†] cannot be cultivated *in vitro*

Fig. 13.6 Replication rates of different microorganisms.

MECHANISMS OF SPREAD THROUGH THE BODY

Spread to lymph and blood

After traversing the epithelium and its basement membrane at the body surface, invading microbes encounter the following defences:
• Tissue fluids
• Local macrophages (histiocytes)
• The physical barrier of local tissue structure
• The lymphatic system.
Antimicrobial substances (antibody, complement) are present in tissue fluids and local tissue macrophages are a threat to microbial survival. Local tissues consist of various cells in a hydrated gel matrix, and although viruses can spread by stepwise invasion of cells, things are more difficult for bacteria – those that spread effectively sometimes possess special spreading factors (e.g. streptococcal hyaluronidase). The rich network of the lymphatic system will soon convey microorganisms to the battery of phagocytic and immunological defences awaiting them in the local lymph node (Fig. 13.7). Macrophages, strategically placed in the marginal and other lymph sinuses, constitute an efficient filtering system for lymph.

The infection may be halted at any stage, but by multiplying locally or in lymph nodes, and by evading phagocytosis, the microorganism can ultimately reach the blood stream. Thus, a minor injury to the skin, followed by a red streak (inflamed lymphatic) and a tender, swollen local lymph node, are classical signs of streptococcal invasion. Most bacteria cause a good deal of inflammation when they invade in this way. In the early stages the lymph flow increases, but eventually if there is enough inflammation and tissue damage in the node itself, the flow of the lymph may cease. By contrast, viruses and other intracellular microorganisms often invade lymph and blood silently and asymptomatically during the incubation period; this is facilitated when they infect monocytes or lymphocytes without initially damaging them.

Spread from blood

Viruses or small numbers of bacteria can enter the blood without causing general bodily disturbance. For instance transient bacteraemias are fairly common in normal individuals (e.g. they may occur after defacation or brushing teeth), but the bacteria are usually filtered out and destroyed in macrophages lining liver and spleen sinusoids. Under certain circumstances the same bacteria have a chance to localize in less well defended sites, such as congenitally abnormal heart valves in the case of viridans streptococci causing infective endocarditis, or in the ends of growing bones in the case of *Staphylococus aureus* osteomyelitis.

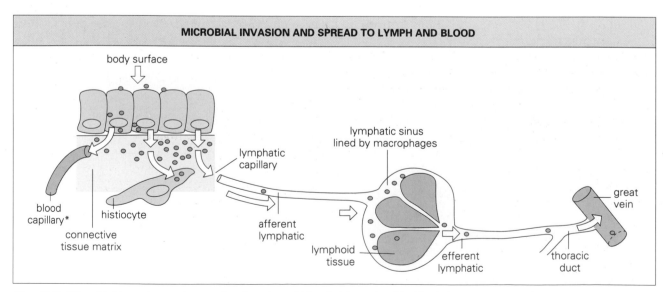

Fig. 13.7 Microbial invasion and spread to lymph and blood. * Invasion by this route is uncommon except following injury or infection by arthropod bite.

CIRCULATING MICROBES THAT INVADE ORGANS VIA SMALL BLOOD VESSELS		
microbe	**disease**	**principal organs invaded***
Viruses		
Hepatitis B	hepatitis B	liver
Rubella	congenital rubella	placenta (fetus)
Varicella-zoster	chicken-pox	skin, respiratory tract
Polio	poliomyelitis	brain, spinal cord
Mumps	mumps	parotid, mammary glands
Bacteria		
Rickettsia rickettsi	rocky mountain spotted fever	skin
Treponema pallidum	secondary syphilis	skin, mucosae
Neisseria meningitidis	Meningitis	meninges
Protozoa		
Trypanosoma cruzi	chagas' disease	heart, skeletal muscle
Plasmodium sp.	malaria	liver
Helminths		
Schistosoma sp. (larvae)	schistosomiasis	veins of bladder, bowel
Ascaris lumbricoides (larvae)	ascariasis	lung
Ankylostoma duodenale (larvae)	hookworm	lung
* in liver, sinusoids; elsewhere, capillaries, venules		

Fig. 13.8 Circulating micoorganisms that invade organs via small blood vessels.

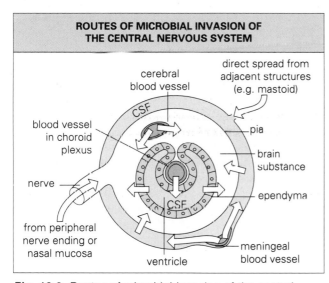

Fig. 13.9 Routes of microbial invasion of the central nervous system.

The fate of microorganisms in the blood depends on whether they are:(a) free in the plasma, and thus exposed to antibodies, phagocytes etc.; or (b) associated with circulating cells. Many viruses (EB virus, rubella) and intracellular bacteria (*Listeria, Brucella*) are present in lymphocytes or monocytes which, if not damaged or destroyed, can protect them from host defences and carry them around the body. Malaria infects erythrocytes, and a few viruses infect platelets.

On entering the blood, microorganisms are exposed to macrophages of the reticuloendothelial system (see Chapter 4). Here in the sinusoids, where blood flows slowly, they are often phagocytosed and destroyed. But certain microorganisms survive and multiply in these cells (*Salmonella typhi, Leishmania donovani*, yellow fever virus). The microorganism may then:(a) spread to adjacent hepatic cells in the liver (hepatitis viruses), or splenic lymphoid tissues (measles virus); or (b) re-invade the blood (*S. typhi*, hepatitis viruses).

If uptake by reticuloendothelial macrophages is not complete within a short time, or if large numbers of microorganisms are present in the blood, there is an opportunity for localization elsewhere in the vascular system. This is likely whenever there is local inflammation because of the slower flow and sticky endothelium in inflamed vessels. Each circulating microorganism, however, invades characteristic target organs and tissues (Fig. 13.8). This 'tropism' is not completely understood but may be due to specific receptors for the microorganism, leading to localization on the vascular endothelium of certain target organs, or to random localization in organs throughout the body, only some of them being suitable for subsequent colonization and replication.

After localization and organ invasion, the replicating microbe is shed from the body, if the organ has a surface with access to the outside world (see Fig. 13.3). It may also be shed back into the bloodstream, either directly or via the lymphatic system.

Spread via nerves

Certain viruses spread from peripheral parts of the body to the CNS, and vice versa from CNS to the periphery, via peripheral nerves. Tetanus toxin reaches the CNS by this route. Rabies, herpes simplex and varicella-zoster viruses travel in axons (see Chapters 11 and 27) and although the rate is slow, being accounted for by axonal flow (up to 10mm per hour), this movement is important in the pathogenesis of these infections. Rabies not only reaches the CNS largely by peripheral nerves, but takes the same route from the CNS when it invades the salivary glands. Few, if any, host defences are in a position to control this type of viral spread, once nerves are invaded. Routes of invasion of the CNS are illustrated in figure 13.9.

An uncommon route of spread to the CNS is via olfactory nerves, whose axons terminate on olfactory mucosa. For instance, certain free living amoeba (e.g. *Naegleria* sp.) found in sludge at the bottom of freshwater pools may take this route and cause meningoencephalitis in swimmers (see Chapter 27). Viruses and bacteria in the nasopharynx (e.g. meningococci, poliovirus) generally spread to the CNS via the blood.

Spread via cerebrospinal fluid

Once microorganisms have traversed the blood–CSF barrier they spread rapidly in the CSF spaces, and can invade neural tissues (echoviruses, mumps virus) as well as multiply locally (*Neisseria meningitidis*, *Haemophilus influenzae*, *Streptococcus pneumoniae*) and possibly infect ependymal and meningeal cells.

Spread via other routes

Rapid spread from one visceral organ to another can take place via the pleural or peritoneal cavity. Both cavities are lined by macrophages, as if in expectation of such events, and the peritoneal cavity contains an antimicrobial armoury, consisting of the omentum (the 'abdominal policeman'), and many lymphocytes, macrophages and mast cells. Injury or disease in an abdominal organ provides a source of infection for peritonitis, as do chest wounds or lung infections for pleurisy.

GENETIC DETERMINANTS OF SPREAD AND REPLICATION

The pathogenicity of a microorganism is determined by the interplay of factors listed in Chapter 11 and as discussed more fully in Chapters 4 and 8. (Note that a distinction is sometimes made between pathogenicity and virulence: virulence implies a quantitative measure of pathogenicity. For instance, it can be expressed as the number of organisms necessary to cause death in 50% of individuals, or lethal dose 50 (LD50).) Nearly all of these pathogenicity factors are controlled by host and microbial genes. It has long been known that there are host genetic influences on susceptibility to infectious disease, and that mutations in microorganisms affect their pathogenicity. Within the past 10 years, however, some of these genetic factors have been revealed by the application of molecular genetics techniques, and as a result it is increasingly possible to identify the specific gene products involved. Progress has also been made, though with greater difficulty, in understanding the mode of action of these gene products.

Genetic determinants in the host

The ability of a microorganism to infect and cause disease in a given host is inevitably influenced by the genetic constitution of the host. At a relatively gross level, some human pathogens either do not infect other species or infect only closely related primates (e.g. measles, trachoma, typhoid, hepatitis B, warts), whereas others infect a very wide range of hosts (rabies, anthrax). Also, within a given host species, there are genetic determinants of sus-

Genetically determined susceptibility to infection

There are several classic examples of susceptibility to infectious disease determined by unidentified but presumably genetic factors in the human host:

The Lubeck disaster – In Lubeck, Germany, in 1926, living virulent tubercle bacilli instead of attenuated (vaccine) bacilli were inadvertently given to 249 babies. There were 76 deaths, but the rest, who developed only minor lesions, survived and were alive and well 12 years later. Each received the same inoculum, and it seems likely that the differences in outcome were largely due to genetic factors in the host.

A military misfortune – In 1942, more than 45 000 US military personnel were vaccinated against yellow fever but were inadvertently injected at the same time with hepatitis B virus present as a contaminant in the human serum used to stabilize the vaccine. There were 914 clinical cases of hepatitis, of which 580 were mild, 301 moderate and 33 severe. Even with a given batch of vaccine the incubation period varied from 10–20 weeks. Serological tests were not then available so the number of subclinical infections is unknown. In this case, physiological, as well as genetic influences on susceptibility may have played a part.

Respiratory tuberculosis in twins – A study was made of tuberculosis in twins, when at least one twin had the disease. With identical twins, the other twin was affected in 87% cases. With non-identical twins the equivalent figure was only 26%. Moreover, the identical twins had a similar type of clinical disease.

ceptibility. The best examples are found in animals, but there are examples from human disease (see above). One example at the molecular level is the sickle cell gene and susceptibility to malaria. Malaria merozoites (see Chapter 29) parasitize red blood cells and metabolize haemoglobin, freeing haem and utilizing globin as a source of amino acids. The sickle cell gene causes a substitution of the amino acid valine for glutamic acid at one point in the beta-polypeptide chain of the hemoglobin molecule. The new haemoglobin (haemoglobin S) becomes insoluble when reduced, and precipitates inside the red cell envelope, distorting the cell into the shape of a sickle. In homozygous individuals there are two of these genes and the individual suffers from the disease sickle cell anaemia, but in the heterozygote (sickle cell trait) the gene is less harmful, and provides resistance to severe forms of falciparum malaria which ensures its selection in endemic malarial regions. The gene would be eliminated from populations after 10–20 generations unless it conferred some advantage. Restriction endonuclease analyses

ATTENUATION OF PATHOGENS *IN VITRO*		
pathogen	**passage**	**attenuated (live) product**
Mycobacterium bovis	10 years of repeated passage in glycerin-bile-potato medium	BCG vaccine
Rubella virus	27 passages in human diploid cells	Rubella vaccine (Wistar RA 27/3)

Fig. 13.10 Examples of attenuation of pathogens following repeated passage *in vitro*.

of the gene in Indian and West African populations have revealed that it arose independently in these malarious countries. Homozygotes, however, show increasing susceptibility to other infections, particularly *Strep. pneumoniae*, as a result of spleen dysfunction following repeated infarcts in this organ.

Recent advances in the study of infection at the molecular genetic level indicate that susceptibility often operates at the level of the immune response. A poor immune response to a given infection can lead to increased susceptibility to disease, whereas too vigorous an immune response may lead to immunopathological disease (see Chapter 16). Of particular importance are the major histocompatibilty complex (MHC) genes on chromosome 6, coding for MHC class II (HLA A–D) antigens and controlling specific immune response (see Chapters 6 and 7). For example, susceptibility to leprosy (see Chapter 28) is strongly influenced by class II genes. People with HLA DR3 are more susceptible to tuberculoid leprosy, whereas those with HLA DQ1 are more susceptible to lepromatous leprosy.

There is evidence from studies of identical twins that genetic determinants affect susceptibility to tuberculosis (see panel). The present day European population shows considerable resistance to this disease. During the great epidemics of pulmonary tuberculosis in Europe in the 17th, 18th and 19th Centuries, genetically susceptible individuals were weeded out. In 1850 mortality rates in Boston, New York, London, Paris and Berlin were over 500 per 100 000, but with improvements in living conditions these fell to 180 per 100 000 by 1900, and they have fallen even more since then. However, previously unexposed populations, especially in Africa and the Pacific Islands, show much greater susceptibility to respiratory tuberculosis. In the Plains Indians living in the Qu'Appelle Valley reservation in Saskatchewan, Canada in 1886, tuberculosis spread through the body, to infect glands, bones, joints and meninges, giving a death rate of 9000 per 100 000.

Microbial genetic determinants

Virulence is determined by numerous factors, such as adhesion, penetration into cells, antiphagocytic activity, production of toxins and interaction with the immune system. Consequently, virulence is likely to be coded for by more than one microbial gene, different gene/gene products being involved at different stages in pathogenesis.

Under natural circumstances microorganisms are constantly undergoing genetic change (especially mutations). The single stranded RNA viruses in particular show very high mutation rates. Some of these mutations affect surface antigens, which undergo rapid selection in the host under immune pressure (antibody, cell mediated immunity), as in the case of the rapidly evolving M proteins of streptococci, and the capsid proteins of picornaviruses. In addition, genetic changes in bacteria are often due to acquisition or loss of extrachromosomal genetic elements called 'plasmids' (see Chapter 3).

Changes in the virulence of a microorganism take place during artificial culture in the laboratory. For instance, in the classical procedure for obtaining a live vaccine (see Chapter 34) a microorganism is repeatedly grown (passaged) *in vitro* and this generally leads to reduced pathogenicity in the host. The new strain is then referred to as 'attenuated' (Fig. 13.10).

Our understanding of the genetic basis for microbial pathogenicity had advanced rapidly in recent years thanks to DNA cloning and genetic manipulation techniques. For instance, by introducing genome segments, the virulence genes can be identified. Examples are shown in figure 13.11 overleaf. For many viruses the nucleic acid sequence of the entire genome has been established and functions are being slowly assigned to specific sequences.

OTHER FACTORS AFFECTING SPREAD AND REPLICATION

Various factors in the host have an influence on susceptibility to infectious disease (Fig. 13.12). In most cases it is not known whether this involves differences in microbial spread and replication, or differences in host immune and inflammatory reponses. Infections in the host suffering from immunological and other defects are described in Chapter 31.

SUMMARY

Infections restricted to the body surfaces (common cold, shigella, dysentery) can be compared with systemic infections (measles, typhoid). The former usually have shorter incubation period and adaptive host responses tend to be less important. Microbes with a slow growth rate (e.g. *M. tuberculosis*) tend to cause more slowly evolving diseases.

Spread through the body takes place primarily via lymph and blood. The fate of circulating microbes depends on whether they are free or present in circulating blood cells. Uptake by reticuloendothelial cells in liver and spleen focusses infection into these organs but specific localization in the vascular bed of other organs (e.g. mumps virus in salivary glands, meningococci in meninges) is not understood. Viruses can spread in either direction along nerve axons, which is important in the pathogenesis of recurrent herpes simplex, zoster and rabies.

Pathogenicty and virulence is strongly influenced by genetic factors in the host (e.g. tuberculosis in identical twins) and by genetic factors in the microbe (e.g sickle cell trait in falciparum malaria).

THE MOLECULAR BASIS OF MICROBIAL PATHOGENICITY		
microorganism	**gene or gene product**	**affect on virulence**
Streptococcus pyogenes	M protein; 60nm long coiled coil extending from bacterial cell wall with N terminal hypervariable domain amino acid sequence overlap with host components (myosin, tropomyosin, keratin, etc.)	antiphagocytic role; exact mechanism unknown autoimmune complication
Yersinia enterocolitica	invasin gene codes for 15kDa protein on bacterial surface	required for uptake of bacteria into epithelial cells and macrophages of Peyer's patches
Shigella sp.	plasmid-encoded haemolysin gene	after shigella have induced their own uptake into vacuoles of colonic epithelial cells, haemolysin mediates lysis of vacuolar membrane and escape of bacteria
Leishmania donovani	Arg-Gly-Asp sequence of gp63 surface protein	binds to C3b receptor on macrophage and thereby infects this cell
Neisseria gonorrhoeae	genes for proteins of pili (fimbriae) and for PII surface proteins	proteins mediate attachment to mucosal cells. Independent control of each gene makes *N. gonorrhoeae* the 'master chameleon', altering its surface antigens to evade host immune responses
Herpes simplex type I	gene for envelope glycoprotein C (gC)	gC acts as receptor for C3b, blocking the classical pathway and enabling virus or virus-infected cell to resist lysis by complement plus antibody

Fig. 13.11 Examples of the molecular basis of microbial pathogenicity.

HOST FACTORS INFLUENCING SUSCEPTIBILITY TO INFECTIOUS DISEASE			
factor	**example**	**alteration in susceptibility**	**mechanism**
Pregnancy	hepatitis viruses urinary infections	more lethal outcome pyelonephritis more common	?increased metabolic burden for liver in pregnancy reduced peristalsis in ureter
Malnutrition	measles	more severe; more lethal	vitamin A deficiency; depressed CMI
Age	respiratory syncytial virus mumps, chicken-pox, EB virus infection	more severe; more lethal in infant more severe in adult	small diameter of airways ?increased immunopathology
Atmospheric pollution	raised SO_2 levels silicosis	excess acute respiratory disease increased susceptibility to tuberculosis	?interference with mucociliary defences ?damage to lung macrophages
Foreign bodies	necrotic bone fragments necrotic tissue	chronic osteomyelitis more common increased susceptibility to *C. perfringens*	antimicrobial defences less effective in necrotic tissue anaerobic necrotic tissues favour bacterial growth

Fig. 13.12 Host factors influencing susceptibility to infectious disease.

Further Reading

Brett-Finlay B, Falkour S. Common themes in microbial pathogenicity. *Microbiol Revs* 1989; **53**: 210–230.

Griffin JW, Watson DF. Axonal transport in neurologic disease. *Ann Neurol* 1988; **23**: 3–13.

Hace TL. Genetic basis of virulence in *Shigella* species. *Microbial Revs* 1991; **55**: 206–224.

Mims CA. *The pathogenesis of infectious disease*. 3rd edn. London: Academic Press, 1987.

Isberg RR, Voorhis DL, Falkour. Identification of invasin: A protein that allows cuteric bacteria to penetrate cultured mammalian cells. *Cell* 1987; **50**: 769–778.

14 ADAPTIVE IMMUNITY IN ACTION

Contents

INTRODUCTION

Foreign organisms which penetrate the external defence barriers, enter the body and survive the natural immune mechanisms, will almost inevitably encounter adaptive immune responses, because they or their antigens will sooner or later make contact with lymphocytes (see Chapters 7 and 12). Nothing illustrates better the value of the adaptive immune mechanism in fighting infection than the generally disastrous results of defects in T and/or B cells, or their products. These are discussed in detail in Chapter 33, but here they may be summed up as follows: antibody deficiencies predispose to uncontrolled infection by extracellular organisms, particularly pyogenic bacteria, whereas T cell deficiencies lead mainly to failure to recover from intracellular infections, whether viral, bacterial, fungal or protozoal. Thus, antibody may be thought of as 'policing' the extracellular spaces of the body while T cells monitor, as far as possible, the intracellular compartment. The crucial role of MHC molecules in the latter activity is described in Chapters 5 and 6.

ANTIBODY-MEDIATED IMMUNITY

The key property of the antibody molecule is to bind specifically to antigens on the foreign organism. In many cases this is followed by secondary binding to other cells or molecules of the immune system (e.g phagocytes, complement). Before these are discussed, some general features that influence the effectiveness of the antibody response should be mentioned.

Speed, amount and duration

Because of the cell interactions involved and the need for proliferation of a small number of specific precursor lymphocytes, a primary antibody response can be dangerously slow in reaching protective levels. The classic example, before penicillin, was lobar pneumonia, where the race between bacterial multiplication and antibody levels was 'neck-and-neck' for about a week, at which point one side

or the other dramatically won. Nowadays, of course, vaccines and antibiotics have intervened to improve the chances of the patient. Experiments with specially bred lines of mice suggest that the speed and size of an antibody response is under the control of a large number of genes, and the same is undoubtedly true in the human.

The rate of replication and spread of the microorganism must also be considered. Replication rates, as indicated by doubling times (see Chapter 13) vary from less than an hour (most viruses, many bacteria) to days or weeks (mycobacteria, *T. pallidum*, scrapie-type agents). Microorganisms tend to grow more slowly *in vivo* than *in vitro*, which shows that the host environment is generally hostile. When the incubation period is only a few days (e.g. rhinovirus and rotavirus infections, cholera) the antibody response is too slow to affect the initial outcome, and rapidly produced factors such as interferon are more important.

Generally speaking, the antibody response continues as long as antigen is present, although some down-regulation may occur in very prolonged responses, presumably in an effort to limit immunopathology (see Chapter 16). The lifelong immunity that follows many virus infections may often be due to regular boosting, e.g. during measles or mumps epidemics, but sometimes (e.g. yellow fever) there is no obvious boost yet antibody levels persist for decades.

Affinity

It seems self-evident that a higher antigen-binding affinity would render antibody more useful, and passive protection experiments have confirmed this. Affinity is determined by both the germ-line antibody gene pool and somatic mutation in individual B lymphocytes, and appears to be under genetic control which is separate from that controlling the total amount of antibody made. A tendency towards a low antibody affinity to the tetanus toxoid vaccine has been found in some patients, particularly those with predominantly IgG4 responses, and there is strong evidence from mouse experiments that failure to develop high affinity antibody responses can predispose to immune complex disease.

Classes and subclasses (isotypes)

The different Fc portions of the antibody molecule are responsible for most of the differences in antibody function (see Chapter 6). Switching from one to another while preserving the same Fab portion allows the immune system to 'try out' different effector mechanisms against the microbial invader. This flexibility is not total. For example, T-independent antigens such as some polysaccharides induce only IgM, T cells being required for the switch to IgG, IgA or IgE. IgG anti-polysaccharide responses tend to be mainly IgG2, whereas anti-protein IgG is mainly IgG1. The poor development of IgG2 in children below the age of about two explains their lack of response to bacteria with polysaccharide capsules (e.g. *Strep. pneumoniae*, *Haemophilus influenzae*) and considerable effort is being made to produce vaccines that incorporate a protein that can induce other subclasses of IgG (see Chapter 36). Antibodies to viruses are predominantly IgG1 and IgG3, and to helminths IgG4 and IgE, while antigens that reach the digestive tract induce mainly IgA, the only type of antibody that can function in the protease-rich intestinal environment; a role for T cells is suspected for all these isotype preferences. Selective immunodeficiency affecting particular isotypes is discussed in Chapter 33.

Blocking and neutralizing effects of antibody

Simple binding of antibody molecules to a microbial structure is often enough to protect the host. It may physically interfere with the receptor interaction necessary for microbial entry (e.g. of a virus into a cell) or with the binding of a toxin to its cell receptor. This is the basis of many life-saving vaccines against viruses or bacterial toxins. The important question of whether a rapid secondary response is sufficient for protection, or whether pre-existing serum antibody levels need to be present before infection, is discussed in Chapter 36.

Blocking of attachment and entry can be effective against all organisms that use specific attachment sites, whether viral, bacterial, or protozoal (see Chapter 11). An important exception is those organisms that parasitize the macrophage, such as the virus of dengue fever; here the presence of a low level of IgG antibody can actually enhance infection by promoting attachment to Fc receptors (see below).

A more subtle blocking effect of antibody is interference with essential surface components of the parasite, particularly if these are enzymes or transport molecules. Needless to say the successful parasite takes steps to protect such components whenever possible, as described in Chapter 15.

Immobilization and agglutination

Immunoglobulin molecules, particularly the large pentameric IgM, are the same order of size as some of the smaller viruses, and larger than the thickness of a bacterial flagellum (Fig. 14.1), so the simple physical attachment of antibody can considerably restrict the activities of motile organisms. In addition, the multivalent design of the antibody molecules enables it to link together two or more organisms, as can readily be demonstrated in the bacterial agglutination tests (Fig. 14.2). The protective value of agglutination *in vivo* is hard to assess; once clumped, most organ-

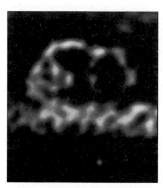

Fig. 14.1 Electron micrograph of an IgM molecule. The crab-like configuration is due to cross-linkage with a single flagellum. Courtesy of A Feinstein.

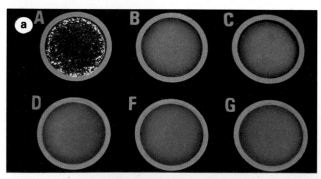

(b) THE WIDAL TEST FOR TYPHOID									
serum dilutions									
antigens	1/20	1/40	1/80	1/160	1/320	1/640	1/1280	1/2560	control
S. typhi O	+	+	+	+	–	–	–	–	–
S. typhi H	+	+	+	+	+	+	+	–	–
S. paratyphi B H	–	–	–	–	–	–	–	–	–
S. paratyphi B O	+[a]	+[a]	–	–	–	–	–	–	–

+ = indicates agglutination
a = weak response probably due to antigenic cross-reactivity

Fig. 14.2 Bacterial agglutination. (a) Agglutination of group A streptococcus with latex particles coated with anti-group A antibodies. (b) The widal test detects typhoid antibody in blood. Here, there are separate antibody responses to the O (somatic) and H (flagellar) antigens 12 days after onset of illness. Courtesy of DK Banerjee.

isms are probably rapidly phagocytosed, but clumps of still motile trypanosomes can be seen in the blood of infected animals with serum antibody levels. Agglutination reactions *in vitro* are very useful in diagnosis (see Chapter 18).

Lysis

Lysis of bacteria in the presence of complement is another convenient assay for the presence of antibody. However, lysis probably plays a major protective role only in a restricted range of infections, notably those caused by *Neisseria* and some viruses (see Chapter 12).

Opsonization

Whether by the direct binding of the CH2 and CH3 regions to Fc receptors, or via the activation of complement to allow C3 to bind to its receptor, opsonization represents the most important overall function of the antibody molecules. Telling evidence for this is the general similarity in the effects on the patient of defects in antibody, complement (up to and including C3) and phagocytic cells (see Chapter 33). It is estimated that the rate of phagocytosis is enhanced by up to a thousand-fold by antibody and complement acting together (Fig. 14.3). Lobar pneumonia due to *Strep. pneumoniae* again provides a good example: IgG antibody against the capsule allows neutrophils to phagocytose the organisms, converting a lung virtually solid with fluid, fibrin and phagocytic cells overnight into the normal breathing apparatus. Note that the later complement components C5–9 are not required, so that deficiencies of these do not predispose to bacterial infection in general (see Chapter 33). Of course, the effectiveness of opsonization depends on the phagocytic cell being capable of finishing off the ingested organism. This is not the case, however, with organisms that inhibit or avoid the normal intracellular killing processes, of which mycobacteria are a typical example (see Chapter 15).

Antibody-dependent cytoxicity

In the case of larger organisms (worms being the most obvious example), phagocytosis is clearly not a possibility. However several types of cell, having made contact with the parasite through antibody and Fc receptors in the same way as phagocytes do, can inflict damage extracellularly. These include most conventional phagocytes (Fig. 14.4), as well as eosinophils and platelets. It must be said, however, that virtually all the evidence for this kind of mechanism comes from experiments done *in vitro*, and here again it is extremely difficult to assess their role *in vivo*.

Indeed, the precise way in which antibody protects against infection is, in the majority of cases, still unknown. For example, the enormous production of IgA in the intestine, which may amount to half of all antibody produced in the body, suggests the vital important of mucosal protection, and yet deficiency of IgA is relatively common and not particularly serious.

Figure 14.5 gives some examples of common infections normally controlled by antibody. Once again, it must be emphasized that the presence of antibody by no means denotes a protective role. They may be directed against irrelevant or non-critical microbial antigens, or the infection may be a type that is not controlled by antibody, as with many intracellular infections (tuberculosis, typhoid, herpes virus). The best indication of the value of antibody comes from antibody-deficiency syndromes (Chapter 33).

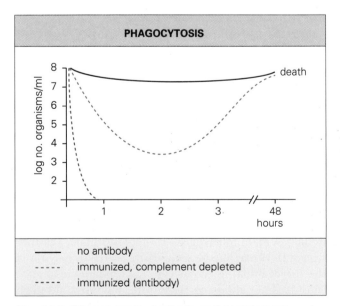

Fig. 14.3 Phagocytosis. Antibody and complement accelerate the clearance of pneumococci from the blood of mice.

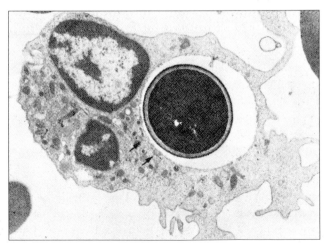
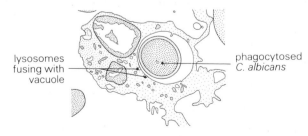

Fig. 14.4 Electron micrograph of neutrophil containing phagocytosed *Candida albicans*. x7000. Courtesy of H Validimarsson.

ANTIBODY AND CMI IN RESISTANCE TO SYSTEMIC INFECTIONS		
type of resistance	**antibody**	**CMI**

Recovery from primary infection	yellow fever
	polioviruses
	coxsackie viruses
	
	streptococci
	staphylococci
	Neisseria meningitidis
	Haemophilus influenzae
	?malaria
	Candida sp.
	Giardia lamblia
		poxviruses
		  e.g. ectromelia (mice)
		      vaccinia (man)
		herpes-type viruses
		  herpes simplex
		  varicella-zoster
		  cytomegalovirus
		LCM virus (mice)
		measles
		tuberculosis
		leprosy
		typhoid
		systemic fungal infections
		?chronic mucocutaneous
		  candidiasis

Resistance to re-infection	nearly all viruses including measles most bacteria	tuberculosis leprosy
Resistance to reactivation of latent infection	?herpes simplex	varicella-zoster cytomegalovirus tuberculosis *Pneumocystis carinii*

Fig. 14.5 Antibody and cell mediated immunity (CMI) in resistance to systemic infections. Either antibody or CMI is known to be the major factor in these examples. But in many other infections there is no information, and sometimes both types of immunity are important.

CELL-MEDIATED IMMUNITY

The term cell-mediated immunity (see Chapter 5) covers two rather different processes: (1) the killing, by CD8$^+$ T cells, of a cell containing a replicating parasite (usually a virus); and (2) the provision of help, usually in the shape of IFN-γ or other cytokines, to enable a macrophage to kill its own intracellular parasite; the latter is the responsibility of CD4$^+$ T cells. In both cases the T cell will not cooperate unless it sees the combination of specific microbial peptide and MHC molecule that it is programmed to recognize.

Although each of these mechanisms has been thoroughly studied *in vitro*, their relative roles *in vivo* are often hard to disentangle, and immunologists still argue over which is more important in, for example, graft rejection or recovery from influenza. Even in mycobacterial infection, where CD4$^+$ cells and cytokines are considered as the principal immune mechanisms, cytotoxic CD8$^+$ cells are now known to develop. In this case, however, such cells may not always be protective, but rather act to release living organisms from the phagocyte and thus spread the infection, though at the same time this may allow more effective anti-microbial cells to take them up (Fig. 14.6). Figure 14.5 lists some well-known examples where cell-mediated immunity is important in protection.

The strikingly different patterns of disease susceptibility seen in different types of T cell deficiency (e.g. primary, or secondary to HIV infection, cyclosporin treatment etc; see Chapter 33) suggest that there are further subdivisions to be made among the two major types of cell-mediated immunity. The separation of CD4$^+$ T cell functions into T_H1 and T_H2 based on preferential cytokine secretion, which at present is better established for the mouse than the human, promises to explain some of these, and is one of the justifications for the study of cytokines in infectious diseases of all kinds. A proper understanding of this may in turn lead to the rational use of cytokines or their antagonists in particular conditions. Figure 14.7 summarizes a few of the more convincing examples of cytokine involvement in infection.

Unfortunately (for science, though fortunately for patients) no cases of total absence of interferons or other cytokines have yet been recorded, so the evidence for their real value in infection is much weaker than for antibody. Nevertheless, they have been successful as treatment for some conditions (see Chapter 37), and the very fact that some viruses appear to have taken steps to evade their action indicates that they have an important function (e.g. hepatitis B does not induce IFN, whereas adenoviruses induce it but are not susceptible to it).

Delayed hypersensitivity

The way in which excessive or inappropriate cell-mediated immune responses may lead to disease is described in Chapter 16. Here it may be remarked that the relationship between delayed (-type) hypersensitivity (DTH) as expressed by skin tests of various kinds, and resistance to infection, is by no means a universal one. To take two examples: a positive DTH (lepromin) skin test in leprosy is found in the tuberculoid form of the disease, in which control of bacterial growth (beneficial) co-exists with severe damage to nerves (harmful), but not in the lepromatous form, in which bacteria multiply without restraint in the tissues. In tuberculosis, on the other hand, a further type of DTH may also be seen, characterized by necrosis at the site of initial injection (the Koch phenomenonon). This does not always correlate with immunity, although Koch's original suggestion that it was a means of sloughing off the infected lesion might be valid for exclusively superficial infections such as *Lupus vulgaris*.

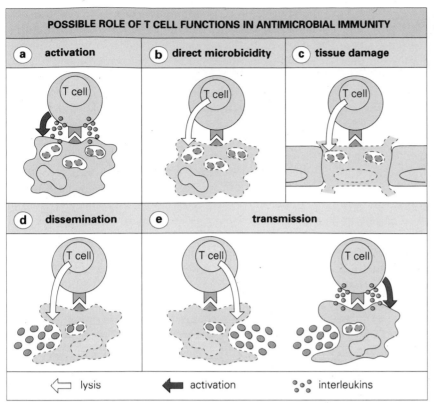

Fig. 14.6 Possible roles for T cells in immunity to intracellular microbes. (a) The T cell activates intracellular killing mechanisms, e.g. in a macrophage. (b) The T cell directly kills cell and parasite. (c) The T cell destroys vital tissue in the process of killing the parasite. (d) By lysing cells the T cell allows still-living parasites to disseminate, e.g. *M. leprae* in Schwann cells. (e) Dissemination as above may allow uptake of the parasite by a more effective host cell. Redrawn from Kaufman, 1989.

Fig. 14.7 Therapeutic role of cytokines in infectious diseases.

THERAPEUTIC ROLE OF CYTOKINES IN INFECTION

organism	cytokine	comments
Viruses		
Herpes	IFN-$_\alpha$	? treatment of reactivation e.g. zoster
	TNF, IL-1, GM-CSF	antiviral in animal experiments
HIV	IFN, IL-2	not effective
Hepatitis B	IFN- α	50% remission of chronic infection
Bacteria		
Pseudomonas, Legionella	IL-1	protective in mice
Listeria	TNF	
Leprosy	IL-2	? treatment
General	IL-3, G-CSF	prevents neutropenia in marrow failure
	IFN-γ	reduces infection in chronic granulomatous disease
	TNF	causes shock in Gram-negative septicaemia; ?antibody protective
Protozoa		
Leishmania	IFN-γ	protective in mice
	IL-3, IL-4	counter-protective in mice
Malaria	TNF	protective in mice
T. cruzi	IFN, TNF	protective *in vitro*
Helminths	IL-4, IL-5	?? contribute to immunity via IgG+ eosinophils

RECOVERY FROM INFECTION

The everyday concept of an infectious disease is one where the patient is ill for a period of days to months and then recovers. In some cases he is subsequently immune to the disease. In such circumstances one can be fairly certain that adaptive (lymphocyte-based) mechanisms have been at work since: (1) the existence of disease symptoms implies that natural defence mechanisms, which act rapidly, did not succeed in eliminating the parasite; (2) a period of days or weeks is typical of the time adaptive mechanisms take to reach maximal levels; and (3) subsequent immunity is a sign of immunological memory that is exclusive to lymphocytes, whose ability to specifically recognize antigens, to proliferate into clones, and to survive as memory cells, allows the host to progressively adapt to the infectious organisms he lives among. Thus, the older an individual is the better he is adapted to his environment - until extreme age begins to debilitate the immune system itself.

In the early stages of an infection, however, the adaptive system can appear somewhat clumsy in its operation. Since lymphocytes are programmed to recognize the shapes of antigenic epitopes, they cannot distinguish virulent from harmless parasites, nor can they 'know' which type of immune response will be most effective. Thus, it is likely that the majority of responses in any individual infection will be irrelevant to recovery, and the demonstration of antibody, cytokines or cytotoxic cells is no proof that they are doing anything useful. Often one mechanism is responsible for recovery and another for resistance to reinfection (e.g. cytotoxic cells and interferon in recovery from measles, antibody in prevention of a second attack). In many infections, notably those by protozoa and helminths, there is still controversy as to which of the numerous responses that can be detected are useful, harmful or neutral. This distinction can only be made by repeated and patient observation and correlation, aided by study of deficiency syndromes if they occur and by animal experiments where good models exist.

Failure to recover from an infection also cannot easily be attributed to a specific cause. If the infection is one from which most people recover (e.g. measles), or from which they do not suffer at all (e.g. pneumocystis), immunodeficiency on the part of the host is considered (see Chapter 33). Infections that are rapidly fatal in normal individuals (e.g. Lassa fever) are frequently those to which the evolving human immune system has not been regularly exposed, since they are normally maintained in animals and only accidentally infect man (see Zoonoses, Chapters 11 and 31). But if the infection normally runs a prolonged course without being either eliminated or killing the host, the parasite could be considered to be successful, and this success will be owed to one or more survival strategies. These are the subject of the next chapter.

SUMMARY

The lymphocyte-based antibody and cell-mediated responses are responsible for recovery from infection in many cases, although the precise mechanism is frequently unknown. Sometimes, as in most common viral infections, cell-mediated immunity is responsible for recovery from initial infection, and antibody for the maintenance of immunity. Failure to recover may be due to some deficiency of host immunity or to successful evasion strategies by the microorganism.

Further Reading ──

Hammerstrom L, Edvard Smith CI. IgG subclasses in bacteria infections. *Monogr in Allergy* 1986; **19:** 122.

Kaufmann, SHE *et al. Curr Opinions in Immunol* 1988;**1(3):** 435.

Kaufmann, SHE. Immunity to bacteria and fungi. *Curr Opinions in Immunol* 1989; **1(3):** 431–440.

Kaufmann, SHE. Immunity to bacteria. *Curr Opinions in Immunol* 1989; **2(3):** 353–359.

Mims CA. *The pathogenesis of infectious disease.* 3rd edn. London: Academic Press, 1987.

Playfair JHL. Principles of immunity to infection. In: Brostoff J, Scadding GK, Male DK, Roitt IM, eds. *Clinical immunology.* London: Gower Medical Publishing, 1991.

Teale JM, Abraham KM. The regulation of antibody class expression. *Immunol Today* 1987; **8:** 122.

15 PARASITE SURVIVAL STRATEGIES AND PERSISTENT INFECTIONS

Contents

INTRODUCTION

So far we have concentrated on the battery of mechanisms available to the host, both natural and adaptive, to keep out and destroy the parasite. Powerful as these are, they are obviously not one hundred percent effective, otherwise healthy people would never suffer from infections. In fact, most of the common infectious organisms described in this book have developed 'answers' to host defences, because their ability to survive as human parasites has depended on this. They successfully infect humans and are of concern to the physician precisely because they have developed strategies for evading or actively interfering with host defences.

The evasive strategies adopted by microbes to avoid natural, non-adaptive defences (phagocytes, complement, etc.) have been outlined in Chapter 12. This includes killing phagocytes, avoiding being killed by phagocytes, producing iron-binding molecules, interfering with ciliary action, and so on. The success of microbes in evading or interfering with adaptive (immune) defences will be discussed here. The strategies involved are somewhat more sophisticated because lymphocytes are programmed in such a way that their cell receptors can recognize virtually any shape (B cells) or amino acid sequence (T cells), provided it is not identical to self. A good illustration of this difference is provided by the polysaccharide capsules of bacteria, which are capable of preventing 'non-specific' contact between phagocytes and the bacterial cell wall. The bacteria thereby avoid non-immune phagocytosis. However, they are quickly recognized as foreign by B cell surface receptors (Ig), leading to the formation of antibody, with consequent opsonization and phagocytosis of the bacteria. In such a case it is clearly much more difficult for the parasite to conceal its presence from lymphocytes than from macrophages.

As another example, many bacteria, fungi etc. can resist intracellular destruction by macrophages, but cannot prevent their peptides being presented in association with MHC molecules on the macrophage surface. This means that their presence is detected by T cells, thus bringing in a new set of cytotoxic and other immune mechanisms which often tip the balance in favour of the host. In both these examples the lymphocytes are behaving like a highly specialized and sharply observant secret police force, in contrast to the everyday activities of the more pedestrian macrophage.

Parasite survival strategies can take as many forms as there are parasites, but they can be usefully classified according to the immune component that is evaded and the means selected to do this (see Chapter 10). As a result, the microbe is able to undergo what are often quite lengthy periods of growth and spread during the incubation period, before being shed and transmitted to the next host (e.g. hepatitis B, tuberculosis). If the microbe is shed for just a few extra days after clinical recovery, when there is more extensive transmission in the community, this is a worthwhile result.

In addition, certain microbes are able to remain (persist) in the host for many years, often for life. From the microbes point of view, persistent is worthwhile only if shedding occurs during the persistence. Persistent microbes fall into two categories: 1. Those that are shed more or less continuously, such as Epstein–Barr virus into saliva, hepatitis B virus into blood, eggs into faeces in various helminth infections; 2. Those that are shed intermittently, such as herpes simplex virus, polyomaviruses, typhoid bacilli, tubercle bacilli, malaria parasites. Persistent infections are discussed more fully later in this chapter.

Viruses are particularly good at thwarting immune defences for a number of reasons. Their invasion of tissues and cells is often 'silent'. Unlike most bacteria they do not form toxins, and as long as they do not cause extensive cell destruction there is no sign of illness until the onset of immune and inflammatory responses, sometimes several weeks after infection (hepatitis B, EB virus). Viruses can also infect cells for long periods without adverse effects on cell viability (rubella virus, wart viruses, hepatitis B virus, EB virus). In addition they establish intimate molecular

15.1

relationships with the infected cell, and they do so to a greater extent and with a greater variety of cells than intracellular bacteria and protozoa. For example, rotaviruses and adenoviruses interfere either with the antiviral action of interferon or with its production in the infected cell.

Virus latency is based on an intimate molecular relationship with the infected cell. The viral genome continues to be present in the host without producing antigens or infectious material, and only does so very occasionally, when the virus reactivates (becomes patent).

The principal strategies employed by parasites to elude the lymphocyte are concealment of antigens, antigenic variation, and immunosuppression, as discussed in the following pages.

CONCEALMENT OF ANTIGENS

A spy in a foreign country can conceal his presence from the police by hiding, by never venturing out of doors, or by adopting the disguise of a native. Parasites have the same choice. Places to hide include the interior of host cells (though the MHC molecules act as 'informers' for this compartment, picking up and transporting microbial peptides to the cell surface where they will be recognized), and particular sites in the body where lymphocytes do not normally circulate ('privileged sites', the equivalent of 'nogo' areas).

The intracellular site

If a microbe can remain inside cells without allowing its antigens to be displayed on the cell surface, it will remain unrecognized ('incognito') as far as immune defences are concerned. Specific antibody and T cell responses may be induced but the microbe inside the cell is unaffected. Persistent latent viruses such as herpes simplex in sensory neurones behave in this way. During reactivation, of course, re-exposure and boosting of immune defences is inevitable.

Other strategies are possible. Several viruses (HIV in macrophages, coronaviruses) display their proteins 'secretly' on the walls of intracellular vacuoles instead of at the cell surface, and bud into these vacuoles. Adenoviruses appear to have taken more active steps to avoid antigen display. One of the adenoviral proteins (E19) combines with class I MHC molecules and prevents their passage to the cell surface, so that infected cells are not recognized by cytotoxic T cells.

Privileged sites

The vast numbers of microbes that colonize the skin and the intestinal lumen, together with those that are shed directly into external secretions, are effectively out of reach of circulating lymphocytes. They are exposed to secretory antibodies which, although able to bind to the microbe and render it less infectious (e.g. influenza virus), are generally unable to kill the microbe or control its replication in or on the epithelial surface (Figs 15.1 and 15.2). A local inflammatory response, however, can enhance host defences.

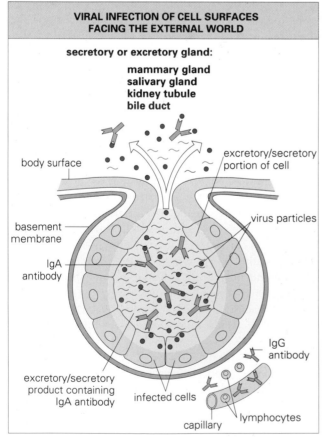

VIRAL INFECTION OF CELL SURFACES FACING THE EXTERNAL WORLD

secretory or excretory gland:
mammary gland
salivary gland
kidney tubule
bile duct

body surface

excretory/secretory portion of cell

basement membrane

virus particles

IgA antibody

IgG antibody

excretory/secretory product containing IgA antibody

infected cells

capillary

lymphocytes

Fig. 15.1 Viral infection of cell surfaces facing the external world. Infection of the surface epithelium of, for instance, a secretory or excretory gland allows direct shedding of the virus to the exterior, as well as avoidance of host immune defences.

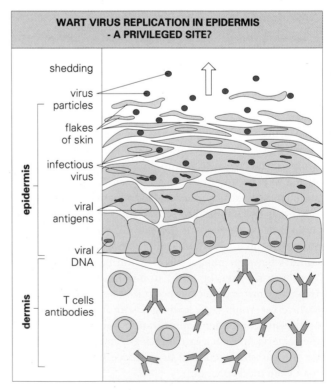

WART VIRUS REPLICATION IN EPIDERMIS - A PRIVILEGED SITE?

shedding

virus particles

flakes of skin

infectious virus

viral antigens

viral DNA

epidermis

dermis

T cells antibodies

Fig. 15.2 Wart virus replication in epidermis - A privileged site? Cell differentiation affects virus replication, and as a result maturing virus is physically removed from immune defences.

Within the body it is more difficult to avoid lymphocytes and antibodies but certain sites are safer than others. These include the CNS, joints, testis and placenta. Here lymphocyte circulation is less intense and there is more restricted access of antibodies and complement. However, as soon as inflammatory responses are induced then lymphocytes, monocytes and antibodies are rapidly delivered and the site loses its privilege.

Additional privileged sites can be created by the infectious organism itself. A good example is the hydatid cyst that develops in liver, lung or brain around growing colonies of the tapeworm *Echinococcus granulosus* (Fig. 15.3) inside which the worms can survive even though the blood of the host contains protective levels of antibody.

Perhaps the most highly privileged site of all is occupied by the retroviruses – host DNA. Retroviral RNA is transcribed by the reverse transcriptase into DNA as a necessary part of the replicative cycle and this then becomes integrated into the DNA of the host cell (see Chapter 24).

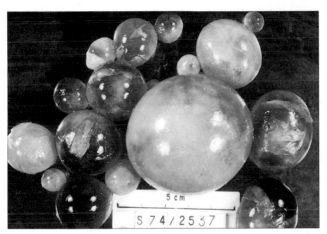

Fig. 15.3 Hydatid cysts. Multiple, thin-walled, fluid-filled cysts in a surgical specimen. The lung is a common site. Courtesy of JA Innes.

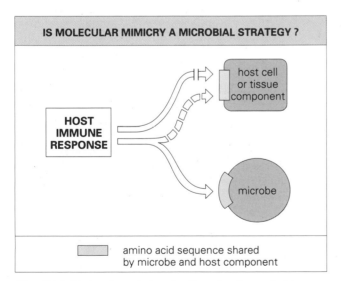

IS MOLECULAR MIMICRY A MICROBIAL STRATEGY ?

amino acid sequence shared by microbe and host component

Fig. 15.4 Molecular mimicry by the microbe probably does not restrain the immune response, but host cells and tissue could then be subject to immune damage; e.g. rheumatic heart disease following streptococcal infection is caused by antibodies reacting with meromyosin, the cross-reacting determinant.

As long as there is no cell damage and viral products are not expressed on the cell surface where they can be recognized by immune defences, the virus enjoys total anonymity. This is what makes complete cure and complete removal of virus in an HIV infected patient such a daunting task. The intragenomic site becomes even more privileged if the egg or sperm is infected. The viral genome will then be present in all embryonic cells and transferred from one generation to another as if it were the host's own DNA. Luckily this does not happen with HIV or with HTLV1 and 2. However, the 'endogenous' retroviruses of humans, present in profusion as DNA sequences in our genome, but not expressed as antigens, come into this category. They are part of our inheritance. This surely represents the ultimate, the final logical step in parasitism, at the borderline between infection and heredity.

Mimicry

If the microbe can in some way avoid inducing an immune response, this can be regarded as a 'concealment' of its antigens.

One method is by mimicking host antigens (Fig. 15.4). Numerous examples are known of parasite-derived molecules that resemble those of the host (Fig. 15.5). In the case of viral proteins, mimicry based on amino acid sequence homology (sharing of 8–10 consecutive amino acids) is seen to be common when computer comparisons

MIMICRY AND UPTAKE OF HOST ANTIGENS		
antigen	parasite	corresponding host antigen
Mimicry	EB virus	human foetal thymus*
	streptococci	cardiac muscle (meromyosin)
	klebsiella	HLA-B27**
	M. tuberculosis	65kDa heat shock protein
	N. meningitidis	embryonic brain
	Treponema	cardiolipin[†]
	Mycoplasma pneumoniae	erythrocytes[††]
	malaria	thymosin-α_1
	Trypanosoma cruzi	heart, nerve
	schistosoma	glutathione transferase
Antigen uptake	cytomegalovirus	β_2-microglobulin
	schistosoma	glycolipids, HLA, Ig etc.
	filarial nematodes	albumin

* also cross-reacts with erythrocytes of certain species and is the basis for the Paul Bunnell (heterophil antibody) test
** possible basis for ankylosing spondylitis
[†] basis for Wassermann-type antibody test for syphilis
[††] basis for cold agglutinin test

Fig. 15.5 Some examples of mimicry or uptake of host antigens by parasites.

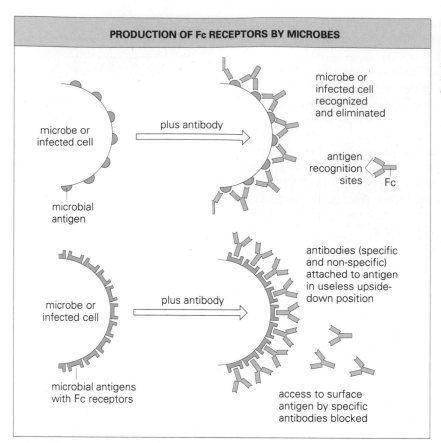

PRODUCTION OF Fc RECEPTORS BY MICROBES

microbe or infected cell

microbial antigen

plus antibody

microbe or infected cell recognized and eliminated

antigen recognition sites

Fc

microbe or infected cell

plus antibody

antibodies (specific and non-specific) attached to antigen in useless upside-down position

microbial antigens with Fc receptors

access to surface antigen by specific antibodies blocked

Fig. 15.6 The production of Fc receptors is of some benefit to the microbe. Examples include staphylococci, streptococci, herpes simplex virus, varicella-zoster virus and cytomegalovirus.

are made between viral and host proteins. Perhaps the most celebrated example, however, is the cross-reaction between group A beta-haemolytic streptococci and human myocardium. This cross-reaction underlies the development of rheumatic heart disease following repeated streptococcal infection, due to antibody made against the cross-reacting determinant meromyosin (see Fig. 15.4). The fact that the host makes such autoantibodies shows that in this case mimicry does not protect the bacteria. The conclusion is that although mimicry sounds like a useful strategy for microbes and occurs quite frequently, it does not prevent the host from making an antimicrobial, autoimmune response.

Uptake of host molecules

Microbes can conceal themselves by taking up host molecules to cover their surface (see Fig. 15.5). A superb example of this is the blood-fluke *Schistosoma* which acquires from the plasma a complete surface coat of host blood-group glycolipids, MHC antigens, immunoglobulin (Ig) molecules, etc. Such a worm must indeed be virtually invisible even to a lymphocyte. For unknown reasons, however, this strategy is essentially restricted to worms.

The uptake of Ig molecules by the microbe seems to be a more widespread phenomenon. A number of viruses and bacteria code for Fc receptors, which are displayed on their surface and bind Ig molecules of all specificities in an immunologically useless upside-down position (Fig. 15.6, and see below). This prevents access of specific antibodies or T cells to the microbe or the infected cell.

Tolerance

An alternative strategy for the microbe seems to be to avoid inducing an immune response in the first place. There are three possible methods:

1. Infection during early embryonic life, before development of the immune system, which could possibly result in immune tolerance. However, in the case of intrauterine infection with CMV, rubella virus and syphilis, the foetus does eventually produce IgM antibody, detectable in cord blood. However, cell-mediated responses are more seriously impaired. Children with congenital CMV or rubella fail to develop lymphoproliferative responses to CMV or rubella antigens and consequently take years to clear virus from the body (see Chapter 26). It is not clear whether infection in the neonatal period is more likely to result in tolerance than infection in later life. This is certainly true in some cases, such as neonatal infection with hepatitis B virus, which frequently results in permanent carriage of the virus, though the mechanism is unknown;

2. Immune tolerance to a given microbial antigen can arise when large amounts of the antigen or of antigen—antibody complexes circulate in the body. For instance anergy, as evidenced by normal antibody but depressed cell-mediated immune responses, is seen in disseminated coccidiomycosis and cryptococcosis, and in visceral and diffuse cutaneous leishmaniasis, in each case associated with large amounts of microbial antigen in the circulation;

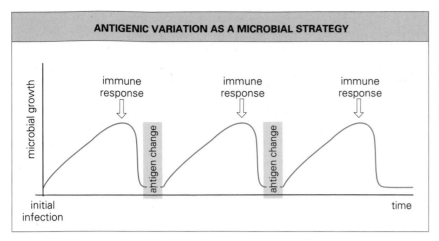

Fig. 15.7 Antigenic variation as a microbial strategy. The change in antigens may take place in the originally infected individual enabling the microbe to undergo renewed growth (e.g. trypanosomiasis), or it may take place as the microbe passes through the host population enabling it to reinfect a given individual (e.g. influenza).

3. There are likely to be certain peptides to which the host makes a poor immune response, based on the nature of the host's MHC class II molecules. These represent genetically determined 'gaps' in the host's immune repertoire, and microbes, as they evolve, might be be expected to match these peptides. In other words, microbes may be constantly 'probing' the immune repertoire of the host, seeking out weaknesses. There is no proof that this occurs but it is conceivable, for instance, that the great susceptibility of African people to tuberculosis is due to a genetically determined, poor cell-mediated immune response to key tubercular antigens. Europeans show greater resistance due to the 'weeding out' of genetically susceptible individuals that has occurred over a period of hundreds of years. It has been estimated that 30% of all adult deaths in Europe in the nineteenth century were due to tuberculosis.

ANTIGENIC VARIATION

Reverting to the image of a spy in foreign territory, there is another way to confuse the enemy – by repeated changes in appearance. The African trypanosome, the causative organism of sleeping sickness, does this, and so do a wide range of viruses, bacteria and protozoa. Antigenic variation can occur during the course of infection of a given individual or during spread of the microbe through the host community (Fig. 15.7). As a strategy for evading host immune responses it depends on the variation occurring in antigens whose recognition is involved in protection. Antigenic variation is common as the microbe passes through the host community and it tends to be more important in longer-lived hosts such as humans, where microbial survival is favoured by multiple reinfections during the lifetime of a given individual. Also it is more common in infections limited to respiratory or intestinal epithelium where the incubation period is less than a week and the microbe can infect, multiply and be shed from the body before a significant secondary immune response is generated. During systemic infections (measles, mumps, typhoid) the incubation period is longer and secondary responses have more opportunity to come into action and control an infection by an antigenic variant. Accordingly, antigenic variation is not an important feature of these systemic infections.

At the molecular level there are three main mechanisms for antigenic variation: mutation, recombination and gene switching.

Mutation

The best known example of this is influenza virus. As the virus spreads through the community there are repeated mutations in the genes coding for the haemagglutinin and the neuraminidase (see Chapter 22), causing small antigenic changes that are sufficient to reduce the effectiveness of B and T cell memory built up in response to earlier infections. This is called 'antigenic drift'. Human rhinoviruses and enteroviruses are evolving rapidly and show a similar drift. During poliovirus epidemics mutations occur at the rate of about two base substitutions per week, some of them involving the main antigenic sites on the virus. HIV (see Chapter 24) undergoes antigenic drift but in this case it occurs during infection of a given individual, which helps to explain the difficulties experienced by the immune system in controlling this infection.

Recombination

More extensive and sudden alterations in antigens can take place by exchange of genetic material between two different microbes. The classic example is genetic 'shift' in influenza A virus, in which human and avian virus strains recombine (see Chapter 22). As a result, a completely new strain of influenza A virus suddenly emerges, brandishing a haemagglutinin or neuraminidase of avian origin. This new virus, not previously experienced by the present population, gives rise to an influenza pandemic.

Gene switching

This represents the most dramatic form of antigenic variation, and was first demonstrated in the African trypanosomes *T. gambiense* and *T. rhodesiense* (see Chapter 30). These organisms carry genes for about 1000 quite distinct surface molecules, known as variant-specific glycoproteins, which cover almost the entire surface and are immunodominant. The trypanosome can switch from the use of one gene to another, much as a B cell does with the immunoglobulin heavy chain constant genes. The effect on the host is a sequence of unrelated infections at approximately weekly intervals. This enables the try-panosome to persist while the immune system is constantly trying to catch up with it. The main stimulus for each gene switch is possibly the antibody response itself but the exact mechanism is not clear. About 10% of the trypanosome genome consists of surface coat genes, but this is a worth-while investment for the parasite.

Gene switching is also thought to be responsible for the relapsing persistent course of certain other infections, including *Borrelia recurrentis* (relapsing fever) and brucel-losis. It is also important in gonorrhoea, not because of antigenic variation but because changes in bacterial prop-erties are desirable at different stages of the infection. For instance, attachment to urethral epithelium is vital early in infection by *Neisseria gonorrhoeae,* but attachment to phago-cytes less desirable. Hence there is a switching of genes coding for the pilin and outer membrane proteins that mediate attachment. However, gonococci also show great antigenic variation as they circulate through the host com-munity and this is achieved by genetic rearrangements and recombinations in the repertoire of pilin genes.

IMMUNOSUPPRESSION

A large variety of microorganisms cause immunosuppres-sion in the infected host. As a subversive strategy this makes sense, but the extent to which the microbe benefits is often debatable. The host shows a depressed immune response to antigens of the infecting microbe (antigen-spe-cific suppression) or, more commonly, both to antigens of the infecting microbe and to unrelated antigens. HIV is one of the most spectacular but by no means the only microbe that interferes with the immune system in this way (Fig. 15.8). The mechanism is generally not understood, but it often involves invasion of the immune system by the microbe – in other words *to evade, invade.*

Clearly it would benefit the microbe most if responses to its own but not to other antigens were suppressed, but this is uncommon. However a general immunosuppression, as long as it was temporary, might give the microbe enough time to grow, spread, and be shed before being eliminated. This is what happens in many virus infections. A lasting general immunosuppression would be detrimental to the microbe because susceptibility to other infections would cause unnecessary damage to the host species. From this point of view HIV has certainly overstepped the mark.

Immunosuppression by microbes often involves actual infection of immune cells, either T cells (HIV, measles), B cells (EB virus), macrophages (HIV, leishmania) or den-dritic cells (HIV). This may result in impaired cell func-tion, such as blocking of cell division, blocking of release of IL-2 or other cytokines, or in cell death.

Additional immunosuppressive actions taken by microbes include the release of immunosuppressive molecules. For instance, the gp41 polypeptide formed by HIV acts as an 'immunological anaesthetic', temporarily blocking T cell function. Other microbes (poxviruses, *T. cruzi*) release molecules that interfere with the action of

DEPRESSED IMMUNE RESPONSES CAUSED BY MICROBIAL INFECTIONS			
parasite		**feature of immunosuppression**	**mechanism**
Viruses	HIV	↓Ab ↓CMI* long-lasting	↓CD4+ T cells immunosuppressive molecule (gp41) ↓ antigen presentation by infected APC polyclonal activation of B cells
	EB virus	↓CMI temporary	includes polyclonal activation of infected B cells
	measles	↓CMI temporary	differentation blocked in infected T and B cells
	CMV	↓CMI temporary	unknown; infection of very occasional mononuclear cells
	V-ZV mumps	↓CMI temporary	infection of T cells
Bacteria	*M. leprae* (lepromatous leprosy)	↓CMI	polyclonal activation of B cells induction of suppressor T cells
Protozoa	Trypanosoma Plasmodia Toxoplasma Leishmania	↓Ab ↓CMI	?
* Ab, antibody; CMI, cell mediated immunity			

Fig. 15.8 Depressed immune responses in microbial infections. In most cases the mechanisms are unclear, but possible important factors are listed. For HIV there are at least nine possible mechanisms involved in immunosuppression, but decreased numbers of CD4+ T cells is probably the most important.

complement, or with immunologically important cytokines such as IL-2 or tumour necrosis factor. There is no doubt that other examples will be discovered in the future.

A particularly dramatic form of immune interference is practised by the staphylococci. Many strains liberate exotoxins (staphylococcal enterotoxin, epidermolytic toxin and toxic shock syndrome toxin) that are responsible for disease. At first sight, producing these toxins seems of no advantage to the staphylococci, but it is now recognized that they have extremely powerful immunomodulatory actions – they are the most potent T cell mitogens known, and act at picomolar concentrations. They function as 'superantigens', and after binding to class II MHC molecules on antigen-presenting cells, act as polyclonal activators of T cells (Fig. 15.9). A large proportion (2–20%) of all T cells respond by dividing and releasing cytokines; only 0.001–0.01% are capable of doing this in response to a regular antigen.

It would be logical to presume that these toxins were acquired (they are coded for by plasmids) by the parasite to upset immune responses and thus help in the eternal battle with host defences. As if to confirm this, it has been found that similar molecules are produced by certain streptococci and mycoplasmas.

Possible mechanisms by which the staphylococcal toxins may interfere with immune defences include:

- Excessive local liberation of cytokines by activated cells, upsetting the delicate balance of immune regulation;
- Killing of T cells or other immune cells;
- Polyclonal activation, diverting T cells of all specificities into immunologically unproductive activity (see Fig. 15.9).

Less dramatic polyclonal activation is seen in many other infections. Microbes may cause polyclonal activation of B cells as well as T cells, for example in EB virus and HIV infections, and this can be interpreted as an 'immuno-diversion' by the infecting microbe. One consequence is that a range of 'irrelevant', sometimes autoimmune antibodies are formed (e.g. heterophil antibodies in EB virus infection).

Local interference with immune defences

Some microbes do not interfere with the development of an immune response, but actively interfere with its expression in tissues. For instance *Neisseria gonorrhoeae*, *Strep. pneumoniae* and many strains of *Haemophilus influenzae* liberate a protease that cleaves human IgA antibody. These bacteria are residents or invaders of mucosae where IgA antibodies operate, and the ability to produce such as enzyme seems unlikely to be an accident.

An equally worthwhile local interference, practised by so many different infectious agents that it is likely to be significant, is the production by the microbe of Fc receptor

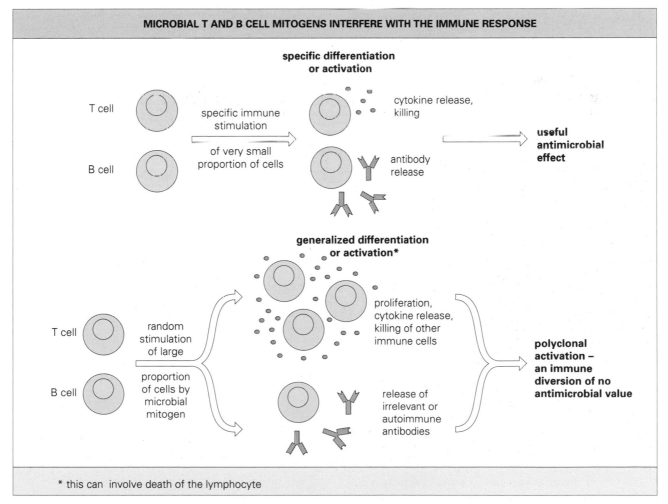

MICROBIAL T AND B CELL MITOGENS INTERFERE WITH THE IMMUNE RESPONSE

* this can involve death of the lymphocyte

Fig. 15.9 Microbial interference with the immune system by production of T or B cell mitogens (polyclonal activators).

molecules (see Fig. 15.6). The best known example is protein A, a cell wall protein excreted from virulent staphylococci, which inhibits the phagocytosis of antibody-coated bacteria, as shown in figure 15.6. Certain herpesviruses (HSV, V-ZV, CMV) code for molecules that act as Fc receptors for IgG, and streptococci produce an Fc receptor for IgA.

Other examples include the production by *Pseudomonas* of an elastase that inactivates the C3b and C5a components of complement and hence tends to inhibit opsonic and other host defence functions of complement. In addition, herpes simplex virus produces a molecule, gC (glycoprotein C), that functions as a receptor for C3b. It is present on the virus particle and on the infected cell, and by interfering with complement activation protects both the virus and the infected cell from destruction by antibody and complement.

Unfortunately, although the above phenomena look convincingly like microbial adaptations for upsetting host defences, it is not always easy to prove that this is the case.

Microbial evasion of interferons can also be considered here. Various viruses either fail to induce adequate amounts of interferons alpha and beta (hepatitis B) or have developed resistance to the antiviral action of these interferons (rotaviruses, adenoviruses).

PERSISTENT INFECTIONS

One way of looking at persistent infections (Fig. 15.10) is to regard them as failures of host defences. Host defences are designed to control microbial growth and spread and to eliminate the microbe from the body. The microbe may persist: 1. In a flagrantly defiant infectious form, as with

PERSISTENT INFECTIONS					
	microorganism	site of persistence	infectiousness of persistent microorganism	consequence	shedding of microorganism to exterior
Viruses	Herpes simplex	dorsal root ganglia salivary glands	– +	activation, cold sore none known	+ +
	Varicella-zoster	dorsal root ganglia	–	activation, zoster	+
	Cytomegalovirus	lymphoid tissue		activation +/- disease	+
	EB virus	lymphoid tissue epithelium salivary glands	– – +	lymphoid tumour nasopharyngeal carcinoma none known	– – +
	Hepatitis B	liver (virus shed into blood)	+	chronic hepatitis: liver cancer	+
	Adenoviruses	lymphoid tissue	–	none known	+
	Polyomaviruses BK and JC (man)	kidney	–	activation (pregnancy, immunosuppression)	+
	T cell leukaemia viruses	lymphoid and other tissues	±	late leukaemia, neurological disease	–
	Measles	brain	±	subacute sclerosing panencephalitis (SSPE)	–
	HIV	lymphocytes, macrophages	+	chronic disease	+
Chlamydia	Trachoma	conjunctiva	+	chronic disease and blindness	?
Rickettsia	*Rickettsia prowazeki*	lymph node	?	activation	+
Bacteria	*Salmonella typhi*	gall bladder, urinary tract	+	intermittent shedding in urine, faeces	+
	Mycobacterium tuberculosis	lung or lymph node (macrophages?)	?	activation, tuberculosis in middle aged	+
	Treponema pallidum	disseminated	±	chronic disease	–
Protozoa	*Plasmodium vivax*	liver	?	activation, clinical malaria	+
	Toxoplasma gondii	lymphoid tissue, muscle, brain	±	activation, neurological disease	–
	Trypanosoma cruzi	blood, macrophages	±	chronic disease	–

Fig. 15.10 Examples of persistent infections in humans. Shedding to be exterior takes place either directly via skin lesions, saliva, urine etc., or indirectly via the blood (hepatitis B, malaria).

15.8

hepatitis B in the blood, or the schistosome in the blood vessels of the alimentary tract or bladder; 2. In a form with low or partial infectivity, for instance adenoviruses in the tonsils and adenoids; or 3. In a completely non-infectious form, often without producing any microbial antigens. Latent virus infections are classic examples of this type of persistence. In the case of herpes simplex virus, viral DNA persists for many years, probably for life, in sensory neurones in the dorsal root ganglia.

The molecular basis for viral latency has still not been elucidated. It involves special adaptations by the virus to the state of latency – in the case of herpes simplex there are 'latency-associated transcripts' produced in infected neurones that are needed to maintain this delicate type of intracellular parasitism.

Latent infections are so-called because they can become patent. This is where they become of immense medical interest. The legacy of latent herpesvirus infections in man is described in Chapter 29. Patterns of acute and persistent infections are illustrated in figure 15.11.

During their persistence, such infections are not important causes of acute illness and, by their nature, cannot be

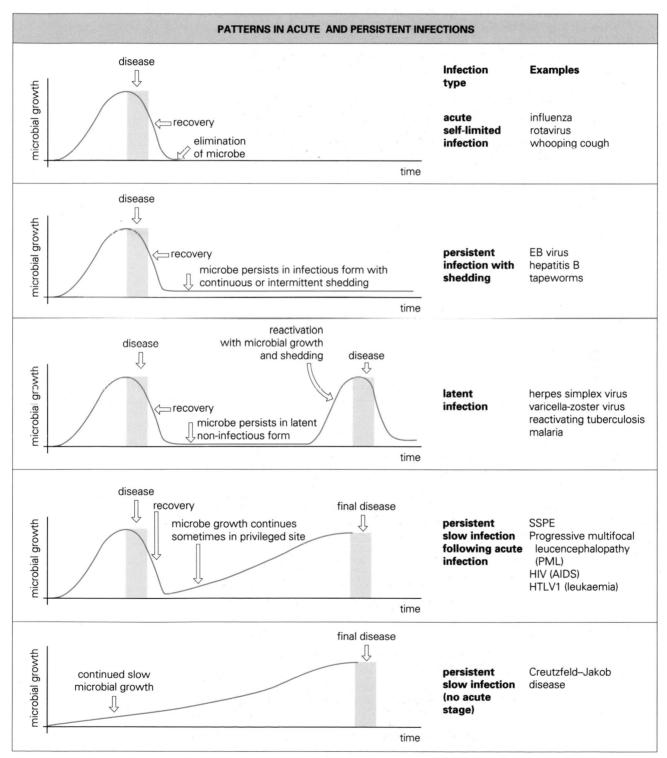

Fig. 15.11 Patterns of acute and persistent infections. For some microbes (e.g. CMV, tuberculosis) the distinction between persistence in infections from and true latency is not clear.

Persistence is of survival value for the microbe

Persistence without any further shedding (e.g. SSPE, PML) is of no survival value, but there are obvious advantages if the microbe is also shed, either continuously or intermittently. This is especially true when the host species consists of small, isolated groups of individuals (Fig. 15.12). Measles, for instance, is not normally a persistent infection. It only infects humans, does not survive for long outside the body, and has nowhere else to go (i.e. there is no animal reservoir). Without a continued supply of fresh susceptible humans the virus could not maintain itself and would become extinct. There has to be, at all times, someone acutely infected with measles. From studies of island communities it is clear that you need a minimum of about 500 000 humans to maintain measles without reintroduction from outside. In palaeolithic times, when humans lived in small, isolated groups, measles could not have existed in its present form.

By contrast, persistent and latent infections are admirably adapted for survival under these circumstances. Varicella-zoster virus can maintain itself in a community of less than a thousand individuals. Children get chickenpox, the virus persists in latent form in sensory neurones and later in life, the virus reactivates to cause shingles. By this time a new generation of susceptible individuals has appeared, and the shingles vesicles provide a fresh source of virus.

Serological studies show that the viral infection prevalent in small, completely isolated Indian communities in the Amazon basin are persistent or latent (adenoviruses, polyomaviruses, papillomaviruses, the seven human herpes viruses, etc.) rather than non-persistent (influenza, measles, polio, etc.) The same applies to those non-viral infections in which there is no animal reservoir for maintenance of the microbe (typhoid, respiratory tuberculosis).

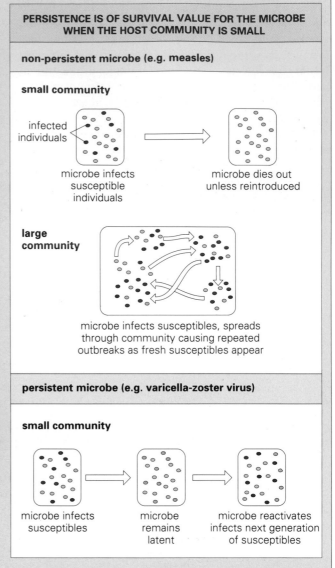

PERSISTENCE IS OF SURVIVAL VALUE FOR THE MICROBE WHEN THE HOST COMMUNITY IS SMALL

non-persistent microbe (e.g. measles)

small community

infected individuals

microbe infects susceptible individuals

microbe dies out unless reintroduced

large community

microbe infects susceptibles, spreads through community causing repeated outbreaks as fresh susceptibles appear

persistent microbe (e.g. varicella-zoster virus)

small community

microbe infects susceptibles

microbe remains latent

microbe reactivates infects next generation of susceptibles

Fig. 15.12 Persistence is a microbial survival strategy.

acutely lethal. Persisting adenoviruses and typhoid bacilli can be compared with non-persistent yet life-threatening infections such as cholera, paralytic poliomyelitis and tetanus.

Persistent infections are important for four main reasons:

- They can be reactivated (Fig. 15.13). This occurs in immunocompromised patients, and is of major clinical importance in those immunosuppressed as a result of chronic disease, tumours (leukaemias, lymphomas), or in those immunosuppressed by the physician following organ transplantation. From the microbe's point of view, latency is an adaptation that allows reactivation, with renewed growth and shedding of the infectious agent during naturally occuring periods of immunocompromise, the most important of these being pregnancy and old age;

- They are sometimes associated with chronic disease, as in the case of chronic hepatitis B infections, subacute sclerosing panencephalitis (SSPE) following measles, and AIDS;

- They are sometimes associated with cancers, such as hepatocellular carcinoma with hepatitis B virus and Burkitt's lymphoma and nasopharyngeal carcinoma with EB virus;

- From the microbial viewpoint, they enable the infectious agent to persist in the host community (see panel above).

Reactivation

Features of reactivation in herpes virus infections are described in Chapters 24, 28 and 29. We still know very little about reactivation mechanisms at the molecular level, as might be expected in view of our ignorance about the latent state itself.

However, it is useful to distinguish two stages in reactivation (Fig. 15.14). The first event (stage A), the resumption of viral activity in the latently infected cell, is the most mysterious one. In the case of herpes simplex virus this can be triggered by sensory stimuli arriving in the neurone (from skin areas responding to sunlight), and also by certain fevers (i.e. during other infections) or by hormonal influences. Little more than this is known!

REACTIVATION OF PERSISTENT INFECTIONS		
Circumstance	**Infectious agent**	**Site of shedding**
Old age	varicella-zoster virus	skin vesicles
	tuberculosis	saliva
Pregnancy	polyomaviruses (BK, JC)	urine
	CMV	cervix
	HSV2	cervix
	EB virus	saliva
Leukaemias, lymphomas (e.g. Hodgkins' disease)	varicella-zoster virus	skin vesicles
	polyomavirus (JC)	CNS (PML)*
Post-transplant immunosuppression	HSV	skin/mucosal lesions
	varicella-zoster virus	skin vesicles
	wart viruses	skin
	CMV	viraemia, pneumonitis*
	EB virus	saliva
	hepatitis B	blood
HIV infection	*Pneumocystis carinii*	lung*
	Toxoplasma gondii	CNS*
	varicella-zoster virus	skin vesicles
	HSV	skin/mucosal lesions
	M. tuberculosis	lung
	polyomavirus (JC)	CNS (PML)*

* No shedding from these sites

Fig.15.13 Reactivation of persistent infections.

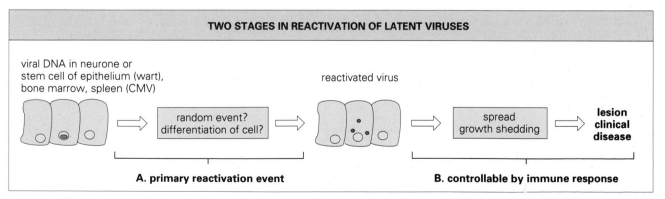

Fig. 15.14 Two stages in reactivation of latent viruses.

The second event (stage B) involves the spread and replication of the reactivated virus. Herpes simplex virus (HSV) must travel down the sensory axon to the skin or mucosal surface, infect and spread in subepithelial tissues and then in the epithelium, finally forming a virus-rich vesicle (more than a million infectious units per ml of vesicle fluid). All this takes at least 3–4 days. Stage B is less mysterious and can be controlled by the immune system. Thus, cold sores

may be associated with poor lymphocyte responses to HSV antigens, and zoster with declining cell-mediated responses (specifically to V-ZV antigens) in old people.

Stage A probably occurs more frequently than stage B, because immune defences often arrest the process during stage B before final production of the lesion. Hence as many as 10–20% of HSV reactivation episodes are thought to be 'non-lesional' with burning, tingling, itching at the site but no signs of a cold sore. Also zoster may involve no more than the sensory prodrome, associated with virus reactivation and replication in sensory neurones; skin lesions are prevented by host defences.

Reactivation of EB virus and CMV, with appearance of the virus in saliva (EBV) or blood (CMV) is generally asymptomatic. In immunologically deficient individuals, however, reactivation may progress to cause clinical disease, either hepatitis and pneumonitis in the case of CMV or the rarer hairy tongue leukoplakia due to EBV (see Chapter 29).

SUMMARY

Parasites survive in the face of immune responses by a variety of strategies. The most important of these are concealment from lymphocytes, resemblance between parasite and host antigens (either by mimicry or actual uptake of host molecules), antigenic variation and immunosuppression. One or more of these strategies is used by the majority of successful parasites to avoid elimination. Some parasites persist for long periods of time, either with or without the production of symptoms, and some of these can be reactivated after many years, thereby increasing the opportunities for further transmission.

Further Reading

Fitzpatrick DR, Bielefeldt-Ohmann H. Mechanisms of herpes virus immuno-evasion. *Microb Pathogenesis* 1991; **10**: 253–259.

Hidaka Y, Sakai Y, Toh Y, Mori R. Glycoprotein C of herpes simplex virus type 1 is essential for the virus to evade antibody-dependant complement-mediated virus inactivation and lysis of virus-infected cells. *J Gen Virol* 1991; **72**: 915–920.

Joiner KA. Complement evasion by bacteria and parasites. *Ann Rev Microbiol* 1988; **42**: 201–230.

Oldstone MBA. Molecular mimicry as a mechanism for the cause and as a probe uncovering etiologic agents of autoimmune disease. *Curr Topics Microbiol Immunol* 1989; **145**: 127

Roizman B, Sears AE. An inquiry into the mechanisms of herpes simplex virus latency. *A Rev Microbiol* 1987; **41**: 543–571

Rosenberg ZF, Fanci AS. Immunopathogenic mechanisms of HIV infection: cytokine induction of HIV expression. *Immunol Today* 1990; **11**: 176–180

16 PATHOLOGICAL CONSEQUENCES OF INFECTION

INTRODUCTION

Symptoms that appear rapidly after the acquisition of an infection are usually due to the direct action of the invading microbe or its secretions. Thus, a virus in a cell may cause metabolic 'shut-down', or lyse the cell. Bacteria, however, provoke most of their acute effects by releasing toxins, but may also cause distress through the induction of inflammation. The inflammatory response is, of course, an important component of host protection, vascular permeability being vital for the rapid mobilization of cells such as neutrophils, and serum components such as complement and antibody. Thus, inflammation is intrinsically a healthy sign and it is interesting that some extremely virulent bacteria (e.g. *Staphylococci*) can to some extent inhibit the inflammatory response.

Often, however, pathological changes are secondary to the activation of immunological mechanisms normally thought of as protective. These may involve the natural or the adaptive immune system or, more usually, both (Fig. 16.1). Tissue damage resulting from adaptive immune responses is usually referred to as 'immunopathology', and is unfortunately quite common in infectious diseases, particularly chronic persistent ones. The immunological basis of these mechanisms of tissue damage is described in Chapter 9.

PATHOLOGY CAUSED DIRECTLY BY THE PARASITE

Organisms which multiply in cells and subsequently spread usually do so by rupturing the cell. Many viruses and some intracellular bacteria and protozoa behave in this way (Fig. 16.2). It is important to realize that many others do not. For example, viruses or bacteria may remain latent (e.g. herpes simplex and varicella in nerve ganglia and *M. tuberculosis* in macrophages), and many viruses can bud from a cell without disrupting it. The type of cell infected may also have an influence on survival of the organism, thus HIV lyses T cells but persists in macrophages. Other direct effects include blockage of major hollow viscera by worms, of the lung alveoli by dense growth of, for example, pneumocystis, and mechanical effect of large cysts (e.g. hydatid).

Exotoxins

A common and serious cause of tissue damage, especially in bacterial infection, is the active secretion of 'exotoxins' by the parasite (Fig. 16.3). In some cases these are clearly part of its strategy for entry, spread, or defence against the host, but sometimes they seem to be of little or no benefit to the parasite.

Most exotoxins are proteins, often coded not by the bacterial DNA but in plasmids (e.g. *E.coli*) or phages (e.g. botulism, diphtheria, scarlet fever). In some cases they consist of two or more subunits, one of which is required for binding and entry to the cell while the other switches on or inhibits some cellular function. Fortunately toxins can often be inactivated (e.g. by formaldehyde) without altering their antigenicity and the resulting toxoids are among the most successful of all vaccines (see Chapter 36), the classic examples being diphtheria and tetanus toxoids. Toxins are generally more highly conserved in their structure than the surface antigens of the organism secreting them. This allows for more effective cross-immunity and, for example, explains why scarlet fever (caused by streptococcal erythrotoxin) usually occurs only once, while streptococcal infections may recur almost indefinitely.

An interesting offshoot of the two-subunit structure of toxins is that by changing the specificity of the part responsible for attachment, the specificity of the toxin for a particular cell type can be changed. An example is the plant toxin ricin, whose A subunit can be attached to a monoclonal antibody to make it a specific poison for tumour cells. The same strategy could obviously be used against

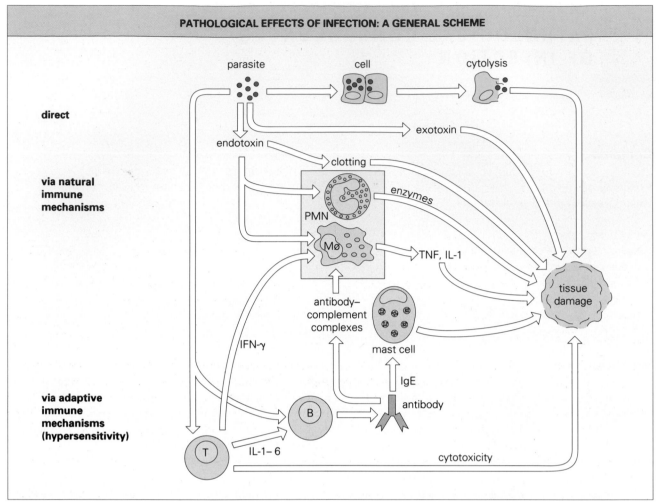

Fig. 16.1 Pathological effects of infection: a general scheme. Infectious parasitic organisms can cause disease directly (top) or indirectly via over-activation of various immune mechanisms, either natural (centre) or adaptive (bottom). Mø, macrophage.

ORGANISMS THAT DIRECTLY DAMAGE TISSUE		
organism	**cell or tissue damaged**	**mechanism**
Viruses polio rhinovirus HIV coxsackie rotavirus	neurones URT mucosa CD4, T cells, macrophages pancreatic β cells, heart enterocytes	cytopathic
Bacteria *Streptococcus mutans* mycobacteria	teeth macrophages	acid production damaged macrophage releases cytokines
Fungi *Histoplasma*	macrophages	damaged macrophage releases cytokines
Protozoa *Plasmodium*	erythrocytes	damaged erythrocyte removed
Helminths *Ascaris* *Echinococcus*	intestinal occlusion biliary occlusion hydatid cyst	mechanical mechanical, inflammation pressure effects

Fig. 16.2 Many organisms directly damage or destroy the tissues they infect. This is especially common with cytopathic viruses. URT, upper respiratory tract.

EXOTOXINS OF IMPORTANCE IN DISEASE				
organism	exotoxin	tissue damaged	action	disease
Bacteria				
Clostridium tetani	tetanospasmin	neurones	spastic paralysis	tetanus
Clostridium perfringens	α-toxin	erythrocytes, platelets leucocytes, endothelium	cell lysis	gas gangrene
Clostridium botulinum	neurotoxin	nerve-muscle junction	flaccid paralysis	botulism
Corynebacterium diphtheriae	diphtheria toxin	throat, heart. peripheral nerve	inhibits protein synthesis	diphtheria
Shigella dysenteriae	enterotoxin	intestinal mucosa	—	dysentery
Escherichia coli	enterotoxin	intestinal epithelium	fluid loss from intestinal cells	gastroenteritis
Vibrio cholerae	enterotoxin			cholera
Staphylococcus aureus	α-toxin	red & white cells (via cytokines)	haemolysis	abcesses
	haemolysin		haemolysis	
	leucocidin	leucocytes	destroys leucocytes	
	enterotoxin	intestinal cells	induces vomiting, diarrhoea	food poisoning
	TSST1	—	release of cytotoxins	toxic shock syndrome
	epidermolytic	epidermis	—	scalded skin syndrome
Streptococcus pyogenes	streptolysin O & S	red and white cells	haemolysis	haemolysis, pyogenic lesion
	erythrogenic	skin capillaries	skin rash	scarlet fever
Bacillus anthracis	cytotoxin	lung	pulmonary oedema	anthrax
Bordetella pertussis	pertussis toxin	trachea	kills epithelium	whooping cough
Legionella pneumophila	numerous	neutrophils	cell lysis	legionnaire's disease
Listeria monocytogenes	haemolysin	leucocytes, monocytes	cell lysis	listeriosis
Pseudomonas aeruginosa	exotoxin A	cell lysis	cell lysis	various infections
Fungi				
Aspergillus fumigatus	aflatoxin	liver	carcinogenic	?liver damage/cancer
Protozoa				
Entamoeba histolytica	enterotoxin	colonic epithelium	cell lysis	amoebic dysentery

Fig. 16.3 Exotoxins of importance in disease. Many bacteria and a few other organisms damage host tissues by the secretion of exotoxins. Some bacterial exotoxins are among the most powerful toxins known. Fortunately vaccination, by inducing antibody, is often very effective in protection.

parasites if desired. The mode of action of toxins (Fig. 16.4), and the consequences for the host, can be considered under four headings:

Toxins promoting survival or spread of bacteria
A number of bacteria release enzymes that break down the tissues or the intercellular substances of the host, allowing the infection to spread freely. Among these enzymes are hyaluronidase, collagenase, DNAase and streptokinase. Some staphylococci release a coagulase which deposits a protective layer of fibrin onto and around the cells, thus localizing them.

Toxins damaging or destroying cells
Cell membranes can be damaged enzymatically by lecithi-nases or phospholipases, or by insertion of pore-forming molecules that destroy the integrity of the cell. The collective term for such toxins is 'haemolysins', although many cells other than red blood cells can be affected. Both staphylococci and streptococci produce pore-forming toxins; pseudomonads release enzymatic haemolysins.

Toxins interfering with cell metabolism
Several toxins enter cells and actively alter some of their metabolic machinery. Characteristically these toxin molecules have two subunits. The A subunit is the active component, whereas the B subunit is a binding component needed to interact with receptors on the cell membrane. When binding occurs the A subunit, or the whole toxin–receptor complex, is taken into the cell by endocytosis, and the A subunit

becomes activated. Two well-studied toxins of this type are those of diphtheria (see Chapter 20) and cholera.

Diphtheria. The toxin is synthesized as a single polypeptide (from bacteriophage *n* genes) and binds by the B subunit to target cells (see Fig. 16.4). Partial cleavage of the polypeptide takes place and then the entire toxin–receptor complex is internalized. The A subunit then splits off and passes into the cytosol, where it inactivates transfer of amino acids from transfer RNA to the polypeptide chain during translation of mRNA by ribosomes. It does this by

catalysing attachment of adenosine diphosphate ribose to the elongation protein (ADP ribosylation), effectively blocking protein synthesis.

Cholera. Here the toxin is released as a complex of five B subunits surrounding the A subunit. The latter is cleaved into two fragments Al and A2 held by disulphide bonds. The B subunits bind to ganglioside receptors on intestinal epithelial cells, leading to internalization of the A subunits which then separate from one another (see Fig. 16.4). The A1 portion then ADP-ribosylates one of the regulatory

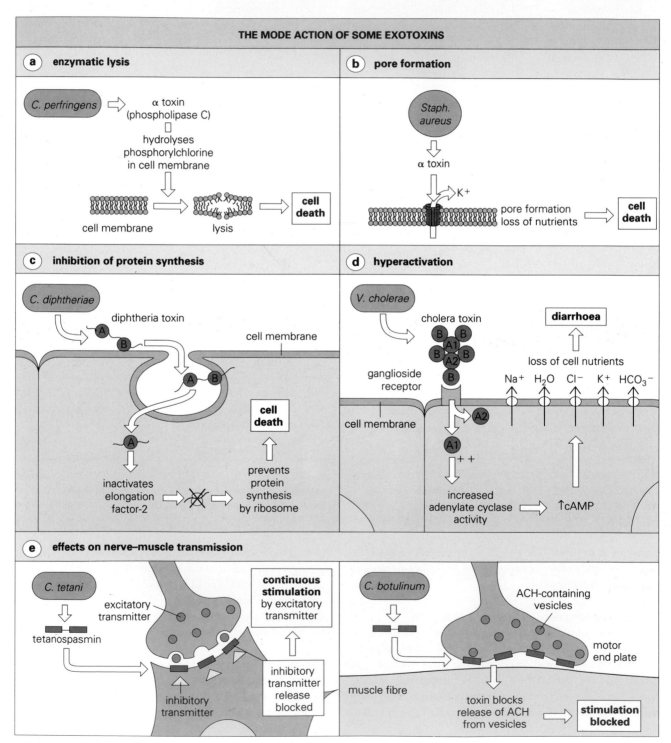

Fig.16.4 The mode of action of some exotoxins. Bacterial toxins act in a variety of ways. Often the toxin is a two-chain molecule, one chain being concerned with entry into cells while the other has inhibitory activity against some vital function.

molecules involved in the production of cyclic AMP. As a result the molecule is unable to turn off production. The increased levels of cAMP in the cell change the Na^+/Cl^- flux across the cell membrane, resulting in a massive outflow of water from the cell and causing the profuse diarrhoea of cholera. The exotoxins of *E. coli* and *Salmonella* have similar actions, as does pertussis toxin.

Toxins affecting passage of nerve impulses

The toxins of tetanus and botulism are among the most potent known, one gram of botulinum toxin being sufficient to kill 10 million people! They have the characteristic A + B structure, the B subunit binding to ganglioside receptors on nerve cells. The internalized A subunit of tetanus is carried by axonal transport from the point of production to the CNS, where it interferes with synaptic transmission in inhibitory neurones by blocking neurotransmitter release. This allows the excitatory transmitter to continuously stimulate the motoneurones, causing spastic paralysis. Botulinum toxin enters the body via the intestine, escaping digestion and crossing the gut wall. The toxin affects peripheral nerve endings at the neuromuscular junction, blocking presynaptic release of acetylcholine. This prevents muscle contraction, causing flaccid paralysis.

Diarrhoea

Diarrhoea, is an almost invariable result of intestinal infections and one of the major causes of death in children world-wide (see Chapter 25). It can be looked at in two ways – as a means for the host to rid itself rapidly of the infectious organism, and as a means for the infection to spread to other hosts.

Diarrhoea is a feature of a wide range of organisms, but in only a few cases is the exact mechanism understood. Damage to the intestinal epithelium is usually the underlying cause, and this may be due directly to infection of the cells (e.g. by rotaviruses) or by the effect of toxins (e.g. cholera, shigella). Many of the organisms causing diarrhoea can be picked up from food, but the term 'food poisoning' is usually reserved for those cases where toxins are already present in the food rather than being generated during the growth of organisms in the intestine. As would be expected, the former causes symptoms earlier, hours after exposure as opposed to days (Fig. 16.5).

PATHOLOGICAL ACTIVATION OF NATURAL IMMUNE MECHANISMS

The very potent natural immune mechanisms discussed in Chapter 12 have in-built safety as far as specificity is concerned. They have had to evolve in the constant presence of the host's 'self' antigens, which they therefore do not respond to. However, they are not so well insured in the quantitative sense, and there are many cases where overactivity in the process of damaging an invading parasite can also damage innocent host tissues.

INFECTIOUS CAUSES OF DIARRHOEA		
food poisoning (due to pre-formed toxin in food)		
	onset	source
Staphylococcus aureus	1–6 hrs	cream, meat, poultry
Clostridium perfringens	8–20 hrs	reheated meat
Clostridium botulinum	12–36 hrs	canned food
Bacillus cereus	1–20 hrs	reheated foods
intestinal infections		
	onset	source
Rotavirus	2–5 days	contact (faecal–oral)
Salmonella	1–2 days	eggs
Shigella	1–4 days	faecal–oral
Campylobacter	1–4 days	poultry, domestic animals
V. cholerae	2 days	faecal–oral
E. coli	1–4 days	traveller's diarrhoea
Yersinia enterocolitica	days–weeks	pets (e.g. dogs)
Giardia lamblia	1–2 weeks	contaminated water
Entamoeba histolytica	days–weeks	
Cryptosporidium	days–weeks	faecal–oral,
Isopora belli		opportunistic (e.g. in AIDS)

Fig.16.5 Infectious causes of diarrhoea. World-wide infectious diarrhoea is the major cause of infant mortality.

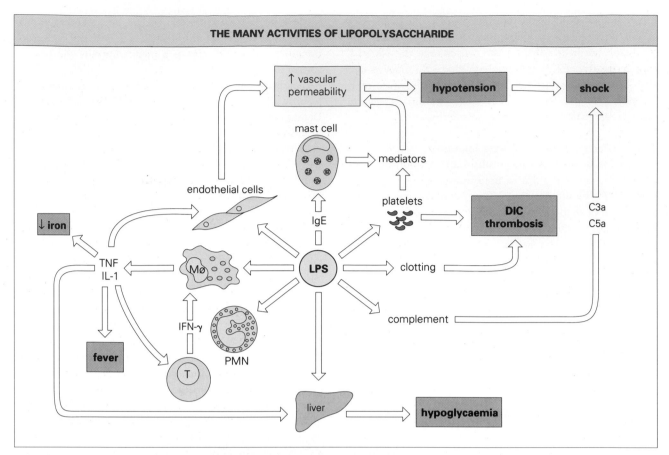

THE MANY ACTIVITIES OF LIPOPOLYSACCHARIDE

Fig.16.6 The many activities of LPS. Bacterial endotoxin (LPS) activates almost every immune mechanism as well as the clotting pathway, which together make LPS one of the most powerful immune stimuli known. DIC, disseminated intravascular coagulation

Endotoxins, macrophages and cytokines

Deceptively similar to exotoxins in name, but profoundly different in their significance, are the 'endotoxins' of bacteria and other microorganisms. Unlike exotoxins, these are integral parts of the microbial cell wall, normally released only when the cell dies. Endotoxins are particularly characteristic of Gram-negative bacteria, and are typically lipopolysaccharides (LPS) composed of a lipid portion (lipid A) inserted into the cell wall, a conserved core polysaccharide, and the highly variable O-polysaccharide, responsible for the serological diversity which is a feature of organisms such as salmonella and shigella.

Lipopolysaccharides stimulate an extraordinary range of host responses, or perhaps one should say a wide range of responses have evolved to respond to LPS. In the words of Lewis Thomas "when we sense lipopolysaccharide, we are likely to turn on every defence at our disposal" (Fig. 16.6). Evidently the body needs to be aware of invading Gram-negative bacteria at the earliest possible stage.

Clinically, the most important effects of LPS are fever and vascular collapse, or shock. As mentioned in Chapter 12, fever may benefit host or parasite or both, and is currently considered to be mainly due to the action on the hypothalamus of two cytokines, interleukin-1 (IL-1) and tumour necrosis factor (TNF), both of which are produced by macrophages in response to LPS (and to analogous molecules from other organisms, see below).

Endotoxin (or 'septic') shock is usually associated with systemic spread of organisms, the commonest example being septicaemia with Gram-negative bacteria such as *E. coli, N. meningitidis*, etc. However, many other organisms also release molecules that stimulate TNF and/or IL-1 production (Fig. 16.7) and thus function in part like LPS, although they are more or less unrelated in structure. For example, in the 'toxic shock syndrome' of young women with staphylococcal infections of the genital tract, the toxin (TSST1) is a protein.

The involvement of cytokines in the pathogenesis of shock is by no means a purely academic concern, because it suggests the possibility of treatment by antagonists of a small number of cytokines (e.g. by monoclonal antibodies or inhibitors) rather than by antibodies to the toxins themselves, which are of enormous antigenic diversity. This idea is discussed further in Chapter 34.

At present the cytokine most closely linked to disease is TNF. Raised levels of TNF in the serum have been shown to correlate with severity in patients with meningococcal septicaemia and with *P. falciparum* malaria. However, animal experiments indicate that in such cases TNF probably synergizes with other cytokines such as IL-1 and IFN-γ to produce its full effects. In meningococcal disease, TNF levels in blood and cerebrospinal fluid can change independently, the former being raised in septicaemia and the latter in meningitis; thus, it appears that the production and/or effects of TNF can be restricted to a particular body compartment.

IMPORTANT ENDOTOXINS AND FUNCTIONALLY RELATED MOLECULES		
organisms	toxin	cytokines induced

Bacteria
Gram-negative
  Salmonella
  Shigella
  E. coli
  N. meningitidis
	LPS	TNF, IL-1

Gram-positive *Staph. aureus*	TSST1	TNF
mycobacteria	lipoarabinomannan	TNF
Bordetella pertussis	endotoxin	TNF
Fungi yeasts	zymosan	TNF
Protozoa *Plasmodium*	phospholipids (exoantigens)	TNF

Fig.16.7 Important endotoxins and functionally related molecules. Most, but not all, endotoxins are lipopolysaccharides, and exert their main effects by stimulating cytokine release.

Complement and neutrophils

The activation of complement is a vital part of immunity to many bacteria, viruses and protozoa (see Chapter 12). However, complement is also involved in several tissue-damaging reactions. One of these, immune complex disease, involves the participation of antibody and is discussed later. Complement also plays an important role in the acute inflammatory response via the generation of the chemotactic factors C3a and C5a (see Chapter 4). Direct activation of complement by LPS may contribute to the shock induced by toxic amounts of this endotoxin, in which the levels of complement components (e.g. C3) drop profoundly; this response appears to involve both the classical and the alternative pathways, activated by the lipid and polysaccharide components respectively. C3a and C5a are produced in large amounts and there is frequently a severe fall in polymorphonucleocytes (PMN), due to aggregation of these cells, adherence to vessel walls, and their activation to release toxic molecules, both oxidative and non-oxidative. When this occurs in the pulmonary capillaries, severe pulmonary oedema may result – the 'adult respiratory distress syndrome' (ARDS).

Platelets and coagulation

A rare but serious feature of bacterial (e.g. meningococcal) septicaemia, seen also in some virus infections, is 'disseminated intravascular coagulation' (DIC). The relative contribution of immune complexes, platelets, and direct activation of the clotting pathway via the effect of LPS on Hageman factor, remain controversial. For example, the haemorrhagic phenomena of yellow fever are probably secondary to coagulation defects due to the extensive liver damage, while in dengue ('haemorrhagic') fever immune complex deposition in blood vessels has been suggested. However, in all these haemorrhagic syndromes the role of cytokines such as TNF also needs consideration.

Mast cells and basophils

Mast cell degranulation in response to LPS is thought to be secondary to IgE antibody formation, though some insect venoms may be able to activate mast cells directly; reactions of this kind are called 'anaphylactoid'.

PATHOLOGICAL CONSEQUENCES OF THE IMMUNE RESPONSE

Adaptive immune responses are vital to defence against infection, as witnessed by the increased susceptibility to infectious disease in immunodeficient patients (see Chapter 33). The antimicrobial effects of lymphocyte responses act mainly by specifically focusing or enhancing non-specific effector mechanisms (see Chapter 5). Unfortunately this may also result in enhancement of the pathological effects outlined above. Such over-reaction of the immune system is known as 'hypersensitivity', and the tissue damaging effects as 'immunopathological'.

The most widely-used classification of hypersensitivity is that of Coombs and Gell, outlined in Chapter 9, which is based on the immunological mechanism underlying the tissue-damaging reaction. Each of the four main types of hypersensitivity can be of microbial or non-microbial origin, but the microbial types include some of the most serious (Fig. 16.8). Organisms of many sorts can be involved, but one common feature is that the infection is prolonged, with continuous or repeated antigenic stimulation.

Allergic reactions (type I)

The most dramatic reaction of this type is that following the rupture of a hydatid cyst. Slow leakage of worm antigens ensures that the patient's mast cells are sensitized with specific IgE, and the massive flood of antigens on rupture may cause acute fatal anaphylaxis, with vascular collapse and pulmonary oedema. Even the small amount of antigen used in diagnostic skin tests can have this effect.

Another worm associated with high levels of IgE is *Ascaris* but here the pathological consequences are mainly respiratory, with eosinophilic infiltrates and asthmatic episodes corresponding to the passage of the parasite through the lung. The itching rashes characteristic of helminth infections, where the worms die in the skin are probably also of this type, an example being 'swimmer's itch' due to animal or avian schistosomes.

Why allergic reactions are such a feature of worm infections is not really clear, but they may be due to some feature of the antigens; moreover, it has been suggested that IgE plays a role in protection against parasites of this type. One would hope so, as in all other respects this class of antibody appears to be nothing but a nuisance.

Cytotoxic reactions and autoantibody (type II)

Strictly speaking, type II reactions are mediated by antibody (usually IgG) leading to cytotoxicity, either extracellular or

HYPERSENSITIVITY OF MICROBIAL ORIGIN		
Coombs & Gell classification	**principal mechanism**	**examples**

Type I (allergic/anaphylactic)	IgE, mast cells	helminths
		  Ascaris
		  hydatid (ruptured cyst)
		? viral skin rash
		? upper respiratory
		  viral infections

Type II (cytotoxic)	IgG to surface complement cytotoxic cells	virus infected cells
		malaria infected erythrocytes
		autoantibodies in:
		  Mycoplasma
		  streptococci
		  T. cruzi

Type III (immune complex-mediated)	immune complexes complement PMN	in tissues:
		  allergic alveolitis
		   actinomycosis
		in blood vessels:
		  glomerulonephritis
		  malaria
		  streptococci
		  hepatitis B
		  syphilis

Type IV (cell mediated)	T lymphocytes cytokines macrophages (and other non-specific cells)	granuloma
		  tuberculosis
		  leprosy (tuberculoid)
		  schistosomiasis (eggs)
		  Histoplasma
		mononuclear infiltration
		  ± cell damage in many
		  virus infections
		  (i.e. tissue delayed-type
		  hypersensitivity responses)
		  with CD4, CD8, cytokines
		  and macrophages playing roles
		viral rashes

Autoimmunity	cross reaction
	  with host
	
	polyclonal B
	  cell activation
		streptococcal myocarditis
		
		African trypanosomiasis

Fig.16.8 Hypersensitivity of microbial origin. All four classic types of hypersensitivity can be induced by infectious organisms, types II and III being the most commonly encountered. Note that some mechanisms that mediate hypersensitivity also take part in protective immunity.

intracellular (e.g. after phagocytosis). Cytotoxicity by T cells is considered under type IV reactions.

An important distinction can be made between antibodies to the (foreign) infectious organism and autoantibodies; the former kill host cells because they display foreign antigens, whereas the latter bind to unaltered host antigens: both types of response are found in infectious disease (see Fig. 16.8). In the latter case, of course, the interesting question is why autoantibodies should be formed during infection; the mechanisms that have been postulated for this are discussed in Chapter 9.

An example of microbial antigens attaching themselves to host cells is blood-stage malaria, where it has been shown that the haemolytic anaemia is due not to autoantibody as previously thought, but to antibodies to parasite-derived antigen that have been picked up by red cells. In some cases it may be the antigen–antibody complex that binds to the cell. A similar reaction can occur following quinine treatment of *P. falciparum* malaria (blackwater fever). Viruses budding from cells are another good example of microbial and host antigens becoming closely associated.

The classic example of an autoantibody triggered by infection is the anti-myocardial antibody of group A beta-haemolytic streptococcal infection, which is due to the presence of the same cross-reacting carbohydrate antigen on the bacterium and the myocardium. However, as more protein sequences are obtained and compared, numerous other similar examples have come to light, and it is possible that cross-reaction between microbial and human antigens may underlie a number of diseases currently of unknown origin. The question whether this mimicry of host antigens has any survival value to the microbe is discussed in Chapter 15.

Immune complexes and disease (type III)

Without the formation of immune complexes, antibody would have a very limited role in protective immunity. However complications occur when the complexes escape

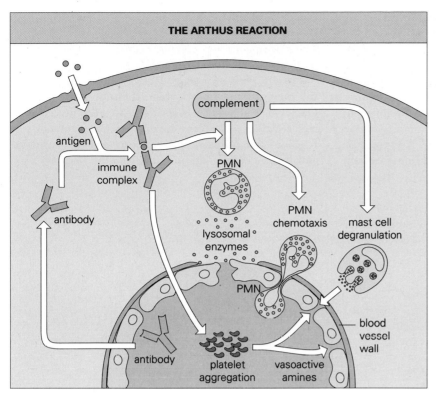

THE ARTHUS REACTION

Fig.16.9 The Arthus reaction. Microbial antigens that enter the tissues (e.g. fungal particles in the lung) encounter antibody and form immune complexes. These activate complement and initiate chemotaxis of PMN, and degranulation of these and tissue mast cells. The resulting inflammatory response is further potentiated by damage induced by PMN-derived lysosomal enzymes.

removal by the phagocytes of the reticulo-endothelial system, and become lodged in the tissues or blood vessels, attracting the attention of complement and of neutrophils. Release of lysosomal enzymes then results in local damage, which is particularly serious in small blood vessels, especially in the renal glomeruli. Immune complex disease is a major cause of both acute and chronic glomerulonephritis, and the majority of cases are probably the result of infection. However, there is also an important group in which autoantigen–autoantibody complexes are responsible (e.g. DNA/anti-DNA in systemic lupus erythematosus), and even these may ultimately be the consequence of virus infection.

Like most other immunopathological conditions, immune complex deposition is usually a feature of chronic infection, for example malaria. However, a persistent antigenic stimulus is not the only prerequisite, indicated by the fact that the most serious form of malarial nephropathy is found in *P. malariae* (quartan) malaria, which progresses despite successful treatment of the infection, whilst the nephropathy of *P. falciparum* (malignant tertian) malaria typically recovers after the infection is cured. Special predisposing factors may include a poor antibody response, in terms of either amount or affinity, a particular tendency of the antigen itself to bind to vascular endothelium, or inhibition of the normal function of phagocytes or complement in removing circulating complexes.

Immune complex deposition in the tissues, made famous by the work of Arthus on antigens injected into the skin of animals with pre-existing antibody (mainly IgG), shows up as a combination of thrombosis in small blood vessels and necrosis in the tissues due to PMN degranulation (Fig. 16.9). Perhaps the best-studied examples are the occupational diseases associated with inhalation of fungi (farmer's lung, pigeon-fancier's disease, maple bark stripper's dis-

ease, etc.) in which chronic inflammation of the lung can lead to a state of destruction and fibrosis known as 'extrinsic allergic alveolitis', an unfortunate name since classical (IgE-mediated) allergy does not seem to be involved.

Another celebrated model of immune complex disease is the serum sickness that follows the repeated injections of foreign protein, leading to circulating complexes which deposit in the kidney (Fig. 16.10), skin, and joint. Common in the pre-antibiotic days of passive serotherapy for infectious disease (see Chapter 37), serum sickness is a possible complication of treatment with monoclonal (usually murine) antibody, an increasingly attractive approach to many conditions, and is one of the reasons why such determined efforts are being made to produce monoclonal antibodies in which as much of the molecule as possible is of the human type.

T cell-mediated reactions and granuloma (type IV)

Despite the examples of antibody-mediated tissue damage discussed above, the antibody response generally achieves its purpose in eliminating invading organisms without any trace of damage to the host. Cell-mediated (type IV) responses are not quite so sure-footed, in that the activation of both cytotoxic T cells and macrophages will invariably cause some tissue destruction, which may be repairable if not too prolonged, but can also lead to fibrosis and even calcification with serious permanent loss of tissue.

Confusion has occurred due to the use of a number of terms to describe and subdivide type IV responses. Some reflect actual pathological conditions while others describe the results of diagnostic skin tests, and none correspond exactly to the processes by which cell-mediated immunity protects against infection (Fig. 16.11). From the medical viewpoint it is granuloma formation that is the most important aspect of these responses, whereas to the immunologist the complex involvement of the cytokine network is currently of major interest. For example, the tendency of some granulomas to undergo necrosis (e.g. caseation in tuberculosis) while others do not (e.g. leprosy, sarcoidosis) may be explained in terms of the different pattern of cytokines involved. TNF, often in association with some microbial products, is especially likely to cause necrosis through its effects on vascular endothelium

(which probably accounts for much of its anti-tumour activity too).

The price paid for protective cell-mediated immunity is particularly well-illustrated by the helminth disease schisto-somiasis. *Schistosoma mansoni* (the blood fluke) lays eggs in the mesenteric venous system, some of which become lodged in small portal vessels in the liver. Strong cell-mediated reactions to secreted enzymes lead to granulomatous reactions around each egg, resulting in egg destruction and sparing of liver parenchyma from the toxic effects of

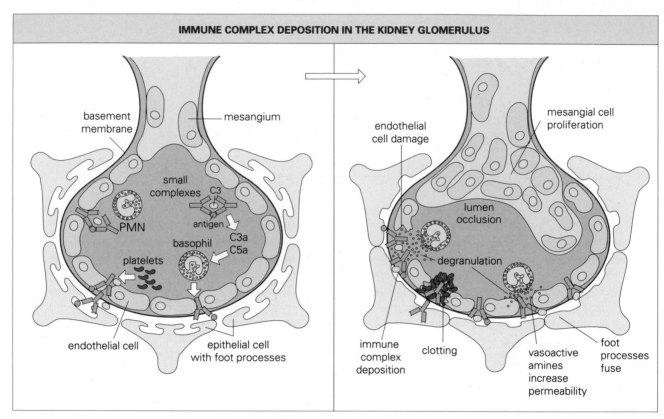

IMMUNE COMPLEX DEPOSITION IN THE KIDNEY GLOMERULUS

Fig.16.10 Immune complex-mediated tissue damage. Type III hypersensitivity results in the deposition of immune complexes in the blood vessel walls, particularly at sites of high pressure, filtration or turbulence such as the kidney.

CELL- MEDIATED RESPONSES			
immune cells or molecules	**protective effect against**	**pathological effect**	**skin test**
Cytotoxic T cells (CD8)	virus infections *Theileria* ? mycobacteria	local tissue loss	–
Basophils T cells	?	inflammation	24 hours (Jones-Mote)
T cells Macrophages Cytokines Giant cells Epithelioid cells Eosinophils	intracellular organisms viruses bacteria fungi protozoa worms	mononuclear cell infiltration granuloma fibrosis calcification (>14 days)	delayed/tuberculin type (>2 days)

Fig.16.11 Cell-mediated immunity in protection and disease. The nomenclature of cell-mediated responses is complicated. Though often described in terms of skin tests, their real significance is related to protective and/or pathological reactions in the tissues.

the egg enzymes. However, the coalescent, calcified granulomas ultimately cause portal cirrhosis, with portal hypertension, oesophageal varices and haematemesis (see chapter 25). An increased cell-mediated response would accelerate the cirrhosis, while a reduction would predispose to toxic parenchymatous liver failure, neither option being at all attractive. In such circumstances the conflict has gone too far for a 'perfect' solution, and the same would be true for tuberculosis and many other persistent intracellular organisms, if the density of infection were comparable.

The rather unexpected effect of malnutrition in reducing the incidence and severity of certain diseases (e.g. typhus, malaria) may be attributable to a reduction in immunopathology, though in the majority of diseases (e.g. measles, meningococcal infection, tuberculosis) the reverse is true. Indeed, poor nutrition is regarded as a major factor predisposing to the greater severity of many common infections in tropical countries.

SKIN RASHES

The ways in which infections can affect the skin are detailed in Chapter 28, but here it should be mentioned that some rashes are considered to be immunologically mediated. For example, the characteristic skin rash of measles is absent in children with T cell deficiency (e.g. thymic aplasia or Di George syndrome), who instead develop a fatal systemic infection, indicating that the skin lesions are T cell mediated and represent some form of successful cell-mediated immunity. By contrast, if the same children are infected with a vaccinia virus (i.e. vaccinated) they develop an inexorable spreading skin lesion; this is clearly due to a direct and not an immunopathological effect. Figure 16.12 lists the commoner skin conditions of immunological origin, in which an infectious organism is thought to be involved. Further details can be found in Chapter 28.

SKIN RASHES AND THEIR IMMUNOLOGICAL BASIS			
organism	disease	character	pathogenic basis
Viruses			
measles	measles	maculopapular rash	T cells; immune complex; allergy
rubella	german measles	maculopapular rash	
varicella-zoster	chicken-pox/ zoster	vesicular rash	viral cytopathic
vaccinia	smallpox	vesicular rash	
hepatitis B	hepatitis B	urticarial	immune complexes
Bacteria			
Strep. pyogenes	scarlet fever	erythematous rash	erythrogenic toxin
Strep. pyogenes	impetigo	vesicular rash	erythrogenic toxin
Staph. aureus			
Treponema pallidum	syphilis	disseminated infectious	immune complexes
Treponema pertenue	yaws	rash in secondary stage	
Salmonella typhi	typhoid, enteric fever	sparse rose spots	immune complexes
Neisseria meningitis	meningitis, spotted fever	petechial or maculopapular lesions	
Mycobacterium leprae	leprosy	–	
Rickettsia prowazeki and others	typhus	maculopapular or haemorrhagic rash	thrombosis
Fungi			
dermatophytes	dermatophytid or allergic rash	–	immune complexes? hypersensitivity to fungal antigens
Blastomyces dermatitidis	blastomycosis	papule or pustule developing into granuloma	immune complexes?
Protozoa			
Leishmania tropica	cutaneous leishmaniasis	papules ulcerating to form crusted infectious sores	organisms growing in skin

Fig.16.12 Many skin rashes represent immunological reactions occuring in the skin. It is suspected that several skin diseases of unknown origin are in fact caused by viruses, either directly or indirectly.

VIRUSES AND CANCER

A variety of RNA and DNA viruses can cause permanent malignant changes within cells (Fig. 16.13). Such malignant transformation by these 'tumour viruses' has been extensively studied. An account of proviruses and oncogenes (genes causing malignancy) is included in Chapter 3. However, only a small number of human cancers have been shown to be associated with such tumour viruses (Fig. 16.14).

MALIGNANT TRANSFORMATION	
changes	**details**
Morphology	loss of shape; rounding; decreased adhesion to surface
Growth, contact	loss of contact inhibition of growth and movement; increased ability to grow from a single cell; increased ability to grow in suspension; capacity for continued growth (immortalization)
Cellular properties	DNA synthesis induced; chromosomal changes; appearance of new antigens (viral or cellular in origin);
Biochemical properties	loss of fibronectin; reduced cyclic AMP

Fig. 16.13 Malignant transformation. These changes occur when tumour viruses cause transformation of cultured cells. Many of these changes are obviously relevant for tumor production *in vivo*.

Human T cell leukaemia viruses

Human T cell leukaemia viruses (HTLV1 and HTLV2) are retroviruses that have no oncogenes (see Chapter 3). Their proviral DNA is detectable in the cellular DNA of certain malignant lymphomas and leukaemias. HTLV1 is known to cause adult T cell laeukemia and lymphoma, particularly in Southern Japan, the Caribbean islands and West Africa. Less is known about the geographical distribution of HTLV2, which can be isolated from a hairy T cell leukaemia. The carcinogenic nature of HTLV1 is not due to activation of a cellular oncogene, but is a result of the *tat* gene product enhancing transcription of host genes involved in cell division. These infections are described in more detail in Chapter 28.

Epstein–Barr virus

Epstein–Barr virus (EBV) is closely linked with the development of nasopharyngeal carcinoma (NPC; see Chapter 29), which is common in Southern China and other parts of Asia (12–30 cases per 100 000 people per year), less common in parts of North Africa, and rare elsewhere in the world. The reason for this restricted geographical distribution is unknown. There is no convincing evidence for specific carcinogenic EBV strains, but these effects could be due to the presence locally of cocarcinogens such as nitrosamines in salted fish. EBV DNA can be demonstrated in the cancer cells but the precise mechanism for tumorigenicity is unknown; cellular oncogenes have not been implicated. People at high risk of developing NPC show high IgA titres to EB viral capsid antigen a year or more before clinical symptoms appear.

Burkitt's lymphoma, a tumour of immature B cells, is seen in parts of East Africa (Uganda) and in Papua New Guinea, occuring in 6–14 year old children, especially males. EBV DNA is present in the tumour cells, but most of the many copies of the EBV gene are not integrated

VIRUSES AND HUMAN CANCER				
viruses	**cancer**	**strength of association**	**viral genome in cancer cells**	**cofactor**
EBV	Burkitt's lymphoma	++	+	malaria
	nasopharyngeal carcinoma	++	+	nitrosamines
	Hodgkin's disease	–	–	–
HPV	cervical cancer	++	+	?cigarettes ?HSV2
	skin cancer	+/–	+	?UV light
HBV	liver cancer	++	+	?aflatoxin ?hepatocyte regeneration
HTLV1, HTLV2	T cell leukaemia	++	+	–
HSV2	cervical cancer	+/–	+/–	–

Fig.16.14 Many viruses transform cells in culture but only a few are important in human cancer. The associations are strongly supported by studies of naturally occuring or experimentally induced cancers in animals.

into the host cell DNA. The tumour is probably caused by the action of EBV on B cells, causing them to proliferate and making activation of cellular oncogenes more likely. The cellular oncogene c-*myc* is translocated from chromosome 8 to the immunoglobulin heavy chain locus on chromosome 14, where it is expressed. As a result of this, the B cell may be prevented from entering the resting stage. There is also down-regulation of adhesion and HLA molecules, so that the EBV-containing cells, normally subject to immune control, develop into tumour cells. The Burkitt's lymphoma cells also show other chromosomal abnormalities, but their role in tumorigenesis is unclear. The fact that EBV is a common world-wide infection, whereas Burkitt's lymphoma, like NPC, is strikingly localized geographically, points once again to the involvement of local cofactors. One hypothesis is that malaria acts as a cofactor, perhaps by decreasing the intensity of T cell surveillance or in some way priming cells for malignant transformation.

EBV does not appear to be associated with non-endemic Burkitt's lymphoma nor with the lymphomas seen in immunosuppressed (e.g. post-renal transplant) patients. It may however be involved in HIV-associated lymphomas. About 3% of AIDS patients develop non-Hodgkin's lymphomas, a fifth of these occurring in the brain. However, there is no good evidence to suggest that Hodgkin's lymphomas are of EBV origin.

Human papillomaviruses

There are clear associations between infection with certain human papillomavirus (HPV) types (16, 18, 31, 33) and the development of cervical cancer (see Chapters 3 and 24). Penile, vulval and rectal cancers are also associated with these types of HPV. HPV types 6 and 11 cause cervical lesions but have a lower risk of progression to malignancy.

In most primary and metastatic cancer cells the HPV genomes are present in integrated form (i.e. within the host genome), and certain viral genes (E6, E7) are transcribed and translated. Integration occurs at different chromosomal locations and the E6 and E7 open reading frames seem to be involved in the transformation of epithelial cells, and in the maintenance of the transformed state, probably by binding to and inactivating cellular proteins concerned with the regulation of the cell cycle. Cervical cancer is an uncommon sequel to infection with these strains of HPV, and cocarcinogens (e.g. cigarette smoke, herpes simplex virus) have been implicated.

There is a link, however, between HPV infection and squamous cell carcinoma of the skin. It is possible that UV light acts as a cocarcinogen, as is known to be the case with papillomaviruses and skin cancers in sheep and cattle. Patients with the rare autosomal recessive disease epidermodysplasia verruciformis are infected with 10–20 different but less common types of HPV, and one-third of patients develop multiple squamous cell carcinomas of the skin. Ninety per cent of these tumours contain HPV 5 or HPV 8 DNA. HPVs may also play a part in the genesis of the skin cancers that appear in immunosuppressed patients (e.g. renal transplant recipients), and cutaneous warts are common in these patients. However, there is no evidence that skin cancers in normal individuals are associated with HPV infection.

Hepatitis B virus

Hepatitis B virus (HBV) is a major cause of hepatocellular carcinoma, with integrated HBV sequences present in the tumour cells. The exact mechanism is unclear, but insertion of HBV sequences may activate cellular oncogenes (e.g. of the *myc* family), or alter cell growth control by transcriptional transactivation.

Hepatocellular carcinoma is commoner in certain parts of the world such as West Africa, and this may be due to the presence of cocarcinogens (e.g. aflatoxin). However, the closely related hepadnavirus of woodchucks (see chapter 25) causes the same tumour in these animals in the apparent absence of cocarcinogens. Perhaps HBV-associated hepatocellular carcinoma in humans could be a sequel to the continuous hepatocyte regeneration that occurs during persistent carriage of this virus.

Miscellaneous viruses

Herpes simplex virus type 2 (HSV2) was once thought to be a possible cause of cervical carcinoma. HSV2 DNA and protein are detectable in cancer cells and HSV2 can transform certain cells *in vitro*. However, HSV2 has now been relegated to a possible cocarcinogenic role. Women with cervical cancer have a higher incidence of antibody to HSV2 but this merely reflects the association of cervical cancer with multiple sexual partners.

Several other DNA viruses can transform cells in which they are unable to replicate, and the viral genome is sometimes integrated into the host cell genome. Extensive studies have been carried out with the conclusion that despite high oncogenicity *in vitro* and in laboratory animals, these viruses do not seem to be important in human cancer. For instance, human adenoviruses transform cells in culture and cause sarcomas experimentally in hamsters. About 10% of the adenovirus genome integrates and the T antigen is expressed. However, adenoviruses are not associated with human cancer.

Polyomavirus (from Latin *poly* many, *oma* tumours), a mouse papovavirus, and simian vacuolating virus 40 (SV40), a monkey papovavirus, both cause tumours in experimentally inoculated hamsters. The viral DNA is integrated into tumour cells and T antigens are expressed. However, neither of these viruses, nor their human equivalents (BK and JC viruses), are linked with human cancers. This is illustrated by an incident that occurred about 30 years ago when thousands of children were accidentally inoculated with SV40 virus present in certain batches of poliovirus vaccine. The formalin inactivation procedure had failed to kill the SV40 virus present in the monkey kidney cells in which the polio vaccine had been grown. There was, however, no consequent increase in tumour incidence in the SV40-infected individuals.

Kaposi's sarcoma is 300-times as common in AIDS patients as in other immunosuppressed groups, but is seen almost entirely in those who acquired HIV by sexual contact. The sarcoma is probably caused by an as yet unidentified but sexually transmitted infectious agent, possibly a virus.

SUMMARY

Tissue damage or disease can be caused by infectious organisms in several ways. They may destroy cells directly, as do cytopathic viruses; they may release toxins that destroy cells or their cellular function (e.g. staphylococcus or tetanus toxins), or that overstimulate normal defence systems (e.g. lipopolysaccharide); or they may stimulate adaptive responses in an excessive or prolonged manner. Such effects may be antibody- or T cell-mediated and are collectively known as 'hypersensitivity reactions' or 'immunopathology'. Finally, some viruses have been shown to be involved in the initiation of tumours, with the viral genome present in the cancer cells. The restricted geographical distribution of some of these tumours may be due to the local presence of cocarcinogens.

Further Reading

Root RK, Saude MA, eds. *Septic shock*. New York: Churchill Livingstone, 1985.

Mims CA. *The pathogenesis of infectious disease*. 3rd edn. London: Academic Press, 1987.

Rees AJ, Andres GA, Peters DK, eds. Symposium on pathogenetic mechanisms in nephritis. *Kidney Int* 1989; **35(4):** 921-1033.

Parkes R. *Occupational lung disease*. Kent: Butterworths Ltd, 1982.

Arbuthnot JR. Host damage from bacterial toxins. *Phil Trans R Soc Lond B* 1983; **303:** 149-165.

DIAGNOSIS AND CLINICAL MANIFESTATIONS

part 1 **Diagnostic Principles**

17 GENERAL PRINCIPLES AND SPECIMEN QUALITY

INTRODUCTION

After the descriptions of the adversaries and their conflicts in the preceding sections, this chapter is concerned with issues which may at first seem mundane. However, it is of fundamental importance to recognize that a microbiological diagnosis is only as reliable as the quality of the specimen on which it is based. With this in mind, we now discuss the role of the clinical microbiology laboratory, with emphasis on the principles of collection and transport of appropriate specimens, and underline the importance of interaction between clinician and microbiologist in the diagnosis of infection.

THE AIMS OF THE CLINICAL MICROBIOLOGY LABORATORY

The aims of the microbiology laboratory are to provide accurate information about the presence or absence in a specimen of microorganisms that may be involved in a patient's disease process and, where relevant, to provide information on the antimicrobial susceptibility of the microorganisms isolated. The precise identification of the causative organism in infection has become increasingly important now that therapeutic intervention is possible. The ability to achieve this depends on a positive interaction between the clinician and the microbiologist; the clinician must be aware of the complexity of the tests and the time required to achieve a result. In turn, the microbiologist must appreciate the nature of the patient's condition and be able to assist the clinician in interpreting the laboratory report. A fundamental step in any diagnosis is the choice of an appropriate specimen, which ultimately depends on an understanding of the pathogenesis of infections.

Laboratory tests are carried out 1) to detect microorganisms or their products in specimens collected from the patient, or 2) to detect evidence of the patient's immune response (production of antibodies) to infection. The tests fall into three main categories:

- *Identification of microorganisms by isolation and culture.* Microorganisms may be capable of growth in artificial media, or in the case of viruses, in cell cultures. In some instances, quantitation is important, e.g. more than 10^5 bacteria per ml of urine is indicative of infection whereas lower numbers are not (see Chapter 23). Once an organism has been isolated in culture, its susceptibility to antimicrobial agents can be determined.

- *Identification of a specific microbial product.* Non-cultural techniques, which do not depend on the growth and multiplication of microorganisms for their detection, have the potential to yield more rapid results. These techniques include the detection of structural components of the cell, e.g. cell-wall antigens, and extracellular products, e.g. toxins. Alternatively, specific gene sequences can be detected by the application of DNA probes to clinical specimens. These techniques are becoming more widely used, especially with the possibilities for amplification of DNA by the polymerase chain reaction (PCR; see Chapter 8). They are potentially applicable to all microorganisms but antimicrobial susceptibilities cannot be determined without culture (although the presence of resistance genes may be detectable by specific probes).

- *Detection of specific antibodies to a pathogen.* This may be the method of choice when the pathogen cannot be cultivated in laboratory media (e.g. *Treponema pallidum*, many viruses) or when to do so would be particularly hazardous to laboratory staff (e.g. the culture of *Francisella tularensis* the cause of tularaemia, or the fungus *Coccidioides immitis*.) The usual method is by detection of a rise (four-fold or greater) in antibody titre between 'paired' sera, collected

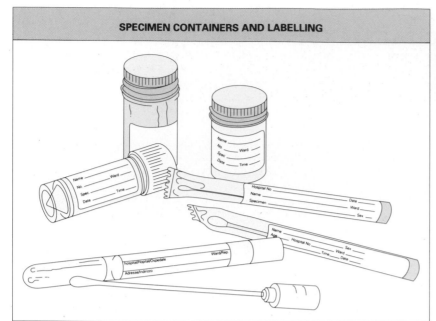

SPECIMEN CONTAINERS AND LABELLING

Fig. 17.1 Specimen containers should be of suitable size for ease of use. Instructions for collection of specimens should be clear and concise. Each specimen should be clearly labelled before it is despatched to the laboratory, and should be accompanied by a request form.

in the acute phase of an infection and in convalescence. Such tests therefore tend to result in a delayed or retrospective diagnosis. However the detection of antibodies in a single serum collected during the acute phase of illness may be helpful in diagnosis, for example of rare diseases such as Lassa fever, or if specific IgM is detected, e.g. in rubella infection.

The methods used in the laboratory for processing patients' specimens are given in detail in Chapter 18.

SPECIMEN COLLECTION

As it is usually impracticable to transport the patient to the laboratory, specimens are collected from the patient in the ward or clinic and sent to the laboratory. Obtaining the specimen is the clinician's responsibility but the laboratory must help by providing suitable containers and instructions (Fig. 17.1). Specimen collection should be performed with care, avoiding harm or unnecessary discomfort to the patient. When the patient is asked to collect a specimen (e.g. of urine or sputum), clear instructions must be given. In order to be useful in the diagnosis and treatment of infection, specimens must be relevant, i.e. representative of the infectious process (see below), of good quality and adequate quantity. Whenever possible, specimens should be collected before antimicrobial therapy is commenced.

Specimens for culture

Specimens intended for isolation and cultivation of microorganisms can be divided into two main types: fluid (including exudate and excreta) and tissue. Swabs may be used to collect samples of fluids (e.g. wound exudate), or for sampling surfaces (e.g. skin), but whenever possible actual fluid should be collected as swabs absorb only a small quantity of sample and provide an arid, unfriendly environment for transport to the laboratory. Many microbiological techniques are relatively insensitive, so it is

important to collect a large enough volume of sample and to maintain viable organisms in the sample while in transit to the laboratory. Important specimens from various sites of infection are listed in figure 17.2. Specimens for culture should be collected in sterile containers and should *not* be put into histological fixatives such as formalin because these are lethal to microorganisms.

Specimens for detection of microbial products

The same specimens are used for this type of test as are used for culture, but maintaining the viability of the organisms is not of prime importance because the detection of microbial products does not depend on the presence of living organisms. However it is important to minimize the risk of contamination by extraneous organisms.

Specimens for detection of antibodies

Samples of sera (and sometimes cerebrospinal fluid) are used to detect antibody responses. 'Paired' sera, collected in the acute and convalescent phases of the disease (ideally 10–14 days apart), are tested in parallel. Serum samples can be stored in the cold (-20°C) for months or years without loss of antibody titre.

Specimen labelling and request forms

All specimens must be properly labelled (see Fig. 17.1) by the person collecting the specimen, as errors in specimen identification can have disastrous consequences. It is equally important that correct identification continues during the specimen's passage through the laboratory. The results of all tests on the specimen should be compiled into a report, which must also be suitably identified so that it is returned to the correct patient's records.

In addition to the label, each specimen should be accompanied by a request form providing the necessary information about the patient, the clinical diagnosis and current antimicrobial therapy. An example is shown in

IMPORTANT SPECIMENS FROM VARIOUS SITES AND TYPES OF INFECTIONS				
site/type of infection	**type of specimen**			
	fluid	**tissue**	**swab**	**other**
Urinary tract Bladder Kidney	urine urine	renal biopsy		
Gastrointestinal tract Intestine Mouth Liver Biliary tract Abdomen	washings bile pus peritoneal aspirate ascitic fluid	liver biopsy	rectal swab	faeces
Respiratory tract Nose Nasopharynx Throat Lung Pleural space Ear Eye	washings (V) sputum alveolar lavage pleural fluid	lung biopsy	nasal swab pernasal swab throat swab ear swab eye swab	'cough plate' - patient coughs directly onto agar plate direct inoculation of culture plates at bedside
Central nervous system Meninges Encephalitis (herpes) Brain abscess	cerebrospinal fluid (CSF) pus; CSF	brain biopsy		
Genital tract Urethra Vagina Cervix Endometrium		endometrial biopsy	urethral swab high vaginal swab cervical swab	direct microscopy and culture in clinic
Skin and soft tissue Skin Wound	vesicle fluid (V) pus	skin biopsy (M) scrapings (F)	skin swab (carriage) wound swab	impression plates
Bone and joint Osteomyelitis Joint	pus aspirate	bone*		
Septicaemia	blood			
Pyrexia of unknown origin	blood			blood films for malarial parasites
Endocarditis	blood	heart valve*		
* collected at operation (V) specimens for virology (F) specimens for fungi (M) specimens for mycobacterium				

Fig. 17.2 Important specimens from various sites and types of infection. Where possible, specimens of fluid (pus, urine, faeces, etc.) or tissue should be sent to the laboratory, as swabs provide an unsatisfactory volume of specimen and a hostile environment for certain organisms.

figure 17.3. The information on the request form allows the laboratory staff to process the specimen in the optimum manner.

Safety

It is sensible to assume that all clinical specimens (including serum samples for antibody detection) are potentially infectious and to handle them with suitable precautions, both while in transit and within the diagnostic laboratory. However specimens known to be of high risk (e.g. those from patients who are hepatitis B or HIV positive) should be clearly labelled as such, both on the specimen and on the request form.

THE REQUEST FORM

LAB REFERENCE NO. **1234**	**Microbiology**	Record number	**1 2 4 9 3 6**

Surname **C O O P E R**

Destination code **1**

Ward/Clinic/Destination **1**
Request made by **RW**

First name **F R E D E R I C K**

Consultant's initials **R W**

Date of birth **01.01.21**
Sex (M or F) **M**
Bed No. **6**

Clinical features
COUGH PRODUCTIVE OF SPUTUM ?Chest Infection

ALL BOXED AREAS MUST BE COMPLETED-OTHERWISE SPECIMEN AND FORM WILL NOT BE ACCEPTED BY THE LABORATORY

Key +++ = profuse S = sensitive ++ = moderate R = resistant

Specimen **SPUTUM** Current antibiotic therapy **NIL**

Precise investigation required **Micros; culture; sens.** Relevant travels **NIL**

SPECIMEN CSF ☐ URINE ☐ SPUTUM ☑ SWAB ☐ HVS ☐ FLUID ☐ FAECES ☐

APPEARANCE **Mucopurulent; blood-stained**

MICROSCOPY Wbc **+++**
Rbc
Epithelial cells **—** Gram-positive cocci **++**
Gram-negative cocci
Gram-positive rods
Gram-negative rods

CULTURE (CO₂) Anaero Ambient temp (24hrs) 48 hrs)
1: **++ Streptococcus pneumoniae**
2:
3:

COMMENT

Signed

ANTIBIOTIC SENSITIVITY	1	2	3
Penicillin	S		
Erythromycin	S		
Flucloxacillin			
Amoxycillin			
Sulphonamide			
Trimethoprim			
Nitrofurantoin			
Nalidixic acid			
Gentamicin			
Mezlocillin			
Tetracycline			
Metronidazole			

Date specimen collected **03.01.93** Time **08.00**

Date specimen in laboratory **03.01.93** Time **10.00**

Fig. 17.3 Every specimen sent to the laboratory should be accompanied by a completed request form, or identified so that it can be linked to a computer-generated request on arrival in the laboratory. Information about the patient, such as **name, date of birth** and **bed number**, will ensure that the report is directed back to the correct patient's notes. Age and sex are important with respect to some infections, and the patient's **clinical features** and any **current antibiotic therapy**, which may make the isolation of the pathogen difficult must be included. This latter information also directs the laboratory to test the appropriate antibiotic if the patient is already on treatment. **Relevant travel** details are also important to indicate possible exposure to pathogens in endemic areas. The **precise investigation required** indicates to the laboratory the type of test the clinician wants, e.g. microscopy, culture, antibiotic sensitivity of any pathogens isolated. Finally the **date** and **time** of specimen collection and of arrival in the laboratory indicate how long ago the specimen was taken. Once the form reaches the laboratory, the relevant tests are carried out and the report completed by the microbiologist (area in grey) including **macro-** and **microscopic reports**, **antibiotic sensitivity** and **culture results** indicating what has grown and in what quantity.

TRANSPORT OF SPECIMENS

Specimens should be transported to the laboratory as quickly as possible. Some samples (e.g. urine, sputum) provide a good medium for growth of non-fastidious bacteria and fungi, so that organisms may multiply during the time between collection and cultivation in the laboratory, giving falsely high results in quantitative cultures (see Chapter 23). With time, the hardy species may overgrow the fastidious, giving a false impression of the balance between species or in fact making it impossible to isolate and identify the less hardy species. In other specimens (e.g. throat swabs, urethral swabs) delicate organisms such as *Neisseria* species survive poorly. Specimens for the detection of viruses may be rendered useless if overgrown by bacteria and fungi, hence the inclusion of antibacterials and antifungals in viral transport media (see below).

Refrigeration for short periods may preserve the organisms in a urine specimen in roughly the same numbers as they occurred in the specimen when it was first collected, but similar conditions will kill certain fastidious organisms and greatly reduce the chances of isolating small numbers of bacteria, from blood cultures for example.

Transport media

Fluids and tissue specimens should be transported to the laboratory in sterile containers, without the addition of preservative. Swabs are better transported in a medium that helps to preserve the organisms in the specimen but prevents them from multiplying, thereby maintaining the ratio of the various species to one another. Transport media often contain a sloppy agar which helps to prevent drying out of the organisms, and charcoal or other absorbant substances to remove toxic agents such as fatty acids. Examples of transport media suitable for swabs destined for bacterial culture are those of Stuart or Amies , or thioglycollate media. If anaerobic bacteria are suspected and a pus sample is obtainable, it should be aspirated into a syringe, the needle removed, the syringe tip capped and the specimen sent without delay to the laboratory to minimize exposure to air.

The optimal virus transport medium is one which preserves the virus in the specimen, prevents loss of the specimen due to bacterial or fungal contamination, is non-toxic to cell cultures, and can be used both for virus isolation and for direct tests to detect and identify virus antigens (e.g. immunofluorescence; enzyme immunoassays).

SAMPLING SITES AND THE NORMAL FLORA

body sites that are normally sterile

blood and bone marrow
cerebrospinal fluid
serous fluids
tissues
lower respiratory tract
urine (if sample is carefully collected)

body sites that have a normal commensal flora

mouth, nose and upper respiratory tract
skin
gastrointestinal tract
female genital tract
urethra

Fig. 17.4 Sampling sites and interpretation of results. Some sites in the body are sterile in health, so that growth of any organism is indicative of infection, provided that the specimen has been properly collected and transported, and examined in the laboratory without delay. The significance of isolates from sites that have a commensal flora depends on the identity of the isolate and the quantity, as well as the immune status of the patient.

AIDE-MEMOIRE FOR SPECIMEN COLLECTION

take the appropriate specimen;
e.g. blood and CSF in suspected meningitis

collect the specimen at the appropriate time, during the acute phase of the disease; e.g. malarial films, virus isolation

if possible collect specimen before patient receives antimicrobials

collect enough material and an adequate number of samples e.g. enough blood/serum for more than one set of blood cultures

avoid contamination
(a) from normal flora; e.g. mid-stream urine
(b) from non-sterile equipment

use the correct containers and appropriate transport media

label specimens properly

complete request form with enough clinical information and a statement of possible aetiology

talk to the microbiologist and inform the laboratory if special tests are required

transport specimens rapidly to the laboratory

Fig. 17.5 Important steps in specimen collection and delivery to the laboratory. The responsibility of the clinician does not end with collection of the specimen and requesting tests. Good communication with the microbiologist is essential.

Several such systems exist, including sucrose-based and broth-based liquid media, and 'transporters' containing a monolayer of human diploid fibroblast cells in buffered serum with added antibiotics. The addition of antibiotics to viral transport media helps to reduce bacterial contamination but means that the same specimen cannot be used for isolation of viruses and bacteria.

SPECIMEN PROCESSING

Specimens intended for the cultivation of microorganisms can be divided into two types: those from sites that are normally sterile and those from sites which usually have a commensal flora (Fig. 17.4; see also Chapter 3). A thorough knowledge of the microorganisms normally isolated from specimens from non-sterile sites, and the common contaminants of specimens collected from sterile sites, is important to ensure that specimens are properly handled and results correctly interpreted. Some specimens from sites that should be sterile, e.g. bladder urine, sputum from the lower respiratory tract, are usually collected after passage through orifices that have a normal flora, which may contaminate the specimens. This needs to be considered when interpreting culture results of these specimens.

Ideally, each specimen arriving in the laboratory should be considered in turn, together with the information provided about the patient on the request form. This would allow the microbiologist to assess which pathogens are likely to be present and to devise an 'individualized' processing plan. In reality this approach is not wholly practicable because of constraints on time and money; specimens tend to be processed by type (i.e. urine, blood, faeces, etc.), so that the microbiologist looks for easily cultivatable pathogens known to be associated with each sample type. However if the laboratory is provided with suitable information, such as a statement of possible aetiology, more fastidious or unusual pathogens can be sought and relevant antibiotic susceptibilities performed. The schemes used for the basic processing of specimens are outlined in the Appendix.

SUMMARY

To obtain a test result that correctly identifies the infection, it is important to collect an appropriate specimen, to use the appropriate transport conditions and to deliver specimens rapidly to the laboratory. These conditions all affect the accuracy of the laboratory report, and therefore its value to the clinician and ultimately to the patient. Good communication between the clinician and the microbiologist is extremely important! The microbiologist can advise the clinician on the collection of optimum specimens, and will be better able to guide the processing of these specimens if the problems have been discussed. The key points to remember about specimen collection are summarized in figure 17.5.

Further Reading ───

Collins CH, Lyne PM, Grange JM, eds. *Collins and Lyne's microbiological methods*. 6th edn. Oxford: Butterworth–Heinemann Ltd, 1989.

Hawkey PM, Lewis DA, eds. *Medical microbiology: a practical approach*. Oxford: IRL Press Ltd, 1989.

Brent Johnson F. Transport of viral specimens. *Clin Microbiol Rev* 1990; **3:** 120–131.

18 MICROBIOLOGICAL TECHNIQUES FOR DIAGNOSIS OF INFECTION

INTRODUCTION

In the previous chapter, we stressed the importance of the specimen in the laboratory diagnosis of infection and discussed types of specimens, their collection and transport to the laboratory . In this chapter we will examine the processing of specimens in the laboratory.

Microbiology differs from other clinical laboratory disciplines in the amount of interpretive input required both in the pre-analytic phase (determining the optimum processing pathway for the specimen) and in the post-analytic phase (interpreting the relevance of the results for each particular specimen and patient). Specimen analysis is less mechanized and automated than in the other disciplines.

Time is a key factor because the conventional methods of microbiological diagnosis depend on growth and identification of the pathogen. Results of culture cannot be achieved in less than 18 hours and may take as long as six weeks for a minority of pathogens, such as the mycobacteria. Thus specimen processing can be categorized according to the time required to achieve a result and the method – cultural or non-cultural. An alternative route to the diagnosis of an infection is an immunological one, relying on the detection in the patient's blood of an antibody response to the putative pathogen. These routes to microbiological diagnosis are summarized in figure 18.1.

NON-CULTURAL TECHNIQUES FOR THE LABORATORY DIAGNOSIS OF INFECTION

Although medical microbiology has long been synonymous with cultivation of microorganisms from patients' specimens, these techniques are labour-intensive and slow to produce results (days rather than hours) because replication of organisms is a necessary but rate-limiting step. In addition there are some microorganisms which cannot be cultured in artificial media, and viable organisms may be difficult to recover from specimens from patients who have received antimicrobial therapy. Non-cultural techniques do not require the multiplication of the microorganism prior to its detection. Some techniques, such as microscopy and detection of microbial antigens in specimens, can provide very rapid results (i.e. within two hours). Other non-cultural methods such as the use of DNA probes and amplification of DNA by the polymerase chain reaction may require up to 1–2 days to complete.

Microscopy

Microscopy plays a fundamental role in microbiology and is an important first step in the examination of all specimens. Although microorganisms show a wide range in size (see Chapters 1 and 3) they are too small to be seen individually by the naked eye and thus a microscope is an essential tool in microbiology. The various types of microscopy are summarized in figure 18.2. The light microscope magnifies objects and thus improves the resolving power of the naked eye from $20\mu m$ to about $0.2\mu m$; the electron microscope can improve this to about $0.001\mu m$.

Light microscopy

Bright field microscopy. Bright field microscopy is used to examine specimens and cultures as wet preparations or as stained preparations. Wet preparations are used to demonstrate blood cells and microbes in fluid specimens such as urine, faeces or cerebrospinal fluid, cysts, eggs and parasites in faeces, fungi in skin and protozoa in blood and tissues. Living organisms can be examined to detect motility.

Dyes are used to stain cells so that they can be seen more easily. Stains are usually applied to dried material that has been fixed (by heat or alcohol) onto the microscope slide. The slide can then be viewed in the light microscope with an oil immersion lens, which improves the resolving power of the microscope.

Differential staining procedures exploit the fact that cells with different properties stain differently and thus can be distinguished. The most important differential staining technique in bacteriology is the 'Gram' stain (Fig. 18.3). Based on their reaction to the Gram stain, bacteria are divided into two broad groups: Gram-positive (stain purple) and Gram-negative (stain pink). This difference is

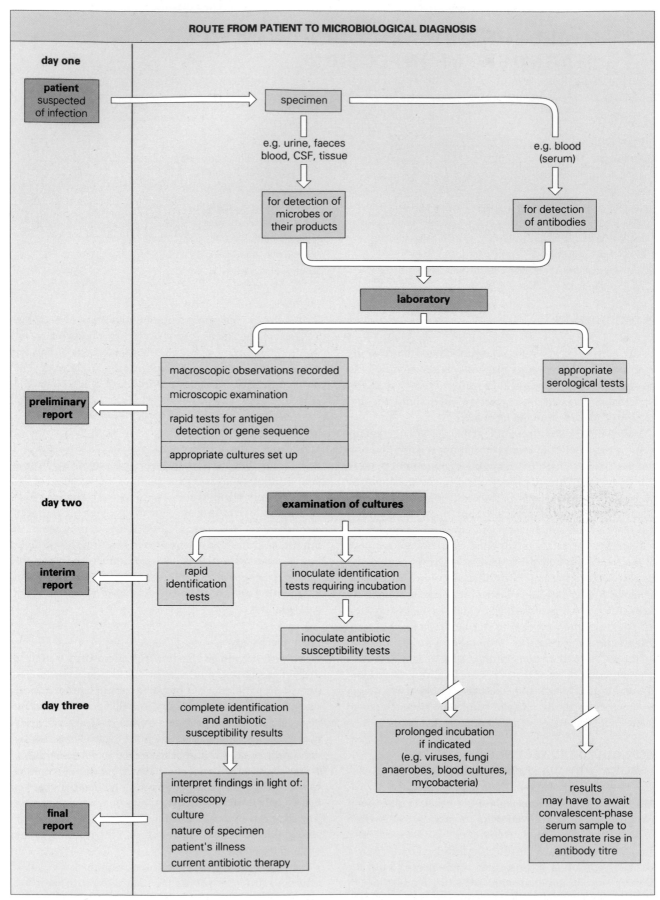

Fig. 18.1 Route from patient to microbiological diagnosis. This scheme shows the key steps in specimen processing. Some tests can be performed on the specimen immediately and yield 'same day' results. Culture of specimens involves a minimum of 18 hours before colonies are visible and can be identified. Antibiotic susceptibility tests involve a further incubation period. Alternatively the diagnosis may be based on the detection of specific antibodies in serum samples.

APPLICATIONS OF MICROSCOPY TO MICROBIOLOGY

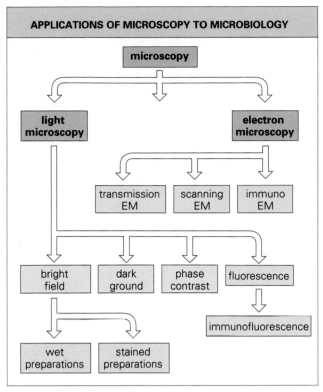

Fig. 18.2 Applications of microscopy to microbiology. The scheme shows the different uses of the light and electron microscopes for looking at microbes.

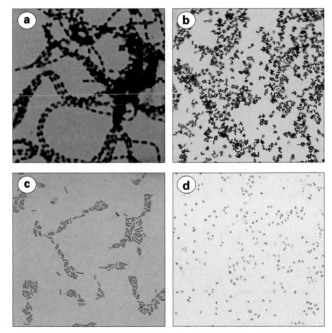

Fig. 18.3 The Gram stain is the most important stain for studying bacteria. The combination of the violet dye (crystal violet) and iodine (acting as a mordant) binds to the cell wall. Gram-positive cells retain the stain when challenged with acetone and remain purple. Gram-negative cells lose the purple stain and appear colourless until stained with a pink counterstain (neutral red or safranin). Examination of Gram-stained films also allows the shape of the cells to be noted. Some examples are shown. (a) Gram-positive cocci in chains (streptococci). (b) Gram-positive rods (*Listeria*). (c) Gram-negative rods (*Escherichia coli*). (d) Gram-negative cocci (*Neisseria*).

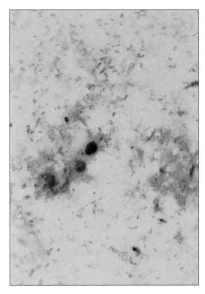

Fig. 18.4 Ziehl-Neelson stained smear of *Mycobacterium tuberculosis*. Pink-stained acid-fast rods show up against a blue background. Because mycobacteria may take several weeks to grow, microscopic examination of specimens stained by this method are important as they can yield a tentative diagnosis on the day of specimen collection.

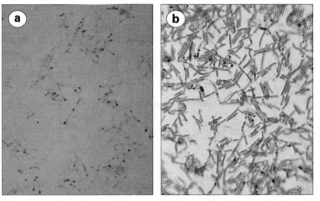

Fig. 18.5 Special staining techniques can be used to demonstrate particular features of bacterial cells. (a) Corynebacteria stained to demonstrate polymetaphosphate storage granules (volutin granules) which appear as dark spots in blue-green cells (Albert's stain). (b) Lipid storage granules in *Bacillus cereus* stained with sudan black (black lipid against red cells).

related to differences in structure of the cell walls of the two groups (see Chapter 3). Some organisms, particularly mycobacteria with their waxy cell walls, do not readily take up the Gram stain and special staining techniques are used to demonstrate their presence. The Ziehl–Neelsen stain (Fig. 18.4) is a differential staining procedure which utilizes heat to drive the fuchsin stain into the cells; mycobacteria stained with fuchsin withstand decolourization with acid and alcohol and hence they are known as 'acid-' and 'alcohol-fast' (other bacteria lose the stain after acid and alcohol treatment). Alternatively, the fluorescent dye auramine, which has a strong affinity for the waxy cell wall of mycobacteria, can be used to demonstrate these organisms by fluorescence microscopy (see below). Other staining techniques can be used to demonstrate particular features of cells, e.g. volutin (polyphosphate) storage granules in *Corynebacterium* spp. or lipid in *Bacillus* spp. (Fig. 18.5) and thus aid identification. Protocols for these staining methods are given in the Appendix.

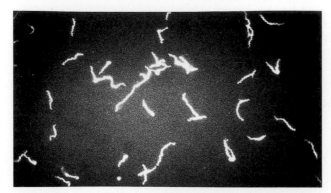

Fig. 18.6 Spirochaetes visualized by dark ground microscopy. Spirochaetes and leptospires are much thinner than most bacterial cells (approximately 0.1 μm in diameter compared with 1 μm *E. coli*) but they appear larger when viewed by dark ground illumination.

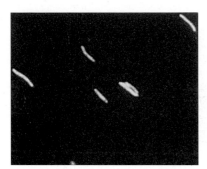

Fig. 18.7 Fluorochrome stain of *M. tuberculosis* with a mixture of auramine O and rhodamine B. Mycobacteria appear fluorescent under UV light. Courtesy of DK Banerjee.

Dark ground (dark field) microscopy. The light microscope may be adapted by modifying the condenser so that the object appears brightly lit against a dark background. Organisms can be examined by dark ground microscopy in the living state and thus motility can be observed. The method is also used for visualizing very thin cells such as spirochaetes because the light reflected from the surface of the cells makes them appear larger and thus more easily visible than they are under bright field. (Fig. 18.6).

Phase contrast microscopy. This technique enhances the very small differences in refractive index and density between living cells and the fluid in which they are suspended and thus produces an image with a higher degree of contrast than that achieved by bright field microscopy. However, phase contrast microscopy is now rarely used in the diagnostic laboratory.

Fluorescence microscopy. If light of one wavelength shines on a fluorescent object, it emits light of a different wavelength. Some biological substances are naturally fluorescent; others can be stained with fluorescent dyes and viewed in a microscope with an ultraviolet light source instead of white light (Fig. 18.7).

Fluorescence microscopy is widely used in microbiology and immunology and has been developed to detect microbial antigens in specimens by 'staining' with specific antibodies tagged with fluorescent dyes (immunofluorescence). Direct or indirect staining methods can be used (see Chapter 8).

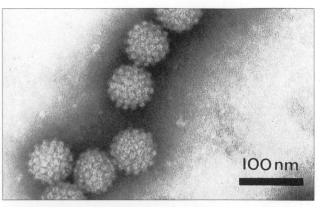

Fig. 18.8 Electronmicrograph of papillomavirus, the human wart virus. Courtesy of the Regional Virus Laboratory, Birmingham.

Electron microscopy

The electron microscope (EM) employs a beam of electrons instead of light and magnets are used to focus the beam in place of the lenses used in a light microscope. The whole system is operated at a high vacuum. Electron beams penetrate poorly and a single microbial cell is too thick to be viewed directly. To overcome this the specimen is fixed and mounted in plastic and cut into thin sections which are examined individually. Electron-dense stains such as osmium tetroxide, uranyl acetate or glutaraldehyde, are applied to the specimen to improve contrast. The electrons pass through the section and produce an image on a fluorescent screen. Images are photographed and enlarged so that the original specimen is magnified many thousand-fold (Fig. 18.8).

Electron microscopy can be used to identify virus particles by direct examination of specimens giving a rapid result and allowing the detection of viruses that are difficult or impossible to cultivate (e.g. rotaviruses, hepatitis A virus). Fluid for examination is dried onto a copper grid and examined. About a million virus particles per ml are needed if they are to be detectable. The sensitivity can be increased by reacting the fluid with antiviral antibody so that clumps of virus particles are visible. This is known as immunoelectron microscopy, a technique analogous to immunofluorescence in light microscopy.

Detection of microbial antigens in specimens

Detection of specific microbial antigens can be a more rapid method for detecting the presence of an organism than attempting to grow and identify the microbe. The methods include those which detect antigens by their interaction with specific antibodies, and those which detect microbial toxins. They are summarized in figure 18.9. For example, the common causative agents of bacterial meningitis (*Streptococcus pneumoniae*, *Haemophilus influenzae* and *Neisseria meningitidis* types A and C) can be detected in cerebrospinal fluid (CSF) by mixing the specimen with specific antibody coated onto latex particles. If the antigen, i.e. the organism or its product, is present the particles will clump together (Fig. 18.10). These tests give results within minutes of receipt of the specimen but their sensitivity is not significantly greater than the Gram stain

NON-CULTURAL TECHNIQUES
non-specific techniques for detection of microbial products
Fatty acid end-products of metabolism of anaerobes can be detected in fluid specimens (e.g. pus, blood) by gas liquid chromatography (GLC)
antigen detection
Detection of soluble carbohydrate antigens by agglutination of antibody-coated latex particles or red blood cells
e.g.
Strep. pneumoniae capsule   *Haemophilus influenzae* type b capsule   *Neisseria meningitidis* capsule   *Cryptococcus neoformans* capsule ⎤ in CSF   ⎦ and urine
Strep. pyogenes group antigen in throat swabs
Detection of particular antigens by binding to antibodies labelled with:
radioisotope,   enzyme or   fluorescent molecule   e.g. ELISA for hepatitis B,   rotavirus
toxin detection
Detection of exotoxins
Clostridium botulinum toxin by injection of patient's serum into mice (unprotected and protected with specific antiserum)
Clostridium difficile cytotoxin in faeces by addition of suspension to cell culture
Clostridium perfringens and *Staph. aureus* enterotoxins in faeces by agglutination of antitoxin-coated latex particles
E. coli toxin genes (LT, ST, vero) in faeces by DNA probes
Detection of endotoxin
Endotoxin from cell walls of Gram-negative bacteria detected by *Limulus* lysate assay (clotting of extracts of amoebocytes of the horseshoe (*Limulus*) crab)

Fig. 18.9 Non-cultural techniques. Identification of specific microbial products can be a more rapid method for the detection of microorganisms than isolation and culture. The available techniques vary in their specificity. Toxins may be detected either by virtue of their antigenic properties or by demonstrating their action.

LATEX AGGLUTINATION OR CO-AGGLUTINATION

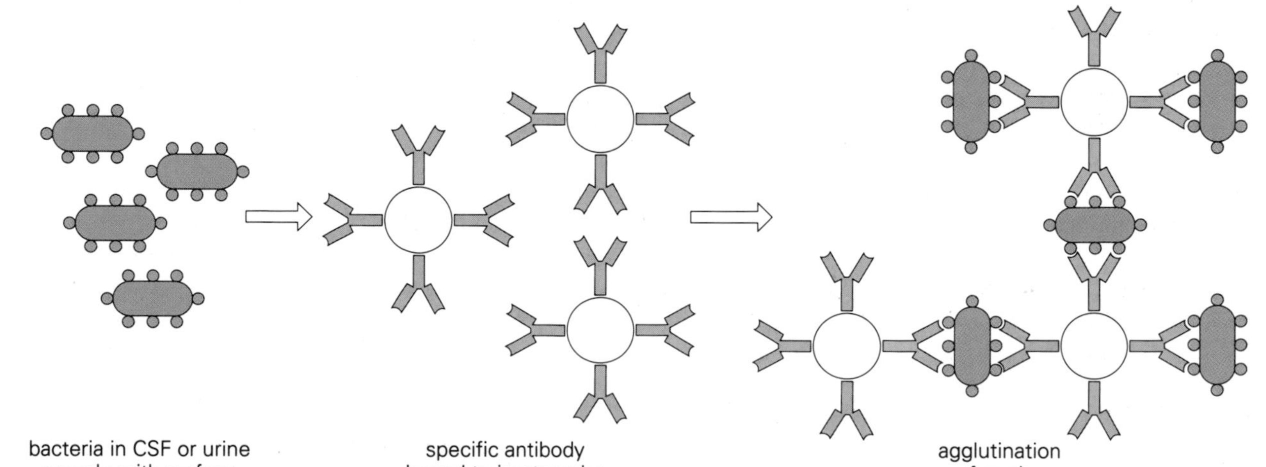

bacteria in CSF or urine sample with surface antigen on bacterial cells

specific antibody bound to inert carrier particles (eg. latex beads)

agglutination of carrier particles

Fig. 18.10 When a specimen of CSF containing bacteria (e.g. *Haemophilus influenzae*) is mixed with a suspension of latex particles coated with specific antibody (e.g. *H. influenzae* anti-capsular antibodies), the interaction between antigen and antibody causes an immediate agglutination of particles which is visible to the naked eye. (See also figure 14.20.)

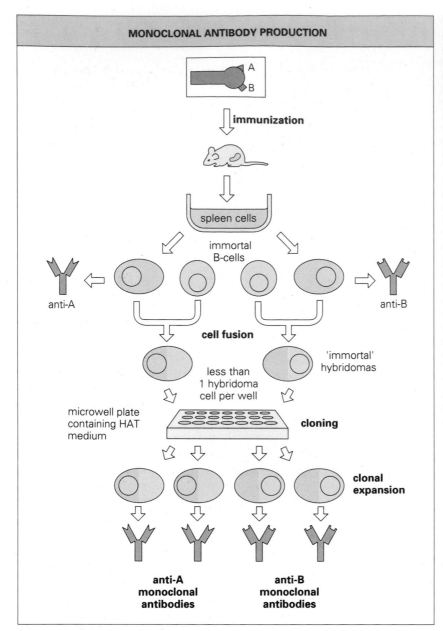

MONOCLONAL ANTIBODY PRODUCTION

immunization

spleen cells

immortal B-cells

anti-A

anti-B

cell fusion

less than 1 hybridoma cell per well

'immortal' hybridomas

microwell plate containing HAT medium

cloning

clonal expansion

anti-A monoclonal antibodies

anti-B monoclonal antibodies

Fig. 18.11 Production of monoclonal antibodies. Mice immunized with an antigen bearing for example, two epitopes, A and B, develop spleen cells making anti-A and anti-B which appear as antibodies in the serum. The spleen is removed and the individual cells fused in polyethylene glycol with constantly dividing (i.e. 'immortal') B-tumour cells selected for a purine deficiency and often for their inability to secrete Ig. The resulting cells are distributed into microwell plates in HAT (hypoxanthine, aminopterin, thymidine) medium which kills off the perfusion partners, at such a high dilution that on average each well will contain less than one hybridoma cell. Each hybridoma being the fusion product of a single antibody-forming cell and a tumour cell will have the ability of the former to secrete a single species of antibody and the immortality of the latter enabling it to proliferate continously, clonal progeny providing an unending supply of antibody with a single specificity–the monoclonal antibody. These monoclonal antibodies can be 'labelled' with enzymes or fluorescent molecules and can then be visualized when they bind to specific antigens, e.g. on virus particles.

and false positive results may occur due to cross-reacting antigens. However they can be a useful diagnostic aid when the patient has received antibiotics and organisms may appear morphologically unidentifiable in the CSF and fail to grow in culture.

Monoclonal antibodies

Monoclonal antibodies (Fig. 18.11) are being used increasingly as diagnostic tools. Because of their specificity, it is possible to use them to distinguish between species and between strains of the same species, on the basis of antigenic differences. Direct ELISA tests (see Chapter 8) frequently employ enzyme-conjugated monoclonal antibodies to detect antigens in specimens from patients. Rotaviruses, HIV, hepatitis B virus, herpesvirus and respiratory syncytial virus (RSV) can all be detected directly with monoclonal antibodies in ELISA tests. *Chlamydia trachomatis* infection can be diagnosed within a few hours by a direct fluorescent antibody test employing a monoclonal antibody labelled with fluorescein (see Chapter 24).

Detection of microbes by probing for their genes

Nucleic acid probes

A gene probe is a nucleic acid molecule which, when in the single stranded state and labelled, can be used to detect a complementary sequence of DNA by hybridizing to it (see Chapter 8). Polynucleotide probes are obtained from naturally occuring DNA by cloning DNA fragments into appropriate plasmid vectors and then isolating the cloned DNA. However, if the sequence of the gene of interest is known, oligonucleotide probes can be synthesized. Probes are labelled either with a radioactive isotope (e.g. ^{32}P) or with compounds which give colour reactions in suitable conditions (e.g. biotin streptavidine or alkaline phosphatase).

By constructing probes for virulence factors such as toxins, organisms carrying these genes can be detected in specimens without the need for culture e.g. probes for enterotoxins of *Escherichia coli* or cholera toxin can be applied directly to faeces. A commercially-available ^{125}I-labelled DNA probe directed against sequences specific for

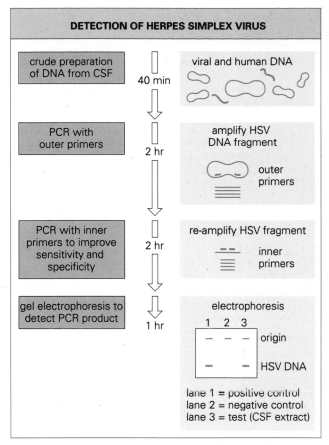

DETECTION OF HERPES SIMPLEX VIRUS

crude preparation of DNA from CSF — 40 min — viral and human DNA

PCR with outer primers — 2 hr — amplify HSV DNA fragment / outer primers

PCR with inner primers to improve sensitivity and specificity — 2 hr — re-amplify HSV fragment / inner primers

gel electrophoresis to detect PCR product — 1 hr — electrophoresis
1 2 3 — origin — HSV DNA

lane 1 = positive control
lane 2 = negative control
lane 3 = test (CSF extract)

Fig. 18.12 Detection of herpes simplex virus (HSV) DNA in cerebrospinal fluid (CSF) from a patient with encephalitis by nested PCR. Nested PCR is a modification of the original PCR technique in which the DNA of interest is amplified first with two primers which recognise sequences some distance apart, and then in a second reaction, with a further pair of primers which recognise sequences within the length of the DNA amplified by the first pair. This technique improves the sensitivity and specificity of PCR.

MICROBES AND SPECIMENS ON WHICH PCR HAS BEEN PERFORMED	
organism	**specimen/tissue**
Bacteria	
Helicobacter pylori	fresh cultures, paraffin embedded gastric biopsies
Legionella pneumophila	water
Mycobacterium tuberculosis	cerebrospinal fluid, sputum
Chlamydia trachomatis	urethral and cervical scrapes conjunctival swabs
Mycoplasma pneumoniae	throat swabs
Viruses	
Coxsackieviruses	endomyocardial biopsies
Cytomegalovirus	urine
Herpes simplex virus	CSF, peripheral white blood cells
Hepatitis B virus	fresh tumour DNA
Hepatitis C virus	serum
Human immuno-deficiency virus	genital ulcer exudate
Measles virus	paraffin-embedded tissue
Human papillomavirus	cervical smears
Rotavirus	faeces
Rubella virus	chorionic villus biopsy placental tissue
Fungi	
Candida albicans	urine, sputum, wound fluid, blood
Protozoa	
Toxoplasma gondii	cerebrospinal fluid
Pneumocystis carinii	bronchoalveolar lavage fluid
Trypanosoma cruzi	extract from vector, blood
Rickettsia	
Rickettsia rickettsiae	blood clots

Fig. 18.13 The polymerase chain reaction has already been used for the diagnosis of a range of infectious diseases, although the technique is still confined to research laboratories. In the future it is likely to play an increasingly important role in diagnostic microbiology. Redrawn from Hayden, *et al.*, 1991.

Mycoplasma pneumoniae ribosomal RNA have been used successfully to detect the organism in sputum specimens.

There is no doubt that gene probes will be developed increasingly for diagnostic purposes but detection of small numbers of organisms (i.e. few copies of the gene) can be a limiting factor and in these circumstances the combination of gene amplification by the polymerase chain reaction (PCR; see below) followed by hybridization with oligonucleotide probes may become the method of choice especially for organisms that are slow or difficult to grow in the laboratory.

The polymerase chain reaction

PCR can be used to amplify a specific DNA sequence to produce millions of copies within a few hours (see Chapter 8). While theoretically PCR can detect a single gene sequence, such sensitivity is seldom achieved in clinical specimens but bacteria present in numbers between 10-100 can be detected by standard PCR techniques and more sophisticated methods can detect one HIV proviral DNA sequence in 10^6 cells. A further advantage is the speed with which this can be achieved. Amplification takes only about five hours although confirmation of the identity of the product by probing or sequencing can add up to 36 hours.

The specificity of PCR is determined by careful choice of primers. These oligonucleotides are complementary to the target DNA and thus in order to synthesize suitable primers, the sequence of the target DNA must be known. At the present time this is one of the limitations of PCR, but this versatile technique will undoubtedly be developed for wider clinical applications. Currently it is used in the research laboratory setting but it seems only a matter of time before the methods become available for routine diagnostic use. Already PCR has been applied to a variety of specimens to diagnose infections (Figs 18.12 and 18.13).

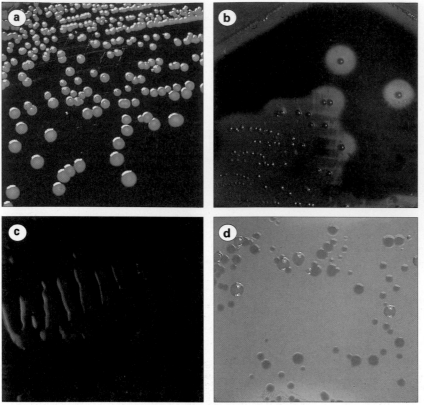

Fig. 18.14 Bacterial colonies. A bacterial cell implanted on a solid nutrient medium will multiply to produce a colony containing millions of cells. Different species produce characteristically different colonies and this feature can be used as a preliminary clue to the identity of the organism. (a) Golden colonies of *Staphylococcus aureus*. (b) Additional features such as the ability to lyse red blood cells can be demonstrated by culturing bacteria on blood-containing media. Here, beta-haemolysis (complete haemolysis) is produced by *Streptococcus pyogenes* on horse blood agar. (c) Culture media can be made selective by including agents that are inhibitory to some species. For example MacConkey agar contains bile salts so only those organisms that are tolerant to bile will grow. In addition it contains lactose and a pH indicator. Species which ferment lactose change the indicator to bright pink (c). Non-lactose fermenting species, such as *Salmonella* and *Shigella* form yellowish colonies (d).

CULTIVATION (CULTURE) OF MICROORGANISMS

Bacteria and fungi grow on the surface of solid nutrient media to produce colonies composed of thousands of cells derived from a single cell implanted on the agar surface. Colonies of different species often have characteristic appearances which can give a clue to their likely identity (Fig. 18.14). It takes 12–48 hours for colonies of most species to become macroscopically visible, but some organisms multiply much more slowly and may take several weeks to produce visible colonies. Cultures can also be made in liquid media (broth) and growth detected by observing the development of turbidity. However it is not possible to tell whether there is more than one species present in a liquid culture nor whether there are few or many organisms, and therefore solid media are more useful in diagnostic microbiology.

It is possible to grow the majority of species of bacteria and fungi of medical importance in artificial media in the laboratory but there is no one universal culture medium which will support the growth of them all, and there are still some species which cannot be grown at all except in experimental animals, e.g. *Mycobacterium leprae* and *Treponema pallidum*. Some bacteria which cannot be cultivated on artificial media, e.g. chlamydia and rickettsia, can be grown in cell cultures (see below).

Many culture media are designed not only to support the growth of the desired organisms but also to inhibit the growth of others, i.e. they are 'selective media'. Constituents common to all bacteriological culture media are shown in figure 18.15. The important media used in the diagnostic laboratory are shown in figure 18.16. Schemes utilizing these media for processing different clinical specimens are outlined in the Appendix (see Protocols for specimen processing).

Specimens collected from body sites which have a normal commensal flora will contain a mixture of organisms from which the pathogen has to be recognized. Specimens are 'plated out' on a carefully chosen range of nutrient and selective media to produce single colonies. These are subcultured to fresh media for identification and antibiotic susceptibility tests (see below). This procedure takes at least 48 hours, and sometimes longer, to yield results (see Fig. 18.1).

Parasites such as *Leishmania*, *Trypanosoma* and *Trichomonas* can be cultivated in liquid media to allow small numbers present in the original specimen (e.g. blood or vaginal secretions) to multiply and thus become easier to detect by microscopical examination. Parasites do not form colonies on solid media in the same way as bacteria and fungi.

Viruses, chlamydia and rickettsia must be grown in cell or tissue cultures because they are incapable of a free-living existence. Most cell cultures used in the diagnostic laboratory are continuous cell lines – human or animal cells adapted to growth *in vitro* and which can be stored at –80°C until required. The specimen is introduced into the cell culture medium and the presence of viruses detected by observation of the cells for a 'cytopathic effect' (CPE).

Cell culture techniques are specialized and labour intensive, and some viruses either cause no CPE (e.g. rubella) or cause a CPE which takes several days to evolve (e.g. cytomegalovirus). Therefore alternative methods such as antigen detection (see above) or antibody detection (see below) to diagnose viral infections are used wherever possible.

CONSTITUENTS OF BACTERIOLOGICAL CULTURE MEDIA

Amino-nitrogen base (digested protein)	e.g. peptone
Growth factors	e.g. blood, serum, yeast extract
Energy source	e.g. sugars, carbohydrates
Buffer salts	e.g. phosphate, citrate
Mineral salts	e.g. calcium, magnesium, iron
Selective agents	e.g. chemicals, dyes, antimicrobials
Indicators	e.g. phenol red
Gelling agent (for solid media)	e.g. agar

Fig. 18.15 Constituents of bacteriological culture media. All culture media share a number of common constituents which are necessary to enable bacteria to grow *in vitro*. Hundreds of different media have been described.

MEDIA IN COMMON USE IN THE CLINICAL DIAGNOSTIC LABORATORY

enriched media

Blood agar (BA)*	in USA, sheep blood is usually used, whereas in UK horse blood is used; it is important to realize that bacterial haemolysins differ in their specificity for different blood cells and that some organisms e.g. *Haemophilus influenzae* grows better on horse than on sheep blood; *Gardnerella vaginalis* prefers human blood
Chocolate agar (CA)*	if blood is heated to 60°C before it is added to the agar medium it decomposes to release extra nutrients from the RBC; this medium is thus richer than blood agar and suitable for growing fastidious organisms

selective media

MacConkey agar (Mac) Cysteine lactose electrolyte deficient media (CLED) Deoxycholate citrate agar (DCA) Eosin methylene blue (EMB)	these media are all selective for enteric organisms; they also contain lactose and an indicator and thus allow the distinction between lactose fermenters and non-fermenters, an important reaction in the identification of the enterobacteria; there are many other selective media

media for isolation of anaerobes

Robertson's cooked meat medium (RCM) Thioglycollate broth Fastidious anaerobe broth (FAB) Wilkins and Chalgren agar (WC)	these media all contain reducing agents which help to keep them anaerobic; anaerobes can grow in the depths of thioglycollate broth or RCM without requiring incubation in an anaerobic environment, whereas FAB and WC are used for culture of anaerobes but require anaerobic incubation i.e. in a jar or chamber from which oxygen has been removed and replaced by nitrogen

special media for particular groups of organisms

Sabouraud dextrose agar	this medium has a low pH which encourages the growth of fungi whilst inhibiting most bacterial species
Lowenstein Jensen agar Middlebrook agar	these media both contain glycerol and malachite green, constituents which favour the growth of mycobacteria but are inhibitory to other bacterial species

* can be made selective by the addition of dyes or antimicrobials, e.g. Thayer-Martin agar contains a mixture of antimicrobials which inhibit normal vaginal flora and make the medium selective for *Neisseria gonorrhoeae*

Fig. 18.16 Media in common use in the clinical microbiology laboratory. From the many media available, the choice of those for routine use will vary from one laboratory to another but the figure shows examples of the most commonly used (and those that are referred to in the specimen processing protocols in the Appendix).

IDENTIFICATION OF MICROORGANISMS GROWN IN CULTURE

A colony or a pure culture is one which consists of only one type of microorganism and is derived from a single cell. Identification tests should always be performed from single colonies or pure cultures. Aseptic techniques must be used to isolate and maintain pure cultures of microorganisms (Fig. 18.17).

Identification of bacteria

A preliminary identification of many of the bacteria of medical importance can be made on the basis of a few simple characteristics of the cells (Fig. 18.18):

- Gram reaction;
- cell morphology (e.g. rod or coccus) and arrangement (e.g. pairs or chains);
- ability to grow under aerobic or anaerobic conditions;
- growth requirements (simple or fastidious).

Further identification is made on the basis of biochemical properties such as:

- ability to produce enzymes that can be detected by simple tests, e.g. coagulase, catalase, oxidase, lecithinase (Fig. 18.19);
- ability to metabolize sugars oxidatively or fermentatively,

e.g. the Hugh and Liefson oxidation/fermentation test (Fig. 18.20);

- ability to utilize a range of substrates for growth e.g. glucose, lactose, sucrose etc. These tests can be done individually e.g. in broth media containing the test sugar, or in commercial kits which allow a range of different tests to be set up simultaneously on each organism (Fig. 18.21).

Some species are identified on the basis of their antigens by reacting cell suspensions with specific antisera. The key tests for species of medical importance are given in the Appendix.

Antibiotic susceptibility tests

When bacteria have been isolated in pure cultures their susceptibility to antibiotics can be determined in the laboratory. This is usually, done by exposing a lawn of the test organism seeded on an agar plate, to antibiotics contained in filter paper discs. During overnight incubation the organisms grow and multiply and the antibiotics diffuse out from the discs and inhibit growth around the disc. Thus after isolation of bacteria from a specimen, a further overnight incubation period is required before antibiotic susceptibility results are available. Methods for antibiotic susceptibility tests are described in more detail in Chapter 33.

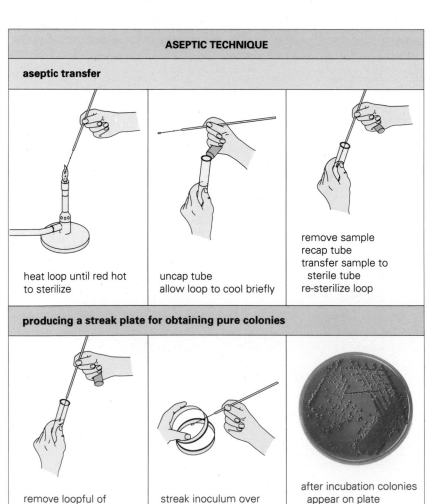

ASEPTIC TECHNIQUE

aseptic transfer

| heat loop until red hot to sterilize | uncap tube allow loop to cool briefly | remove sample recap tube transfer sample to sterile tube re-sterilize loop |

producing a streak plate for obtaining pure colonies

| remove loopful of inoculum from culture tube | streak inoculum over agar plate to spread organisms | after incubation colonies appear on plate pure cultures can be made from this |

Fig. 18.17 Aseptic technique. Because culture media provide excellent conditions for microbial growth, bacteria and fungi from the air and the environment that settle on the medium will grow and contaminate the cultures. It is vital to prevent this occuring if we are to be sure that the organisms growing in the cultures actually originated from the specimen. Therefore culture media are sterilized before use and handled with aseptic techniques. Likewise, aseptic techniques are an important part of patient care in operating theatres and wound dressing to prevent surgical wounds becoming contaminated (see Chapter 39).

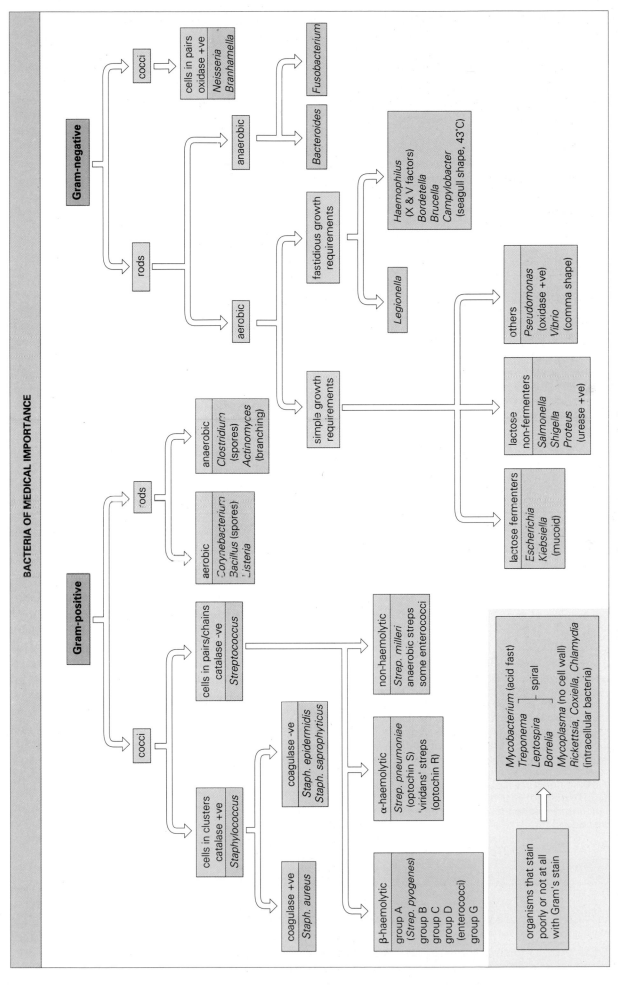

Fig. 18.18 Identifying bacteria. The preliminary investigation of the bacteria of medical importance can be made on the basis of a few key characteristics (see text). Further identification is made on the basis of biochemical and serological tests.

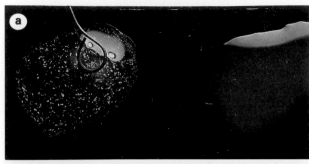

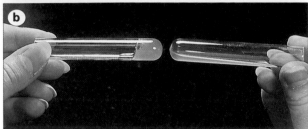

Fig. 18.19 Once bacteria have been isolated in pure cultures they can often be identified by their biochemical reactions. For example the ability to produce certain enzymes can be easily demonstrated. The production of coagulase distinguishes *Staphylococcus aureus* from *Staph. epidermidis*. The slide test (a) demonstrates bound coagulase by its ability to cause staphylococcal cells to clump within a few seconds when mixed with plasma. The tube test (b) detects free coagulase by its ability to cause plasma to clot after incubation at 37°C for about 4 hours.

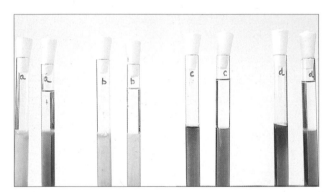

Fig. 18.20 Oxidation/fermentation test. The distinction between fermentative and non-fermentative bacteria is important in the identification of the Gram-negative rods. Some species can utilize sugars such as glucose and produce acid (shown by the indicator change from green to yellow) by both aerobic (oxidative) and anaerobic (fermentative) pathways (b). Others can only grow aerobically (a). Some species cannot metabolize glucose but break down the peptone (peptides) in the medium producing alkaline end-products as shown by the indicator turning blue (d). Other species are non-reactive in an oxidation/fermentation test and the green indicator remains unchanged (c).

Identification of fungi

Fungi are identified from colonies or pure cultures largely on the basis of colonial characteristics e.g. colour etc., and the morphology of the individual cells viewed under the microscope (Fig. 18.22). Biochemical tests (substrate assimilation) can be used for detailed identification of yeasts of medical importance. In general, fungi grow more slowly than bacteria and final identification may take up to two weeks.

Identification of protozoa and parasites

Protozoa are identified on the basis of their morphological characteristics; different stages of the life cycle may be visible in different specimens from the same patient and at different stages in the disease (Fig. 18.23).

Helminths

Helminths are identified by the macroscopic appearance of the worm (e.g. *Ascaris* or *Enterobius*) or by microscopic examination of specimens (e.g. faeces or urine) for eggs of, for example, schistosomes (see Chapter 25).

Many protozoa and parasites can be identified by direct examination of specimens without resort to culture and thus the results can be obtained on the day of receipt of the specimen in the laboratory.

Identification of viruses

Viruses may be identifiable by their cytopathic effect in cell culture, and their morphology in electron microscopic preparations (see Fig. 18.7) but diagnosis is more often made by detecting viral antigens or by testing for the presence of specific antibodies in the patient's serum (see below).

ANTIBODY DETECTION METHODS FOR THE DIAGNOSIS OF INFECTION

Serological tests (the study of antigen–antibody interactions) are used to diagnose infections, to identify microorganisms (see above), to type blood for blood banks and tissues for transplantation. The major disadvantage of diagnosis based on serology is that it is retrospective, as 2–4 weeks must elapse before IgG antibodies, produced in response to the infection, are detectable in the serum. What is more, a positive result indicates only that the patient has come into contact with the infection at some time in the past. IgM antibodies may be detected earlier in the infection (7–10 days) and are usually indicative of active, as opposed to past, infection. It is desirable to show that the patient has 'seroconverted' by demonstrating a

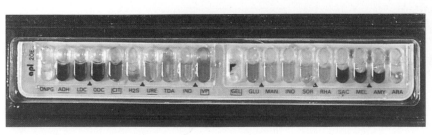

Fig. 18.21 Multitest systems. Commercially available kits allow 20 or more miniaturized biochemical tests to be set up simultaneously on one isolate. After incubation the results are scored as positive or negative and the score compared with a database which gives the 'best-fit' identification for the isolate.

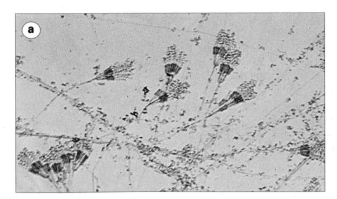

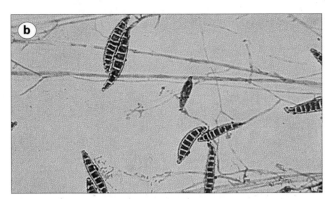

Fig. 18.22 Fungi under the microscope. Fungi can be grown on agar culture media in the same way as bacteria but most species grow much more slowly than bacteria and it may take up to two weeks for a colony to form. Colonial characteristics (such as colour) are helpful in the identification of fungi but confirmation depends on microscopic examination of the hyphae and sporing structures. (a) *Penicillium* in a wet preparation showing the conidiophores and free conidia. (b) Macroconidia of *Microsporum canis* stained with lactophenol cotton blue.

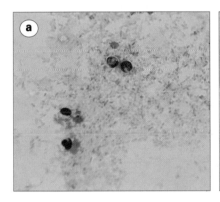

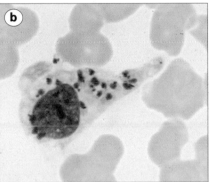

Fig. 18.23 Although some parasites can be cultivated in the laboratory, identification is usually based on microscopic appearances in the specimen. (a) Acid-fast stain of *Cryptosporidium* in faeces. Like mycobacteria, this organism is able to retain the pink carbol fuchsin stain when challenged with acid alcohol.(b) *Leishmania donovani* (Donovan bodies) in a stained preparation from a specimen of bone marrow.

four-fold or greater rise in antibody titre between sera collected in the acute and convalescent phases of the disease.

Despite these drawbacks, antibody detection can be invaluable if the microbe involved is slow or difficult to grow in the laboratory. It is still the main method for the laboratory diagnosis of viral infections. The techniques employed often allow several different infections to be screened for simultaneously (e.g. causes of atypical pneumonia; see Chapter 22). Sera should be collected during the acute phase of the disease and stored at −20°C until a convalescent phase serum is available and the two sera then tested in parallel. Few diagnoses can be made with any confidence on the results of single serum samples, but sometimes early testing is justified when there is clinical suspicion of an infection which is rare and which the patient is unlikely to have encountered before e.g. legionellosis. The possibility of prior immunization makes the interpretation of some serological tests difficult if not impossible because one cannot tell whether the antibodies detected are present as a result of immunization or infection (e.g. the Widal test for the serologic diagnosis of enteric fever; see Chapter 25).

The common serological tests used in the laboratory for the diagnosis of infection include:
- precipitation (see Chapter 8);
- haemagglutination (see Chapter 8);
- haemagglutination inhibition (Fig. 18.24);
- complement fixation (CF; Fig. 18.25);
- agglutination or flocculation (Fig. 18.26);
- fluorescent antibody techniques (Fig. 18.27);
- ELISAs (enzyme-linked immunosorbent assays; see Chapter 8).

The important applications of these methods are referred to in the appropriate systems chapters (see Chapters 19–33).

Antibodies to some viruses can be detected by the ability of the patient's serum to prevent virus infectivity, i.e. to prevent the development of a cytopathic effect. Radioimmunoassays (see Chapter 8) are being superseded by other techniques where possible to avoid the use of radioactive reagents in the diagnostic laboratory.

PROTOCOLS FOR SPECIMEN PROCESSING

Basic protocols used in the diagnostic laboratory for processing specimens of the following types are given in the Appendix:
- Urine;
- Faeces;
- Genital tract specimens;
- Skin and soft tissue specimens;

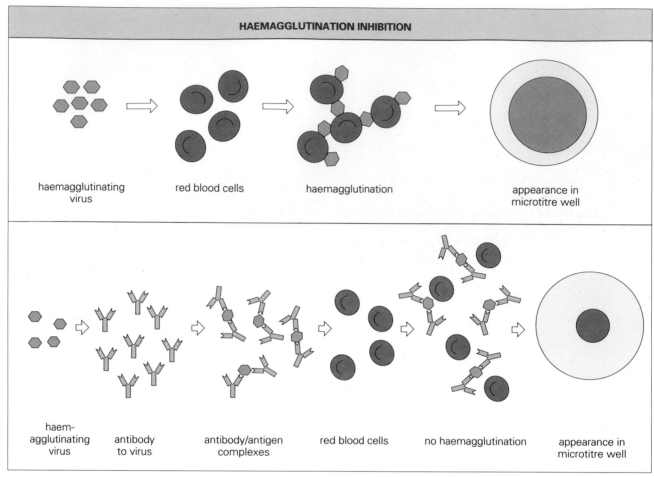

HAEMAGGLUTINATION INHIBITION

haemagglutinating virus

red blood cells

haemagglutination

appearance in microtitre well

haem-agglutinating virus

antibody to virus

antibody/antigen complexes

red blood cells

no haemagglutination

appearance in microtitre well

Fig. 18.24 Haemagglutination inhibition (HAI). Some viruses (e.g. influenza) have haemagglutinin molecules on their outer surface, and when virus particles are mixed with red blood cells they cause haemagglutination (see Chapter 8). In the presence of specific antibody, however, haemagglutination is inhibited. This test can therefore be used to detect the presence of antibodies to influenza virus in a patient's serum.

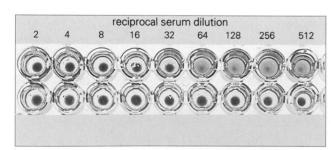

reciprocal serum dilution

2 4 8 16 32 64 128 256 512

Fig. 18.25 Complement fixation tests (CFTs) are available for the serological diagnosis of a range of infections. The basis of the test is described in Chapter 8. This figure shows a CFT for antibodies to *Coxiella burnetii* (a cause of atypical pneumonia). Dilutions of acute and convalescent sera are shown. In the top row complement has been fixed only in the first 5 wells i.e. the antibody titre is 1/32, whereas in the second row there is no lysis of the red blood cells at any dilution of serum and this the antibody titre is equal to, or greater than, 1/512. This demonstrates a four-fold rise in titre between acute-and convalescent-phase sera, indicating infection with *Coxiella burnetii*. CFTs are rather complicated and time-consuming to perform and there is a tendency to replace them with other more modern tests such as ELISAs.

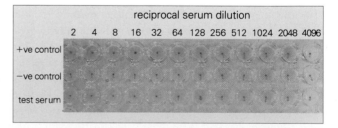

reciprocal serum dilution

2 4 8 16 32 64 128 256 512 1024 2048 4096

+ve control

−ve control

test serum

Fig. 18.26 The ability of antibodies to *Legionella* in a patient's serum to agglutinate a standardized preparation of *Legionella* antigen can be demonstrated by the rapid microagglutination test (RMAT). Doubling dilutions of the patient's serum are mixed with the antigen preparation in a microtitre tray. After a brief incubation period (10 min) the tray is centrifuged and then left to stand propped on its side. Agglutination (a positive result) is indicated by a tight button at the bottom of each well; in a negative test the stained antigen has streaked down the well giving a 'tear-drop' appearance. In this test the serum has an antibody titre of 1/32. A titre of 1/8 or greater in an acute phase serum is suggestive of infection, although the result should be confirmed by demonstrating a rising titre between acute and convalescent sera. Positive and negative control sera are included (upper two rows) to show that the test is working satisfactorily.

- Eye swabs;
- Respiratory tract specimens including nose, throat and ear swabs, and sputum;
- Cerebrospinal fluid (CSF);
- Pus;
- Other fluids such as pleural, pericardial fluids and joint aspirates;
- Blood;
- Bone marrow and other biopsy specimens;
- Autopsy and forensic specimens.

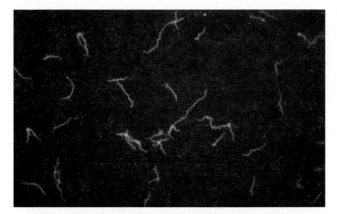

Fig. 18.27 Immunofluorescent tests for diagnostic purposes. The fluorescent treponemal antibody test (FTA) is an example of the use of an antigen labelled with fluorescent dye (in this case *Treponema pallidum* labelled with fluorescein) to detect the presence of antitreponemal antibodies in a patient's serum.

SUMMARY

In this chapter, we have outlined the techniques that are used for the laboratory diagnosis of infections. For many years confirmation of a clinical diagnosis of a bacterial or fungal infection has been based largely on the isolation of the pathogen from the patients' specimens. This allows the complete identification of the organism, and tests for susceptibility to antimicrobial agents to be performed. However, cultural methods are time consuming and labour intensive, and are unavailable or hazardous for some organisms. Thus, serological methods are also important.

The application of molecular techniques to diagnostic microbiology has the potential to increase the sensitivity, specificity and speed of laboratory diagnosis, but it will be some time before the techniques are sufficiently versatile to hunt for all 'unknown' organisms in patients' specimens.

Further Reading

Collins CH, Lyne PM, Grange JM. *Microbiological methods.* 6th edn. Oxford: Butterworths, 1989.

Hayden JD, Ho SA, Hawkey PM, Taylor GR, Quirke P. The promises and pitfalls of PCR. *Rev Med Microbiol* 1991; **2**: 129–137.

Lennette EH, Balows A, Hausler WJ, Shadomy J, eds. *Manual of clinical microbiology.* 5th edn. Washington: American Society for Microbiology, 1990.

section 3

DIAGNOSIS AND CLINICAL MANIFESTATIONS

part 2 **System Infection**

19 THE CLINICAL MANIFESTATIONS OF INFECTION – AN INTRODUCTION

As there are at least 150 different infectious diseases to describe, a system of classification is essential. In this section (Chapters 20 to 28), infections are classified according to the bodily system primarily involved at the clinical level. For example, rhinoviruses specifically cause infection of the upper respiratory tract, and bacillary or amoebic dysentery are gastrointestinal tract infections. Other infections characteristically cause damage predominantly to one part of the body, although other parts may be affected. Thus, tuberculosis is considered in Chapter 32 (lower respiratory tract infections) and typhoid in Chapter 25 (gastrointestinal tract infections), these being the sites primarily affected. Again, when microbes are transmitted as a result of certain states or activities, they can be grouped together with others acquired in the same way, even though more than one system may be involved. Hence syphilis and AIDS are dealt with in Chapter 24 (sexually transmitted diseases) and rubella in Chapter 26 (obstetric and perinatal infections).

The systems approach is useful because it includes under a given heading infections caused by a wide variety of microbes on the basis of the clinical syndrome produced. As with any system of classification, however, there are grey areas and overlaps. Referral to the Appendix, where definitive accounts of the most important infectious organisms are given, will help to clarify any ambiguities.

The following section (Chapters 29 to 33) deals with those infections which cannot be so readily pigeon-holed into systems. These include multisystem infections, i.e. infections that are not obviously localized to any one system of the body. Some of these are virus infections which occur world-wide and are exclusively human (e.g. measles, herpes simplex, Epstein-Barr virus infections; see Chapter 29). However, many multisystem infections are also multihost, in that they can be transmitted: 1) from person to person by an intermediate vector (usually an arthropod), their distribution depending on climate, ecology, and the presence of adequate numbers of the required arthropod (see Chapter 30); and 2) directly to humans from other vertebrates, in which case they are known as 'zoonoses' (see Chapter 31), with distributions ranging from highly restricted (Rocky Mountain spotted fever, Lassa fever) to widespread (Q fever, leptospirosis).

Finally there are two further disease groupings, founded on clinical presentation: those presenting as 'pyrexias of unknown origin' (see Chapter 32), and those seen in the compromised host (see Chapter 33). The latter category has become increasingly important because of the large number of patients whose defences are impaired as a result of disease (cystic fibrosis, diabetes), infection (AIDS), immunosuppressive therapy (transplant patients), or other causes (burns, catheters, etc.).

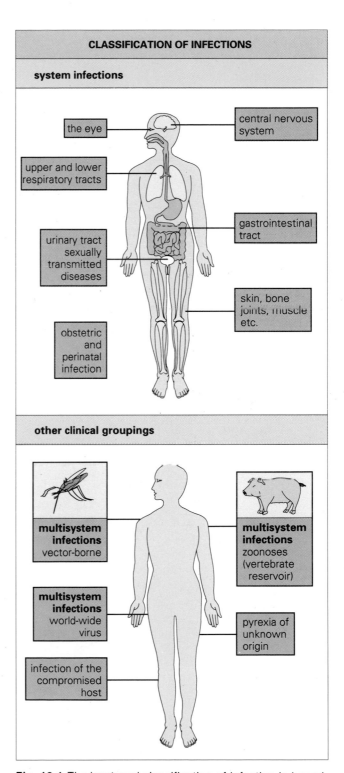

Fig. 19.1 The 'systems' classification of infection is based upon the clinical manifestations of the diseases. Many infections are, however, multisystem in effect, and some are vector-borne or are zoonoses. These can be considered as separate groupings. In addition, pyrexias of unknown origin (PUO) and infections of the compromised host are important clinical groupings.

20 UPPER RESPIRATORY TRACT INFECTIONS

Contents

INTRODUCTION

The air we inhale contains millions of suspended particles, including microorganisms. Nearly all these microorganisms are harmless, but in the vicinity of infected individuals the air may contain large numbers of pathogenic microorganisms. Efficient cleansing mechanisms (see Chapters 4 and 11) are therefore essential to keep the respiratory tract clean, and are vital components of the defence against infection of the upper as well as the lower respiratory tract.

It is against the background of these natural defence mechanisms that infection takes place, and it is then fitting to ask why the defences have failed. In the nasopharynx the mucociliary system is important, and in the oropharynx the flushing action of saliva. As on other surfaces of the body (see Chapter 2), a variety of microorganisms live harmlessly in the upper respiratory tract and oropharynx (Fig. 20.1). They colonize the nose, mouth, throat, teeth and are well adapted to life in these sites. Normally they are well behaved guests, not invading tissues and not causing disease. However, as in other parts of the body, resident microorganisms may cause trouble when host resistance is weakened.

Although in these chapters we distinguish between upper and lower respiratory tract infections, the respiratory tract, from nose to alveoli, is a continuum as far as infectious agents are concerned (Fig. 20.2). There may be a preferred 'focus' of infection (e.g. nasopharynx for coronaviruses and rhinoviruses) but parainfluenza viruses, for instance, can infect the nasopharynx to give a cold, as well as the larynx and trachea (croup, laryngotracheitis), and occasionally the bronchi and bronchioles (bronchitis, bronchiolitis, pneumonia).

NORMAL FLORA OF THE RESPIRATORY TRACT	
type of resident*	**microorganism**
Common residents (>50% of normal people)	Viridans streptococci Neisseria sp., *Branhamella* Corynebacteria Bacteroides Anaerobic cocci (*Veillonella*) Fusiform bacteria** *Candida albicans*** *Streptococcus mutans* *Haemophilus influenzae*
Occasional residents (<10% normal people)	*Streptococcus pyogenes* *Streptococcus pneumoniae* *Neisseria meningitidis*
Uncommon residents (<1% normal people)	*Corynebacterium diphtheriae* *Klebsiella pneumoniae* *Pseudomonas* ⎤ especially after *E. coli* ⎬ antibiotic *Candida albicans* ⎦ treatment

Residents in latent state in tissues:***
  Lung
  Lymph nodes etc.
  Sensory neurone/glands
    connected to mucosae
	P. carinii, M. tuberculosis
	Cytomegalovirus
	Herpes simplex virus,
	  Epstein–Barr virus

* All except tissue residents are present in oronasopharynx or on teeth
** Present in mouth; also *Entamoeba gingivalis*, *Trichomonas tenax*, micrococci, *Actinomyces* sp.
*** All except *M. tuberculosis* are present in most humans

Fig. 20.1 The normal flora of the respiratory tract.

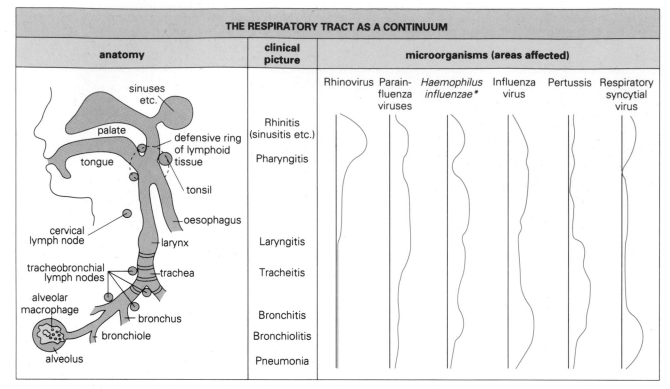

Fig 20.2 The respiratory tract as a continuum. * asymptomatic nasopharyngeal colonization is common.

	TWO TYPES OF RESPIRATORY INFECTION	
type	**examples**	**consequences**
Restricted to surface	common cold viruses influenza streptococci in throat chlamydia (conjunctivitis) diphtheria pertussis *Candida albicans* (thrush)	local spread local (mucosal) defences important adaptive (immune) response sometimes too late to be important in recovery short incubation period (days)

Spread through body	measles, mumps, rubella
	EB virus, CMV
	Chlamydia psittaci
	Q fever
	cryptococcosis
		little or no lesion at entry site
		microbe spreads through body, returns to surface for
		  final multiplication and shedding e.g. salivary gland
		  (mumps, CMV, EB virus), respiratory tract (measles)
		adaptive (immune) response important in recovery
		longer incubation period (weeks)

Fig. 20.3 After entry via the respiratory tract, microbes either stay on the surface epithelium or spread through the body.

Two useful generalizations can be made about upper and lower respiratory tract infections:

1) Many microorganisms are restricted to the surface epithelium, but others spread to other parts of the body, before returning to the respiratory tract, oropharynx, salivary glands etc. (Fig. 20.3);

2) Two groups of microbes can be distinguished. First, the 'professional' invaders, those which successfully infect the normally healthy respiratory tract (Fig. 20.4). They generally possess specific properties that enable them to evade local host defences, such as the attachment mechanisms of respiratory viruses (Fig. 20.5) and the other devices shown in figure 20.4. The others are the 'secondary' invaders, those which cause disease only when host defences are already impaired (see Fig. 20.4).

THE COMMON COLD

Aetiology, transmission, pathogenesis and clinical features

Viruses are the commonest invaders of the nasopharynx. There is a great variety of types (see Fig. 20.5), though

RESPIRATORY INVADERS - PROFESSIONAL OR SECONDARY		
type	**requirement**	**examples**
Professional invaders (infect healthy respiratory tract)	adhesion to normal mucosa (in spite of mucociliary system)	respiratory viruses (influenza, rhinoviruses) *Strep. pyogenes* (throat) *Strep. pneumoniae* *Mycoplasma pneumoniae* chlamydia (psittacosis, chlamydial conjunctivitis and pneumonia, trachoma)
	ability to interfere with cilia	*B. pertussis, Mycoplasma pneumoniae* *Strep. pneumoniae* (pneumolysin)
	ability to resist destruction in alveolar macrophage	*Legionella, M. tuberculosis*
	ability to damage local (mucosa, submucosal) tissues	*Corynebacterium diphtheriae* (toxin) *Strep. pneumoniae* (pneumolysin)
Secondary invaders (infect when host defences impaired)	initial infection and damage by respiratory virus (e.g. influenza virus)	*Staph. aureus; Strep. pneumoniae* pneumonia complicating influenza
	local defences impaired (e.g. cystic fibrosis)	*Staph. aureus, Pseudomonas*
	chronic bronchitis local foreign body or tumour	*H. influenzae, Strep. pneumoniae* etc.
	depressed immune responses e.g. AIDS, neoplastic disease	*P. carinii,* CMV, *M. tuberculosis* etc.
	depressed resistance e.g. elderly, alcoholism, renal or hepatic disease	*Strep. pneumoniae, Staph. aureus, H. influenzae* etc.

Fig. 20.4 Two types of respiratory invader.

VIRUSES CAUSING COMMON COLDS			
virus	**types involved**	**attachment mechanism**	**disease**
Rhinoviruses (>100 types)*	several at any given time in the community	capsid protein binds to ICAM-1 type molecule on cell**	common cold
Coxsackie virus A (24 types)	especially A21	capsid protein binds to ICAM-1 type molecule on cell**	common cold; also oropharyngeal vesicles (herpangina) and hand, foot and mouth disease (A16)
Influenza viruses	several	haemagglutinin binds to neuraminic acid-containing glycoprotein on cell	may also invade lower respiratory tract
Parainfluenza virus (4 types)	1,2,3,4	viral envelope protein binds to glycoside on cell	may also invade larynx
Respiratory syncytial virus	(1 type)	—	may also invade lower respiratory tract
Coronaviruses (several types)	all	viral envelope protein, binds to glycoprotein receptors on cell	common cold
Adenovirus (41 types)	5–10 types	penton fibre binds to cell receptor	mainly pharyngitis; also conjunctivitis, bronchitis
Echoviruses (34 types)	11, 20	—	common cold

* A given type shows little or no neutralization by antibody against other types
** ICAM-1: intercellular adhesion molecule, expressed on a wide variety of normal cells; member of immunoglobulin superfamily, coded on chromosome 19

Fig. 20.5 Common cold viruses and their mechanisms of attachment.

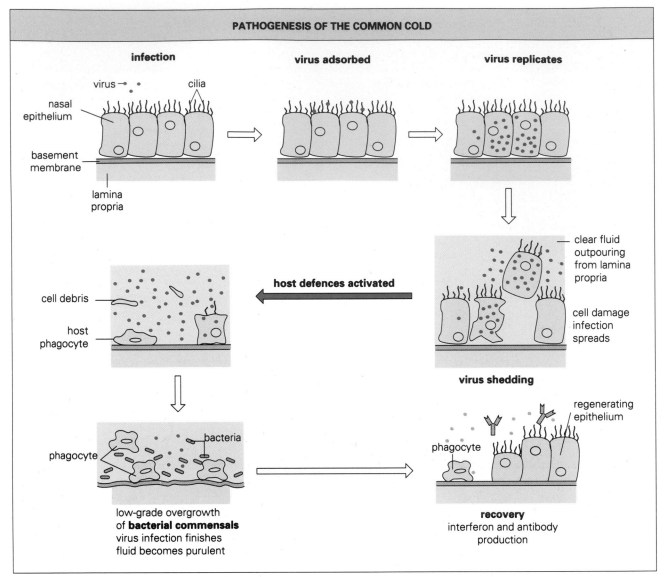

Fig. 20.6 The pathogenesis of the common cold. For simplification, the epithelium is represented as one cell thick.

rhinoviruses and coronaviruses together cause more than 50% of colds. They induce a flow of virus-rich fluid from the nasopharynx, and when the sneezing reflex is triggered, large numbers of virus particles are discharged into the air. Transmission is therefore by aerosol and also by virus-contaminated hands (see Chapter 11). Most of these viruses possess surface molecules which bind them firmly to host cells, or to cilia or microvilli protruding from these cells. As a result they are not washed away in secretions and are able to initiate infection in the normal individual. Virus progeny from the first infected cell then spreads to neighbouring cells and, via surface secretions, to new sites on the mucosal surface. After a few days, damage to epithelial cells and the secretion of fluid containing inflammatory mediators such as bradykinin leads to the common cold type symptoms (Fig. 20.6).

Laboratory diagnosis

Common cold virus infections are diagnosed by clinical appearance. Because of the large variety of viruses, and because the illness is generally mild and self-limiting with no systemic spread, laboratory tests are not worthwhile. Diagnosis becomes important when the lower respiratory tract is involved, as for instance with influenza viruses or in children with respiratory syncytial virus (RSV) infection. The antigens of these viruses can be detected in exfoliated cells present in nasopharyngeal aspirates from children, and a rise in virus-specific antibodies may give a (generally retrospective) diagnosis. Virus isolation is tedious and can be difficult, but is usually carried out for public health purposes by central laboratories when, for instance, a new pandemic strain of influenza virus has arisen.

Treatment and prevention

It is often said that if vigorous treatment with anticongestants, analgesics and antibiotics is undertaken, the common cold may resolve in 48 hours; untreated it will take two days! There are no worthwhile vaccines for the common cold viruses and treatment is for the most part symptomatic. There are, however, vaccines for influenza virus.

CAUSE OF ACUTE PHARYNGITIS		
organisms	examples	comments
Viruses	rhinoviruses, coronaviruses	a mild symptom in the common cold
	adenoviruses (types 3, 4, 7, 14, 21)	pharyngoconjunctival fever
	parainfluenza viruses	more severe than common cold
	influenza viruses	not always present
	coxsackie A and other enteroviruses	small vesicles (herpangina)
	EB virus	occurs in 70–90% of glandular fever patients
	herpes simplex types 1 and 2	can be severe, with palatal vesicles or ulcers
Bacteria	*Streptococcus pyogenes*	causes 10–20% cases of acute pharyngitis; sudden onset; mostly in 5–10 year old children
	Neisseria gonorrhoeae	often asymptomatic; usually via orogenital contact
	Corynebacterium diphtheriae	pharyngitis often mild, but toxic illness can be severe
	Haemophilus influenzae	epiglottitis
	Borrelia vincenti plus fusiform bacilli	vincent's angina; commonest in adolescents and adults

Fig. 20.7 Microorganisms that cause acute pharyngitis.

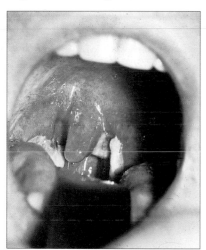

Fig. 20.8 Infectious mononucleosis caused by EB virus. The tonsils and uvula are swollen and covered in white exudate. There are petechiae on the soft palate. Courtesy of JA Innes.

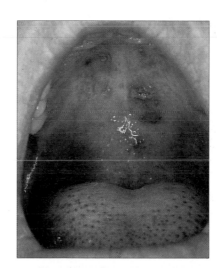

Fig. 20.9 Ulcers on the hard palate and tongue in hand, foot and mouth disease due to coxsackie A virus. Courtesy of JA Innes.

PHARYNGITIS AND TONSILLITIS

Aetiology, pathogenesis and clinical features

About 70% of acute sore throats are caused by viruses (Fig. 20.7). Common cold and other upper respiratory tract viruses inevitably encounter the submucosal lymphoid tissues that form a defensive ring round the oropharynx (see Fig. 20.2). Either because the overlying mucosa is infected or because of inflammatory and immune responses in the lymphoid tissues themselves, the throat becomes sore (pharyngitis). Adenoviruses are common causes, often infecting the conjunctiva as well as the pharynx to give pharyngoconjunctival fever. Epstein-Barr (EB) virus multiplies locally in the pharynx to produce a characteristic type of sore throat (Fig. 20.8), and herpes simplex virus and certain coxsackie A viruses multiply in the oral mucosa to produce a painful local lesion or ulcer. Certain enteroviruses (e.g. coxsackie A16) can cause additional vesicles

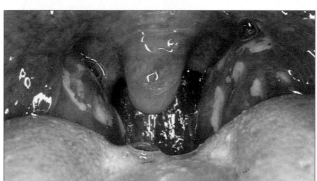

Fig. 20.10 Streptococcal tonsillitis due to group A, beta-haemolytic *Strep. pyogenes*, with intense erythema of the tonsils and a creamy-yellow exudate. Courtesy of JA Innes.

on hands, feet and in the mouth ('hand, foot and mouth disease'; Fig. 20.9).

Bacteria responsible for pharyngitis include: (1) *Streptococcus pyogenes* (Group A, beta-haemolytic; Fig. 20.10), the commonest and the most important to diagnose because it can lead to complications, (see below); it can readily be treated with penicillin; (2) *Corynebacterium diphtheriae* (see page 20.9); (3) *Haemophilus influenzae* (type B), which occasionally causes severe epiglottitis with obstruction of the airway, especially in young children; (4) *Borrelia vincenti* together with certain fusiform bacilli, which can cause throat or gingival ulcers; and (5) *Neisseria gonorrhoeae*. Each of these bacteria attach to the mucosal surface, sometimes invading local tissues.

Laboratory diagnosis and treatment

There are many possible viruses, and generally the clinical condition is not serious enough to seek laboratory help. EB virus infection is diagnosed by the presence of lymphocytosis, atypical lymphocytes, and heterophil antibodies (detected by the Paul Bunnell test). Herpes simplex virus is readily isolated in the laboratory but clinical diagnosis is usually adequate. Bacteria are identified by culturing throat swabs (see Chapter 18). It is especially important to diagnose streptococcal infection because of the possible complications (see below) and because it can be treated with penicillin. Although during winter months up to 20% of schoolchildren can carry group A streptococci in the throat without symptoms, treatment is recommended.

Complications of *Streptococcus pyogenes* throat infection

These are important enough to be listed separately although most are uncommon in developed countries where there is good access to medical care and probably less exposure to streptococci:

- Untreated streptococcal sore throats can lead to a peritonsillar abcess ('quinsy'), but this is uncommon;
- *Strep. pyogenes* may spread locally to give otitis media, sinusitis, etc. (see below);
- Certain strains of *Strep. pyogenes* produce an erythrogenic toxin, coded for by a lysogenic phage. The toxin spreads through the body and localizes in the skin to induce a punctate erythematous rash (scarlet fever; Fig. 20.11).

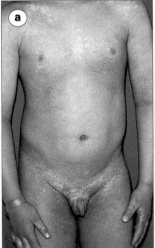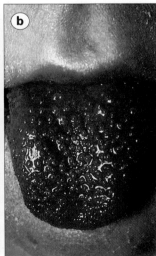

Fig. 20.11 Scarlet fever. (a) Punctate erythema is followed by peeling for 2–3 weeks. (b) The tongue, furred at first, becomes raw with prominent papillae. Courtesy of W E Farrar.

The tongue is initially furred, but later red. The rash begins as facial erythema and then spreads to involve most of the body, except the palms and soles. The face is generally flushed, with circumoral pallor. The rash fades over the course of a week and is followed by extensive desquamation. The skin lesions themselves are not a serious matter but they signal infection by a potentially harmful streptococcus, which in pre-antibiotic days could sometimes spread through the body to cause cellulitis and septicaemia;

- *Rheumatic fever.* This is an indirect complication. Antibodies are formed to antigens in the streptococcal cell wall which cross-react with the sarcolemma of human heart, and with tissues elsewhere. Granuloma are formed in the heart (Aschoff's nodules) and 2–4 weeks after the sore throat the patient (usually a child) develops myocarditis or pericarditis, perhaps subcutaneous nodules, polyarthritis and rarely chorea, a disease of the central nervous system that can be caused by anti-streptococcal antibodies reacting with neurones;

- *Rheumatic heart disease.* Repeated attacks of *Strep. pyogenes* with different M types (see Appendix) can result in damage to the heart valves. Certain children have a genetic predisposition to this immune-mediated disease. If a primary attack is accompanied by rising or high anti-streptolysin O (ASO) antibody levels (see Appendix), future attacks must be prevented by penicillin prophylaxis throughout childhood. In many developing countries rheumatic heart disease is the commonest type of heart disease;

- *Acute glomerulonephritis.* Antibodies to streptococcal components combine with these components to form circulating immune complexes, which are then deposited in glomeruli. Here, the complement and coagulation systems are activated, resulting in local inflammation. Blood appears in the urine (red cells, protein), with signs of an acute nephritis syndrome (oedema, hypertension) one to two weeks after the sore throat. ASO antibodies are usually elevated. Only 4–5 of the 65 M types of *Strep. pyogenes* give rise to this condition, and repeated infection with different 'nephritogenic' types is unlikely. Penicillin prophylaxis therefore is not given. In contrast to rheumatic fever, second attacks are rare.

OTITIS AND SINUSITIS

Aetiology and pathogenesis

Many viruses are capable of invading the air spaces associated with the upper respiratory tract (sinuses, middle ear, mastoid). Mumps virus or respiratory syncytial virus for instance, can cause vestibulitis or, generally temporarily, deafness. The range of secondary bacterial invaders is the same as in other upper respiratory tract infections, that is *Strep. pneumoniae, H. influenzae,* sometimes with anaerobes such as *Bacteroides fragilis.* Brain abscess is a major complication (see Chapter 27). Blockage of the eustachian (auditory) tube or the opening of sinuses due to allergic swelling of the mucosa, prevents mucociliary clearance of the infection, and the local accumulation of inflammatory bacterial products cause further swelling and blockage.

Acute otitis media

This condition is extremely common in infants and small children, partly because the eustachian (auditory) tube is more widely open at this age. A recent study in Boston showed that 83% of three year olds had had at least one episode, and 46% three or more episodes since birth. At least half of the attacks are viral in origin and the bacterial invaders are nasopharyngeal residents, most commonly *Strep. pneumoniae* or *H. influenzae*, and sometimes *Strep. pyogenes* or *Staph. aureus*. There may be general symptoms, and acute otitis media should be considered in any child with unexplained fever, diarrhoea or vomiting. The ear drum shows dilated vessels with bulging of the drum at a later stage (Fig. 20.12). Fluid often persists in the middle ear for weeks or months ('glue ear') regardless of therapy, and in infants and small children contributes to impaired hearing and learning difficulties. If acute attacks are inadequately treated there may be continued infection, with chronic discharge through a perforated drum and impaired hearing. This is 'chronic suppurative otitis media.'

Otitis externa

Infections of the outer ear can cause irritation and pain, and must be distinguished from otitis media. In contrast to the middle ear, the external canal has a bacterial flora similar to the skin (staphylococci, corynebacteria, and to a lesser extent propionibacteria), and the pathogens responsible for otitis media are rarely found in otitis externa. The warm moist environment favours *Staph. aureus, Candida albicans* and Gram-negative opportunists such as *Proteus* and *Pseudomonas aeruginosa*. Ear drops containing polymyxin or other antibiotics are usually effective.

ACUTE SINUSITIS

Aetiology and pathogenesis are similar to otitis media. Clinical features include facial pain and localized tenderness. It may be possible to identify the causative bacteria by microscopy and culture of pus aspirated from the sinus, but sinus puncture is not often carried out and, as in the case of otitis media, the patient is usually treated empirically with ampicillin or amoxycillin.

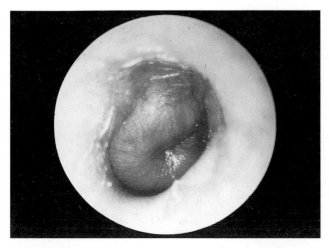

Fig. 20.12 Acute otitis media with bulging ear drum. Courtesy of M Chaput de Saintonge.

ACUTE EPIGLOTTITIS

Aetiology and pathogenesis

Acute epiglottitis is most often seen in young children, and is generally due to *Haemophilus influenzae* capsular type B. For unknown reasons the bacteria spread from the nasopharynx to the epiglottis, causing severe inflammation and oedema. Bacteraemia is usually present.

Clinical features, diagnosis and treatment

This condition must be considered as an emergency. There is difficulty with breathing because of respiratory obstruction, and until the airway has been secured (intubation), extreme care must be taken with examination of the throat in case the swollen epiglottis is sucked into the oedematous airway to cause total obstruction. Treatment is begun immediately with antibiotics effective against *H. influenzae* (cefuroxime, chloramphenicol). The clinical diagnosis is confirmed by isolating bacteria from blood and possibly the epiglottis.

Respiratory obstruction due to diphtheria (see below) is rare in developed countries, but the characteristic false membrane and local swelling can extend from the pharynx to involve the uvula.

ORAL CAVITY INFECTIONS

General features

The oral cavity is continuous with the pharynx, but is dealt with separately because of the presence of teeth, which are subject to a particular set of microbiological problems. The normal mouth contains commensal microorganisms, some of them more or less restricted to the mouth (see Fig. 20.1). Most of them make specific attachments to teeth or mucosal surfaces, and as they multiply are shed into the saliva. The litre or so of saliva secreted each day mechanically flushes the mouth. It also contains secretory antibodies, polymorphs, desquamated mucosal cells and antibacterial substances such as lysozyme and lactoperoxidase. When salivary flow is decreased for a few hours, as between meals, there is a four-fold increase in the number of bacteria in saliva, and in dehydrated patients or in severe illnesses such as typhoid or pneumonia, the mouth becomes foul because of microbial overgrowth.

Oral candidiasis

The presence of commensal bacteria makes it more difficult for invading microorganisms to become established, and changes in oral flora upset the balance. For instance, prolonged administration of broad spectrum antibiotics allows the normally harmless *C. albicans* to flourish, penetrating the epithelium with its pseudomycelia, and causing thrush. Oral thrush (candidiasis; Fig. 20.13) is also seen when immunity is impaired, as in HIV infection, malignancy, and occasionally in newborn infants and in the elderly. It sometimes spreads to involve the oesophagus. Diagnosis is readily confirmed by gram stain and culture of scraped material which shows large gram-positive budding yeasts. Topical antifungal agents such as nystatin serve as an effective treatment, together with attention to any predisposing factors.

As another example of the shifting boundary between harmless coexistence and tissue invasion by resident microbes, vitamin C deficiency reduces mucosal resistance and allows residents to cause gum infections.

Caries

The microorganisms specifically adapted for life on teeth form a film called dental plaque on the tooth surface. This is a complex mass containing about 10^9 bacteria per gram embedded in a polysaccharide matrix (Fig. 20.14). The film, visible as a red layer when a dye such as erythrocin is taken into the mouth, is largely removed by thorough brushing, but reestablishes itself within a few hours. The clean teeth become covered with salivary glycoproteins to which certain streptococci (especially *Strep. mutans* and *Strep. sobrinus*) become attached and multiply. In the USA and western Europe, 80–90% of people are colonized by *Strep. mutans*. *Strep. mutans* itself synthesizes glucan (a sticky high molecular weight polysaccharide) from sucrose and this forms a matrix between these streptococci. Certain other bacteria, including anaerobic filamentous fusobacteria and actinomyces are also present. When the teeth are not cleaned for several days plaque becomes thicker and more extensive, a tangled forest of microorganisms.

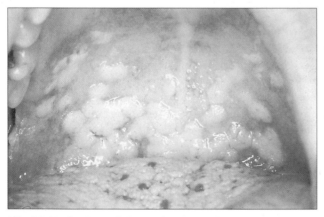

Fig 20.13 Oral candidiasis. Courtesy of JA Innes.

The bacteria in plaque utilize dietary sugar and form lactic acid, which decalcifies the tooth locally. Proteolytic enzymes from the bacteria help to break down other components of the enamel to give a painful cavity in the tooth (caries). The pH in an active caries lesion may be as low as 4.0. Thus caries develops, usually in crevices on the tooth, when suitable bacteria *(Strep. mutans)* are in the plaque and there is a regular supply of sucrose. It may legitimately be regarded as an infectious disease – one of the most prevalent infectious diseases in western man, with his closely placed bacteria-coated teeth and his sugary, often fluoride-deficient diet.

Periodontal disease

The space between the gums and tooth margin, the gingival crevice, may be considered as an oral backwater. It normally contains polymorphs, complement, IgG and IgM antibodies, but readily becomes infected. Gingival crevices in healthy adults contain an average of 2.7×10^{11} microbes per gram, three-quarters of them anaerobes. Bacteria such as *Actinomyces viscosus*, *Actinobacillus* and *Bacteroides* species are commonly involved. There is local inflammation, with an increasing number of polymorphs and a serum exudate. The inflamed gum bleeds readily and later recedes, while the multiplying bacteria cause halitosis. Finally the structures supporting the teeth are affected, with reabsorption of ligaments and weakening of bone, causing the teeth to loosen. Periodontal disease, with gingivitis is almost universal, although its severity varies greatly. It is a major cause of tooth loss in adults.

LARYNGITIS AND TRACHEITIS

Aetiology

Viral infections of the upper respiratory tract may spread downwards to involve the larynx and the trachea. In adults laryngeal infection (laryngitis) and tracheitis causes hoarseness, and a burning retrosternal pain on breathing in and out. The larynx and trachea have non-expandable rings of cartilage in the wall, which in children are easily

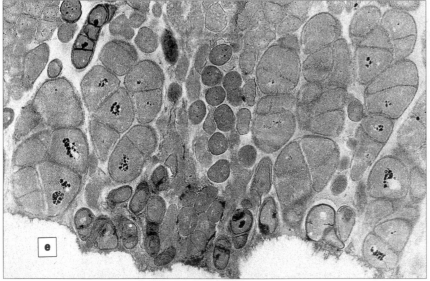

Fig 20.14 Dental plaque on the deep surface of a child's tooth. e, enamel. x20 000. Courtesy of H N Newman.

obstructed due to their narrowness. Swelling of the mucous membrane may lead to *croup*, which consists of a dry cough and inspiratory stridor ('crowing'). Difficulty with respiration may lead to hospital admission. Parainfluenza viruses, especially types I and III, are common causes, and sometimes respiratory syncytial virus or influenza virus. Diphtheria(see below) may involve the larynx or trachea.

DIPHTHERIA

Aetiology, pathogenesis and clinical features

Diphtheria is caused by toxin-producing strains of *Corynebacterium diphtheriae*. The infection is now rare in developed countries due to widespread immunization with toxoid (see Chapter 34) but it is still common in developing countries. Non-toxigenic strains occur in the normal pharynx, but to cause disease toxigenic bacteria must be present. They can colonize the pharynx (especially the tonsillar regions), the larynx, the nose, occasionally the genital tract, or the skin (in the tropics or in indigent people with poor skin hygiene). Adhesion mechanisms are not understood but the bacteria multiply locally without invading deeper tissues or spreading through the body. The toxin destroys epithelial cells and polymorphs and an ulcer forms, which is covered with a necrotic exudate, forming a 'false membrane'. This soon becomes dark and

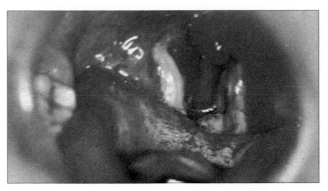

Fig. 20.15 Pharyngeal diphtheria with dirty-white exudate over tonsils and severe local inflammation and swelling. Courtesy of K Nye.

malodourous, and bleeding occurs when there is an attempt to remove it. There is much local inflammation and swelling (Fig. 20.15) and the cervical lymph nodes may be enlarged to give a 'bull neck' appearance. Nasopharyngeal diphtheria is the most severe form of the disease. When the larynx is involved it can result in life-threatening respiratory obstruction. Anterior nasal diphtheria, if it occurs on its own, is a mild form of the disease because toxin is less well absorbed from this site, and a nasal discharge may be the main symptom. The patient will, however, be highly infectious.

Diphtheria toxin

The genes encoding toxin production are carried by a temperate bacteriophage which, during the lysogenic phase, is integrated into the bacterial chromosome. The toxin is synthesized as a single polypeptide (mol. wt 62 000; 535 amino acids), consisting of fragment B (binding) at the carboxyterminal end, which attaches the toxin to the host cells (or to any eucaryotic cell), and fragment A (active) at the aminoterminal end, which is the toxic fragment. Toxic fragment A is only formed (by protease cleavage and reduction of disulphide bonds) after uptake of the toxin into the cell. Fragment A inactivates elongation factor-2 (EF-2) by ADP ribosylation, and thereby inhibits protein synthesis (Fig. 20.16). Procaryotic and mitochondrial protein synthesis is not affected because a different elongation factor is involved. A single bacterium can produce 5000 toxin molecules per hour and the toxic fragment is so stable within the cell that a single molecule can kill a cell. For unknown reasons myocardial and peripheral nerve cells are particularly susceptible.

Fig 20.16 Diphtheria toxin – mechanism of action.

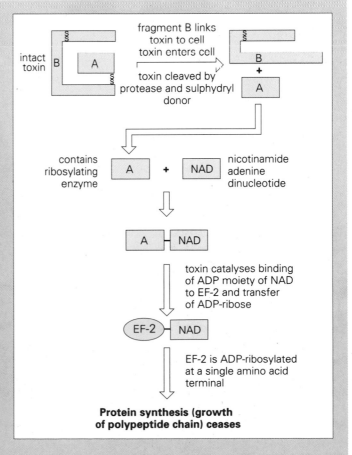

The toxin (see panel above) is absorbed into the lymphatics and blood, and has several effects:

* Constitutional upset, with fever, pallor, exhaustion;
* Myocarditis, usually within the first two weeks. ECG changes are common and cardiac failure can occur. If this is not lethal, complete recovery is usual;
* Polyneuritis may occur, usually not until many weeks after the onset of illness. It may for instance affect the 9th cranial nerve, resulting in paralysis of the soft palate and regurgitation of fluids.

Diagnosis and treatment

Diphtheria is a life threatening disease and clinical diagnosis is a matter of urgency. As soon as the diagnosis is suspected clinically the patient is isolated to reduce the risk of the toxigenic strain spreading to other susceptible individuals, and treatment with antitoxin is begun. The antitoxin is produced in horses, and tests for hypersensitivity to horse serum should be carried out. Penicillin or erythromycin is given as an adjunct. Laryngeal diphtheria may require tracheotomy. The diagnosis is confirmed in the laboratory by isolation and identification of the organism (see Appendix and Chapter 18), and demonstrating toxin production by a gel-diffusion precipitin reaction (Elek test). Contacts should be tested for carriage of toxigenic *C. diphtheriae* and if necessary be given chemoprophylaxis or immunization. Toxigenic bacteria may be carried and transmitted by asymptomatic convalescents or by normal individuals.

Prevention

Diphtheria has almost disappeared from developed countries, due to immunization of children with a safe, effective vaccine, consisting of diphtheria toxoid plus aluminium hydroxide as adjuvant (for details see Chapter 36).

SUMMARY

The respiratory tract, from nose to alveoli, is a continuum, and any given microbe can cause disease in more than one segment. Some respiratory infections are restricted to the surface epithelium (influenza, diphtheria, pertussis), while others spread throughout the body (measles, rubella). 'Professional' invaders infect the healthy respiratory tract (e.g. common cold viruses, influenza viruses, *M. tuberculosis*), and can be distinguished from 'secondary' invaders that cause disease when host defences are impaired (e.g. *Staph. aureus, P. carinii, Pseudomonas*). In the oral catvity the teeth and neighboring structures are sites of very prevalent diseases (caries, periodontal disease) that are of microbial aetiology. Diphtheria, a life threatening disease caused by a biochemically defined bacterial toxin is completely preventable by vaccination.

Further Reading

Congoni B, Rizzo C, Congeni J *et al*. Outbreak of acute rheumatic fever in northeast Ohio. *J Pediatr* 1987; **111**: 176–179.

Dixon JMS. Diphtheria in North America. *J Hyg* (Camb) 1984; **93**: 419–432.

Fischetti VA. Streptococcal M protein: molecular design and biological behaviour. *Clin Microb Revs* 1989; **2**: 285–314.

Henderson FW, Collier AM, Sanyal MA *et al*. A longitudinal study of respiratory viruses and bacteria in the etiology of acute otitis media with effusion. *N Engl J Med* 1982; **366**: 1377.

McCain LG. Group syndrome. *Am Fam Physician* 1987; **36**: 202–214.

McMillan JA, Sandstrom C, Weiner LB *et al*. Viral and bacterial organisms associated with acute pharyngitis in a school-aged population. *J Pediatr* 1986; **109**: 747–752.

Pappinheimer AM. The diphtheria bacillus and its toxin; a model system. *J Hyg* (Camb) 1984; **93**: 397–440.

Shaw JH. Causes and control of dental caries. *N Engl J Med* 1987; **317**: 996.

Turner RB, Hendley JO, Gwaltney JM. Shedding of infected ciliated epithelial cells in rhinovirus colds. *J Infect Dis* 1982; **145**: 849.

White JM, Littman DR. Viral receptors of the immunoglobulin superfamily. *Cell* 1989; **56**: 725–728.

21 INFECTIONS OF THE EYE

Contents

INTRODUCTION

The outer surface of the eye is exposed to the external world and is therefore open to contact with infective organisms. The conjunctiva is particularly susceptible. Not only is it a vulnerable epithelial surface, but it is covered by the eyelids, which create a warm, moist, enclosed environment in which contaminating organisms may quickly establish and set up a focus of infection. The eyelids and tears, however, also serve to protect the external surfaces of the eye, both mechanically and biologically; any interference with their function increases the chances that pathogens may become established.

The conjunctiva can be invaded by other routes, such as the blood or nervous systems (Fig. 21.1) and the deeper tissues of the eye can also be invaded from within, particularly by protozoan and worm parasites (Fig. 21.2). Eyelid infections are generally due to *Staphylococcus aureus*, with involvement of lid margins (blepharitis) or eyelid glands and follicles (stye, hordeolum).

MICROBIAL INFECTIONS OF THE CONJUNCTIVA	
organism	**comments**
Adenovirus	especially types 3,7,8,19
Measles virus	infection of conjunctiva via blood
Herpes simplex virus	virus reactivating in ophthalmic division of trigeminal ganglia causes corneal lesion (dendritic ulcer)
Varicella-zoster virus	may involve conjunctiva
Enterovirus 70 Coxsackie virus A 24	acute haemorrhagic conjunctivitis
Chlamydia trachomatis (types A-C)	cause of trachoma and commonly blindness
(types D-K)	cause of 'trachoma', inclusion conjunctivitis (TRIC); infection via fingers etc. or, in newborn, via birth canal
Neisseria gonorrhoeae	infection of newborn via birth canal
Staphylococcus aureus	cause of eyelid infection (styes) and 'sticky eye' in neonates

Fig. 21.1 Microbial infections of the conjunctiva.

INFECTIONS OF THE DEEPER LAYERS OF THE EYE		
organism	**disease**	**route of infection**
Rubella	cataracts, microphthalmia	infection *in utero*
Cytomegalovirus	chorioretinitis	infection *in utero*; may occur in AIDS
Pseudomonas aeruginosa	serious inner eye infection	after trauma foreign bodies in eye eye operations bacteria can contaminate eye drops
Toxoplasma gondii (toxoplasmosis)	chorioretinitis	infection *in utero*
Echinococcus granulosus (hydatid disease)	distortion of the eye by growth of larval tapeworm in hydatid cyst	transmission by eggs passed by dogs
Toxocara canis (ocular toxocariasis)	chorioretinitis, blindness	transmission by eggs passed by dogs
Onchocerca volvulus (river blindness)	sclerosing keratitis chorioretinitis	larvae transmitted by blood-feeding *Simulium* flies

Fig. 21.2 Infections of the deeper layers of the eye.

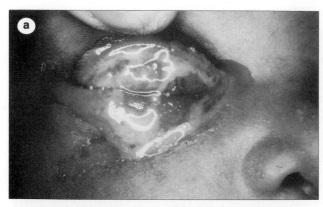
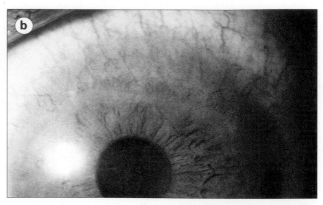

Fig. 21.3 Chlamydial conjunctivitis (a) is the commonest form of neonatal conjunctivitis. Courtesy of G Ridgway. Trachoma (b), showing formation of trachomatous pannus with new vessel formation and hazy corneal margin. Courtesy of MJ Wood.

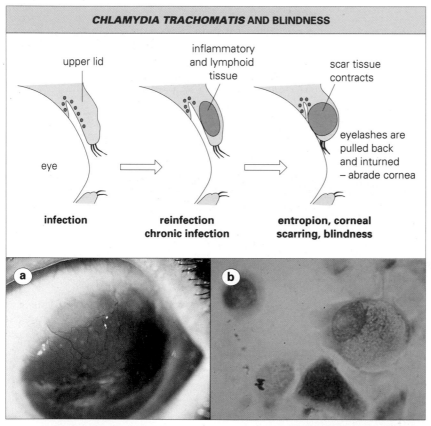

CHLAMYDIA TRACHOMATIS AND BLINDNESS

upper lid

inflammatory and lymphoid tissue

scar tissue contracts

eye

eyelashes are pulled back and inturned – abrade cornea

infection

reinfection chronic infection

entropion, corneal scarring, blindness

Fig. 21.4 *Chlamydia trachomatis* and blindness. Scarring of the cornea (a) results from long-standing ocular trachoma. Courtesy of RC Barnes. Giemsa stain of an ocular scraping from trachoma (b) shows *C. trachomatis* as an intracellular inclusion. Courtesy of G Ridgeway.

CONJUNCTIVITIS

Aetiology and pathogenesis

To establish infection on the conjunctiva, microorganisms must avoid being rinsed and wiped away in tears. The best way of achieving this is to have a specific mechanism of attachment to conjunctival cells. Chlamydia, for example, have surface molecules that bind specifically to receptors on host cells. This is one of the reasons that, of all the organisms which infect the conjunctiva (see Fig. 21.1), they are among the most successful. There are at least fifteen different serotypes of chlamydia responsible for inclusion conjunctivitis (Fig. 21.3), and also for trachoma the most important eye infection in the world. More than 600 million people, are infected by *Chlamydia trachomatis* and 10–20 million are blinded by it, while many others suffer visual impairment. Transmission of *C. trachomatis* is by contact with contaminated flies, fingers, towels, etc. Trachoma itself is the result of chronic repeated infections (Fig. 21.4), especially prevalent when there is poor access to water, preventing regular washing of hands and face. Under these circumstances spread of chlamydia from one conjunctiva to another is frequent, and can be referred to as 'ocular promiscuity', comparable with the spread of genital secretions in non-specific urethritis (see Chapter 24). Some chlamydial serotypes can infect the urinogenital tract (see Chapter 24) as well as the conjunctiva, and the conjunctiva or lungs of a newborn infant may become infected after passage down an infected birth canal (see Chapter 26). Systemic treatment with erythromycin is generally needed.

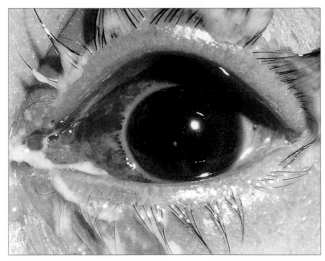

Fig. 21.5 Purulent discharge in bacterial conjunctivitis, often associated with infections by *Streptococcus pnemoniae*, *Haemophilus influenzae* and *Staphylococcus aureus*. Courtesy of M Tapert.

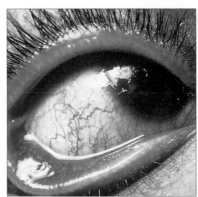

Fig. 21.6 Herpes simplex keratitis. Dendritic ulcers, seen here on the cornea, are common in recurrent herpes simplex infections. Courtesy of MJ Wood.

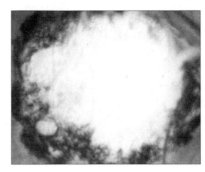

Fig. 21.7 Congenital toxoplasmosis. Fundus photograph showing scar left after healed chorioretinitis. Courtesy of MJ Wood.

Chlamydia – diagnosis, treatment and prevention.

Laboratory diagnosis of chlamydial infections (see Appendix) can be carried out using conjunctival fluid or scrapings. Because infection and reinfection is facilitated by overcrowding, shortage of water and abundant fly populations, the disease can be prevented by improvements in standards of hygiene. For example, a study in Mexico showed that a daily face wash reduced the incidence of trachoma in children from 48% to 10%. In spite of many decades of research there are still no vaccines for chlamydial infections. This is partly because immunopathology itself makes a major contribution to the disease.

Other conjunctival and surface infections

Several bacteria (e.g. *Streptococcus pneumoniae*, *Haemophilus influenzae* and *Leptospira*) may cause conjunctivitis (Fig. 21.5). Infection by *Neisseria gonorrhoeae* is a hazard of birth through an infected birth canal and can result in a severe purulent condition. It is seen on the first or second day of life (ophthalmia neonatorum) and requires urgent treatment with penicillin, but can be prevented by applying erythromycin ointment shortly after birth. *Staphylococcus aureus* also produces infections in newborns as well as in adults. The eyes of infants may be invaded by this organism if there is transfer from the child's own body or from infected adults.

Direct infection of the eye may also be associated with the use of contact lenses. Excessive wearing can lead to a reduction in effectiveness of the eye's defence mechanisms, allowing pathogens to become established, but more likely hazards are the use of contaminated eye drops or cleaning solutions and the insertion of contaminated lenses. A number of bacteria can be transmitted directly in this way. The free-living amoeba *Acanthamoeba* can multiply in unchanged lens cleaning fluids, be transferred when the lens is inserted and cause corneal damage.

Several organisms invade the superficial tissues of the eye after transport through the bloodstream or, in the case of herpes simplex virus, by movement along the trigeminal nerve. Reactivation of the virus in previously infected patients can result in the development of a keratitis with formation of dendritic ulcers (Fig. 21.6). Inadvertent use of topical steroids may aggravate this condition, and the resultant severe ulceration may lead to corneal destruction.

INFECTION OF THE DEEPER LAYERS OF THE EYE

Trauma to the eye may result in the establishment of *Pseudomonas aeruginosa*, giving rise to serious inner eye infection. This organism may also be introduced via contaminated eye drops. Rubella and cytomegalovirus may invade the fetal eye *in utero*, the former causing cataracts and microphthalmia, the latter a severe chorioretinitis. Congenital syphilis produces a retinopathy with quiescent lesions, and keratitis may appear in later life. Secondary syphilis is also associated with ocular inflammation.

Toxoplasmosis

Chorioretinitis is also associated with toxoplasmosis. Although infection with this protozoan (*Toxoplasma gondii*) is widespread (see Chapter 3) it is not serious unless: 1) acquired *in utero*, when the organism invades all tissues, especially the central nervous system, or 2) acquired (or reactivated) under immunosuppression. Infection occurs by swallowing oocysts released by infected cats (the primary host) or by eating meat containing tissue cysts. Women who become infected in pregnancy may transmit the infection to the foetus, as tachyzoites can cross the placenta. Tissue cysts can form in the retina of the foetus and undergo continuous proliferation, producing progressive lesions, particularly when levels of immunity are low. These lesions may also involve the choroid (Fig. 21.7) and lead ultimately to blindness.

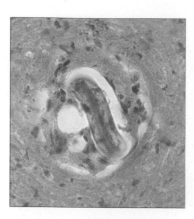

Fig. 21.8 *Toxocara canis.* Granuloma in the posterior pole of an infected eye. The larval nematode is clearly visible in the centre of the granuloma. Courtesy of D Spalton.

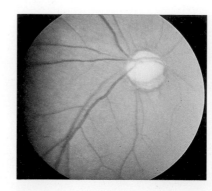

Fig. 21.9 Onchocerciasis. Sclerosis of the choroidal vessels caused by invading microfilaria of *O. volvulus.* Courtesy of J Anderson.

Worm infections

A number of worm parasites are known to invade the eye, preferentially or accidentally. Larval tapeworms (e.g. the hydatid cyst stage of *Echinococcus granulosus* transmitted by eggs passed from infected dogs), occasionally enter the eye, the growth of the cysts causing severe mechanical damage. More common is invasion by migratory larvae of the nematode *Toxocara canis.* This parasite occurs naturally in the intestines of dogs, releasing thick-shelled resistant eggs into the environment. The eggs can hatch if swallowed by humans, the larvae initiating, but failing to complete their customary migration through the tissues. In the canine host, migration results in the worm regaining the intestine where they become mature. In humans larvae can enter almost any organ, often CNS or eye (Fig. 21.8) triggering an intense inflammatory response. In the eye, localized lesions in the retina may cause detachment. The misdiagnosis of such ocular lesions as retinoblastoma has led to enucleation. Anthelmintic treatment is beneficial.

The other major worm infection associated with ocular damage is *Onchocerca volvulus,* the cause of river blindness in Africa and Central America. This infection is transmitted by the bites of *Simulium* flies. These take up microfilaria larvae from the skin of infected hosts and, after the larvae have become infective, reintroduce them when next feeding. Adult worms live in subcutaneous nodules, and are comparatively harmless. The microfilaria, released by the females in enormous numbers for uptake by other flies, induce intense inflammatory reactions in the skin. This causes severe itching and eventually degenerative changes; lymphadenitis, lymphoedema and elephantiasis may also occur. The larvae migrate through subcutaneous tissue, and invasion of the eye is particularly common in certain regions of Africa, as well as Central America. The inflammatory responses in the eye cause a number of pathological changes, which may affect both the anterior and posterior chambers (Fig. 21.9). These include punctate and sclerosing keratitis, iridocyclitis, chorioretinitis and optic atrophy. The disease is called 'river blindness' because the *Simulium* flies develop in rivers and those living near rivers are most affected. Blindness rates may reach 40% of the adult population in endemic areas. Microfilariae can be seen in biopsies of affected skin. Anthelmintic treatment (ivermectin) may reduce microfilarial levels and block transmission, but the blindness is irreversible.

SUMMARY

Because the nature of the conjunctiva makes the eye particularly vulnerable to infectious organisms it is well protected against external invasion. The number of organisms responsible for infection of the conjunctiva is relatively small, but the consequences of infection are always potentially serious, given that sight is dependent upon the presence of an intact, transparent cornea. Inflammatory responses to surface infections, though 'designed' to limit invasion and repair damage, have the capacity to alter conjunctival and corneal surfaces irreversibly. Similarly, the structure–function relationships of the retina make this vulnerable to the consequences of infection and inflammation. Again, although relatively few organisms invade the retina, those that do are potentially dangerous. It is striking that some of the most serious infection-related diseases of the eye involve invasion by protozoan or helminth parasites. Unfortunately, the biology of these organisms is such that diagnosis of ocular infections often follows, rather than precedes, the development of visual impairment.

Further Reading

Levin RM, Ticknor W, Jordan C. *et al.* Etiology of conjunctivitis. *J Pediatr* 1981; **99**: 831.

Tight RR. Gonococcal conjunctivitis. *J Am Med Assoc* 1982; **247**: 2499.

Holmes KK. The chlamydia epidemic. *J Am Med Assoc* 1981; **245**: 1718.

D'Angelo LJ, Hierholzer JC, Holman RC *et al.* Epidemic keratoconjunctivitis caused by adenovirus type 8. Epidemiology and laboratory aspects of large outbreak. *Am J Epidemiol* 1981; **113**: 44.

Molk R. Ocular toxocariasis. A review of the literature. *Ann Ophthalmol* 1983; **15**: 216.

22 LOWER RESPIRATORY TRACT INFECTIONS

Contents

INTRODUCTION

Although the respiratory tract is continuous from nose to alveoli, it is convenient to distinguish between infections of the upper and lower respiratory tract, even though the same microorganism may be implicated in infections throughout the continuum. Infections of the upper respiratory tract and associated structures are the subject of the previous chapter. Here, we discuss infections of the lower respiratory tract. These infections tend to be more severe and the choice of appropriate antimicrobial therapy is important and may be life saving.

Broadly speaking the infections can be divided into acute and chronic. Among the acute infections four major syndromes can be identified; acute bronchitis, acute exacerbations of chronic bronchitis, bronchiolitis and pneumonia. Influenza is a specific infection which, if severe, may proceed to bronchitis or pneumonia. Whooping cough will be considered in this chapter as a serious and acute infection of the lower respiratory tract. The latter part of the chapter deals with chronic infections, including specific infections such as tuberculosis and aspergillosis and conditions such as lung abscesses and empyema. Infections in cystic fibrosis patients are also covered in the section on chronic infections.

ACUTE INFECTIONS OF THE LOWER RESPIRATORY TRACT

Whooping cough

Aetiology and pathogenesis

Whooping cough or pertussis is a severe disease of childhood caused by the bacterium *Bordetella pertussis*. This species of *Bordetella* is confined to humans and is spread from person to person by airborne droplets. The organisms attach to and multiply in the ciliated respiratory mucosa but do not invade deeper. Surface components such as filamentous haemagglutinin and fimbrial agglutinogens play an important role in specific attachment to respiratory epithelium. Several toxic factors have been identified, some of which affect inflammatory processes, while others damage ciliary epithelium. These are:

- Pertussis toxin – this resembles diphtheria and other toxins (see Chapter 16) in being a subunit toxin with an active (A) unit and a binding (B) unit. The A unit is an ADP-ribosyl transferase which catalyses the transfer of ADP-ribose from NAD to host cell proteins. The functional consequence of this is a disruption of signal transduction to the affected cell, but the toxin probably has other effects on the cell surface as well;
- Adenylate cyclase toxin – this is a single peptide which can enter host cells and cause them to increase their cyclic AMP to supraphysiologic levels. In neutrophils this results in an inhibition of defence functions such as chemotaxis, phagocytosis and bactericidal killing. This toxin may also be responsible for the haemolytic properties of *B. pertussis*;
- Tracheal cytotoxin – this is a cell wall component derived from the peptidoglycan of *B. pertussis* which kills tracheal epithelial cells specifically;
- Endotoxin – the structure of the cell wall lipopolysaccharide in *Bordetella* differs from the classic endotoxin in other Gram-negative rods but has functional similarities and may play a role in the pathogenesis of infection.

Clinical features

After an incubation period of 1–3 weeks, infection is manifest first as a catarrhal illness with little to distinguish it from other upper respiratory tract infections. This is followed up to a week later by a dry, non-productive cough which becomes paroxysmal. A paroxysm is characterized by a series of short coughs productive of copious mucus, followed by a 'whoop'; a characteristic sound produced by an inspiratory gasp of air. Despite the severity of the cough, the symptoms are confined to the respiratory tract; lobar or segmental collapse of the lungs can occur (Fig. 22.1). Complications include central nervous system anoxia, exhaustion and secondary pneumonia due to invasion of other pathogens into the damaged respiratory tract.

Diagnosis

The early clinical picture is non-specific and the true diagnosis may not be suspected until the paroxysmal phase. The organisms can be isolated on suitable media from throat swabs or on 'cough plates' (see Chapter 18 and Appendix) but they are fastidious and do not survive well outside the host's environment.

Treatment

Supportive care is of prime importance. Infants are at greatest risk of complications and admission to hospital should be considered for children under one year of age.

For specific antibacterial treatment to be effective it must penetrate the respiratory mucosa and inhibit or kill the infecting organism. Erythromycin is the drug of choice. Although treatment is often not begun until the disease is recognized in the paroxysmal phase, it does appear to reduce the severity and duration. It also reduces the numbers of organisms in the throat (thereby helping to reduce the infectivity of the patient) and helps to reduce the number of secondary infections.

Erythromycin prophylaxis of close contacts of active cases is helpful in controlling the spread of infection.

Prevention

Whooping cough can be prevented by active immunization. For many years a whole cell vaccine comprising a killed suspension of *B. pertussis* cells has been used. It is usually combined with purified diphtheria and tetanus toxoids and administered as 'DPT' or 'triple' vaccine. The efficacy of pertussis vaccine is generally high but variable, and recent years have seen major concern about side effects. These take the form of (a) fever, malaise and pain at the site of administration, which may occur in up to 20% of infants and are not serious; (b) convulsions, thought to be associated with the vaccine in about 0.5% of vaccinees; (c) encephalopathy and permanent neurologic sequelae associated with vaccination, with an estimated rate of 1 in 100 000 vaccinations (<0.001%). The concern

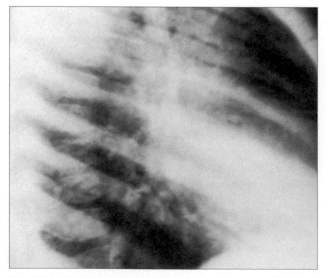

Fig. 22.1 Chest radiograph showing patchy consolidation and collapse of the right middle lobe in whooping cough. Courtesy of JA Innes.

about side effects led to a marked fall in uptake of the vaccine and subsequently to a marked increase in the incidence of whooping cough (see Chapter 36). Efforts are now being concentrated on the production of a subunit vaccine containing only the 'protective' antigens. The difficulty has been in identifying those antigens, but a combination of inactivated pertussis toxin and filamentous haemagglutinin appears to be promising and such vaccines have already been used in Japan.

Acute bronchitis

This is an inflammatory condition of the tracheobronchial tree usually associated with infection. Causative agents include viruses (rhinoviruses, coronaviruses) which are also found infecting the upper respiratory tract, and lower tract pathogens such as influenza virus, adenoviruses and *Mycoplasma pneumoniae*. Secondary bacterial infection with *Streptococcus pneumoniae* and *Haemophilus influenzae* may also play a role in pathogenesis. The degree of damage to the respiratory epithelium varies with the infecting agent; with influenza virus infection it may be extensive and leaves the host prone to secondary bacterial invasion (post-influenza pneumonia; see below). With *Mycoplasma pneumoniae* infection, the specific attachment of the organism to receptors on the bronchial mucosal epithelium (Fig. 22.2) and release of toxic substances by the organism results in sloughing off of affected cells.

A cough is the most prominent presentation and treatment is largely symptomatic. The value of antibiotics is uncertain but they are usually recommended.

Acute exacerbations of chronic bronchitis

Chronic bronchitis is a condition in which cough and excessive secretion of mucus are present in the tracheo-bronchial tree and are not attributable to specific diseases such as bronchiectasis, asthma, or tuberculosis. Infection appears to be only one component of the syndrome, the others being cigarette smoking and inhalation of dust or fumes from the workplace. Bacterial infection does not appear to initiate the disease but is probably significant in perpetuating it and in producing the characteristic acute exacerbations. *Strep. pneumoniae* and unencapsulated strains of *H. influenzae* are the organisms most frequently isolated, but interpretation of their presence in sputum is difficult because they are also commonly found in the normal throat flora and thus can contaminate expectorated sputum. Other bacteria such as *Staphylococcus aureus* and *Mycoplasma pneumoniae* are less commonly associated with infection and exacerbation. Viruses are frequent causes of acute infection.

Antibiotic therapy may be helpful in the treatment of acute exacerbations although efficacy is difficult to assess.

Bronchiolitis

Bronchiolitis is a disease restricted to childhood and usually to children of less than 2 years. The bronchioles of a young child have such a fine bore that if their lining cells are swollen by inflammation the passage of air to and from the alveoli may be severely restricted. Infection results in necrosis of the epithelial cells which line the bronchioles and leads to peribronchial infiltration which may spread into the lung fields to give an interstitial pneumonia (see below). As many as 75% of these infections are caused by respiratory syncytial virus (RSV); most of the remaining 25% are also of viral aetiology although *Mycoplasma pneumoniae* is implicated occasionally.

Respiratory syncytial virus infection

Aetiology and transmission

This is a typical paramyxovirus and there is only one antigenic type. Its surface spikes are fusion proteins (not haemagglutinins or neuraminidases) which fuse host cells to form 'syncytia'.

The infection is transmitted by droplets and to some extent via hands. RSV is the most important cause of bronchiolitis and pneumonia (see below) in infants, about one in a hundred cases requiring admission to hospital. Outbreaks occur each winter (Fig. 22.3), and during the RSV season infection can spread in hospitals as well as in the community. Nearly all individuals have been infected by two years of age.

Clinical features and pathogenesis

After inhalation the virus establishes infection in the nasopharynx and lower respiratory tract. Clinical illness appears after an incubation period of four to five days. The illness can be particularly severe in young infants (peak mortality at 3 months of age), the virus invading the lower respiratory tract by direct surface spread to cause bronchiolitis or pneumonia. In young children and adults, however, the virus is restricted to the upper respiratory tract, causing a less severe common cold-type illness. Young infants develop a cough, rapid respiratory rate, and cyanosis. Otitis media is quite common. Secondary bacterial infection is rare and the disease appears to have an immunopathological basis. Maternal antibodies present in the infant react with virus antigens, perhaps together with the liberation of histamine and other mediators from the host's cells. In early trials a killed vaccine was used and the fact that this often resulted in more severe disease supports the idea of immunopathology.

Neutralizing antibodies are formed (lower levels in younger infants) but cell-mediated immunity is needed

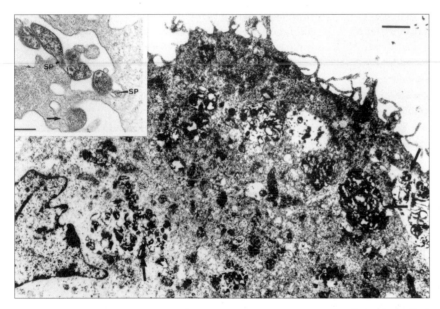

Fig. 22.2 Osponized *M. pneumoniae* cells (arrowed) phagocytosed by an alveolar macrophage (bar, 2μm). The insert shows *M. pneumoniae* cells adhering with the tip organelle (SP) to macrophage surfaces. Reproduced from Jacobs E, 1991; with permission from Churchill-Livingstone Medical Journals.

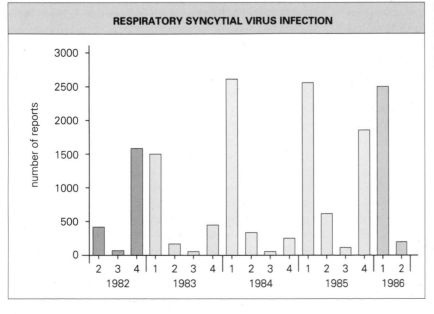

RESPIRATORY SYNCYTIAL VIRUS INFECTION

Fig. 22.3 Acute bronchiolitis in respiratory syncitial virus infection. Seasonal variation in quarterly reports of RSV infection in England and Wales. Redrawn from CDSC data.

for termination of the infection. In children lacking cell-mediated immunity the virus continues to be shed from the lungs for many months. Normal children, even a year or two after apparent recovery, may continue to show depressed pulmonary function or wheezing. Recurrent infections are common although they are less severe. The reason for this, which is also seen with parainfluenza viruses, is unknown.

Diagnosis

RSV-specific antigens are detectable by immunofluorescence (Fig. 22.4) or ELISA methods (see Chapter 18), in smears of exfoliated cells obtained by nasopharyngeal lavage. Virus isolation is less commonly useful and success depends on inoculating respiratory secretions as soon as possible into cell cultures.

Treatment and prevention

The antiviral agent ribavirin used as an aerosol has occasionally been successful in severe cases. At present there is no vaccine.

Pneumonia

Pneumonia has long been known as 'the old man's friend'; it is the most common cause of infection-related death in USA and UK and is caused by a wide range of microorganisms giving indistinguishable symptoms. The challenge lies not in the clinical diagnosis of pneumonia (except perhaps in children, where it may be more difficult) but in the laboratory identification of the microbial cause (see Appendix). In the absence of this, the choice of antimicrobial therapy may not be optimal.

Pathogenesis

Microorganisms gain access to the lower respiratory tract by inhalation of aerosolized material or by aspiration of the normal flora of the upper respiratory tract. The size of inhaled particles is important in determining how far down into the respiratory tract they can travel, only those less than about 5μm diameter reaching the alveoli. Less frequently, the lungs become seeded with organisms as a result of spread via the blood from other infected sites. Perfectly healthy individuals are susceptible to infection by a range of pathogens possessing adhesins which allow them to attach specifically to the respiratory epithelium (see Chapter 10). In addition, the host with impaired defences (immunocompromise, preceding viral damage, cystic fibrosis, etc.) may suffer infection with organisms which do not cause infections in the healthy person (e.g. *Pneumocystis carinii* is an important cause of pneumonia in AIDS patients).

The respiratory tract is limited in the number of ways in which it can respond to infection. The host's responses can be defined by their pathological and radiological findings but the terms can be confusing because they are applied differently in different situations. However four descriptive terms are in common use (Fig. 22.5):
- Lobar pneumonia refers to involvement of a distinct region of the lung. The polymorphonuclear exudate formed in response to infection clots in the alveoli and

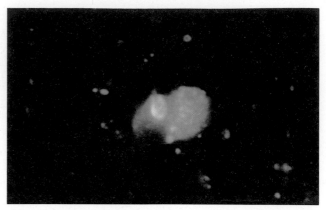

Fig. 22.4 Immunofluorescent preparation from the nasopharynx showing RSV-infected cells (bright green). Courtesy of H Stern.

renders them solid. Infection may spread to adjacent alveoli until constrained by anatomic barriers between segments or lobes of the lung. Thus one lobe may show complete consolidation;
- Bronchopneumonia refers to a more diffuse, patchy consolidation which may spread throughout the lung as a result of the original pathologic process in the small airways;
- Interstitial pneumonia involves invasion of the lung interstitium and is particularly characteristic of viral infections of the lungs;
- Lung abscess, sometimes referred to as necrotizing pneumonia, is a condition in which there is cavitation and destruction of the lung parenchyma.

The outcome common to all these conditions is respiratory distress resulting from the interference with air exchange in the lungs and systemic effects such as result from infection in any part of the body.

Causative organisms

A very wide range of microorganisms is capable of causing pneumonia. Age is an important determinant (Fig. 22.6). Most childhood pneumonia is caused either by viruses or by bacteria invading the respiratory tract secondary to viral infection, e.g. after measles infection. Neonates born to mothers with genital *Chlamydia trachomatis* infection may develop a chlamydial interstitial pneumonitis (see Chapter 24) resulting from colonization of the respiratory tract during birth. In the absence of underlying abnormality such as cystic fibrosis, pneumonia is unusual in older children. Children and young adults with cystic fibrosis are very prone to lower respiratory tract infection caused characteristically by *Staph. aureus*, *H. influenzae* and *Pseudomonas aeruginosa*. The cause of pneumonia in adults depends on a number of risk factors such as age, underlying disease and particular exposure to pathogens through occupation, travel or contact with animals. Pneumonia acquired in hospital tends to be caused by a different spectrum of organisms, particularly Gram-negative bacteria. The causative agents of adult pneumonia are summarized in figure 22.7. Although clinical and epidemiological clues

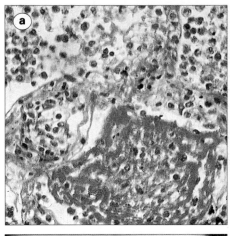
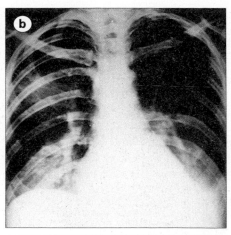
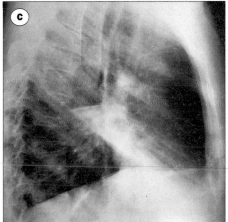
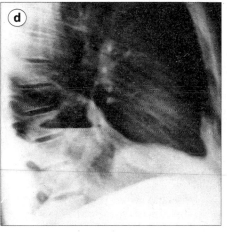

Fig. 22.5 Four types of pneumonia. (a) Pneumococcal lobar pneumonia, showing consolidated alveoli filled with neutrophils and fibrin. H & E stain. Courtesy of ID Starke and ME Hodson. (b) *Mycoplasma* bronchopneumonia, with patchy consolidation in several areas of both lungs. Courtesy of JA Innes. (c) Interstitial pneumonia due to influenza virus. Courtesy of ID Starke and ME Hodson. (d) Lung abscess, showing abscess cavity in lower lobe of the right lung. Courtesy of JA Innes.

CAUSES OF PNEUMONIA RELATED TO AGE	
children	**adults**
Mainly viral e.g. RSV, parainfluenza, or bacterial secondary to viral respiratory infection e.g. after measles Neonates may develop interstitial pneumonitis caused by *Chlamydia trachomatis* acquired from mother at birth	Bacterial causes more common than viral. Aetiology varies with age, underlying disease, occupational and geographical risk factors

Fig. 22.6 Pneumonia in children is more often viral in origin, or bacterial secondary to a viral respiratory infection. In adults, bacterial pneumonia is more common.

help to suggest the likely cause, microbiological investigations are essential to confirm the diagnosis and ensure optimal antimicrobial therapy.

It is often difficult to distinguish on clinical grounds between bacterial and viral pneumonias, although the latter more often show a characteristic interstitial pneumonia on chest x-ray (see Fig. 22.5). For the sake of clarity they are described separately below. Infections with RSV have been described earlier in this chapter and opportunist pathogens (such as *Pneumocystis carinii*) associated specifically with pneumonia in the immunocompromised are described in Chapter 33.

Bacterial pneumonia

The classic bacterial cause of acute, community-acquired pneumonia is *Strep. pneumoniae* (the 'pneumococcus'). In the past, 50–90% of cases were caused by *Strep. pneumoniae* but in recent years the relative importance of this pathogen has decreased and it now causes only 25–60% of cases (Fig. 22.8). *Haemophilus influenzae* is estimated to be the cause of 5–15% of cases but the true incidence is difficult to determine because this organism frequently colonizes the upper respiratory tract of bronchitic patients (see above).

When effective antibiotic treatment (penicillin) for the pneumococcus became widely available it was clear that a significant proportion of cases of pneumonia failed to respond to this treatment and were labelled 'primary atypical pneumonia'. 'Primary' refers to pneumonia occurring as a new event, not secondary to influenza for example, and 'atypical' because *Strep. pneumoniae* is not isolated from sputum from such patients, the symptoms are often general as well as respiratory, and because of failure to respond to penicillin or ampicillin therapy. The causes of atypical pneumonia include *Mycoplasma pneumoniae*, *Chlamydia pneumoniae* and *C. psittaci*, *Legionella pneumophila* and *Coxiella burnetii*. The relative importance of these pathogens varies in different studies (see Fig. 22.8). *Mycoplasma pneumoniae* and *C. pneumoniae* appear to be solely human pathogens whereas *C. psittaci* and *Coxiella burnetii* are acquired from infected animals, and *L. pneumophila* is acquired from contaminated environmental sources (see Fig. 22.7).

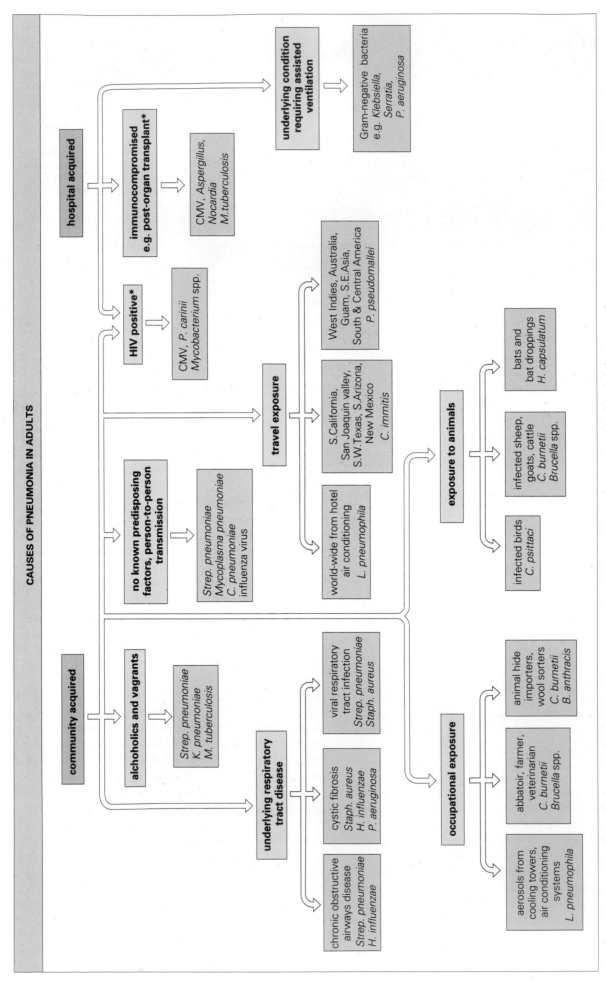

Fig. 22.7 There are many pathogens capable of causing pneumonia in adults, and the aetiology is related to risk factors such as the exposure to pathogens through occupation, travel, and contact with animals. The elderly are more likely to be infected and tend to be more severely ill than young adults. * These infections are often reactivating endogenous infections rather than community or hospital acquired.

COMMON CAUSES OF PNEUMONIA IN COMMUNITY-BASED STUDIES IN THREE COUNTRIES			
pathogen	percentage* of cases from whom a pathogen was identified		
	Sweden	Denmark	Canada
Streptococcus pneumoniae	66	26	11
Legionella pneumophila	4	30	5
Mycoplasma Chlamydia	9	8	10
Haemophilus influenzae	13	32	8
Moraxella catarrhalis	3	0	1
Staphylococcus aureus	0	7	6
Viral cause (not specified)	15	13	21

*note that more than one possible cause was isolated from some patients, therefore accounting for totals greater than 100%

Fig. 22.8 Despite the numerous possible pathogens, the vast majority of infections are caused by just a few. *Streptococcus pneumoniae* is the classic cause of lobar pneumonia but has been declining in incidence in recent years in comparison with the so-called atypical causes of pneumonia such as *Mycoplasma* and *Legionella*. Data from TJ Marrie *et al.*, 1987 and SS Pedersen, 1989.

Moraxella catarrhalis (previously *Branhamella catarrhalis*) is increasingly recognized as a cause of pneumonia, particularly in patients with carcinoma of the lung or other underlying lung disease. Other aetiologic agents of pneumonia associated with particular underlying disease, occupations or exposure to animals and travel are summarized in figure 22.7 and described in other chapters. It is important to note that in as many as 35% of lower respiratory tract infections a causative organism is not isolated.

Clinical features
Patients usually present feeling unwell and with a fever. They may have signs and symptoms of a chest infection; chest pain (which may be pleuritic), a cough which may be productive of sputum, shortness of breath and difficulty and pain on breathing. Some infections result in symptoms confined mainly to the chest, whereas others e.g. Legionnaires disease (caused by *Legionella pneumophila*) have a much wider systemic involvement and the patient may present with mental confusion, diarrhoea, and evidence of renal or liver derangement. However, the distinction between localized and systemic symptoms is not usually reliable enough for an accurate diagnosis.

Chest examination may reveal 'rales' (abnormal crackling sounds) and evidence of consolidation even before changes become evident on x-ray. The chest x-ray is an important adjunct to the clinical diagnosis. Patients with pneumonia usually have shadows in one or more areas of the lung indicating consolidation (see above for descrip-

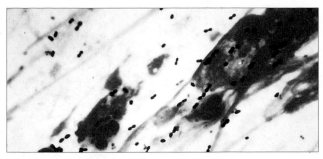

Fig. 22.9 Gram-stained smears of sputum can help the physician to make a rapid diagnosis if, like this, they contain abundant Gram-positive diplococci characteristic of pneumococci, as well as polymorphs. However it is important to remember that many of the important causes of pneumonia will not be stained by Gram's stain.

tions of lobar, broncho- and interstitial pneumonia). However, careful interpretation is required to differentiate between infection and non-infective processes such as tumours.

Complications
Pneumonia is not only the most common cause of death from infection in the elderly, but it is also an important cause in the young and previously healthy. Complications of infection include spread of the infecting organisms directly to extra-pulmonary sites such as the pleural space, giving rise to empyema (see below), or indirectly via the bloodstream to other parts of the body. For example, the majority of patients with pneumococcal pneumonia have positive blood cultures and pneumococcal meningitis not infrequently follows pneumonia in the elderly.

Laboratory diagnosis
Microscopic examination and culture of expectorated sputum remain the mainstays of respiratory bacteriology, despite doubts about the value of these procedures. Collection of sputum is non-invasive but more invasive techniques, such as transtracheal aspiration, bronchoscopy and broncho-alveolar lavage, and open lung biopsy, may yield more useful results.

Sputum samples are best collected in the morning because sputum tends to accumulate while the patient is lying in bed, and before breakfast to reduce contamination by food particles and bacteria from food. It is important that the specimen submitted for examination is truly sputum and not simply saliva. A physiotherapist can be of great assistance to ill patients who may be unable to cough unaided. The usual laboratory procedures are Gram stain and culture (see Chapter 18). Examination of the Gram-stained sputum can give a presumptive diagnosis within minutes if the film reveals a host response in the form of abundant polymorphs and the putative pathogen (for example, Gram-positive diplococci characteristic of *Strep. pneumoniae*; Fig. 22.9). The presence of organisms in the absence of polymorphs is suggestive of contamination of the specimen rather than infection, but is is important to remember that immunocompromised patients may not be able to mount a polymorphonuclear leucocyte response.

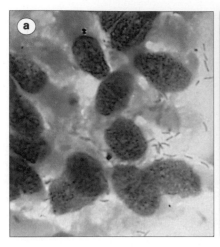
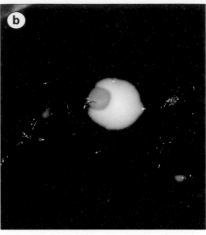

Fig. 22.10 *Legionella pneumophila.* (a) Gram-stain of a specimen from bronchial biopsy in a patient with fulminant Legionnaire's disease. Courtesy of S Fisher-Hoch. (b) Culture plate showing white colonies on buffered charcoal yeast extract medium. Courtesy of I Farrell.

SEROLOGICAL DIAGNOSIS OF 'ATYPICAL' PNEUMONIA		
pathogen	**test**	**significant titre**
Mycoplasma pneumoniae	complement fixation test (CFT)	1/16
	IgM by latex agglutination or ELISA	positive*
Legionella pneumophila	rapid microagglutination test	1/16
Chlamydia pneumoniae *Chlamydia psittaci*	microimmunofluorescence or ELISA using species-specific antigens	positive*
Coxiella burnetii	CFT (phase I and phase II antigens)	1/200
*any positive reaction is considered indicative of infection		

Fig. 22.11 Several of the bacterial causes of pneumonia are difficult to grow in the laboratory, so that examination of the patient's serum for specific antibodies is the usual method of diagnosis. It is always better to demonstrate a rising titre between acute and convalescent phase sera than to rely on a single sample, but the titres shown here give an indication of infection.

Also remember that the causative agents of atypical pneumonia, with the exception of *L. pneumophila* (Fig. 22.10), will not be seen in Gram-stained smears.

Standard culture techniques will allow the growth of the bacterial pathogens such as *Strep. pneumoniae, Staph. aureus, H. influenzae* and *Klebsiella pneumoniae* and other non-fastidious Gram-negative rods. Special media or conditions are required for the causative agents of atypical pneumonia, including *Legionella pneumophila* (see Fig. 22.10; also see Appendix).

Rapid non-cultural techniques have been applied successfully to the diagnosis of pneumococcal pneumonia. Detection of pneumococcal antigen by agglutination of antibody-coated latex particles (see Chapter 18) can be used both on sputum and urine specimens (antigen is excreted in the urine). Use of this technique means the result is available within an hour of receipt of the specimen, but antibiotic susceptibility tests cannot be performed unless the organisms are isolated.

As mentioned above, there are several important causes of pneumonia that will not be revealed in Gram-stained sputum smears and cannot be grown on the simple routine culture media. For these reasons the diagnosis is usually confirmed by serological tests rather than by culture. A single high titre of specific antibodies or preferably demonstration of a titre rising between the acute and convalescent phase of the disease is required and thus serological diagnosis is often retrospective. The important serological tests are shown in figure 22.11.

Treatment

Once the cause of the infection has been identified, selection of appropriate antimicrobial therapy is relatively straightforward (Fig. 22.12). However, the choice of treatment is more difficult when sputum is not produced or does not reveal the pathogen; hence the importance of taking a full history and employing invasive diagnostic techniques when appropriate in order to improve the chances of establishing the cause.

Prevention

Respiratory infections are usually transmitted by airborne droplets, so that person-to-person spread is virtually impossible to prevent, although less crowding and better ventilation help to reduce the chances of acquisition of infection. Infections acquired from sources other than humans may be more amenable to prevention, e.g. by avoiding contact with sick animals (Q fever), or birds (psittacosis). The contamination of cooling systems and hot water supplies by legionellae has been the subject of intense study and regulations are now in force to provide guidance for maintenance engineers.

Prevention by immunization is available for few of the respiratory pathogens. A pneumococcal vaccine incorporating the polysaccharide capsular antigens of the most common types of *Strep. pneumoniae* is recommended for those at particular risk, e.g. post-splenectomy or in individuals with sickle-cell disease, as these patients are unable to deal effectively with capsulate organisms.

ANTIBACTERIAL AGENTS FOR PNEUMONIA	
initial treatment of community-aquired pneumonia	
First choice	ampicillin+erythromycin
unless clinical picture clearly indicates lobar pneumonia; if so	ampicillin
Pneumonia secondary to viral respiratory tract infection	ampicillin+flucloxacillin
Pneumonia in chronic bronchitic	augmentin or cefuroxime
Pneumonia in vagrants, alchoholics, drug addicts and others who may have aspirated	ampicillin+gentamicin
treatment of choice when pathogen has been identified	
Streptococcus pneumoniae	ampicillin or penicillin (erythromycin if allergic to beta-lactams)
Mycoplasma pneumoniae Legionella pneumophila Chlamydia pneumoniae Chlamydia psittaci Coxiella burnetii	erythromycin
Staphylococcus aureus	flucloxacillin
Haemophilus influenzae	ampicillin*, augmentin or cefuroxime
Klebsiella pneumoniae	gentamicin, chloramphenicol or ciprofloxacin
*if non-beta-lactamase producer	

Fig. 22.12 Penicillin-resistant pneumococci are now present in many countries, but their incidence is still generally low and penicillin (or ampicillin) remains the agent of choice. It is important to recognize that penicillin and ampicillin are not active against the other common causes of pneumonia. Hence for initial therapy a combination is often recommended.

Viral pneumonia

Viruses can invade the lung from the bloodstream as well as directly via the respiratory tract. Many viruses cause pneumonia (Fig. 22.13) and, as in the case of viruses in the upper respiratory tract, generally accomplish this in the face of normal host defences. Perfectly healthy individuals are susceptible, and most of these viruses have surface molecules that attach specifically to the respiratory epithelium.

Sometimes the virus fails to spread significantly to air spaces but remains in interstitial tissues to cause interstitial pneumonia (e.g. CMV in immunodeficient patients). Even when viruses of this group do not themselves cause pneumonia they may, by damaging respiratory defences, lay the ground for secondary bacterial pneumonia.

Note that respiratory syncytial virus can cause pneumonia in infants and is described earlier in this chapter.

Parainfluenza virus infection
As with RSV these viruses are more likely to cause lower respiratory tract disease (croup and pneumonia) in children.

Aetiology and pathogenesis. The surface spikes of this virus are composed of haemagglutinin plus neuraminidase on one type of spike and fusion proteins on another. There are four types of parainfluenza viruses, differing in their clinical effects as well as in their antigens. After infec-

tion by respiratory droplets these viruses spread locally on respiratory epithelium.

Clinical features. Parainfluenza viruses 1 and 2 cause pharyngitis, and croup is seen in children under five years of age, consisting of acute laryngotracheobronchitis, with harsh cough and hoarseness. Parainfluenza virus 3 infection is often subclinical. Parainfluenza virus 4 usually gives rise to a common cold-type illness.

Diagnosis, treatment and prevention. Virus-specific antigens can often be detected in cells in respiratory washings. The virus can be isolated, and rises in antibody titre demonstrated.

Neither antivirals nor vaccines are available.

Adenovirus infection
There are 41 antigenic types of adenovirus, some of which cause upper and lower respiratory tract infections. (Pharyngoconjunctival fever, sore throat, etc. are referred to in Chapter 20.) Adenoviruses cause about five per cent of acute respiratory tract illness, generally with non-specific symptoms under the age of five. As maternal antibody fades, lower respiratory tract illnesses become more frequent, especially with adenovirus 7. Types 3, 4 and 7 have caused outbreaks of respiratory illness ranging from

VIRAL PNEUMONIA		
virus	**clinical condition**	**comments**
Influenza A or B	primary viral pneumonia or pneumonia associated with secondary bacterial infection	pandemics (type A) and epidemics (type A or B); increased susceptibility in elderly or in certain chronic diseases
Parainfluenza (types 1–4)	croup, pneumonia in children less than 5 yrs old; upper respiratory illness (often subclinical) in older children and adults	antivirals and vaccines not available
Measles	secondary bacterial pneumonia common; primary viral (giant cell) pneumonia in immuno-deficient subjects	adult infection rare but severe; King and Queen of Hawaii both died of measles when they visited London in 1824
RSV	pneumonitis pneumonia (infants); common cold syndrome (adults)	peak mortality in 3–4 month old infants; secondary bacterial infection rare
Adenovirus	pharyngoconjunctival fever, pharyngitis, atypical pneumonia (military recruits)	no antivirals; vaccines not generally available
CMV	interstitial pneumonia	in immunodeficient patients (e.g. AIDS)
Varicella-zoster virus	pneumonia in young adults suffering primary infection	uncommon; recognized 1–6 days after rash; lung lesions may eventually calcify

Fig. 22.13 Several different groups of viruses cause infection of the lower respiratory tract, particularly in children. Some such as influenza and measles, leave the patient particularly prone to secondary bacterial infection.

pharyngitis to atypical pneumonia in military recruits, with crowding and stress as possible cofactors. Recovery is generally uneventful but adenoviruses may persist in the body because they can be recovered from at least 50% of surgically-removed tonsils. An enteric-coated vaccine for types 4 and 7 has been used to prevent infection in military recruits.

Influenza virus infection

These are classic respiratory viruses, causes of endemic, epidemic and pandemic influenza.

Aetiology and pathogenesis. The structure of a typical myxovirus (ssRNA) is shown in figure 22.14, and the budding process in figure 22.15. The internal ribonucleoprotein (RNP) is a group-specific antigen, which distinguishes influenza A, B and C viruses. Influenza A viruses cause epidemics, occasionally pandemics, and there is an animal reservoir, notably in birds. Influenza B viruses cause only epidemics and do not involve animal hosts, while influenza C viruses do not cause epidemics and give rise to only minor respiratory illness.

The viral envelope has haemagglutinin (H) and neuraminidase (N) spikes (see Fig. 22.14). In the case of influenza A, the H and N are type-specific antigens and are used to characterize different strains of influenza A virus (Fig. 22.16). Current strains are H3N2 and H1N1. In

giving the full nomenclature, the influenza group, the location and year of isolation is also included (for example A/Phillipines/82/H3N2).

The ssRNA genome is segmented, and when virus particles of more than one strain infect a cell simultaneously, these segments can be reassorted during virus replication to give progeny virus with a novel combination of H and N antigens.

Influenza viruses undergo genetic change as they spread through the host species. These changes are of two types:

Antigenic drift. Small mutations, affecting the H and N antigens are constantly occurring. When changes in these antigens (Fig. 22.17) enable the virus to multiply significantly in individuals with immunity to preceding strains, then the new subtype can reinfect the community. Antigenic drift is seen with all types of influenza.

Antigenic shift. Less commonly, and only with influenza A, there is a sudden major change (shift) in antigenicity of the H or N antigens. This is based on recombination between different virus strains when they infect the same cell. The major change in H or N means that the new strain can spread through population immune to pre-existing strains and the stage is set for a new pandemic (see Fig. 22.16). Associated with the change in H and N are other genetic changes which may or may not confer increased

a STRUCTURE OF INFLUENZA A VIRUS PARTICLE

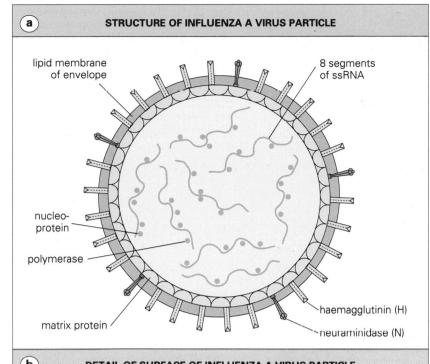

lipid membrane of envelope

8 segments of ssRNA

nucleo-protein

polymerase

matrix protein

haemagglutinin (H)

neuraminidase (N)

b DETAIL OF SURFACE OF INFLUENZA A VIRUS PARTICLE

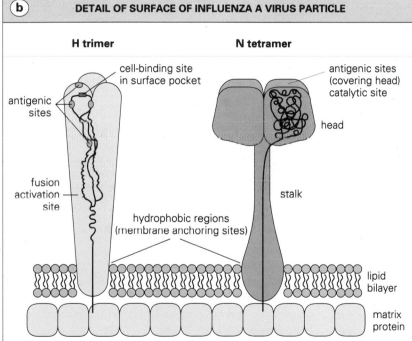

H trimer

N tetramer

cell-binding site in surface pocket

antigenic sites

antigenic sites (covering head) catalytic site

head

fusion activation site

stalk

hydrophobic regions (membrane anchoring sites)

lipid bilayer

matrix protein

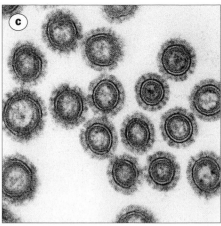

Fig. 22.14 The influenza A virus particle (a), with detail enlarged (b) to show surface haemagglutinin (H) and neuraminidase (N). Each particle has approximately 500 H spikes which bind to the host cell and fuse the viral envelope to the cell's plasma membrane to initiate infection, and approximately 100 N spikes which function to release the virus from the cell surface. Nucleoprotein and polymerase proteins are closely associated with RNA segments to form ribonuclease protein (RNP). The N tetramer is propeller-shaped as viewed from the end; details of only one unit of H trimer and N tetramer are shown. The 3-dimensional structure is known from x-ray crystallographic analysis. Electronmicrograph (c) shows sectioned influenza virus particles. x300 000. Courtesy of D Hockley.

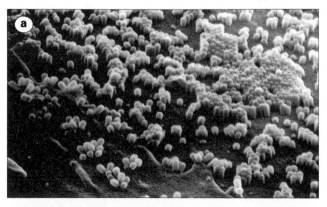

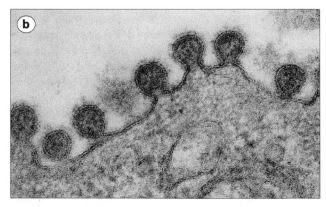

Fig. 22.15 Influenza virus budding from the surface of an infected cell. (a) Scanning electronmicrograph, x27 000. (b) In section, x350 000. Courtesy of D Hockley.

HUMAN INFLUENZA VIRUSES				
type	subtype*	year	clinical severity	prototype virus
A	H3N2 (?)	1889	moderate	⎤ designation based on serological studies, viruses not isolated
	H1N1 (swine)	1918	severe	⎦
	H1N1	1977	mild	A / USSR / 77
	H2N2 (Asian)	1957	severe	A / Japan / 57 / H2N2
	H3N2 (Hong Kong)**	1968	moderate	A / Hong Kong / 68 / H3N2
B	none	1940	moderate	B / Lee / 40
C	none	1947	very mild	C / Taylor / 47

* antigenic shift in influenza A virus is shown by appearance of novel combination of H and N antigens
** amino acid and base sequence analysis suggests that recombination between H3N8 (from ducks) and H2N2 gave rise to H3N2

Fig. 22.16 Human influenza viruses. Novel strains of virus arising in one continent spread rapidly to other continents, causing outbreaks during appropriate times of the year (winter months in temperate climates). There is a World Health Organisation global surveillance system for influenza involving more than 100 laboratories in 79 different countries.

ANTIGENIC DRIFT OF INFLUENZA A (H3N2) VIRUSES								
Virus strain	A/Hong Kong/1/68	A/England/42/72	A/Port Chalmers/1/73	A/Scotland/840/74	A/Victoria/3/75	A/Texas/1/77	A/Bangkok/1/79	A/Philippines/2/82
A / Hong Kong /1 / 68	2560	2560	320	80	<20	<20	<20	<20
A / England / 42 / 72	80	1280	320	160	40	<20	<20	<20
A / Port Chalmers / 1 / 73	20	640	640	160	40	40	<20	<20
A / Scotland / 840 / 74	<20	40	40	640	<20	320	40	<20
A / Victoria / 3 / 75	<20	<20	<20	20	1280	320	160	160
A / Texas / 1 / 77	<20	<20	<20	<20	80	1280	640	160
A / Bangkok / 1 / 79	<20	<20	<20	<20	20	320	2560	160
A / Philippines / 2 / 82	<20	<20	<20	<20	20	160	80	640

Fig. 22.17 Antigenic drift of influenza A (H3N2) between1968 and 1982. Haemagglutination-inhibition (HI) tests (see Chapter 18) were carried out using viral antigens plus antibodies (produced in ferrets) from various H3N2 strains of influenza virus. The figures show H1 antibody titres. A given virus strain is inhibited by homologous antibody, and also to a lesser extent by antibody to closely related viruses. A gradual change in viral antigen is seen between the years 1968 and 1982. After recovery from infection, specific immunity could prevent infection by a neighbouring virus in the series, but not by a more distantly related (2-3 steps away) virus. Data from Stuart-Harris C *et al.*, 1985.

pathogenicity or changes in the ability to spread rapidly from person to person.

There are thirteen types of H and nine types of N, most of them occurring in birds. This gives 117 possible combinations of H and N. Seventy-one combinations have been found in birds (especially in ducks, sometimes leading to severe epidemics in chickens and turkeys) but so far only three in man. Evidently only some of the combinations are successful, from the virus's point of view, in man. Influenza A viruses also infect pigs, horses, seals, and other mammals, but it seems less likely that these species play a part as sources of human infection.

Transmission of influenza is by droplet inhalation and almost everyone in a given society is affected. Influenza occurs throughout the world and except in the tropics is almost entirely restricted to the coldest months of the year. This is largely because during cold weather people spend more time inside buildings with limited air space, which favours transmission, and perhaps also because of decreased host resistance (diet, depressed mucociliary activity). Influenza activity within a community is reflected

not only in the numbers of people becoming ill and consulting doctors, but also in excess mortality due to acute respiratory disease (pneumonia), which affects elderly people especially (Fig. 22.18).

Epidemics and pandemics are due to the appearance of new strains of viruses, so that a given individual is regularly reinfected with different strains. This is in contrast to viruses that undergo minimal antigenic variation (monotypic viruses) such as measles or mumps, one infection conferring life-long immunity.

Clinical features and pathogenesis. The virus enters the respiratory tract in droplets and attaches to sialic acid receptors on epithelial cells via the H components of the virus envelope. Fewer virus particles are needed to infect the lower respiratory tract than the upper respiratory tract. One to three days after infection the cytokines liberated from damaged cells and from infiltrating leucocytes cause symptoms such as chills, malaise, fever and muscular aches. There are also respiratory symptoms – runny nose, cough, etc. The virus remains restricted to the respiratory

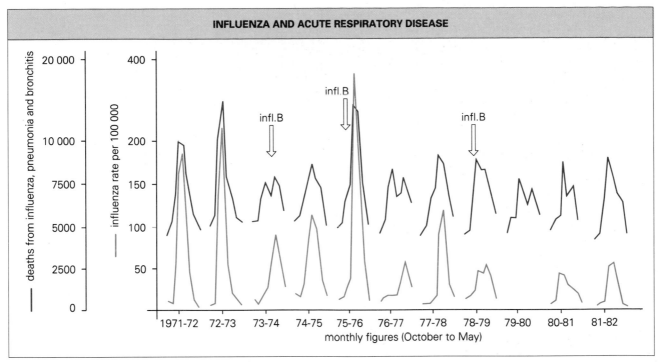

Fig. 22.18 Outbreaks of influenza within a community are reflected by a general increase in deaths from acute respiratory disease. Notifications of new cases of clinical influenza are paralleled by an increase in deaths attributed to influenza, pneumonia and bronchitis. Monthly figures from October to May for England and Wales (1971–1983) are shown. The peaks are due to the spread in the community of different strains of influenza A (H3N2 and H1N1) and influenza B (arrows) viruses. Data from the Office of Population, Censuses and Surveys.

tract and there is no viraemia. Although the initial symptoms are due to direct viral damage and associated inflammatory responses these can be severe enough to cause bronchitis and interstitial pneumonia. Damage to the respiratory epithelium also gives opportunities to secondary bacterial invaders, especially staphylococci, pneumococci, and *H. influenzae*. In fact life-threatening influenza is often due to secondary bacterial infection, the viral infection being brought under control by antibody and cell-mediated immune responses to the infecting virus. Interferon probably plays a part during the early stages of the infection. Although antiviral antibodies may not be detected within serum for a week or two they are produced at an earlier stage but are complexed with viral antigens in the respiratory tract.

Complications. Mortality due to secondary bacterial pneumonia is higher in apparently normal individuals over the age of 60 years, and in those with impaired resistance due to chronic cardiorespiratory disease (emphysema, etc.) renal disease and so on. Pregnant women are also more susceptible. CNS complications occur rarely and include encephalomyelitis, polyneuritis (Guillain–Barré syndrome, GBS). These appear to be indirect immunopathological complications, rather then due to CNS invasion by the virus. The GBS syndrome occurred as a significant but rare (1 per 100 000) sequel to the widespread vaccination of US citizens with the inactivated H3N2 influenza virus in 1976.

Diagnosis. During epidemics a clinical diagnosis can generally be made. Influenza-infected cells are seen after fluorescent antibody or immunoperoxidase staining of cells obtained from nasal aspirates. A rise in specific antibodies can be detected (by haemagglutination inhibition, complement fixation or ELISA) in paired serum samples taken within a few days of illness and 7 to 10 days later. The virus can also be isolated from throat washings taken within a day or two of onset, after inoculation into eggs or into certain cell cultures. This takes several days and is more important for public health authorities following infection with new virus strains rather than for diagnosis in individual patients.

Treatment and prevention. Amantidine HCl inhibits the replication of influenza A viruses. It can reduce the severity of the infection, but only if given within 1 to 2 days of disease onset and is more valuable when used for prophylaxis. Individuals at high risk can be protected if given 200 mg per day during epidemics.

Vaccines. Influenza virus vaccines in regular use are: 1) those consisting of egg-grown virus, purified, then formalin-inactivated; 2) the less reactogenic purified H and N antigens prepared from virus that has been disrupted ('split') by lipid solvents. Influenza A (currently H3N2 and H1N1) and influenza B are included in the vaccine. The exact virus strains are reviewed annually in relation to the viruses circulating in the previous year. The vaccines are given by parenteral injection, and provide protection against disease in up to 70% of individuals. Vaccination of high risk individuals, especially those over 65 years of age and those with chronic cardiopulmonary disease, is recommended. It might be expected that the respiratory route would be a better way of inducing respiratory immunity, and trials with live attenuated virus vaccines administered intranasally are in progress.

Measles

Aetiology and pathogenesis. Measles is dealt with in detail as a multisystem infection in Chapter 29. It is mentioned here because 1) it can cause 'giant cell' pneumonia in those with impaired immune responses, and 2) the virus replicates in the lower respiratory tract and, under certain circumstances, causes enough damage to lead to secondary bacterial pneumonia. This is now uncommon in developed countries. However, in children in developing countries secondary bacterial pneumonia is a frequent complication, and measles remains a major cause of death in childhood. Depressed immune responsiveness, inadequate vaccination programmes, malnutrition (especially vitamin A) and poor medical care to deal with complications, tip the host–parasite balance markedly in favour of the virus.

Clinical features. After an incubation period of 10 to 14 days, there is fever, a runny nose, conjunctivitis and cough. Koplik's spots and then the characteristic rash appear a day or two later. The virus replicates in the epithelium of the nasopharynx, middle ear and lung, interfering with host defences and enabling bacteria such as pneumococci, staphylococci and meningococci to establish infection. Pneumonia is what generally brings measles cases to hospital, but otitis media is also common. In children with severely impaired cell-mediated immune defences virus replication continues unchecked to give a giant cell pneumonia – a rare and usually fatal manifestation (Fig. 22.19). Other complications are referred to in Chapter 29, and the neurological complications in Chapter 27.

Diagnosis, treatment and prevention. The diagnosis is made on clinical grounds. Virus isolation and detection of specific antibody responses is rarely necessary.

No antiviral treatment is available, but antibiotics are needed for secondary bacterial complications. Children with severe measles generally have very low levels of serum retinol; recovery is hastened and death is made less likely when they are given 400 000 IU vitamin A. The disease is prevented by a highly effective, live, attenuated vaccine, given with mumps and rubella (MMR; see Chapter 36).

Cytomegalovirus infection

This multisystem virus is described in Chapter 29. The virus does not normally replicate on respiratory epithelium or cause respiratory illness, but in immunocompromised patients (bone marrow transplant recipients, AIDS patients) it can give rise to an interstitial pneumonia. In AIDS, for instance, pneumonia is associated with reactivation of persistent CMV infection. Virus can be isolated and

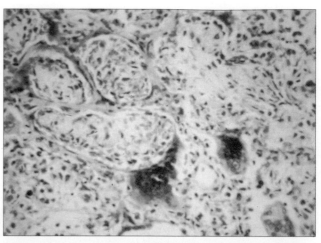

Fig. 22.19 Lung biopsy in measles pneumonia, showing inflammatory cell infiltrate, proliferation of the alveolar lining cells and large, darkly staining, multinucleate giant cells. H & E stain. Courtesy of ID Starke and ME Hodson.

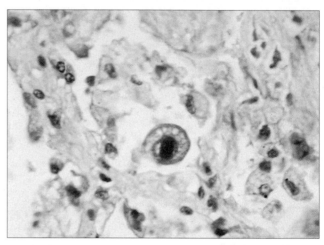

Fig. 22.20 Owl's eye inclusion body in cytomegalovirus infection. Large numbers of virus particles accumulate in the nucleus of the enlarged infected cell to produce a single dense inclusion. H & E stain. Courtesy of ID Starke and ME Hodson.

characteristic inclusions demonstrated in lung tissue (Fig. 22.20), but *Pneumocystis carinii* is also commonly present, contributing to the pathological picture.

CHRONIC INFECTIONS OF THE LOWER RESPIRATORY TRACT

Tuberculosis

Tuberculosis is a killer and ranks as one of the most serious infectious diseases of the developing world and wherever poverty, malnutrition and poor housing prevail. It affects the apparently healthy as well as being a serious disease of the immunocompromised. This has become particularly obvious in patients with AIDS. Tuberculosis is primarily a disease of the lungs but may spread to other sites or proceed to a generalized infection ('miliary' tuberculosis). It is also referred to in Chapters 23, 27 and 28.

Aetiology and transmission

Tuberculosis is caused by *Mycobacterium tuberculosis* but other species of mycobacteria also cause infection in the

MYCOBACTERIA ASSOCIATED WITH HUMAN DISEASE	
species	**clinical disease**
***slow growers**	
M. tuberculosis	tuberculosis
M. bovis	bovine tuberculosis
M. leprae	leprosy
M. avium M. intracellulare } **	disseminated infection in AIDS patients
M. kansasii	lung infections
M. marinum	skin infections and deeper infections, e.g. arthritis, osteomyelitis, associated with aquatic activity
M. scrofulaceum	cervical adenitis in children
M. simiae	lung, bone, kidney infections
M. szulgai	lung, skin and bone infections
M. ulcerans	skin infections
M. xenopi	lung infections
M. paratuberculosis	? association with Crohn's disease
***rapid growers** M. fortuitum M. chelonae	opportunist infections with introduction of organisms into deep subcutaneous tissues; usually associated with trauma or invasive procedures.

*slow growers require >7 days for visible growth from a dilute inoculum; rapid growers require <7 days for visible growth from a dilute inoculum

**M. avium complex; recent studies show that the two species are distinct. Of the M. avium complex, serovars 1–6 and 8–11 are assigned to M. avium, serovars 7, 12–17, 19, 20 and 25 assigned to M. intracellulare

Fig. 22.21 Many species of mycobacteria are associated with occasional disease but the major pathogens of the genus are *M. tuberculosis*, *M. bovis* and *M. leprae*.

lungs (Fig. 22.21). These are called the 'atypical' mycobacteria, 'mycobacteria other than tuberculosis' (MOTT) or 'non-tuberculous mycobacteria' (NTM).

Infection is acquired by inhalation of *M. tuberculosis* in aerosols and dust. Airborne transmission of tuberculosis is efficient because infected people cough up enormous numbers of mycobacteria, projecting them into the environment, where their waxy outer coat (see Chapter 3) allows them to withstand drying and thus survive for long periods of time in air and house dust.

Pathogenesis

The pathogenesis of the disease depends on the history of previous exposure to the organism. In primary infection, i.e. infection in individuals 'seeing' *M. tuberculosis* for the first time, the organisms are engulfed by the alveolar macrophages where they can both survive and multiply. Non-resident macrophages are attracted to the site and these also ingest the mycobacteria and carry them via the lymphatics to the local (hilar) lymph nodes. In the lymph nodes the immune response – predominantly a cell-mediated response – is stimulated. The CMI response is detectable

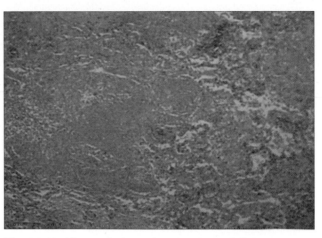

Fig. 22.22 Histopathology showing dense inflammatory infiltration, granuloma formation and caseous necrosis in pulmonary tuberculosis. Courtesy of R Bryan.

4–6 weeks after infection by introducing PPD (purified protein derivative) of *M. tuberculosis* into the skin. A positive result is shown by local induration and erythema, 48–72 hrs later. The CMI response helps to curb the further spread of organisms, although some may have already escaped to set up foci of infection in other body sites. Sensitized T cells release lymphokines that activate macrophages and increase their ability to destroy the mycobacteria. The body reacts to contain the organisms within 'tubercles', small granulomas consisting of epithelioid cells and giant cells (Fig. 22.22). The lung lesion plus the enlarged lymph nodes is often called the Ghon (or primary) complex. After a time the material within the granuloma becomes necrotic and caseous (cheesy). In persons who are otherwise healthy the tubercles may heal spontaneously, become fibrotic or calcified and persist as such for a lifetime. They will show up on a chest x-ray as radio-opaque nodules (Fig. 22.23). However in a small percentage of people with primary infection, and particularly in the immunocompromised, the mycobacteria are not contained within the tubercles but invade the bloodstream and cause disseminated disease ('miliary' tuberculosis; Fig. 22.24).

Secondary tuberculosis is due to reactivation of dormant mycobacteria usually as a consequence of impaired immune function resulting from some other cause such as malnutrition, infection (e.g. AIDS), chemotherapy for treatment of malignancies or corticosteroids for treatment of inflammatory diseases.

Tuberculosis nicely illustrates the dual role of the immune response in infectious disease. On the one hand, CMI controls the infection, and when it is inadequate the infection disseminates or reactivates. On the other hand nearly all the pathology and disease is a consequence of this CMI response, *M. tuberculosis* causing little or no direct or toxin-mediated damage.

Reactivation occurs most commonly in the apex of the lungs. This site is more highly oxygenated and allows the mycobacteria to multiply more rapidly to produce caseous necrotic lesions which spill over into other sites in the lung, and from whence organisms spread to more distant sites in the body.

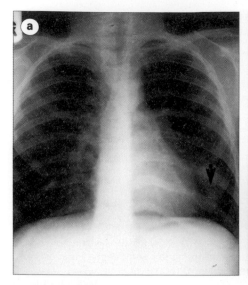
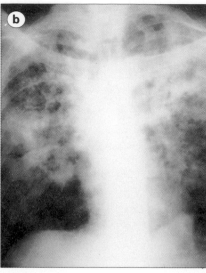

Fig. 22.23 Chest radiographs of (a) Primary tuberculosis, showing Ghon focus (arrow) in lower left lung, and (b) post-primary pulmonary tuberculosis showing far advanced disease. Courtesy of JA Innes.

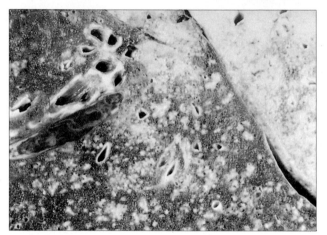

Fig. 22.24 Miliary tuberculosis. Gross specimen of lung showing cut surface covered with white nodules, which are the miliary foci of tuberculosis. Courtesy of JA Innes.

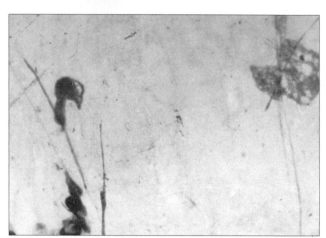

Fig. 22.25 Pulmonary tuberculosis. Sputum preparation showing large numbers of pink-staining, acid-fast tubercle bacilli. Ziehl-Neelson stain. Courtesy of JA Innes.

Clinical features

In contrast to pneumonia, which is usually an acute infection, the onset of tuberculosis is insidious, infection proceeding for some time before the patient becomes sufficiently ill to seek medical attention. Primary tuberculosis is usually mild and often asymptomatic, and in 90% of cases does not proceed further. However, in the remaining 10% clinical disease develops.

Secondary infection may occur in almost any organ as the mycobacteria have the ability to colonize almost any site in the body. The clinical manifestations are variable; fatigue, weight loss, weakness and fever are all associated with tuberculosis. When infection occurs in the lungs there is characteristically a chronic cough productive of sputum, which may be blood-stained as a result of tissue destruction, and necrosis may erode blood vessels which can rupture and causes death through haemorrhage.

Complications

The complications of *M. tuberculosis* infection of the lungs arise either from local spread or from dissemination of the organism via the lymphatics and bloodstream to other parts of the body. This usually occurs at the time of primary infection, and in this way chronic foci are established which

may proceed to necrosis and destruction in, for example, the kidney. Alternatively spread may be by extension to a neighbouring part of the lung, for instance when a tubercle erodes into a bronchus and discharges its contents, or into the pleural cavity, resulting in a pleural effusion.

Although the number of cases of pulmonary tuberculosis has been declining in developed countries since the beginning of the twentieth century, hastened since the advent of specific chemotherapy, the incidence of extrapulmonary tuberculosis has stayed roughly constant for a number of years and thus makes up a greater proportion of the tuberculosis caseload in developed than in developing countries.

Diagnosis

The diagnosis of tuberculosis is suggested by the clinical signs and symptoms referred to above, supported by characteristic chest x-ray changes (see Fig. 22.23) and positive skin test reactivity in the tuberculin (Mantoux) test (see Chapter 9). These tests are confirmed by microscopic demonstration of acid-fast rods and culture of *M. tuberculosis*. Microscopic examination of a smear of sputum stained by Ziehl–Neelsen's method or by auramine (see Chapter 18 and Appendix) often reveals masses of acid-fast rods (Fig. 22.25). This result can be obtained within an

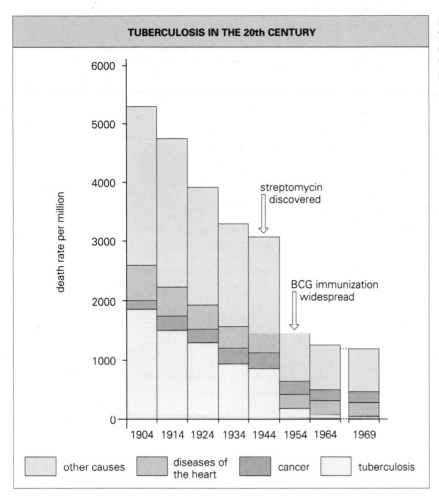

TUBERCULOSIS IN THE 20th CENTURY

death rate per million

6000
5000
4000
3000
2000
1000
0

streptomycin discovered

BCG immunization widespread

1904 1914 1924 1934 1944 1954 1964 1969

other causes | diseases of the heart | cancer | tuberculosis

Fig. 22.26 The death rate from tuberculosis in England and Wales had already fallen by half during the 20th Century before specific treatment and prevention became available.

hour of receipt of the specimen in the laboratory. This is important because *M. tuberculosis* can take up to six weeks to grow in culture (although radiometric methods may reduce the time required for detection; see Appendix) and thus confirmation of the diagnosis is necessarily delayed. Further tests are required to identify the species of *Mycobacterium* and to establish susceptibility to antituberculous drugs.

Treatment

Mycobacteria are innately resistant to most antibacterial agents and specific antituberculous drugs have to be used (these are reviewed in Chapter 35). The key features of treatment are the use of combination therapy (usually three drugs, e.g. isoniazid, rifampin, ethambutol) to prevent emergence of resistance, and prolonged therapy (minimum 6 months) which is necessary to eradicate these slow-growing intracellular organisms.

Prevention

A review of the steady decline in incidence of tuberculosis since the beginning of the twentieth century, and before specific preventive measures were available, underlines the importance of improvements in social conditions in the prevention of this and many other infectious diseases (Fig. 22.26).

Immunoprophylaxis. Immunization with a live attenuated vaccine, the so-called BCG (bacille Calmette-Guérin) vaccine, has been used effectively in situations where tuberculo-

sis is prevalent. Immunization, which confers positive skin test reactivity, does not prevent infection but it allows the body to react quickly to limit proliferation of the organisms. In areas of low prevalence of disease immunization has largely been replaced by chemoprophylaxis.

Chemoprophylaxis. Prophylaxis with isoniazid for one year is recommended for people who have had close contact with a case of tuberculosis. It is also advocated for individuals who show recent conversion to skin test positivity; this is essentially early treatment of subclinical infection rather than prophylaxis.

Aspergillosis

The genus *Aspergillus* contains many species of fungi which are ubiquitous in the environment. They do not form part of the normal flora of man but some species, notably *Aspergillus fumigatus*, are able to cause a range of conditions. These include allergic bronchopulmonary aspergillosis which is, as its name suggests, an allergic response to the presence of aspergillus antigen in the lungs and occurs in patients with asthma. In other patients with pre-existing lung cavities or chronic pulmonary disorders, *Aspergillus* may colonize a cavity and grow to produce a fungal ball, a mass of entangled hyphae, called an 'aspergilloma' (Fig. 22.27). The fungi do not invade the lung tissue but the presence of a large aspergilloma can cause respiratory problems. In the immunosuppressed patient the fungus may invade from the lungs to produce

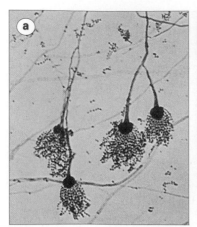
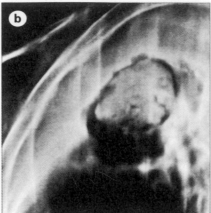
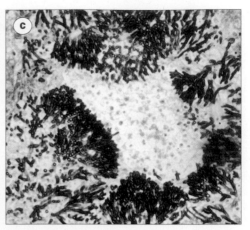

Fig. 22.27 *Aspergillus fumigatus.* (a) Lactophenol cotton blue stained preparation showing the characteristic conidiophores. (b) Aspergilloma. Tomogram showing fungus ball contained within the lung cavity, outlined by air space. Courtesy of JA Innes. (c) Invasive aspergillosis. Histological section showing fungal hyphae invading the lung parenchyma and blood vessels. Grocott stain. Courtesy of C Kibbler.

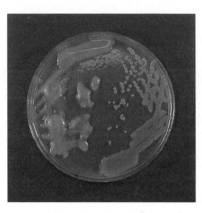

Fig. 22.28 *Pseudomonas aeruginosa* isolated from the sputum of patients with cystic fibrosis characteristically grows in a very mucoid colonial form (shown here on the left of the picture, with the normal colonial form on the right for comparison).

disseminated disease. The limited number and toxic nature of antifungal agents active against *Aspergillus* (see Chapter 35) and the lack of functional host defences make treatment of invasive aspergillosis very difficult.

Cystic fibrosis

Cystic fibrosis (CF) is the most common lethal inherited disorder among Caucasians, with an incidence of approximately 1 in 2500 live births. The disease is characterized by pancreatic insufficiency, abnormal sweat electrolyte concentrations and production of very viscid bronchial secretions. The latter tend to lead to stasis in the lungs and this predisposes to infection. In children with cystic fibrosis the respiratory mucosa presents a different environment for potential pathogens from that found in normal individuals and the common infecting organisms and the nature of infection differ from other lung infections. The first invader is *Staph. aureus* which causes respiratory distress and lung damage. This can be well controlled by specific anti-staphylococcal chemotherapy. *Pseudomonas aeruginosa* is the pathogen of paramount importance. It is uncommon in those less than 5 years old but colonizes the lungs of almost all patients of 15–20 years of age, often encouraged by its intrinsic resistance to antistaphylococcal agents. Early in the course of infection normal colony types are grown from sputum cultures but as infection progresses the organism changes to a highly mucoid form, almost mimicking the mucoid secretions of the patient (Fig. 22.28). These mucoid forms are thought to grow in micro-colonies in the lung but most of the lung damage is due to immunological responses to the organisms and to the algi-nate which forms the mucoid material (Fig. 22.29). *Pseudomonas aeruginosa* rarely invades beyond the lung even in the most severely infected individuals.

The third pathogen characteristically associated with cystic fibrosis is *H. influenzae*, typically non-encapsulated strains. These organisms may be found in association with *Staph. aureus* and *P. aeruginosa*; their pathogenic significance is unclear but they appear to contribute to the respiratory exacerbations experienced by CF patients.

Although specific antibacterial chemotherapy can reduce the symptoms of infection and improve the quality of life, infections, particularly with *P. aeruginosa*, are impossible to eradicate and are frequently the cause of death in these patients. Heart–lung transplantation has offered a successful alternative to treatment in some patients.

Lung abscess

This is a suppurative infection of the lung, sometimes referred to as 'necrotizing pneumonia'. The most common predisposing cause is aspiration of respiratory or gastric secretions as a result of altered consciousness. Thus the infection is endogenous in origin and cultures often reveal a mixture of bacteria, with anaerobes such as *Bacteroides* and *Fusobacterium* playing an important role (Fig. 22.30). Patients with lung abscesses may have been ill for at least two weeks prior to presentation. They usually produce large amounts of sputum which if foul-smelling gives a strong hint of the presence of anaerobes and often suggests the diagnosis. Most diagnoses are made from chest x-rays (see Fig. 22.5) and the cause confirmed by microbiological investigation. Because of the likely presence of anaerobes, a suitable anti-anaerobic agent such as metronidazole should be part of the treatment regimen and treatment may need to be continued for 2–4 months to prevent relapse. If diagnosis and treatment are delayed, infection may spread to the pleural space giving rise to empyema (see below).

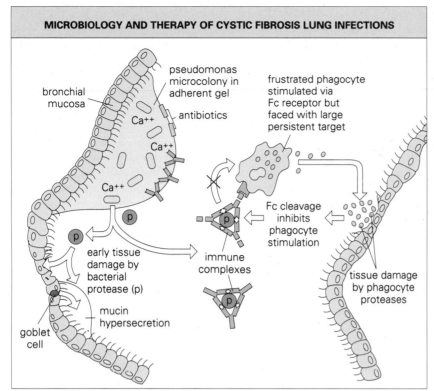

MICROBIOLOGY AND THERAPY OF CYSTIC FIBROSIS LUNG INFECTIONS

Fig. 22.29 *Pseudomonas* infection in the lung of cystic fibrotics is chronic but rarely invasive beyond the bronchial mucosa. The organisms are thought to grow in microcolonies embedded in a Ca++-dependant mucoid alginate gel, which contains DNA and tracheobronchial mucin, and which attaches to the bronchial mucosa. This protects the organisms from the host defences and provides a physical and electrolyte barrier to antibiotics. Much of the damage to tissue is thought to be due to slow release of bacterial proteases, which disrupt the mucosa and cause mucin hypersecretion, and immunopathologic mechanisms exacerbated by the size, antigenicity and persistence of the alginate matrix, as well as the indirect action of immune complexes associated with pseudomonas antigens. Tissue damage is also caused by phagocyte proteases. Intermittent exacerbations can be explained by the Fc cleavage of immune complexes by these proteases and consequent inhibition of further phagocyte stimulation. Redrawn from JRW Govan, 1990.

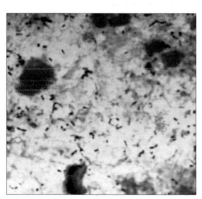

Fig. 22.30 Gram-stain of pus from a lung abscess, showing Gram-positive cocci and both Gram-negative and Gram-positive rods. Courtesy of JR Cantey.

Pleural effusion and empyema

Pleural effusions may arise in a variety of different diseases and may be found in up to 50% of patients with pneumonia. Sometimes the actual organisms infecting the lung spread to the pleural space and give rise to a purulent exudate or 'empyema'. Pleural effusions can be demonstrated radiologically but detection of empyema can be difficult, particularly in a patient with extensive pneumonia. Aspiration of pleural fluid provides material for microbiological examination. Nowadays *Staph. aureus*, Gram-negative rods and anaerobes are commonly involved. Treatment should be directed at drainage of pus, eradication of infection and expansion of the lung.

PARASITIC INFECTIONS OF THE LOWER RESPIRATORY TRACT

A number of parasitic infections may localize to the lung, or involve the lung at some stage in their development. Nematodes such as *Ascaris* and the hookworms (see Chapter 25) migrate through the lungs as they move to the small intestine, breaking out of the capillaries around the alveoli to enter the bronchioles. The damage caused by this process, and the development of inflammatory responses can lead to a transient pneumonitis. Mild respiratory symptoms may also accompany the migration of schistosome larvae through the lungs (see Chapter 30).

The microfilaria larvae of filarial nematodes such as *Wuchereria* or *Brugia* appear in the peripheral circulation with a regular diurnal or nocturnal periodicity, their appearance coinciding with the time at which the vector bloodsucking insects are likely to feed. Outside these periods the larvae becomes sequestered in the capillaries of the lung. Under certain conditions, as yet undefined, and in certain individuals, the presence of the larvae triggers a condition known as 'tropical pulmonary eosinophilia' (TPE or Weingartner's syndrome). This is characterized by cough, respiratory distress and high eosinophilia; microfilaria are usually absent from the blood. Infections with *Ascaris* and *Strongyloides* may also trigger a pulmonary eosinophilia, although the condition is distinct from TPE.

In a proportion (20–30%) of cases, larvae of the tapeworm *Echinococcus granulosus* localize in the lungs. There they develop into hydatid cysts (see Chapter 16) which may reach a considerable size, causing respiratory distress, largely as a consequence of the mechanical pressure exerted on lung tissue. Involvement of the lung can also be a rare complication of extra-intestinal infection with the protozoan *Entamoeba histolytica*.

Very few adult parasites live in the lung, the most important being *Paragonimus westermanii*, the oriental lung fluke. Infection is acquired by eating crustacea whose tissues contain the infective metacercariae. These migrate from the intestine across the body cavity and penetrate into the lungs. The adults develop within fibrous cysts that connect with bronchi to provide an exit for the eggs (Fig. 22.31). Infections cause chest pain, difficulty in breathing, and can cause bronchopneumonia when large numbers of parasites are present. Praziquantel is an efficient anthelminthic for this infection.

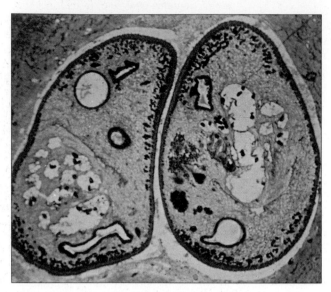

Fig. 22.31 Two adult *Paragonimus* contained within a fibrous cyst in the lung. Courtesy of H Zaiman.

SUMMARY

Respiratory tract infections are among the most common infections seen in people attending their family doctor and account for considerable morbidity and absence from school and work. Infections of the upper respiratory tract, covered in Chapter 20, are usually mild and self-limiting. In contrast, infections lower in the respiratory tract, sometimes caused by the same pathogens, tend to be severe and may be life-threatening. The spectrum of pathogens is wide but the most common causes of lower respiratory tract infection tend to be viral in children and bacterial in adults. Precise identification of the aetiology is important to ensure optimal therapy. Many of the infectious agents are spread from person to person in aerosols and thus prevention of infection is difficult to achieve, although improvements in living conditions and reduction in overcrowding undoubtedly play an important role. The recognition of the risk of *Legionella* infection associated with aerosols from cooling towers and air conditioning systems has led to recommendations for the maintenance of such systems. The association between exposure to particular animals or travel in certain areas of the world and specific pathogens is well-documented and stresses the importance of taking a full history from the patient whenever possible.

Further Reading

Couch RB, Kasel JA, Glezen WP, *et al*. Influenza: Its control in persons and populations. *J Infect Dis* 1986; **153:** 431–447.

Department of Health and Welsh Office. *The control of legionellae in health care premises.* London: HMSO, 1988.

Gillespie SH. Aspects of pneumococcal infection including bacterial virulence, host response and vaccination. *J Med Microbiol* 1989; **28:** 237–248.

Goven JRW, Glass S. The microbiology and therapy of cystic fibrosis lung infections. *Rev Med Microbiol* 1990; **1:** 19–28.

Henderson FW, Collier AM, Clyde WA. Respiratory syncytial virus infections, reinfections and immunity. A prospective, longitudinal study in young children. *New Engl J Med* 1979; **300:** 530–534.

Howe GM. *Man, environment and disease.* London: Penguin books, 1972.

Hutchinson DN. Nosocomial legionellosis. *Rev Med Microbiol* 1990; **1:** 108–115.

Jacobs E. *Mycoplasma pneumoniae* virulence factors and the immune response. *Rev Med Microbiol* 1991; **2:** 83–90.

Kawaoka Y, Webster RG. Molecular mechanisms of acquisition of virulence in influenza virus in nature. *Microb Pathogenesis* 1988; **5:** 311–318.

Marrie TJ, Grayston JT, Wang-P, Kuo C-C. Pneumonia associated with the TWAR strain of *Chlamydia. Ann Intern Med* 1987; **106:** 507–511.

Moser MR, Bender TR, Marelolis NS, Noble GR, Kendal AP, Ritter DG. An outbreak of influenza aboard a commercial airliner. *Am J Epidemiol* 1979; **110:** 1–7.

Pedersen SS. Clinical efficacy of ciprofloxacin in lower respiratory tract infections. *Scand J Infect Dis* 1989; Suppl 60: 89–97.

Stuart-Harris C, Schild GC, Oxford JS. *Influenza, the virus and the disease.* 2nd edn. Littleton, Ma. Publishing Sciences Group, 1985.

Wayne LG, Sramek HA. Aspects of newly recognized or infrequently encountered mycobacterial diseases. *Clin Microbiol Rev* 1992; **5:** 1–25.

23 URINARY TRACT INFECTIONS

Contents

INTRODUCTION

The urinary tract is one of the most common sites of bacterial infection, particularly in females; 10–20% of women have a urinary tract infection (UTI) at some time in their life and a significant number have recurrent infections. Although the majority of infections are acute and short-lived, they contribute to a significant amount of morbidity in the population. Severe infections result in loss of renal function and serious long-term sequelae. In females a distinction is made between cystitis, urethritis and vaginitis, but the genitourinary tract is a continuum and the symptoms often overlap.

ACQUISITION AND AETIOLOGY

Bacterial infection

Bacterial infection is usually acquired by the ascending route from the urethra to the bladder and may proceed to the kidney. Occasionally bacteria infecting the urinary tract invade the bloodstream to cause septicaemia. Less commonly infection may result from haematogenous spread of an organism to the kidney, with the renal tissue being the first part of the tract to be infected.

Ascending infections of the urinary tract are most commonly caused by the Gram-negative rod *Escherichia coli* (Fig. 23.1). Other members of the Enterobacteriaceae are also implicated; *Proteus mirabilis* is often associated with urinary stones (calculi), probably because this organism produces a potent urease which acts on urea to produce ammonia, rendering the urine alkaline. *Klebsiella, Enterobacter, Serratia* species and *Pseudomonas aeruginosa* are more frequently found in hospital-acquired UTI because their resistance to antibiotics favours their selection in hospital patients (see Chapter 39).

Among the Gram-positive species, *Staphylococcus saprophyticus* seems to have a particular propensity for causing infections in young, sexually active women. *Staphylococcus*

epidermidis, and *Enterococcus* species are more often associated with UTI in hospitalized patients. More recently, capnophilic species (organisms which grow better in air enriched with CO_2) including corynebacteria and lactobacilli, have been implicated as possible causes of UTI. On the other hand, obligate anaerobes are very rarely involved.

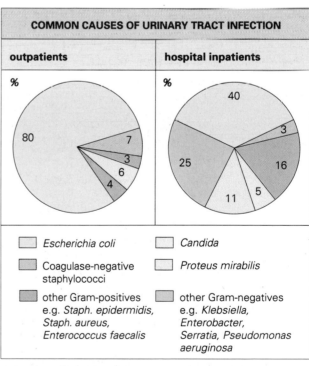

Fig. 23.1 Common causes of urinary tract infection. The percentage of infections caused by different bacteria in outpatients compared with hospital inpatients is shown. *Escherichia coli* is by far the most common isolate in both groups of patients, but note the difference in the percentage of infections caused by other Gram-negative rods. These isolates often carry multiple antibiotic resistance and colonize patients in hospital, especially those receiving antibiotics.

When haematogenous spread to the urinary tract has occurred, other species may be found e.g. *Salmonella typhi*, *Staphylococcus aureus* and *Mycobacterium tuberculosis* (renal tuberculosis).

Viral infection

Viral causes of urinary tract infection appear to be rare, although certain viruses may be recovered from urine in the absence of urinary tract disease. The human polyomaviruses JC and BK enter the body via the respiratory tract, spread through the body and infect epithelial cells in the kidney tubules and ureter, where they establish latency with persistence of the viral genome but not infectious virus. About one-third of kidneys from healthy individuals contain polyomavirus DNA sequences. However, during normal pregnancy the viruses may reactivate asymptomatically, with the appearance of large amounts of virus in the urine. Reactivation also occurs in immunocompromised patients (see Chapter 33). High titres of cytomegalovirus may be shed asymptomatically in the urine of congenitally-infected infants (see Chapter 26). In contrast to asymptomatic shedding, some serotypes of adenoviruses have been implicated as a cause of haemorrhagic cystitis.

Other types of infection

Non-bacterial causes of urinary tract infection include the fungi *Candida* spp. and *Histoplasma capsulatum*. Very few parasites are responsible for infections in the urinary tract. The protozoan *Trichomonas vaginalis* (see Chapter 24) can cause urethritis in both males and females, but is most often considered as a cause of vaginitis. Infections with *Schistosoma haematobium* (see Chapter 30) result in inflam-mation of the bladder and commonly haematuria. The eggs penetrate the bladder wall (Fig. 23.2), and in severe infections large granulomatous reactions can occur and the eggs may become calcified. Malignant changes are associated with chronic infections, although the cause of such changes is uncertain. Obstruction of the ureter as a result of egg-induced inflammatory changes can also lead to hydronephrosis.

PATHOGENESIS OF URINARY TRACT INFECTIONS

Factors predisposing to infection

Mechanical factors are important. Anything that disrupts normal urine flow or complete emptying of the bladder, or facilitates access of organisms to the bladder, will predispose an individual to infection (Fig. 23.3). The shorter female urethra is a less effective deterrent to infection than the male urethra (see Chapter 11). Sexual intercourse facilitates the movement of organisms up the urethra, particularly in females, so that the incidence of UTI is higher among sexually active than celibate women. Preceding bacterial colonization of the periurethral area of the vagina is perhaps important (see below). In male infants, urinary tract infections are more common in the uncircumcised and this is associated with colonization of the inside of the prepuce and urethra with faecal organisms.

Pregnancy, prostatic hypertrophy, renal calculi, tumours and strictures of any sort, are the main causes of obstruction to complete bladder emptying. When there is residual urine of more than 2–3ml, infection is more likely. Infection, superimposed on urinary tract obstruction may

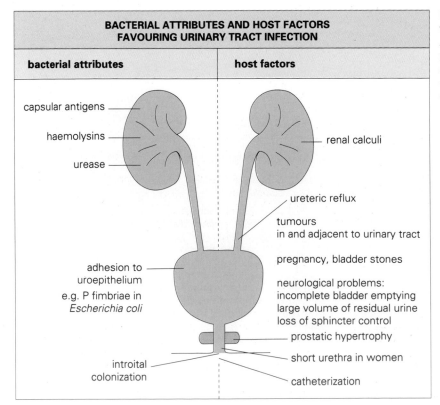

BACTERIAL ATTRIBUTES AND HOST FACTORS FAVOURING URINARY TRACT INFECTION	
bacterial attributes	**host factors**

capsular antigens

haemolysins

urease

renal calculi

ureteric reflux

tumours in and adjacent to urinary tract

pregnancy, bladder stones

adhesion to uroepithelium e.g. P fimbriae in *Escherichia coli*

neurological problems: incomplete bladder emptying large volume of residual urine loss of sphincter control

prostatic hypertrophy

introital colonization

short urethra in women

catheterization

Fig. 23.2 Bacterial attributes and host factors favouring urinary tract infection. Abnormalities of the urinary tract tend to predispose to infection. Bacterial adherence factors have been studied in detail but relatively little is known about other bacterial virulence factors in UTI.

lead to ascent to the kidney and then rapid destruction of renal tissue. Loss of neurological control of the bladder and sphincters (e.g. in spina bifida, paraplegia or multiple sclerosis) and the resultant large residual volume of urine in the bladder causes a functional obstruction to urine flow and such patients are particularly prone to recurrent infections.

Vesicoureteral reflux (reflux of urine from the bladder cavity up the ureters, sometimes into the renal pelvis or parenchyma) is common in children with anatomical abnormalities of the urinary tract and may predispose to ascending infection and kidney damage. Reflux may also occur in association with infection in children without underlying abnormalities but tends to disappear with age.

Despite reports that pyelonephritis (infection of the kidney) is a common finding in diabetics at post mortem, clinical surveys have failed to produce convincing evidence that there is a significant difference in the prevalence of UTI in diabetic and non-diabetic persons of the same age. However, diabetics may suffer more severe urinary infections and when diabetic neuropathy interferes with normal bladder function, persistent urinary infections commonly occur.

Catheterization is another major predisposing factor for UTI. During insertion of the catheter, bacteria may be carried directly into the bladder, and while *in situ* the catheter facilitates bacterial access to the bladder either via the lumen of the catheter or by tracking up between the outside of the catheter and the urethral wall (Fig. 23.3). The catheter disrupts normal bladder function and potentiates the effect of small numbers of bacteria.

Bacterial virulence factors

The conflict between host and parasite in the urinary tract has been discussed in Chapter 10. It is surprising that despite the frequent occurrence of urinary tract infections, relatively little is known about the virulence factors of the causative organisms (see Fig. 23.2).

Most urinary tract pathogens originate in the faecal flora but only the aerobic and facultative species such as *E. coli* possess the attributes required to colonize and infect the urinary tract. The ability to cause infection of the urinary tract is limited to certain serogroups of *E. coli* (e.g. 01, 02, 04, 06, 07 and 075; these serotypes differ from those associated with gastrointestinal tract infection, see Chapter 25). The success of these strains may be attributable in part to their ability to colonize the periurethral areas. Some *E. coli* have been shown to have particular types of fimbriae (pili) which enable them to adhere to urethral and bladder epithelium. Studies with other species of urinary tract pathogens have confirmed the presence of adhesins for uroepithelial cells (Fig. 23.4).

Other features of *E. coli* appear to assist in localization of organisms in the kidney and in renal damage. The capsular acid polysaccharide (K) antigens are associated with the ability to cause pyelonephritis and are known to enable *E. coli* strains to resist host defences by inhibiting phagocytosis. Haemolysin production by these species may also be linked with the capacity to cause kidney damage; many haemolysins act more generally as membrane-damaging toxins. The production of urease by organisms such as *Proteus* spp. has been correlated with their ability to cause pyelonephritis.

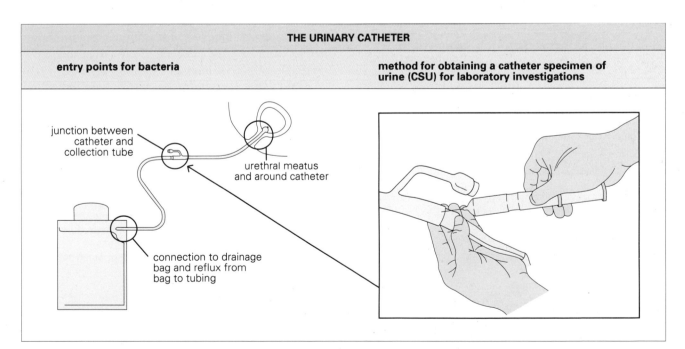

THE URINARY CATHETER

entry points for bacteria

method for obtaining a catheter specimen of urine (CSU) for laboratory investigations

junction between catheter and collection tube

urethral meatus and around catheter

connection to drainage bag and reflux from bag to tubing

Fig. 23.3 The urinary catheter. Catheterization is an important predisposition to infection. Bacteria can be pushed into the bladder as the catheter is inserted. While the catheter is in place, bacteria reach the bladder by tracking up between the outside of the catheter and the urethra. Contamination of the catheter drainage system by bacteria from other sources can also result in infection. Specimens of bladder urine for laboratory investigations can be collected from catheterized patients as shown. The second port above is for the instillation of fluids into the bladder. Urine from the drainage bag should not be tested because it may have been standing for several hours.

Host defence mechanisms

With the exception of the urethral mucosa, the normal urinary tract is resistant to bacterial colonization and usually eliminates microorganisms rapidly and efficiently (see Chapter 10). The pH, chemical content and flushing mechanism of urine helps to dispose of organisms in the urethra. Although urine is a good culture medium for most bacteria, it is inhibitory to some, and anaerobes and other species (non-haemolytic streptococci, corynebacteria and staphylococci) that comprise most of the normal urethral flora do not multiply readily in urine.

The role of humoral immunity in the host's defence against infection of the urinary tract is poorly understood. After infection of the kidney, IgG and secretory IgA antibodies can be detected in urine, but the protective role of these antibodies against subsequent infection is unclear. Infection of the lower urinary tract is usually associated with a low or undetectable serological response reflecting the superficial nature of the infection; the bladder and urethral mucosa are rarely invaded in urinary tract infections.

CLINICAL FEATURES AND COMPLICATIONS

Lower urinary tract

Acute infections of the lower urinary tract are characterized by a rapid onset of dysuria (burning pain on passing urine), urgency (the urgent need to pass urine) and frequency of micturition. However, urinary tract infections in the elderly and those with indwelling catheters are usually asymptomatic. The urine is cloudy, due to the presence of pus cells (pyuria) and bacteria (bacteriuria), and may contain blood (haematuria). Examination of urine specimens in the laboratory is essential to confirm the diagnosis. Patients with genital tract infections such as vaginal thrush or chlamydial urethritis may present with similar symptoms (see Chapter 24).

Pyuria in the absence of positive urine cultures can be due to chlamydiae or tuberculosis (see below) and is also seen in patients receiving antibacterial therapy for urinary tract infection; the bacteria are inhibited or killed by the antibacterial agent before the inflammatory response has died away.

Recurrent infections of the lower urinary tract occur in a significant proportion of patients. They may be relapses, caused by the same strain of organism or reinfections by a different organism. Recurrent infections can result in chronic inflammatory changes in the bladder, prostate and periurethral glands.

Acute bacterial prostatitis gives rise to systemic symptoms (fever) as well as local ones (perineal and low back pain, dysuria and frequency). It may arise from ascending or haematogenous infection and those people lacking the antibacterial substances normally present in prostatic fluid are perhaps more susceptible. Chronic bacterial prostatis, however, although usually caused by *E. coli*, is difficult to cure and can be a source of relapsing infection within the urinary tract.

Upper urinary tract

Although it may be important to know whether an infection is restricted to the bladder (lower urinary tract) or has ascended to the upper urinary tract and kidney, there are no satisfactory methods for distinguishing the two other than by examing urine obtained directly from the ureter by ureteric catheterization.

Patients presenting with pyelonephritis (infection of the kidney; Fig. 23.5), complain of lower tract symptoms and usually have a fever. Staphylococci are a common cause and renal abscesses are generally present. Recurrent episodes of pyelonephritis result in loss of function of renal tissue which may, in turn, cause hypertension, itself a cause of

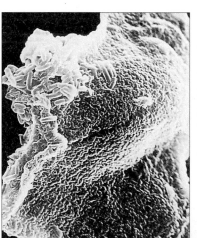

Fig. 23.4 Scanning electron micrograph showing bacteria attached to an exfoliated uroepithelial cell from a patient with acute cystitis. Courtesy of Dr TSJ Elliot and the editor of *British Journal of Urology.*

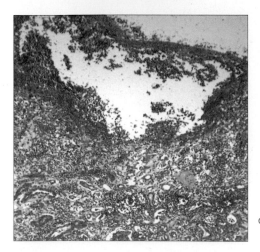

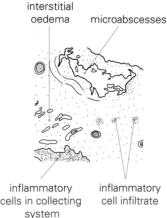

interstitial oedema   microabscesses

inflammatory cells in collecting system

inflammatory cell infiltrate

Fig. 23.5 Histological appearance of the kidney in acute pyelonephritis showing the intense inflammatory reaction and microabscesses. H & E Stain. Courtesy of MJ Wood.

renal damage. Infection associated with stone formation can result in obstruction of the renal tract and septicaemia.

Haematuria is a feature of endocarditis and a manifestation of immune complex disease as well as a result of infections of the kidney, and its presence warrants careful investigation. Pyuria may be associated with kidney infection with *Mycobacterium tuberculosis*. This organism cannot be grown by normal urine culture methods (see Appendix) and thus the patient may appear to have a sterile pyuria.

Asymptomatic infection (i.e. significant numbers of bacteria in the absence of symptoms; see below) can be detected only by screening urine samples in the laboratory. It is important in pregnant women and young children, where failure to treat may result in chronic renal damage, and in people undergoing instrumentation of the urinary tract in whom bacteriuria may proceed to bacteraemia.

LABORATORY DIAGNOSIS OF URINARY TRACT INFECTIONS

Methods for the processing of urine specimens in the laboratory are summarized in the Appendix. A key feature is the detection of significant bacteriuria.

Significant bacteriuria

In health the urinary tract is sterile, although the distal region of the urethra is colonized with commensal organisms which may include periurethral and faecal organisms. Because urine specimens are usually collected by voiding a specimen into a sterile container they become contaminated with the periurethral flora during collection. Infection can be distinguished from contamination by quantitative culture methods. Bacteriuria is defined as 'significant' when a properly collected midstream urine specimen is shown to contain >10^5 organisms per ml. Infected urine usually contains only a single bacterial species.

Contaminated urine usually has <10^4 organisms per ml and often contains more than one bacterial species (Fig. 23.6). Distinguishing infection from contamination when counts are between 10^4 and 10^5 organisms per ml can be difficult. Careful collection and rapid transport of urine specimens to the laboratory is essential (see below and Chapter 17).

It is important to recognize that the criteria for 'significant bacteriuria' do not apply to urine specimens collected from catheters or nephrostomy tubes, or by supra-pubic aspiration directly from the bladder, in which any number of organisms may be significant because the specimen is not contaminated by periurethral flora. In addition, infection of sites in the urinary tract below the bladder, and by organisms which are not members of the normal faecal flora, may not produce significant numbers in the urine.

Specimen collection

The usual specimen submitted for microbiological examination is a midstream urine (MSU) sample (see Chapter 17). This should be collected into a sterile, wide-mouthed container after careful cleansing of the labia or glans with soap (not antiseptic) and water, and after allowing the first part of the urine stream to be voided (this helps to wash out contaminants in the lower urethra). After suitable instruction the majority of adult patients can collect satisfactory samples with minimum supervision. With elderly and bedridden patients the problems are much greater and consideration should be given to these difficulties when interpreting results.

Collection of MSU samples from babies and young children is obviously difficult. 'Bag urine' may be collected by sticking a plastic bag to the perineum in girls or to the penis in boys, but such specimens are frequently heavily contaminated with faecal organisms. These problems may be overcome by suprapubic aspiration of urine directly from the bladder (Fig. 23.7).

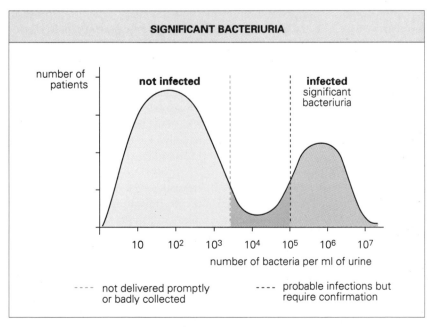

SIGNIFICANT BACTERIURIA

number of patients

not infected

infected significant bacteriuria

number of bacteria per ml of urine
10 10^2 10^3 10^4 10^5 10^6 10^7

- - - - not delivered promptly or badly collected

- - - - probable infections but require confirmation

Fig. 23.6 Significant bacteriuria. Voided specimens of urine are rarely sterile because the urine is contaminated with organisms from the periurethral area during collection. Even well-collected specimens from healthy individuals may contain up to 10^3 bacteria per ml of urine. Studies by Kass (see further reading) suggested that a count of 10^5 bacteria per ml was a reliable indicator of infection. However, there are various reasons, discussed in the text, why lower counts may sometimes be significant.

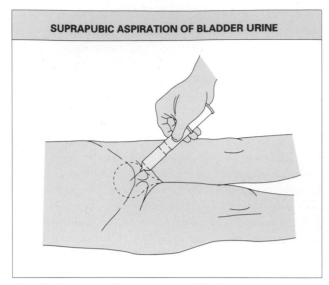

SUPRAPUBIC ASPIRATION OF BLADDER URINE

Fig. 23.7 Suprapubic aspiration of bladder urine. Urine samples can be collected directly from the bladder by insertion of a needle. This method is useful in young children from whom uncontaminated midstream urine (MSU) specimens are difficult to obtain.

Patients should not be catheterized simply to obtain a urine sample but in patients who have a catheter *in situ*, urine samples should be obtained by withdrawing a sample with a syringe and needle from the catheter tube (see Fig. 23.3). Urine that has been standing in the catheter drainage bag for hours is unsuitable because organisms may have multiplied to give much greater numbers than those present in the patient.

Special samples are required for the detection of certain pathogens. For *M. tuberculosis* three early morning urine samples should be sent on consecutive days. These do not require the same precautions during collection as a MSU because the culture technique prohibits the growth of organisms other than mycobacteria. For detection of *S. haematobium* the last few millilitres of a morning urine sample collected after exercise should be examined.

Ideally, samples should be collected before antimicrobial therapy is started. However if the patient is receiving therapy, or has done within the last 48 hours, this should be stated clearly on the request form.

Specimen transport
Urine specimens should be transported to the laboratory with minimum delay because urine is a good growth medium for many bacteria and multiplication of organisms in the specimen between collection and culture will distort the results (see Chapter 17).

Laboratory investigations
Urine specimens should be examined macroscopically and microscopically and should be cultured by quantitative or semiquantitative methods, as summarized in Chapter 18.

Microscopic examination allows a rapid preliminary report to be issued, but the presence of red and white blood cells, although abnormal, is not necessarily indicative of urinary tract infection. Haematuria may be present in infection both of the urinary tract and elsewhere (e.g. bacterial endocarditis), in renal trauma, when there are calculi, urinary tract carcinomas, clotting disorders and thrombocytopenia. Occasionally red blood cells may contaminate a urine specimen in menstruating women.

White blood cells are present in the urine in very small numbers (e.g. <10 per ml) in health; a count of >10 per ml is considered abnormal but is not always associated with bacteriuria. Sterile pyuria is an important finding which may reflect concurrent antibiotic therapy, other diseases such as neoplasms or urinary calculi, or infection with organisms that are not detected by routine urine culture methods (see Appendix). Renal tubular cells, seen in the urine of aspirin abusers, may be confused with white blood cells. Urinary casts are also indicative of renal tubular damage.

Bacteria may be seen on microscopy when present in the specimen in large numbers. However they are not necessarily indicative of infection but may be the result of a poorly collected specimen or one which has been left at room temperature for a prolonged period of time.

Detection of significant bacteriuria
As discussed above, the laboratory diagnosis of significant bacteriuria requires quantitation of the bacteria in a urine specimen. Culture media and methods are outlined in the Appendix. Conventional methods produce results within 18–24 hours but rapid methods based on bioluminescence, turbidometry and flow cytometry are also available. In some laboratories the detection of abnormal numbers of white blood cells or bacteria on microscopy prompts the setting up of direct antibiotic susceptibility tests so that both culture and susceptibility result are available within 24 hours.

Interpretation of the significance of the culture results is subject to several provisos:
- Collection – specimen collection must be carried out properly;
- Storage – the urine must be cultured within 1 hour of collection or held at 4°C for not more than 18 hours before culture;
- Antibiotics – in a patient receiving antibiotics, smaller numbers of organisms may be significant and may represent an emerging resistant population. Simple laboratory methods are available for the detection of antibacterial substances in urine;
- Fluid intake – the patient may be taking more or less fluid than usual and this will clearly influence the quantitative result;
- The specimen – the quantitative guidelines are valid for MSU specimens; they do not apply to catheter specimens, suprapubic aspirates or nephrostomy samples.

TREATMENT OF URINARY TRACT INFECTIONS

Uncomplicated urinary tract infection (cystitis) should be treated with antibacterial agents taken by mouth as a single dose or for 3 days depending on the drug. The com-

ORAL ANTIBACTERIALS FOR URINARY TRACT INFECTIONS		
antibacterial	class of agent*	comments
Ampicillin Amoxycillin	β-lactam β-lactam	note that >50% of Gram-negative rods causing UTI are β-lactamase producers and are therefore resistant
Augmentin	β-lactam + β-lactamase inhibitor	active against most Gram-negative rods resistant to ampicillin by virtue of β-lactamase production
Cephalexin Cefaclor	β-lactam β-lactam	relatively β-lactamase stable, therefore wider spectrum than ampicillin not active against enterococci
Trimethoprim	nucleic-acid synthesis inhibitor	incidence of resistant strains increasing
Cotrimoxazole	combination of trimethoprim with sulphamethoxazole (also nucleic-acid synthesis inhibitor)	may be useful in 'blind' treatment but more toxic than trimethoprim alone
Nitrofurantoin	urinary antiseptic	for uncomplicated UTI only not active at alkaline pH (therefore not useful for *Proteus* infections)
Nalidixic acid	quinolone	for uncomplicated UTI Gram-negative infections only not active against Gram-positive
Ciprofloxacin	quinolone	very broad spectrum only oral agent active against *Pseudomonas aeruginosa* not active against enterococci

Fig. 23.8 Oral antibacterials for urinary tract infections. Several different classes of antibacterials are available in oral formulations and suitable for treatment of UTI. Nitrofurantoin and nalidixic acid are useful only for lower urinary tract infections as they do not achieve adequate serum and tissue concentrations to treat upper urinary tract infections. Ciprofloxacin is an example of the new generation of quinolones; others may be preferred in different countries. *For details see Chapter 35.

monly prescribed agents are shown in figure 23.8. The choice of agent should be based on the results of susceptibility tests. However, for uncomplicated urinary tract infection in patients in the community, therapy is often 'best guess', at least until laboratory results are available. This requires a knowledge of the likely pathogens and their antibiotic susceptibility patterns in the locality. Follow-up cultures should be done after treatment has been completed (at least 2 days later) to confirm eradication of the infecting organism. In addition to antibacterial therapy, the patient should be advised to drink large volumes of fluid to help the normal flushing-out process.

Children and pregnant women with asymptomatic bacteriuria should be treated with antibacterials and followed up to check for eradication of the infection. Instrumentation of the urinary tract should be delayed in patients with significant bacteriuria until appropriate treatment has rendered the urine sterile.

Complicated UTI (pyelonephritis) should be treated with a systemic antibacterial agent to which the organism is known to be susceptible until signs and symptoms subside. This can then be replaced by oral therapy. The usual length of treatment is ten days but longer treatment may be necessary to sterilize the kidney.

Hospital-acquired infections or recurrent infections, particularly in catheterized patients, may be caused by antibiotic resistant organisms and the agent of choice will depend on the antibacterial susceptibility pattern. Wherever possible the catheter should be removed; eradication of infection in catheterized patients is extremely difficult to achieve and some would advocate treatment only when the patient complains of symptoms or prior to invasive procedures. Guidelines for catheter care and for the prevention of catheter-associated UTI are shown in figure 23.9.

Infections acquired by haematogenous spread require specific antibacterial therapy, as described in Chapter 22 for tuberculosis, Chapter 25 for *Salmonella typhi*, Chapter 28 for *Staphylococcus aureus* and Chapter 30 for schistosomiasis.

PREVENTION OF URINARY TRACT INFECTIONS

Many of the features of the pathogenesis of urinary tract infection and host predispositions are not understood clearly, but it has been shown that recurrent infections in otherwise healthy women can be prevented by encouraging regular emptying of the bladder, particularly following intercourse, to wash bacteria out of the urinary tract. The prophylactic use of antibiotics may also prevent recurrent infections, but in the presence of underlying abnormalities there is a tendency to select antibiotic-resistant strains which subsequently cause infections that are more difficult to treat.

GUIDELINES FOR CATHETER CARE
avoid catheterization whenever possible
keep duration of catheterization to a minimum
use intermittent, rather than continuous, catheterization when feasible
insert catheters with good aseptic technique
use a closed sterile drainage system
maintain a gravity drain
use topical antiseptics around the meatus in women
wash hands before and after inserting catheters and collecting specimens, and after emptying drainage bags

Fig. 23.9   Guidelines for catheter care. Catheters that drain into open collecting vessels are particularly conducive to infection. Virtually every patient who has such a catheter in place for more than 4 days becomes infected. Nowadays closed drainage systems are used in most hospitals but even then bacteriuria occurs in 10–25% of patients. Hospitals with active catheter care programmes can keep this rate below 10%.

Infection in catheterized patients is very common but can be reduced by good catheter care procedures (see Fig. 23.10 and Chapter 39). Whenever possible catheterization should be avoided or kept to a minimum duration.

SUMMARY

Urinary tract infections are the cause of a considerable amount of morbidity, especially in the female population. They are important, and often asymptomatic, in pregnancy and some studies have shown a correlation between UTI in pregnancy and low birth weight babies. When associated with underlying structural or neurological abnormalities, UTI is difficult to treat effectively and results in severe incapacity and fatal infection. Antibacterial agents play an important role in treatment and prevention of UTI, but in the absence of laboratory investigations may be inappropriate or unnecessary.

Further Reading

Association of Clinical Pathologists. *Estimation of bacteria and white cells in the urine.* Broadsheet 80: August 1973.

Kass E H. Asymptomatic infections of the urinary tract. *Trans Assoc Am Phys* 1956; **69:** 56–64.

Komeroff AL, Friedland G. The dysuria–pyuria syndrome. *N Eng J Med* 1980; **303:** 452–453.

Kunin CM. *Detection, prevention and management of urinary tract infections.* Maryland: Lea & Febiger, 1972.

24 SEXUALLY TRANSMITTED DISEASES

Contents

INTRODUCTION

Sexually transmitted infections (STIs) usually, but not always (e.g. asymptomatic gonorrhoea in females, the early stages of HIV infection), cause sexually transmitted diseases (STDs). These are of major medical importance throughout the world. Unfortunately, most STDs are increasing rather than decreasing in occurrence, due to a number of factors, including:

- increasing density and mobility of human populations;
- the difficulty of engineering changes in human sexual behaviour;
- the absence of vaccines for any of these infections.

The last two items may well alter. There is already evidence for changes in male homosexual behaviour, leading to decreased transmission of STDs in this group, and vaccines for certain infections (herpes simplex, gonorrhoea, HIV) will eventually come.

Recently, the emergence of HIV infection and AIDS has overshadowed other STDs. Nevertheless, despite its immense impact as a new and highly lethal infectious disease for which there is so far no satisfactory treatment or vaccine, it is still uncommon in developed countries compared with other STDs.

The general principles of entry, exit and transmission of the microorganisms that cause STDs are set out in Chapter 11. The spread of STDs is inextricably linked with sexual behaviour, and as such there are far greater opportunities for the control of such infections than in the case of, for instance, respiratory infections. Infected but asymptomatic individuals play an important role. Promiscuity (having diverse and frequent sexual relationships) and details of sexual practice, such as the actual orifices or mucosal surfaces brought into contact with body fluids (see Chapter 11), are important determinants. Transmission between heterosexuals or male homosexuals can take place following oral or anal intercourse. The gonococcus, for instance, causes pharyngitis and proctitis, although it infects stratified squamous epithelium less readily than columnar epithelium. Condom usage is another major determinant. Condoms have been shown to retain gonococci, herpes simplex virus, HIV and chlamydia in simulated coital tests of the syringe and plunger type (even when the 'infected' plunger was left in place for an extra eight hours!). Further discussion of the control of STDs is included in Chapter 38.

Various host factors influence the risk of acquiring STDs. It is not surprising that the type of sexual activity is important, or that genital lesions or ulcers increase the risk of acquiring infections such as HIV. Other factors are less well understood, such as the numerous observations that uncircumcized men have a higher risk of infection.

STDs do not necessarily come singly, and the possibility of multiple infection must always be borne in mind. For instance, syphilis can accompany gonorrhoea, and there is evidence that genital herpes may be reactivated during an attack of gonorrhoea.

The 'top ten' STDs are listed in figure 24.1, while those that are less common are listed in figure 24.2; Figure 24.3 gives examples of the strategies used by the microorganisms to overcome host defences.

SYPHILIS

Aetiology and transmission

Syphilis is caused by the spirochaete *Treponema pallidum* (see Appendix), an organism that is closely related to treponemes which cause the non-venereal infections pinta and yaws (see Fig. 24.4). *Treponema pallidum* has a worldwide distribution, but syphilis is now uncommon in the USA and in the UK (approximately 1000 new cases per annum) and is much less prevalent than other STDs. Despite this, syphilis remains a problem, especially in developing countries, because of the serious sequelae and the risk of congenital infection.

THE TOP TEN SEXUALLY TRANSMITTED DISEASES				
organism	**disease**	**comment**	**treatment**	**vaccine available**
Papillomaviruses (6 of the 70 types)	genital warts, dysplasias	the commonest of all STDs; associated with cancer of cervix, penis, etc.	*	no
Chlamydia trachomatis (D–K serotypes)	non-specific urethritis	increasing incidence	+ (tetracycline)	no
Candida albicans	vaginal thrush, balanitis	very common; predisposing factors	+ (nystatin, fluconazole)	no
Trichomonas vaginalis	vaginitis, urethritis	very common	+ (metronidazole)	no
Herpes simplex viruses types 1and 2	genital herpes	? increasing problem of latency and reactivation	± (acyclovir)	no
Neisseria gonorrhoeae	gonorrhoea	decreasing incidence in developed countries	++ (penicillin, cefotaxime, spectinomycin)	no
Human immuno-deficiency virus	AIDS	highly lethal; incidence increasing world-wide	± (retrovir)	no
Treponema pallidum	syphilis	decreasing incidence in developed countries	++ (penicillin)	no
Hepatitis B virus	hepatitis	especially male homosexuals (? decreasing incidence)	−	yes
Chlamydia trachomatis (L1, L2, L3 serotypes)	lymphogranuloma venereum	mainly tropical countries	+ (tetracycline)	no

Fig. 24.1 The 'Top Ten' of sexually transmitted diseases. * Podophyllin, surgical removal; no chemotherapy available.

OTHER SEXUALLY TRANSMITTED DISEASES				
organism	**disease**	**comment**	**treatment**	**vaccine available**
Calymmato-bacterium granulomatis	granuloma inguinale	tropical	+ (tetracycline)	no
Haemophilus ducreyi	chancroid	mainly tropical	+ (erythromycin, ceftriaxone, cotrimoxazole)	no
Sarcoptes scabiei	genital scabies	common	+ (benzyl benzoate)	no
Phthirus pubis	pediculosis pubis	common	+ (malathion)	no
Mycoplasma (T strains)	non-specific urethritis	less important than chlamydia	+ (tetracycline)	no
Gardnerella vaginalis	vaginitis	acts together with anaerobes	+ (metronidazole)	no

Fig. 24.2 Other sexually transmitted diseases.

STRATEGIES ADOPTED BY SEXUALLY TRANSMITTED MICROORGANISMS TO COMBAT HOST DEFENCES		
host defences	microbial strategies	examples
integrity of mucosal surface	specific attachment mechanism	gonococcus or chlamydia to urethral epithelium
urine flow (for urethral infection)	specific attachment; induce its own uptake and transport across urethral epithelial surface in phagocytic vacuole infection of urethral epithelial or sub-epithelial cells	gonococcus herpes simplex, chlamydia
Phagocytes (especially polymorphs) Complement Inflammation	induce negligible inflammation C3d receptor on microbe binds C3b/d and reduces C3b/d-mediated polymorph phagocytosis induce strong inflammatory response, yet evade consequences	*T. pallidum*; mechanism unclear, perhaps poorly activates alternative complement pathway due to sialic acid coating *Candida albicans* gonococcus, *C. albicans*, herpes simplex, chlamydia; mechanism unknown
Antibodies (especially IgA) Cell mediated immune response (T cells, lymphokines, NK cells etc.)	produce IgA protease antigenic variation; allows re-infection of a given individual with an antigenic variant antigenic variation within a given individual unknown factors cause ineffective cell-mediated immune response	gonococcus gonococcus, chlamydia, papillomaviruses (not herpes simplex or *T. pallidum*) HIV *T. pallidum*, HIV

Fig. 24.3 Strategies adopted by sexually transmitted microorganisms to combat host defences.

SPIRAL ORGANISMS OF MEDICAL IMPORTANCE				
family	genus	species	sub-species	disease
Spirochaetales	*Treponema*	*pallidum* *pallidum* *carateum*	*pallidum* *pertenue* –	syphilis yaws pinta
	Borrelia	*recurrentis* *burgdorferi*	– –	relapsing fever Lyme disease
Leptospiraceae	*Leptospira*	*icterohaemorrhagiae* *hardjo*	– –	leptospirosis (Weil's disease)

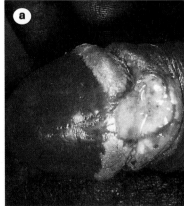
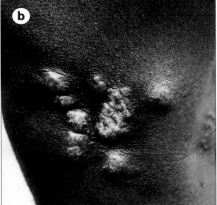
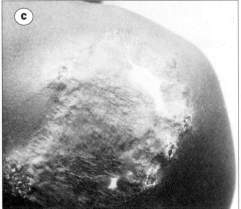

Fig. 24.4 Spiral organisms of medical importance. (a) Typical penile chancre of primary syphilis. Courtesy of RD Catterall. Yaws (b) and pinta (c) are endemic in tropical and sub-tropical countries and are spread by direct contact. Courtesy of PJ Cooper and G Griffin.

THE PATHOGENESIS OF SYPHILIS		
stage of disease	**signs and symptoms**	**pathogenesis**
initial contact ⇩ 2–10 weeks (depends on inoculum size) ⇩	primary chancre* at site of infection	multiplication of treponemes at site of infection; associated host response
primary syphilis ⇩ 1–3 months ⇩	enlarged inguinal nodes spontaneous healing	proliferation of treponemes in regional lymph nodes
secondary syphilis ⇩ 2–6 weeks ⇩	flu-like illness myalgia, headache, fever mucocutaneous rash* spontaneous resolution	multiplication and production of lesions in lymph nodes liver joints muscles skin and mucous membranes
latent syphilis ⇩ 3–30 years ⇩		treponemes dormant in ?liver and spleen re-awakening and multiplication of treponemes
tertiary syphilis	neurosyphilis; general paralysis of the insane, tabes dorsalis cardiovascular syphilis; aortic lesions, heart failure progressive destructive disease	further dissemination and invasion and host response (cell-mediated hypersensitivity) gummas in skin, bone, testis

* Live treponemes can be seen in dark-ground microscopy of fluid from lesions; patient highly infectious

Fig. 24.5 The pathogenesis of syphilis. A feature of *T. pallidum* infection is its chronic nature which seems to involve a delicately balanced relationship between pathogen and host.

Transmission requires close personal contact because the organism survives poorly outside the body and is very sensitive to drying, heat and disinfectants. Horizontal spread (see Chapter 11) occurs through sexual contact, vertical spread via transplacental infection of the foetus (see Chapter 26).

Pathogenesis

The organism enters the body through minute abrasions on the skin or mucous membranes. Local multiplication leads to plasma cell polymorph and macrophage infiltration, with later endarteritis. Bacteria multiply very slowly, and the average incubation period is three weeks. Classically, the course of the infection is divided into three stages – primary, secondary, and tertiary syphilis (Fig. 24.5). However, not all patients go through all three stages; a substantial proportion remains permanently free of disease after suffering the primary or secondary stages of infection. The secondary stage may be followed by a latent period of some 3–30 years, after which the disease may recur – the tertiary stage. Unlike most bacterial pathogens, *T. pallidum* can survive in the body for many years despite a vigorous immune response. It has been suggested that the healthy treponeme evades recognition and elimination by the host by maintaining a cell surface, rich in lipid, that is antigenically unreactive, and it is only in dead and dying organisms that antigens are uncovered and the host responds.

Despite many years of effort, *T. pallidum* still cannot be cultivated in the laboratory in artificial media. It has not, therefore, been possible to study possible virulence factors at a molecular level, although a number of major proteins have now been characterized.

Clinical features

The clinical features of syphilis are summarized in figure 24.5, and the lesion of primary syphilis illustrated in figure 24.4.

FALSE–POSITIVES IN SYPHILIS SEROLOGY	
test	**conditions associated with false–positive result**
Non-specific (non-treponemal) VDRL RPR	viral infection, collagen-vascular disease, acute febrile disease, post-immunization, pregnancy, leprosy, malaria
Specific (treponemal) FTA-ABS TPHA	diseases associated with increased or abnormal globulins, lupus erythematosus, skin diseases, anti-nuclear antibodies, drug addiction, pregnancy

Fig. 24.6 Serological tests for syphilis and conditions associated with false-positive results.

Congenital syphilis

An infected woman can transmit *T. pallidum* to her baby *in utero* after the first three months of pregnancy. The manifestations of the disease range from serious infection resulting in intrauterine death to congenital abnormalities which may be obvious at birth, or to silent infection which may not be apparent until about two years of age (facial and tooth deformities).

Laboratory diagnosis

As *T. pallidum* cannot be grown *in vitro*, laboratory diagnosis hinges on microscopy and serology.

Microscopy

Exudate from the primary chancre should be examined by dark-ground microscopy immediately after collection, or by UV microscopy after staining with fluorescein-labelled anti-treponemal antibodies. The organisms have tightly wound, slender coils with pointed ends and are sluggishly motile in unstained preparations. *T. pallidum* is very thin (about 0.2 μm in diameter, compared with *E. coli* which is about 1 μm) and cannot be seen in Gram-stained preparations. Silver impregnation stains can be used to demonstrate the organisms in biopsy material.

Serology

Serological tests for syphilis are the mainstay of diagnosis and are divided into non-specific and specific tests for the detection of antibodies in patients' serum:

* *Non-specific tests (non-treponemal tests).* The term 'non-specific' is used because the antigens are not treponemal in origin but are from extracts of normal mammalian tissues. Cardiolipin, from beef heart, allows the detection of anti-lipid IgG and IgM formed in the patient in response to lipoidal material released from cells damaged by the infection as well as to lipids in the surface of *T. pallidum.* The two tests in common use today are the 'Venereal Disease Research Lab' (VDRL) test and 'Rapid Plasma Reagin' (RPR) tests; both are available in kit form. Non-

specific tests become positive within 4–6 weeks of infection (or 1–2 weeks after the primary chancre appears) and decline in positivity in tertiary syphilis or after effective antibiotic treatment of primary or secondary disease. Thus, these tests are useful for screening. However, the tests are non-specific and may give positive results in conditions other than syphilis (biological false positives; Fig. 24.6). All positive results should, therefore, be confirmed by a specific test.

* *Specific tests.* These tests use treponemal antigens extracted from *T. pallidum.* Two tests are in common use: 'Fluorescent Treponemal Antibody Absorption' (FTA-ABS) in which the patient's serum is first absorbed with non-pathogenic treponemes to remove cross-reacting antibodies, prior to reaction with *T. pallidum* antigens; and the '*Treponema pallidum* Haemaglutination Assay' (TPHA). These tests should be used to confirm that a positive result with a non-specific test is truly due to syphilis. Also, because they become positive earlier in the course of the disease, they can be used for confirmation when the clinical picture is strongly indicative of syphilis. They tend to remain positive for many years and may be the only positive test in patients with late syphilis. However, they remain positive after appropriate antibiotic treatment and thus cannot be used as indicators of therapeutic response. Unfortunately, they can also given false positive reactions (see Fig. 24.6).

Positive results in serological tests from babies born to infected mothers may represent passive transfer of maternal antibody or the baby's own response to infection. These two possibilities can be distinguished by testing for IgM and retesting at six months of age, by which time maternal antibody levels have waned. Antibody titres remain elevated in babies with congenital syphilis.

Thus, at present, the confirmation of a diagnosis of syphilis depends on several serological tests. None of these tests distinguish syphilis from the non-sexually transmitted treponematoses, yaws and pinta. In future, monoclonal antibodies may be useful in detecting specific treponemal protein antigens and in the development of competition assays for the host's antibody.

Treatment

Penicillin is very active against *T. pallidum* (see Fig. 24.1) and is the drug of choice for treatment. For patients who are allergic to penicillin, treatment with tetracycline, doxycycline or erythromycin should be given. Only penicillin therapy reliably treats the foetus when administered to a pregnant mother.

Prevention

Prevention of secondary and tertiary disease depends on early diagnosis and adequate treatment. Contact tracing, with screening and treatment is also important. Several STDs may be present in one patient concurrently, and patients with other STDs should be screened for syphilis.

Congenital syphilis is completely preventable if women are screened serologically early in pregnancy (less than three months) and those who are positive treated with penicillin.

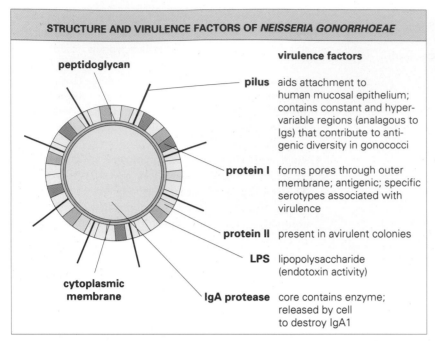

STRUCTURE AND VIRULENCE FACTORS OF *NEISSERIA GONORRHOEAE*

peptidoglycan

cytoplasmic membrane

virulence factors

pilus — aids attachment to human mucosal epithelium; contains constant and hyper-variable regions (analogous to Igs) that contribute to antigenic diversity in gonococci

protein I — forms pores through outer membrane; antigenic; specific serotypes associated with virulence

protein II — present in avirulent colonies

LPS — lipopolysaccharide (endotoxin activity)

IgA protease — core contains enzyme; released by cell to destroy IgA1

Fig. 24.7 The spread of *Neisseria gonorrhoeae* is facilitated by various virulence factors. Changes in the surface structure of the gonoccus render the organism avirulent.

BACTERIAL FEATURES ASSOCIATED WITH DISSEMINATION

resistance to bactericidal action of serum

marked susceptibility to penicillin

require arginine, uracil and hypoxanthine for growth in laboratory

Fig. 24.8 Characteristics of *N. gonorrhoeae* strains associated with disseminated disease.

GONORRHOEA

Aetiology and transmission

Gonorrhoea is a bacterial infection caused by the Gram-negative coccus *Neisseria gonorrhoeae* (the 'gonococcus'). This organism is a human pathogen and does not cause natural infection in other animals. Thus, its reservoir is human and transmission is direct, usually through sexual contact, from person to person. The organism is sensitive to drying and survives poorly outside the human host, so intimate contact is required for transmission to occur. It is thought that a woman has a 50% chance of becoming infected after a single intercourse with an infected man, and a man has a 20% chance of acquiring infection from an infected woman.

Asymptomatically infected individuals (almost always women; see below) form the major reservoir of infection. Infection may also be transmitted 'vertically' from an infected mother to her baby during childbirth. Infection in babies are usually manifested as ophthalmia neonatorum (see Chapter 21).

Pathogenesis

The usual site of entry of gonococci into the body is into the vagina or the urethral mucosa of the penis, but other sexual practices may result in the deposition of the organisms in the throat or the rectal mucosa. Special adhesive

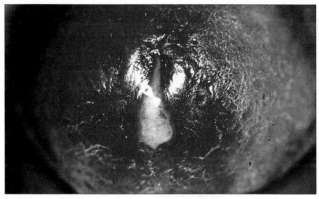

Fig. 24.9 Gonococcal urethritis. Typical purulent meatal discharge with inflammation of the glans. Courtesy of J Clay.

mechanisms (Fig. 24.7) attach the bacteria to mucosal cells and prevent them from being washed away by the tide of urine or by vaginal discharges. Following attachment the gonococci multiply rapidly and spread through the cervix in women and up the urethra in men. Spread is facilitated by various virulence factors (see Fig. 24.7) although the organisms do not possess flagella and are non-motile. Production of an IgA protease helps to protect them from the host's secretory antibodies.

The gonococci invade non-ciliated epithelial cells which internalize the bacteria and allow them to multiply within intracellular vacuoles, protected from phagocytes and antibodies. These vacuoles move down through the cell and fuse with the basement membrane, discharging their bacterial contents into the sub-epithelial connective tissues. Damage to the host results from the inflammatory responses elicited by the organism; *N. gonorrhoeae* does not produce a recognized exotoxin. Persistent untreated infection can result in chronic inflammation and fibrosis.

Infection is usually localized, but the bacteria can invade the bloodstream and thence spread to other parts of the body. Strains of *N. gonorrhoeae* that are associated with

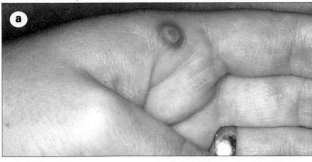

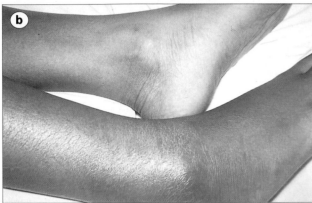

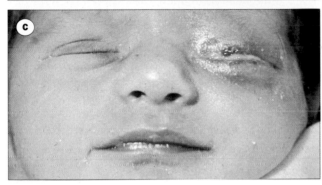

COMPLICATIONS OF GONOCOCCAL INFECTION

systemic spread　　　　　　　local spread

skin lesions (a)

endocarditis

female
damage to
fallopian tubes
pelvic inflammatory
disease
ano-rectal infection

male
occasional
epididymitis

arthritis (b)

ophthalmia
neonatorum (c)

Fig. 24.10 Local and systemic complications in gono-coccal infection. (a) Skin lesions start as erythematous papules which often become pustular and haemorrhagic with necrotic centres. (b) Septic arthritis of the ankle with marked erythema and swelling of the ankle and leg. (c) Ophthalmia neonatorum usually appears 2–5 days after delivery down an infected birth canal. (a) and (c) Courtesy of JS Bingham; (b) Courtesy of TF Sellers, Jr.

disseminated disease have particular characteristics, includ-ing resistance to the bactericidal action of serum (Fig. 24.8).

Clinical features

Symptoms develop within 2–7 days of infection and are characterized in the male by urethral discharge (Fig. 24.9) and pain on passing urine (dysuria), and in the female by vaginal discharge. However, infection is not necessarily symptomatic. At least half of all women infected have only mild symptoms or are completely asymptomatic. Hence, they do not seek treatment and will continue to infect others. Asymptomatic infection, however, is not the usual course of events in men. Women may not be alerted to their infection unless or until complications arise such as pelvic inflammatory disease (PID), chronic pelvic pain, or infertility resulting from damage to the fallopian tubes.

Ophthalmia neonatorum is characterized by a sticky dis-charge. Infection of the throat may result in a sore throat (see Chapter 22) and infection of the rectum also results in a purulent discharge.

Complications

In men local complications of urethral infection are rare (Fig. 24.10). Invasive gonococcal disease is much more common in women than in men, but prompt treatment is also important in containing local infection. Again the common occurrence of asymptomatic infection in women is an important factor. In 10–20% of untreated infected women, infection spreads up the genital tract to cause PID and damage to the fallopian tubes. Disseminated infection occurs in 1–3% of women but is less common in men. It is a function not only of the strain of gonococcus (see Fig. 24.8) but also of ill-understood host factors. About 5% of people with disseminated infection have deficiencies in the late-acting components of complement (C5–C8).

Diagnosis

Diagnosis rests on microscopy and culture of urethral and vaginal discharge, and of other specimens where indicat-ed. Although a purulent discharge is a characteristic of local gonococcal infection, it is not possible clinically to distinguish reliably between gonococcal discharge and that caused by other pathogens such as *Chlamydia trachomatis*.

With experience, the finding of Gram-negative intra-cellular diplococci in smear of urethral discharge from a symptomatic male patient is a highly sensitive and specific test for the the diagnosis of gonorrhoea. Culture is essential for the investigation of infection in women and asymptomatic men, and for specimens taken from sites other than the urethra. Specimens from symptomatic men should also be cultured, for the following reasons:

- to confirm the identify of the isolate; misinterpretation of microscopy or culture results can cause severe distress and may result in litigation;
- to perform antibiotic susceptibility tests (see Chapter 18);
- to aid in the distinction between treatment failure and reinfection.

Because of the organism's sensitivity to drying, cultures should be made in the clinic or at the bedside onto warmed media and transported to the laboratory without delay. Blood cultures should be collected if disseminated disease is suspected, and joint aspirates may yield positive cultures.

Treatment and prevention

The antibacterial agents of choice are shown in figure 24.1. Resistance is increasing in incidence and has severely compromised the effective treatment of gonorrhoea in some parts of the world such as South–East Asia. Prophylactic use of antibacterials has no effect in preventing sexually-acquired infection, but application of antibacterial eye drops to babies born to mothers known or suspected to be infected is effective.

Infection can be prevented by the use of condoms. Follow-up of patients and contact tracing are vital to control the spread of gonorrhoea. At present effective vaccines are not available, but the possibility of using some of the pilus proteins or other outer membrane components of the gonococcal cell as antigens is under investigation. However, immunization may prevent symptomatic disease without preventing infection, and the dangers of asymptomatic infection have been stressed above.

CHLAMYDIA INFECTION

Aetiology and transmission

The chlamydiae are very small bacteria which are obligate intracellular parasites. They have a more complicated life cycle than free-living bacteria because they can exist in different forms; the elementary body (EB) is adapted for extracellular survival and for initiation of infection, the reticulate body (RB) for intracellular multiplication (Fig. 24.11).

Three species of chlamydia are currently recognized: *C. trachomatis*, *C. psittaci* and *C. pneumonia* (Fig. 24.12). *Chylamydia psittaci* and *C. pneumoniae* infect the respiratory tract and have been discussed in Chapter 22. The species *C. trachomatis* can be subdivided into different serotypes (also known as serovars) and these have been shown to be linked characteristically with different infections. Serotypes A, B and C are the causes of the serious eye infection trachoma (see Chapter 21). Serotypes D–K are the cause of genital infection and associated ocular and respiratory infections (Fig. 24.13), and serotypes L1, 2 and 3, cause the systemic disease lymphogranuloma venereum (LGV; see below). *Chlamydia trachomatis* serotypes D–K have a world-wide distribution whereas the LGV serotypes are more restricted in their distribution.

The majority of infections are genital and are acquired during sexual intercourse. Asymptomatic infection is common, especially in women. Ocular infections in adults are probably acquired by auto-inoculation from infected genitalia or by ocular–genital contact. Ocular infections in neonates are acquired during passage through an infected maternal birth canal, and the infant is also at risk of developing *C. trachomatis* pneumonia (see Chapter 22).

Pathogenesis and clinical features

Chlamydia enter the host through minute abrasions in the mucosal surface. They bind to specific receptors on the host cells and enter the cells by 'parasite-induced' endocytosis (see Chapter 11). Once inside the cell, fusion of the chlamydia-containing vesicle with lysozomes is inhibited by an unknown mechanism and the EB begins its developmental cycle (see Fig. 24.11). Within 9–10 hours of cell invasion the EBs differentiate into metabolically active

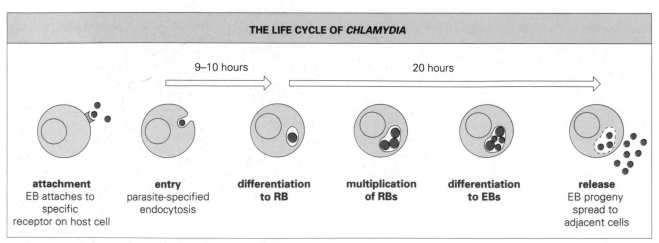

Fig. 24.11 The life cycle of *Chlamydia*. EB, elementary body; RB, reticulate body.

reticulate bodies (RBs); these divide by binary fission and produce fresh EB progeny which are released into the extracellular environment within a further 20 hours. It is not yet clear whether release involves host-cell rupture or exocytosis, but the clinical manifestations of infection indicate that damage results from a combination of cell destruction and the host's inflammatory response. The released EBs invade adjacent cells or, if carried in lymph or blood, can invade cells distant from the site of infection. Growth of *C. trachomatis* serotypes D–K seems to be restricted to columnar and transitional epithelial cells, but serotypes L1, L2 and L3 cause systemic disease (lymphogranuloma venereum). The site of infection determines the nature of clinical disease (see Fig. 24.13).

Diagnosis (non-LGV serotype infections)

Chlamydial urethritis and cervicitis cannot be distinguished reliably from other causes of these conditions on clinical grounds alone and laboratory tests are essential. The methods available include cell culture and direct antigen detection. Most infected patients develop antibodies, but serology is unreliable for diagnostic purposes. Because chlamydia are obligate intracellular parasites, isolation must be performed in cell cultures. The specimen is suspended in fluid and centrifuged onto a monolayer of tissue culture (McCoy) cells pretreated with cycloheximide, which enhances uptake of chlamydia. After 48–72 hours *C. trachomatis* forms characteristic cytoplasmic inclusions which stain with iodine (because they contain glycogen; Fig. 24.14), or can be visualized by immunofluorescent stains.

Chlamydia trachomatis can be detected directly in smears of clinical specimens made on microscope slides, stained with fluorescein-conjugated monoclonal antibodies and viewed by UV microscopy – the 'direct fluorescent antibody' (DFA) test. The EBs stain as bright green dots (Fig. 24.15). Results can be obtained within a few hours. When compared with culture, this method is extremely specific, but often not sensitive enough in patients with asymptomatic infections. Chlamydial antigens can also be detected in specimens using an enzyme-linked immunosorbent assay (ELISA), but this test also suffers from reduced sensitivity in asymptomatic patients.

MEDICALLY IMPORTANT SPECIES OF CHLAMYDIA

species	serotype (serovar)	natural host	disease in humans
C. trachomatis	A,B,C	humans	trachoma
	D–K	humans	cervicitis urethritis proctitis conjunctivitis pneumonia (in neonates)
	L1,L2,L3	humans	lymphogranuloma venereum
C. psittaci	?	birds and non-human mammals	pneumonia
C. pneumoniae	1	humans	acute respiratory disease

Fig. 24.12 Medically important species of *Chlamydia*. *C. trachomatis* is the species associated with sexually transmitted disease.

CHLAMYDIA TRACHOMATIS: CLINICAL SYNDROMES AND THEIR COMPLICATIONS

infection in:	clinical syndromes	complications
Men	urethritis epididymitis proctitis conjunctivitis	systemic spread Reiter's syndrome*
Women	urethritis cervicitis bartholinitis salpingitis conjunctivitis	ectopic pregnancy infertility systemic spread: perihepatitis arthritis dermatitis
Neonates	conjunctivitis	interstitial pneumonitis

Fig. 24.13 Clinical syndromes and complications caused by *C. trachomatis*, serovars D–K. * Urethritis, conjunctivitis, polyarthritis, mucocutaneous lesions.

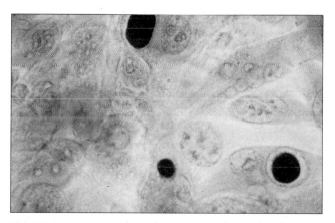

Fig. 24.14 *Chlamydia* inclusion bodies (stained dark brown with iodine).

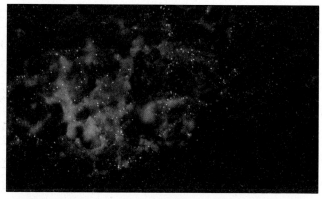

Fig. 24.15 DFA test for *C. trachomatis*. Elementary bodies (EBs) can be seen as bright green dots under the UV microscope. Courtesy of JD Treharne.

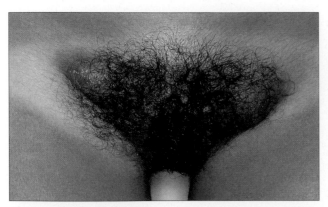

Fig. 24.16 Lymphogranuloma venereum. Bilateral enlargement of inguinal glands. Courtesy of JS Bingham.

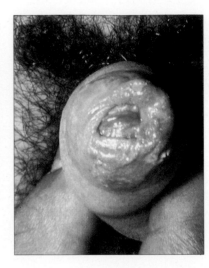

Fig. 24.17
Chancroid. Several irregular ulcers on the prepuce. Courtesy of L Parish.

Treatment

Treatment for chlamydial infection is with tetracycline (see Fig. 24.1). It is important to remember that these organisms are not susceptible to the beta-lactam antibiotics which are the drugs of choice for treatment of gonorrhoea and syphilis. It is recommended that patients receiving treatment for gonorrhoea are also treated with tetracycline for possible concurrent chlamydial infection. In addition, patients with clinically diagnosed chlamydial genital infections, their sexual contacts, and babies born to infected mothers, should be treated. For babies erythromycin should be used.

Prevention

Prevention depends on recognizing the importance of asymptomatic infections. Early diagnosis and treatment of cases and of their sexual partners is important. Remember that STDs are not mutually exclusive and patients may have concurrent infections with quite different pathogens.

OTHER CAUSES OF INGUINAL LYMPHADENOPATHY

Among sexually active people, genital infections are common causes of inguinal lymphadenopathy (swelling of lymph nodes in the groin). Syphilis and gonorrhoea have been discussed above. Lymphogranuloma venereum, chancroid and donovanosis are rare in Europe and USA, but are much more common in tropical and sub-tropical countries, and may be imported by travellers who have acquired the disease through sexual contact in these areas.

Lymphogranuloma venereum

Lymphogranuloma venereum (LGV) is a serious disease which is common in Africa, Asia and South America and occurs sporadically in Europe, Australia and North America, particularly among homosexual males. The prevalence appears to be higher in males than females, probably because symptomatic infection is more common in men.

LGV is caused by *Chlamydia trachomatis* serotypes L1, L2 and L3, which cause a systemic infection involving lymphoid tissue, rather than the more restricted infection seen with serotypes D–K (see above). The primary lesion is an ulcerating papule at the site of inoculation (after an incubation period of 1–4 weeks) and may be accompanied by fever, headache and myalgia. The lesion heals rapidly, but the chlamydia proceed to infect the draining lymph nodes, causing characteristic inguinal buboes (Fig. 24.16) which gradually enlarge. *Chlamydia* may disseminate from the lymph nodes via the lymphatics to the tissues of the rectum to cause proctitis. Other systemic complications include fever, pain hepatitis, pneumonitis and meningoencephalitis. The infection may resolve untreated, but abscesses may form in lymph nodes, which suppurate and discharge through the skin, and chronic granulomatous reactions in lymphatics and neighbouring tissues can give rise eventually to fistula *in ano* or genital elephantiasis.

Diagnosis and treatment

Cell culture methods are available (see above), but the chlamydia isolation rate is reported to be low (24–30%). Classically, the 'Frei' skin test was used in diagnosis. This involves intradermal injection of the LGV antigen, but it is unreliable, lacking sensitivity in early disease and lacking specificity because the Frei antigen is only genus specific. Treatment with tetracycline (see Fig. 24.1) is recommended.

Chancroid (soft chancre)

This is a sexually transmitted disease caused by the Gram-negative bacterium *Haemophilus ducreyi*. Infection is manifest as painful, non-indurated genital ulcers and local lymphadenitis (Fig. 24.17). Note the different between this and the chancre of primary syphilis which is painless, but the ulcers may be confused with those of genital herpes, although they are usually larger and have a more ragged appearance. The disease is rare in the USA but has a world-wide distribution, and outbreaks within communities have been reported. This epidemiological information is important because the diagnosis is usually clinical as the organism is difficult to grow in the laboratory. Chancroid may also be confused with donovanosis (see below).

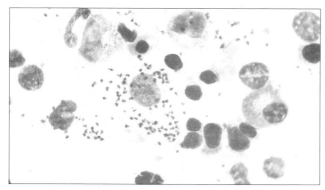

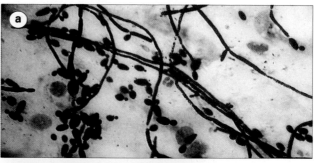

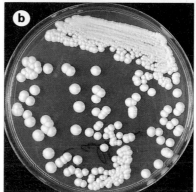

Fig. 24.18 Donovan bodies in cytoplasm of mononuclear cells.

Fig. 24.19 *Candida albicans.* (a) Light microscopical appearance and (b) culture of vaginal discharge.

Diagnosis and treatment

Gram-stained smears of aspirates from the ulcer margin or enlarged lymph node characteristically show large numbers of short Gram-negative rods and chains, often described as having a 'school of fish' appearance, within or outside polymorphs. Aspirates should be cultured on a rich medium (chocolate agar with 1% isovitalex) at 30–34°C. *Haemophilus ducreyi* will not tolerate higher temperatures. Growth is slow and it may take 2–9 days for colonies to appear. Treatment with erythromycin, ceftriavone or cotrimoxoazole (see Fig. 24.2) is recommended.

Donovanosis

Donovanosis (granuloma inguinale or granulomavenereum) is rare in temperate climes but common in tropical and sub-tropical regions such as the Caribbean, New Guinea, India and central Australia. The infection is characterized by nodules, almost always on the genitalia, which erode to form granulomatous ulcers that bleed readily on contact. The infection may extend and the ulcers may become secondarily infected. The pathogen is a Gram-negative rod called *Calymmatobacterium granulomatis.* The bacteria invade and multiply within mononuclear cells and are liberated when the cells rupture. The diagnosis of donovanosis is made by examining a smear from the lesion stained with Wright or Geimsa stain. 'Donovan bodies' appear as clusters of blue- or black-stained organisms in the cytoplasm of mononuclear cells (Fig. 24.18). Treatment with tetracycline is recommended (see Fig. 24.2).

The role of sexual transmission of this infection is still controversial. The disease is often absent in sexual contacts of infected individuals and, in a study in New Guinea, was present in young children and adults but not in 5–15 year olds.

MYCOPLASMAS – ANOTHER CAUSE OF NON-GONOCOCCAL URETHRITIS?

Although *Mycoplasma pneumoniae* has a proven role in the causation of pneumonia (see Chapter 22), the role of *Mycoplasma hominis* in non-gonococcal urethritis is uncertain.

Mycoplasma hominis and the related organism *Ureaplasma urealyticum,* are frequently found colonizing the genital tracts of normal, sexually active men and women. They are less common in sexually inactive populations, which supports the view that they may be sexually transmitted. It is difficult to prove that they cause infection of the genital tract, but *M. hominis* may cause pelvic inflammatory disease, post–abortal and post-partum fevers; *U. urealyticum* has been associated with urethritis and prostatitis in men.

Fortunately, both *M. hominis* and *U. urealyticum* are susceptible to tetracycline which is also the treatment of choice for chlamydial infections.

OTHER CAUSES OF VAGINITIS AND URETHRITIS

Candida infection

Candida albicans causes a range of diseases from mild, superficial, localized infections in an otherwise healthy individual, to disseminated, often fatal, infection in the immunocompromised. This yeast is a normal inhabitant of the female vagina but in some women, and in circumstances which are not clearly understood, the load of *Candida* increases and causes an intensely irritant vaginitis with a cheesy vaginal discharge. This may be accompanied by urethritis and dysuria and may present as a urinary tract infection (see Chapter 23). The diagnosis can be confirmed by microscopy and culture of the discharge (Fig. 24.19). Treatment with an oral antifungal, such as fluconazole, or a topical preparation such as nystatin, is recommended, but recurrence is frequent in a small proportion of women. Balanitis is seen in up to 10% of male partners of females with vulvo–vaginal candidiasis, but urethritis in men is uncommon and rarely symptomatic.

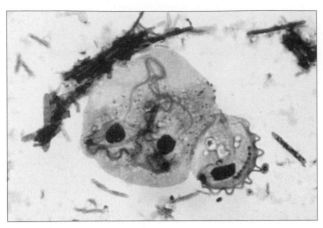

Fig. 24.20 Motile trophozoites in vaginal discharge in *T. vaginalis* infection. Giemsa stain. Courtesy of R Muller.

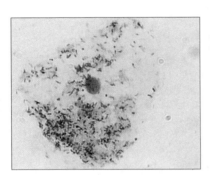

Fig. 24.21 Clue cells in bacterial vaginosis.

Trichomonas vaginalis infection

Trichomonas vaginalis is a protozoan parasite that inhabits the vagina in women and the urethra (and sometimes the prostate) in men, and is transmitted during sexual intercourse. In women, heavy infections cause vaginitis, with a characteristic copious, foul-smelling discharge. There is an associated rise in the vaginal pH; the infection should be distinguished from bacterial vaginosis (see below) by microscopical examination of the discharge, which shows actively motile trophozoites (Fig. 24.20). Treatment with metronidazole is recommended for symptomatic infections. In men, *T. vaginalis* is rarely pathogenic but sometimes causes a mild urethritis. However, regular sexual partners of symptomatic women should also be treated to prevent reinfection.

BACTERIAL VAGINOSIS

Bacterial vaginosis (non-specific vaginitis) is a syndrome in women characterized by at least three of the following signs and symptoms:
• Excessive malodorous vaginal discharge;
• Vaginal pH greater than 4.5;
• Presence of clue cells (vaginal epithelial cells coated with bacteria; Fig. 24.21);
• A fishy, amine-like odour.
There is a significant increase in the numbers of the bacterium *Gardnerella vaginalis* in the vaginal flora and a concomitant increase in numbers of obligate anaerobes such as *Bacteroides*.

Gardnerella vaginalis is consistently found in association with vaginosis, but is also found in 20–40% of healthy women. It is generally present in the urethra of male partners of women with vaginosis, indicating that it can be sexually-transmitted. *Gardnerella vaginalis* has also been isolated from blood cultures from women with postpartum fever.

The organism has had a chequered taxonomic history (first classified as a *Haemophilus*, then as a *Corynebacterium*) which reflects the fact that it tends to be Gram-variable (sometimes appearing Gram-negative, sometimes Grampositive). It grows in the laboratory on human blood agar in a moist atmosphere enriched with CO_2.

The pathogenesis of bacterial vaginosis is still unclear, but appears to be related to factors that disrupt the normal acidity of the vagina and the equilibrium between the different constituents of the normal vaginal flora. Whether any of these or other unknown factors are sexually transmissible is also unclear.

GENITAL HERPES

Aetiology and transmission

Herpes simplex virus type 1 (HSV1) is generally transmitted via saliva, causing primary oropharyngeal infection in children and later in life, after reactivation, cold sores. However, a separate virus strain, HSV2, has emerged as a result of independent transmission by the venereal route. HSV2 shows biological and antigenic differences from the original (HSV1) strain, but special laboratory techniques are needed to distinguish them. There is little cross-immunity. Although originally recovered from separate sites, orogenital sexual practices have become prevalent enough to obscure the topographical difference between the strains, so that both HSV1 and HSV2 are sometimes recovered from oral and genital sites.

Clinical aspects and pathogenesis

The primary genital lesion is seen is on penis, vulva etc., 3–7 days after infection. It consists of vesicles that soon break down to form painful shallow ulcers (Fig. 24.22). Local lymph nodes are swollen, and there may be constitutional symptoms (fever, headache, malaise). Occasionally the lesions are on the urethra, causing dysuria. Healing takes up to 2 weeks, but the virus in the lesion travels up sensory nerve endings to establish latent infection in dorsal root ganglion neurones (see also Chapter 27). From this site it can reactivate, travel down nerves to the same area, and cause recurrent lesions ('genital cold sores').

Aseptic meningitis or encephalitis occurs in adults as a rare complication, and spread of infection from mother to the infant at the time of delivery can give rise to disseminated herpes or encephalitis in the neonatal period.

Diagnosis and treatment

Diagnosis is generally possible by clinical appearance. Virus can be isolated from vesicle fluid or ulcer swabs, and viral antigens detected by the ELISA method. Topical acyclovir can be worthwhile for severe or early lesions, and this drug may need to be given intravenously when there

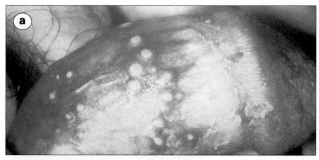

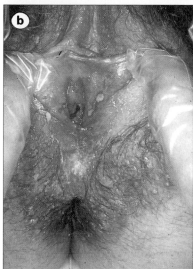

Fig. 24.22 Genital herpes. Vesicles on (a) the penis in male and (b) in the peri-anal area and vulva in female. Those on the labia minora and fourchette have ruptured to reveal characteristic herpetic erosions. Courtesy of JS Bingham

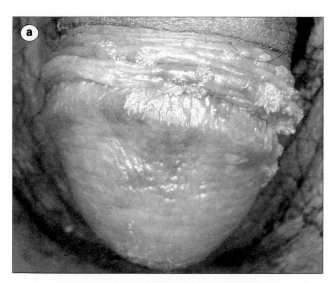

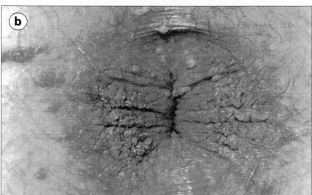

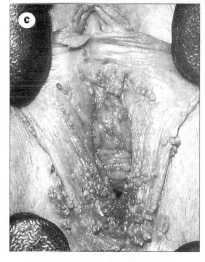

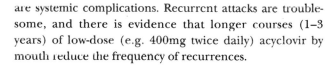

Fig. 24.23 Genital warts. (a) Warts on the penis are usually multiple, and on the shaft are often flat and kera-tinized. (b) Warts in the perianal area often extend into the anal canal. (c) Warts in the vulvo-perineal area can enlarge dramatically and extend into the vagina. Courtesy of JS Bingham.

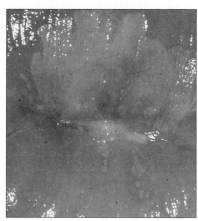

Fig. 24.24 Cervical dysplasia caused by papillomavirus should be removed by laser. Courtesy of A Goodman.

are systemic complications. Recurrent attacks are trouble-some, and there is evidence that longer courses (1–3 years) of low-dose (e.g. 400mg twice daily) acyclovir by mouth reduce the frequency of recurrences.

PAPILLOMAVIRUS INFECTION

Aetiology

There are now about 70 distinct types of human papillo-maviruses, all infecting skin or mucosal surfaces, and the DNA of each showing less than 50% cross-hybridization with that of others. Evidently these are ancient viral associ-ates of man that have evolved extensively, and many of the different types are adapted to specific regions of the body. Types 6, 12, 16, 18 and 31 are regularly transmitted by the venereal route.

Pathogenesis, clinical features, diagnosis and treatment

Warts (condylomata accuminata) appear on penis, vulva and perianal regions (Fig. 24.23) after an incubation period of 1–6 months (see also Chapter 27). They may not regress for many months, and can be treated with podophyllin. On the cervix the lesion is a flat area of dys-plasia, visible by colposcopy as a white plaque (Fig. 24.24) after the local application of 5% acetic acid. Because of the association with cervical cancer (especially types 16 and 18) cervical lesions are best removed by laser.

HUMAN RETROVIRUSES	
virus	**comment**
HTLV1	endemic in W Indies and SW Japan; transmission via blood, human milk; can cause adult T-cell leukaemia, and HTLV1–associated myelopathy and tropical spastic paraparesis
HTLV2	uncommon, sporadic occurrence; transmission via blood; can cause hairy T-cell leukaemia
HIV1, HIV2	transmission via blood, sexual intercourse; responsible for ARC, AIDS, AIDS dementia etc.; HIV2 W African in origin; closely related to HIV1 but antigenically distinct
Human foamy virus	causes foamy vacuolation in infected cells; little is known of its occurrence or pathogenic potential
Human placental virus(es)	detected in placental tissue by electron microscopy and by presence of reverse transcriptase
Human genome viruses	nucleic acid sequences representing endogenous retroviruses are common in the vertebrate genome, often in well-defined genetic loci; acquired during evolutionary history; not expressed as infectious virus; function unknown; perhaps should be regarded as mere parasitic DNA

Fig. 24.25 Human retroviruses. HTLV1, HTLV2, HIV1 and HIV2 have been cultivated in human T cells *in vitro*. The human placental and genome viruses are not known as infectious agents. Retroviruses are also common in cats (FAIDS), monkeys (MAIDS) and mice (mouse leukaemia), and other vertebrates.

HUMAN IMMUNODEFICIENCY VIRUS INFECTION

Aetiology

The human immunodeficiency virus (HIV) is a retrovirus (Fig. 24.25), so called because this ssRNA virus contains a *pol* gene that codes for a reverse transcriptase (Latin *retro*, backwards). In 1981, the Communicable Disease Centre, Atlanta, USA noted an increase in requests to use pentamidine for *Pneumocystis carinii* infection in previously well individuals who also suffered severe infections by other normally harmless microorganisms. These included *Candida albicans* oesophagitis, mucocutaneous herpes simplex, toxoplasma CNS infection or pneumonia, and cryptosporidial enteritis; Kaposi's sarcoma was often also present. Patients had evidence of impared immune function, as shown by skin test anergies, and depletion of CD4-positive T helper lymphocytes. This immunodeficiency syndrome, appearing in an individual without a known cause, such as treatment with immunosuppressive drugs, was referred to as 'Acquired Immune Deficiency Syndrome' (AIDS). An internationally agreed definition of AIDS soon followed. Epidemics subsequently occurred in San Francisco, New York and other US cities, and in Britain and Europe a few years later (see Chapter 38).

In 1983, the causative virus, HIV, was isolated from blood lymphocytes and recognized as belonging to the lentivirus (slow virus) group of retroviruses, related to similar agents in monkeys, and to visna virus in sheep and goats. The structure of the viral particle and its genome is illustrated in figure 24.26 and its replication mechanism in figure 24.27.

Virus replication is regulated by the products of six genes. The replication cycle is often halted after integration of the provirus, so that the infection remains latent in the cell. The *tat* and *rev* genes, for instance, function as trans-activating factors, and can increase production of viral RNAs and proteins when latently infected cells are stimulated to differentiate (e.g. T helper cells by antigen) or stimulated by infection with certain other viruses (e.g. HSV, cytomegalovirus).

The molecular biological evidence (in terms of nucleic acid sequence) indicates that both HIV1 and the closely related HIV2, seen in West Africa, probably arose from closely related primate viruses. HIV1 may have been present in humans in Central Africa for many years, but in the late 1970s it began to spread rapidly (Fig. 24.28), possibly with changed biological properties, as a result of increased transmission following major socio-economic upheavals and migrations of people from central to east Africa. Female prostitutes and mobile male soldiers and workers played a major part. The disease soon appeared in Haiti and the USA, followed by Europe and Australasia.

Pathogenesis

HIV infects cells bearing the CD4 antigen, including T helper cells (T_H), monocytes and dendritic cells (Figs 24.29 and 24.30). The CD4 molecule acts as a binding site for the gpl20 envelope glycoprotein of the virus. Productive replication and cell destruction does not occur until the T helper cell is activated. T cell activation is greatly enhanced not only in attempts to respond to HIV antigens, but also as a result of the secondary microbial

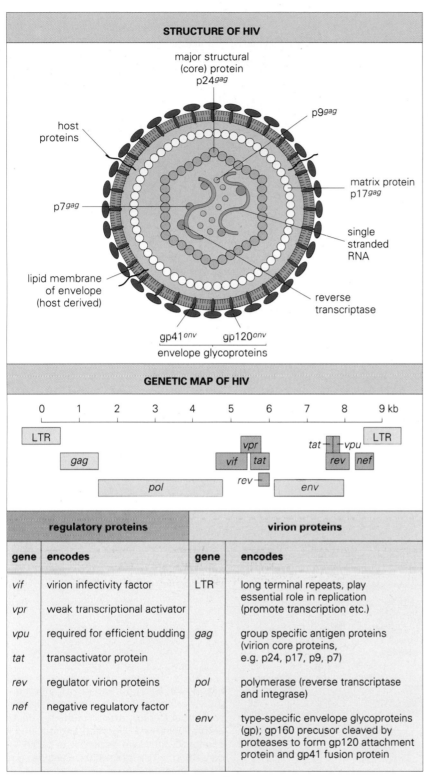

Fig. 24.26 The structure and genetic map of HIV. The *rev* and *tat* genes are divided into non-contiguous pieces and the gene segments spliced together in the RNA transcript. Occasional host proteins (e.g. MHC molecules) are present in the envelope.

infections seen in patients. Monocytes and macrophages, Langerhans' cells and follicular dendritic cells also express the CD4 molecule and are infected but are not generally destroyed, although there is a remarkable disruption of histological pattern in lymphoid follicles. Infected cells bear the fusion protein gp41 and may therefore fuse with other infected or uninfected cells. This helps the virus to spread, and accounts for the multinucleated cells seen especially in the brain.

As a result of the decreased numbers of CD4-positive T helper cells and defects in antigen presentation, together with other factors such as the production of virus coded immunosuppressive molecules (gp120, gp41), there are depressed immune responses. Skin test (dth) responses are absent, NK activity is reduced, and there are various other immunological abnormalities, including polyclonal activation of B cells. Functional changes in lymphocytes (reduced responses to mitogens, reduced IL-2 and IFN-γ

HIV REPLICATION CYCLE

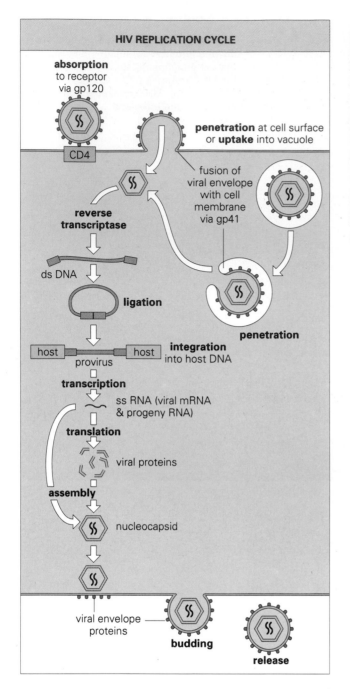

absorption
to receptor
via gp120

CD4

penetration at cell surface
or **uptake** into vacuole

fusion of
viral envelope
with cell
membrane
via gp41

**reverse
transcriptase**

ds DNA

ligation

penetration

host   host   **integration**
into host DNA

provirus

transcription

ss RNA (viral mRNA
& progeny RNA)

translation

viral proteins

assembly

nucleocapsid

viral envelope
proteins

budding

release

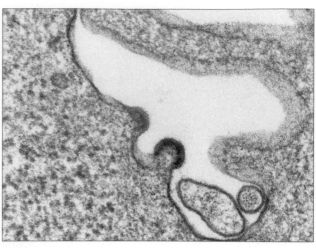

Fig. 24.27 The HIV replication cycle. The virus enters the cell either by fusion with the cell membrane at the cell surface, or via uptake into a vacuole and release within the cell. The electron micrograph above shows of HIV budding from the cell surface prior to release. Courtesy of D Hockley.

EARLY SPREAD OF HIV INFECTION

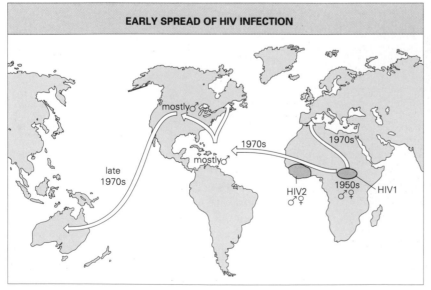

mostly ♂

mostly ♂

1970s

1970s

late
1970s

HIV2
♂♀

1950s

HIV1
♂♀

Fig. 24.28 Early spread of HIV infection (now world-wide). HIV1 may have been present in Central Africa for many years before increased migration and socio-economic upheaval caused it to begin spreading in the late 1970s. Outside Africa, most infections occurred in males.

production, etc.) are greater than would be explained by the T helper cell loss. Only a proportion of circulating T helper cells are actually infected and it is possible that virus-triggered autoimmune responses to CD4 antigens, or immune responses to otherwise normal CD4-positive cells which have bound HIV antigens, may contribute to the loss of T helper cells. The immunosuppression is permanent, the patient remains infectious, and the virus persists in the body. The eventual mortality, due to opportunist infections, tumours etc., approaches 100%.

Although neutralizing antibodies are eventually formed, and virus specific T cells, including CD8-positive Tc cells, are detectable, the cell mediated immune response, as judged by lymphoproliferation to viral antigens, is poor. It is detectable only in about half of infected but otherwise healthy patients, in spite of normal numbers of circulating T helper cells, whereas responses to other antigens are normal. Perhaps the virus engineers a specific suppression of protective responses to itself. Later on, as AIDS develops, responses to HIV are further depressed, and also responses to unrelated antigens. The host response is further handicapped by antigenic variation in the 'hypervariable' region of gp120. This occurs during infection, so that different antigenic variants can be isolated from a given individual. Some of the variants show resistance to currently circulating Tcs, i.e. are immune escape variants. Others show increased pathogenicity.

HIV is present in peripheral blood mononuclear cells, the major source of transmitted virus. Titres are, however, quite low, about 10 000 infectious doses per ml of blood, so that the blood is much less infectious than in hepatitis B virus infections. The amount present tends to fall after seroconversion, and rises again during the development of AIDS related complex (ARC) and AIDS. Smaller amounts of virus are also present in semen and saliva, and probably even smaller amounts in colostrum, the human cervix and tears. Infection is reported in CD4-positive submucosal cells in the rectum and large bowel and could be a route for entry in homosexuals.

A subacute encephalitis, often with dementia, is seen in infected patients. Viral invasion of the CNS and CNS disease occurs in infected patients independently of AIDS. Multiple small nodules of inflammatory cells are seen, and most of the infected cells appear to be microglia or infiltrating macrophages. These cells express the CD4 antigen, and it has been suggested that infected monocytes carry the virus into the brain. Most AIDS patients develop neurological disease, and the picture is complicated by the various persistent infections that are activated and give rise to their own CNS pathology. These include herpes simplex virus, varicella-zoster virus, *Toxoplasma gondii*, JC virus (prog-ressive multifocal leucoencephalopathy), and *Cryptococcus neoformans*.

The origin of the type of Kaposi's sarcoma seen in AIDS patients is not understood. Although 21% of homosexual or bisexual males with AIDS develop the tumour, it is seen in only 10% of haemophiliacs who were infected by contaminated blood (factor VIII) products. The tumour could be due to another virus whose pathogenic effect is promoted by AIDS. Some of the B cell lymphomas are attributable to reactivating Epstein–Barr virus.

Studies of pathogenicity of HIV2 are in progress. It is not yet clear whether this virus differs significantly from HIV1 in transmission, progression to AIDS, or the occurrence of the AIDS dementia complex.

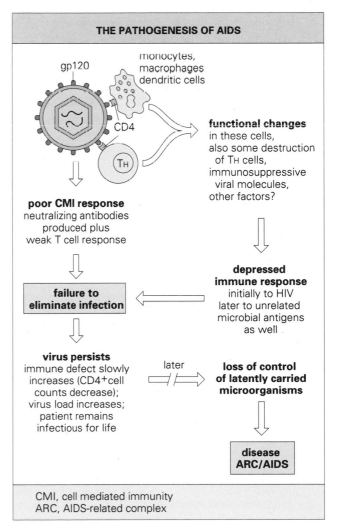

Fig. 24.30 The pathogenesis of AIDS.

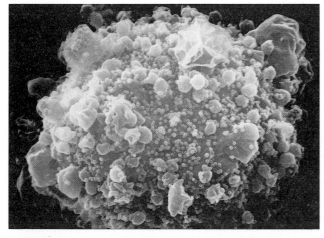

Fig. 24.29 Scanning electron micrograph of an HIV-infected T helper cell (x20 000). Courtesy of D Hockley.

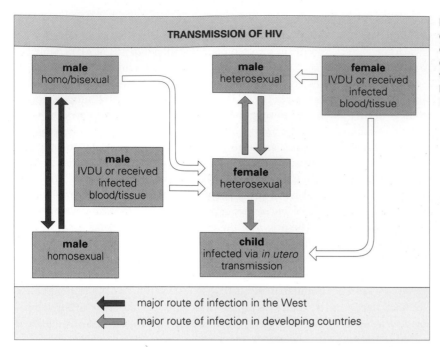

Fig. 24.31 Major routes of transmission of HIV. Although the heterosexual route of transmission has, so far, been well established only in developing countries, there is evidence that this route is becoming more important in the West. IVDU, intravenous drug user.

Transmission

In developed countries homosexual men have so far been the group most vulnerable to HIV infection and AIDS, especially the passive partner in anal intercourse. Haemophiliacs who received contaminated blood products have also been contaminated, though less commonly, as well as intravenous drug abusers. Infection is transmitted primarily from male to male and from male to female (Fig. 24.31), although not very efficiently compared with other sexually transmitted diseases. Transmission from female to male, however, is a common and well established feature of HIV in Africa. In randomly selected rural communities in parts of Central and East Africa seropositivity rates of up to 40% are encountered, mostly in young adults. The demographic predictions are for a disastrous mortality, with major economic and political implications in these countries.

So far, heterosexual transmission has not been notable in developed countries. One possible explanation for the greater heterosexual spread in Africa is that ulcers and other lesions due to other sexually transmitted agents are very common on the cervix of African females, and could be a source of infected lymphocytes and monocytes. But there are signs that transmission by heterosexual intercourse is beginning to be more important in developed countries. It is not clear whether HIV can infect males by the urethra or whether pre-existing genital skin breaks are necessary. There is evidence that those possessing a foreskin are more likely to be infected.

HIV can also be transmitted vertically from infected mother to offspring. Little is known about this but it occurs in about 20% of cases, especially *in utero* but also peri- and postnatally. At least half of the infected offspring develop AIDS within the first year of life, but at this age there are fewer latent infections available for reactivation. So far about 1 million infants have been infected, mainly in subsaharan Africa, and it is predicted that paediatric AIDS will be a major cause of death, with 10 million infants affected, by the year 2000.

The fact that infection in Africa does not generally occur until after the onset of sexual maturity indicates that arthropod transmission probably does not occur. Transmission by close contact, aerosols, kissing and so forth is virtually unknown.

Clinical features

Initial infection may be accompanied by a mild mononucleosis-type illness with fever, malaise, etc. (Fig. 24.32). Antibodies often take many months to become detectable, and cytotoxic T cells are formed. There is probably some curtailment of viral replication, and the individual remains well. Infected cells, however, are still present, and at a later stage the infected individual may show weight loss, fever, persistent lymphadenopathy, oral candidiasis and diarrhoea. This is the AIDS-related complex (ARC). Further viral replication takes place until finally, some years after initial infection, there is development of full-blown AIDS (see Fig. 24.32).

It is not understood what determines progression through the cycle of seropositivity to ARC and AIDS. The virus exercises complex control over its own replication (see Fig. 24.27). Replication is also influenced during the response to other infections which act as antigenic stimuli, and some of them directly as transactivating agents.

A subacute encephalitis, sometimes with dementia may occur, as described above, and also a variety of reactivating infections of the CNS (see Fig. 24.32). In infants the CNS picture may include arrested CNS development with microcephaly. Some patients, especially in Africa, develop a wasting disease ('slim' disease), possibly due to unknown intestinal infections or infestations, and perhaps also to the direct effects of the virus infecting cells of the intestinal wall. The disease AIDS consists of the microbial diseases

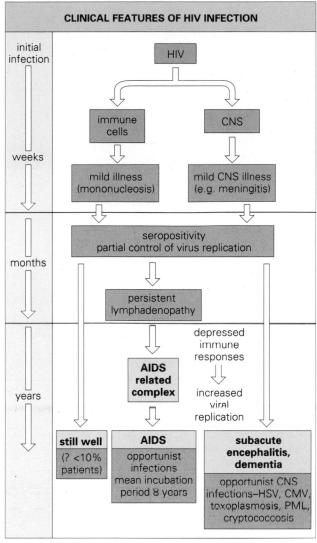

CLINICAL FEATURES OF HIV INFECTION

initial infection

weeks

HIV

immune cells

CNS

mild illness (mononucleosis)

mild CNS illness (e.g. meningitis)

seropositivity
partial control of virus replication

months

persistent lymphadenopathy

AIDS related complex

depressed immune responses

increased viral replication

years

still well
(? <10% patients)

AIDS
opportunist infections
mean incubation period 8 years

subacute encephalitis, dementia
opportunist CNS infections–HSV, CMV, toxoplasmosis, PML, cryptococcosis

Fig. 24.32 The clinical features and progression of HIV infection.

acquired or reactivated as a result of the underlying immunosuppression due to HIV (Fig. 24.33). In other words, the entire disease picture is an indirect result of infection with HIV, which by itself causes only a minor clinical illness. The neurological disease is an independent and direct result of neural invasion by HIV, although complicated by reactivation or infection with other infectious agents.

In New York, 80% of patients are dead 5 years after the onset of the disease and the average survival time after hospital admission is 242 days.

Diagnosis

Laboratory tests for HIV infection depend on the demonstration of specific antibodies. AIDS itself is a clinical definition and in the presence of antibodies to HIV any of the conditions listed in figure 24.34, regardless of the presence of other causes of immunodeficiency, indicate AIDS.

Initially an ELISA test is carried out (see Chapter 18). A positive result is confirmed on a further blood sample, by either western blotting, radioimmunoassay or immunofluorescence testing. This is done (a) because the ELISA test very occasionally gives a false positive report, and (b) to eliminated possible clerical errors in the clinic or laboratory. Tests for the infectious virus, for viral antigens, or for viral nucleic acids, are not yet routinely available, requiring specialized and expensive technology. Tests to distinguish between antibodies to HIV1 and HIV2 are also available only in specialized laboratories.

Diagnosis of HIV infection in newborn infants is a problem. If IgG antibodies are present they are presumably of maternal origin, and tests for virus specific IgM antibodies, which would signify *in utero* infection (see Chapter 26), are not yet available. Hopefully, reliable tests for HIV antigens or nucleic acid sequences will soon be developed.

Prevention

In many developed countries there have been widespread measures to reduce the chances of spread of HIV. In these countries, unlike in Africa, most cases so far have been in male homosexuals or bisexuals (Fig. 24.35), although the picture is changing. All blood donors are tested for antibodies and they are discouraged from volunteering if they belong to high risk HIV groups. Also, all donors of blood for factor VIII and other blood products are screened for HIV antibody. Heat treatment of factor VIII is carried out as a further precaution before this product is used to treat haemophiliac patients. HIV has a delicate outer envelope and is highly susceptible to heat and chemical agents – much more susceptible than hepatitis B. HIV is inactivated under pasteurization conditions and also by hypochlorites, even at concentrations as low as 1 in 10 000 ppm; 2.5% glutaraldehyde and ethyl alcohol are also effective against the virus.

The main effort in the prevention of HIV infection concerns mass public education programmes. These involve inducements to change sexual behaviour, particularly reduction in promiscuous behaviour, and the use of barrier contraceptives (condoms). In developed countries there are clear signs that gay communities, by altering their behaviour in these ways, are controlling the spread of STDs. Infection rates for gonorrhoea, syphilis and hepatitis B are already falling. The problem of transmission between intravenous drug abusers is being tackled in some areas by originally controversial measures such as the free distribution of clean needles and syringes.

The biggest risk for the future in developed countries is that heterosexual transmission becomes more common, following the African pattern. Unfortunately, the determinants of heterosexual transmission are not understood, but the means for prevention are nevertheless clear – condoms and decreased promiscuity. So far it has proved difficult to induce changes in sexual behaviour of heterosexuals by means of public health educational programmes both in the press and on the television. If these changes in heterosexual behaviour can take place, then a dramatic reduction in the incidence of all STDs would be assured.

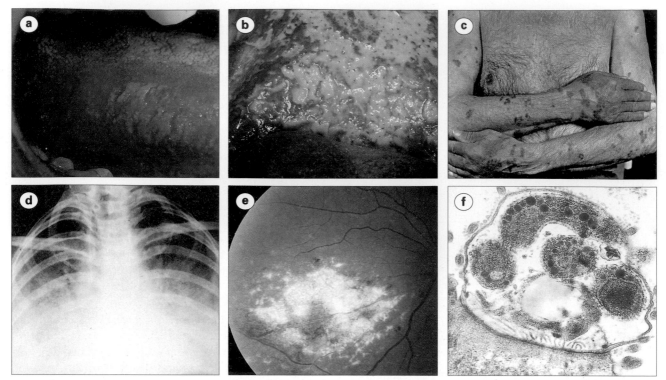

Fig. 24.33 Opportunist infections and tumours associated with HIV infection. (a) Hairy leukoplakia. Raised white lesions of oral mucosa, predominently along the lateral aspect of the tongue, due to Epstein–Barr virus. Courtesy of HP Holley. (b) Extensive oral candidiasis. Courtesy WE Farrar. (c) Kaposi's sarcoma. Brown pigmented lesions on the upper extremities. Courtesy of E Sahn. (d) *Pneumocystis* pneumonia, with extensive infiltrates in both lungs. Courtesy of JA Innes. (e) Cytomegalovirus retinitis showing scattered exudates and haemorrhages, with sheathing of vessels. Courtesy of CJ Ellis. (f) Cryptosporidiosis. Electron micrograph showing mature schizont with several merozoites attached to intestinal epithelium. Courtesy of WE Farrar.

Protection of health care staff has been thoroughly investigated. The risk of transmission is much less than with hepatitis B and extensive studies have shown that there is less than a 1% chance of HIV transmission following needle stick injuries involving HIV-infected patients. Otherwise regular precautions such as the wearing of gloves, especially by dentists, will minimize the chances of infection.

So far the prospects for a successful vaccine are limited, partly because of antigenic variation of the virus even in a given infected patient. On the other hand, intensive work is in progress and various subunit, envelope glycoprotein and whole virus vaccines are being developed and tested. Trials are being carried out in animal (monkey) models and also preliminary trials in humans. The danger of inducing antibodies that enhance infectivity has been noted. Enhancing antibodies are known to be important in the haemorrhagic shock syndrome caused by dengue virus. They combine with the virus without neutralizing it, and the complex then attaches to the Fc receptor present on monocytes, which ingest the complex and thus become infected. In other words, the antibody not only fails to protect but is responsible for carrying the virus into the susceptible cell! The fact that there is a successful killed virus vaccine for a feline retrovirus (feline leukaemia), and that a similar vaccine protects monkeys from simian AIDS does, however, give some hope for the development of an HIV vaccine. Peptide vaccines seem less likely because of the general problem of immunogenicity (e.g. carrier proteins, adjuvants, see Chapter 36), and because numerous T cell epitopes would have to be included, in view of the extensive class II MHC antigen variations in human populations.

Treatment

The opportunist infections are treated in the appropriate way (e.g. pentamidine for *P. carinii*; gancyclovir for CMV). So far azidothymidine (AZT; see Chapter 35) is the only anti-HIV drug licensed for AIDS. The frequency of opportunist infections is reduced and there are increases in T helper cells. Unfortunately the drug is expensive at present, and appears to be needed indefinitely by the patient, as latent infection is not eliminated and recurrence occurs when the drug is stopped. The important question of whether administration of the drug will prevent the progression from HIV seropositivity to ARC, AIDS, and the neurological disease, has not yet been answered. The search continues for more effective or cheaper antiviral agents. Possibilities have included soluble CD4 molecules, acting as 'molecular decoys' which block attachment of the virus to cells by combining with gp120. Numerous trials with combinations of drugs (AZT and derivatives, human IFN-α, soluble CD4) are in progress.

OPPORTUNIST INFECTIONS AND TUMOURS IN AIDS	
Viruses	disseminated CMV (including lungs, retina, brain) HSV (lungs, intestinal tract, CNS, skin) JC papovavirus (brain–progressive multifocal leukoencephalopathy) EB virus (hairy leukoplakia)
Bacteria*	mycobacteria, e.g. *M. avium, M. tuberculosis* (disseminated, extrapulmonary) *Salmonella* (recurrent, disseminated) septicaemia
Protozoa	*Pneumocystis carinii* (pneumonia) *Toxoplasma gondii* (disseminated, including CNS) *Cryptosporidium* (chronic diarrhoea) *Isospora* (with diarrhoea, persisting more than one month)
Fungi	*Candida albicans* (oesophagitis, lung infection) *Cryptococcus neoformans* (CNS) histoplasmosis (disseminated, extrapulmonary) *Coccidioides* (disseminated, extrapulmonary)
Tumours	Kaposi's sarcoma** B cell lymphoma (e.g. in brain, some are EB virus induced)
Other	wasting disease (cause unknown) HIV encephalopathy (AIDS dementia complex)

* also pyogenic bacteria (*Haemophilus, Streptococcus, Pneumococcus etc.*) causing septicaemia, pneumonia, meningitis, osteomyelitis, arthritis, abscesses etc.; multiple or recurrent infections, especially in children.

** probably due to independently but sexually transmitted agent; 300-times as frequent in AIDS as in other immunodeficiencies

Fig. 24.34 Opportunist infections and tumours in AIDS. AIDS is defined as the prescence of antibodies to HIV plus one of the conditions in this table.

AIDS AND ITS CONTROL					
risk group	male		female		control*
	US	UK	US	UK	
Homosexual/bisexual	124961	4421	–	–	++
Intravenous drug users (IVDU)	36962	187	11350	76	+
IVDU and homosexual	13823	88	–	–	+
Haemophiliacs	1939	304	46	4	+++
Received infected blood or tissue	2935	32	1902	47	++
Heterosexual contact with high risk person or overseas contact	5100	297	7781	194	?
Children infected via mother	1560	24	1573	34	±
Other (undetermined)	6646	64	1727	10	?
Totals	193926	5417	24379	398	

Fig. 24.35 Total numbers of AIDS cases reported in the USA and UK to March 1992. Five- to ten-times as many are infected (HIV-seropositive) and infectious. Data courtesy of PHLS Communicable Disease Surveillance Centre, London.

OPPORTUNIST STDS

Although STDs are classically transmitted during regular heterosexual intercourse, they can also be transmitted whenever two mucosal surfaces are brought together (see Fig. 11.18). Anal intercourse, especially in male homosexuals, allows transfer of microorganisms from penis to rectal mucosa or to anal perianal regions. Gonococci or papillomavirus lesions, for instance, may occur in any of these sites. A few microorganisms (hepatitis B, HIV) are transmitted more regularly across rectal mucosa. When there is oro–anal contact, a variety of intestinal infections are given the opportunity to spread as STDs and can then be regarded as 'opportunist STDs'. These include *Salmonella, Shigella,* hepatitis A virus, *Giardia lamblia* and *Entamoeba histolytica* (for details of intestinal infections caused by these organisms see Chapter 25). Together with persistent infections such as CMV and cryptosporidiosis, they contribute to intestinal symptoms and diarrhoea in AIDS patients.

Hepatitis B virus (see also Chapter 25) is often transmitted by the sexual route, especially in male homosexuals. The virus and its surface antigen, HBs, is detectable in semen, saliva and vaginal secretions, although infectivity titres in these fluids are probably low. Hepatitis B virus transmission among male homosexuals parallels the transmission of HIV, with passive anal intercourse as a high risk factor. Infection rates have also fallen, following reduction in promiscuous, condom-free sexual activity in this group of individuals.

ARTHROPOD INFESTATIONS

Pediculosis pubis infection

The 'crab louse', *Phthirus pubis*, is distinct from the other human lice, *Pediculosis corporis* and *P. capitis*. The crab louse is nicely adapted for life in the genital region, clinging tightly to the pubic hairs (see Chapter 3). Occasionally hairs on the eyebrows or in the axilla are colonized. It takes up to 10 blood feeds a day and this causes itching at the site of the bites. Eggs called 'nits' are seen attached to pubic hairs and the characteristic lice, up to 2 mm long, are visible (often at the base of a hair), under a hand lens or by microscopy. Infestation is common, with more than 10 000 cases per year in the UK. Treatment is by the application of malathion to all affected hair sites.

Genital scabies

Sarcoptes scabiei (see Chapter 28) may cause local lesions on the genitalia, and can be spread as a sexually transmitted disease. Patients may have evidence of scabies elsewhere on the body, with burrows between fingers or toes. Treatment is by application of 10% benzyl benzoate or 1% benzene hexachloride.

SUMMARY

Microorganisms transmitted by the sexual route in humans include representatives from all groups (apart from the rickettsia, protozoa and helminths). With the exception of hepatitis B, there are no vaccines for these infections, and although chemotherapy is often available, the best method of control at the moment is prevention. Transmission, however, depends on human behaviour, which is notoriously difficult to influence. The longer the interval between onset of infectiousness and disease, and the less incapacitating the disease, the greater the chances of transmission.

Unfortunately, STDs are becoming more widespread in the community, rather than remaining confined to high risk groups. Genital warts and chlamydial urethritis are by far the most common of all the STDs, but HIV infection has had a major impact, eclipsing all the other well known STDs such as gonorrhoea and HSV. This is perhaps because it is generally, in the end, lethal.

Further Reading

Greene WC. The molecular biology of human immunodeficiency virus type 1 infection. *New Eng J Med* 1991; **324:** 308–317.

Hook EW, Holmes KK. Gonococcal infections. *Ann Intern Med* 1985; **102:** 229–243.

Kelly GE, Stanley BS, Weller, IVD. The natural history of human immunodeficiency virus infection; a five year study in a London cohort of homosexual men. *Genitourin Med* 1990; **2:** 238–243.

Mindell A, ed. Sexually transmitted diseases. *Curr Opin Infect Dis* 1990; **3:** 1–38.

Morrison PRP, Belland RJ, Lyng K *et al.* Chlamydial disease pathogenesis. *J Exp Med* 1989; **170:** 1271–1283.

Plummer FA, Brunham RC. Gonococcal recidivism, diversity and ecology. *Rev Inf Dis* 1987; **9:** 846.

Sande MA, ed. HIV infection and AIDS. *Curr Opin Infect Dis* 1990; **3:** 67–112.

Treharne JD, Ballard RC. The expanding spectrum of the *Chlamydia* – a microbiological and clinical appraisal. *Rev Med Microbiol* 1990; **1:** 10–18.

25 GASTROINTESTINAL TRACT INFECTIONS

Contents

INTRODUCTION

Ingestion of pathogens can cause many different infections. These may be confined to the gastrointestinal tract or initiated in the gut before spreading to other parts of the body. In this chapter we consider the important bacterial causes of diarrhoeal disease and summarize the other bacterial causes of food-associated infection and food poisoning. Viral and parasitic causes of diarrhoeal disease are discussed, as well as infections that are acquired via the gastrointestinal tract and cause disease in other body systems, including typhoid and paratyphoid fevers, listeriosis, and some forms of viral hepatitis. For the sake of clarity, all types of viral hepatitis are included in this chapter. Infections of the liver can also result in liver abscesses and several parasitic infections cause liver disease. Peritonitis and intra-abdominal abscesses can arise from seeding of the abdominal cavity by organisms from the gastrointestinal tract. Several different terms are used to describe infections of the gastrointestinal tract; those in common use are shown in figure 25.1

A wide range of microbial pathogens is capable of infecting the gastrointestinal tract and the important bacterial and viral ones are listed in figure 25.2. They are acquired by the faecal–oral route, from faecally-contaminated food, fluids or fingers. Infection associated with consumption of contaminated food is often termed 'food poisoning', but 'food-associated infection' is a better term. True food poisoning occurs after consumption of food containing toxins; these may be chemical, e.g. heavy metals, or bacterial in origin, e.g. from *Clostridium botulinum* or *Staphylococcus aureus*. The bacteria multiply and produce toxin within contaminated food. The organisms may be destroyed during food preparation but the toxin is unaffected, consumed and acts within hours. In food-associated infections, the food may simply act as a vehicle for the pathogen (e.g. *Campylobacter*) or provide conditions in which the pathogen can multiply to produce numbers large enough to cause disease (e.g. *Salmonella*).

For infection to occur, the pathogens must be ingested in adequate number and/or possess particular attributes to elude the host defences of the upper gastrointestinal tract and reach the intestine (Fig. 25.3; see also Chapter 10). Here they remain localized and cause disease as a result of multiplication and/or toxin production, or they may invade through the intestinal mucosa to reach the lymphatics or the bloodstream (Fig. 25.4). The damaging effects resulting from infection of the gastrointestinal tract are summarized in figure 25.5.

TERMS USED TO DESCRIBE GASTROINTESTINAL TRACT INFECTIONS

gastroenteritis
a syndrome characterized by gastrointestinal symptoms including nausea, vomiting, diarrhoea and abdominal discomfort

diarrhoea
abnormal faecal discharge characterized by frequent and/or fluid stool; usually resulting from disease of the small intestine and involving increased fluid and electrolyte loss

dysentery
an inflammatory disorder of the gastrointestinal tract often associated with blood and pus in the faeces and accompanied by symptoms of pain, fever, abdominal cramps; usually resulting from disease of the large intestine

enterocolitis
inflammation involving the mucosa of both the small and large intestine

Fig. 25.1 As well as many colloquial expressions, several different clinical terms are used to describe infections of the gastrointestinal tract. Diarrhoea without blood and pus is usually the result of enterotoxin production, whereas the presence of blood and/or pus cells in the faeces indicates an invasive infection with mucosal destruction.

IMPORTANT BACTERIAL AND VIRAL PATHOGENS OF THE GASTROINTESTINAL TRACT

pathogen	animal reservoir	foodborne	waterborne
Bacteria			
Escherichia coli	+?	+(VTEC)	+(ETEC)
Salmonella	+	+++	+
Campylobacter	+	+++	+
Vibrio cholerae	–	+	+++
Shigella	–	+	–
Clostridium perfringens	+	+++	–
Bacillus cereus	–	++	–
Vibrio parahaemolyticus	–	++	–
Yersinia enterocolitica	+	+	–
Viruses			
Rotavirus	–	–	–
Small round viruses (SRV)	–	++	+

Fig. 25.2 Many different pathogens cause infections of the gastrointestinal tract. Some are found in both humans and animals while others are strictly human parasites. This difference has important implications for control and prevention. VTEC, verocytotoxin-producing *E. coli*; ETEC, enterotoxigen *E. coli*.

DEFENCES AGAINST INFECTION IN THE GASTROINTESTINAL TRACT

mouth
flow of liquids
saliva
lysozyme
normal bacterial flora

oesophagus
flow of liquids
peristalsis

stomach
acid pH

small intestine
flow of gut contents
peristalsis
mucus; bile
secretory IgA
lymphoid tissue
(Peyer's patches)
shedding and replacement
of epithelium
normal flora

large intestine
normal flora
peristalsis
shedding and replication
of epithelium
mucus

Fig. 25.3 Every day we swallow large numbers of microorganisms. Because of the body's defence mechanisms, however, they rarely succeed in surviving the passage to the intestine in large enough numbers to cause infection.

DIARRHOEAL DISEASE

Infections of the gastrointestinal tract range in their effects from a mild, self-limiting attack of 'the runs' to severe, sometimes fatal, diarrhoea. There may be associated vomiting, fever and malaise. Diarrhoea is the result of an increase in fluid and electrolyte loss into the gut lumen, leading to the production of unformed or liquid faeces. It is the most common outcome of infection of the gastrointestinal tract, and can be thought of as the method by which the host forcibly expels the pathogen (and in doing so, aids its dissemination). However, diarrhoea also occurs in many non-infectious conditions, and an infectious cause should not be assumed.

In the developing world, diarrhoeal disease is a major cause of morbidity and mortality, particularly in young children. In the developed world it remains a very common complaint but is usually mild and self-limiting except in the very young, the elderly, and in immunocompromised patients. Most of the pathogens listed in figure 25.2 are found throughout the world but some, e.g. *Vibrio cholerae*, have a more limited geographical distribution. However, such infections may be acquired by travellers to these areas and imported into their home countries.

Many cases of diarrhoeal disease go undiagnosed either because they are mild and self-limiting and the patient does not seek medical attention, or because medical and laboratory facilities are unavailable, particularly in developing countries. It is generally impossible to distinguish on clinical grounds between infections caused by the different pathogens. However, information on the patient's recent food and travel history and macroscopic and microscopic examination of the faeces for blood and pus may provide helpful clues. A precise diagnosis can only be achieved by laboratory investigations. This is especially important in outbreaks, because of the need to instigate appropriate epidemiological investigations and control measures.

Bacterial causes of diarrhoea

Escherichia coli

This is one of the most versatile of all bacterial pathogens. Some strains are important members of the normal gut flora in man and animals (see Chapter 3), whereas others possess virulence factors which enable them to cause infections in the intestinal tract or at other sites, particularly the urinary tract (see Chapter 23). Strains that cause diarrhoeal disease do so by several distinct pathogenic mechanisms and differ in their epidemiology (Fig. 25.6).

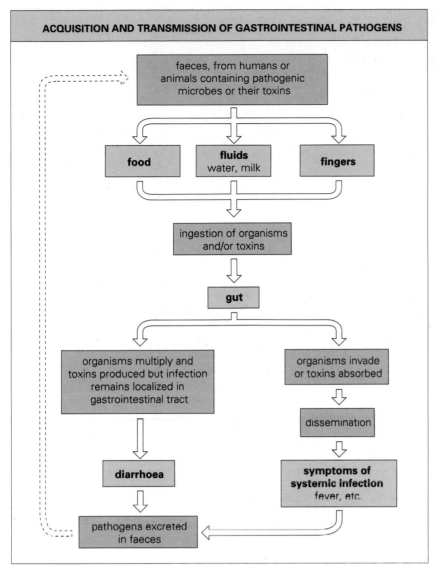

ACQUISITION AND TRANSMISSION OF GASTROINTESTINAL PATHOGENS

faeces, from humans or animals containing pathogenic microbes or their toxins

food

fluids
water, milk

fingers

ingestion of organisms and/or toxins

gut

organisms multiply and toxins produced but infection remains localized in gastrointestinal tract

organisms invade or toxins absorbed

dissemination

diarrhoea

symptoms of systemic infection
fever, etc.

pathogens excreted in faeces

Fig. 25.4 Infections of the gastrointestinal tract can be grouped into those which remain localized in the gut and those which invade beyond the gut to cause infection in other sites in the body. In order to spread to a new host, pathogens are excreted in large numbers in the faeces and must survive in the environment for long enough to infect another person directly, or indirectly, through contaminated food or fluids.

DAMAGE RESULTING FROM INFECTION OF THE GASTROINTESTINAL TRACT

pharmacological action of bacterial toxins, local or distant to site of infection
e.g. cholera, staphylococcal food poisoning

local inflammation in response to superficial microbial invasion
e.g. shigellosis, amoebiasis

deep invasion to blood or lymphatics dissemination to other body sites
e.g. hepatitis A, enteric fevers

perforation of mucosal epithelium after infection, surgery or accidental trauma
e.g. peritonitis, intra-abdominal abscesses

Fig. 25.5 Infection of the gastrointestinal tract can cause damage locally or at distant sites.

Pathogenesis. Enterotoxigenic *Escherichia coli* (ETEC) possess colonization factors which bind the bacteria to specific receptors on the intestinal cell membrane (Fig. 25.7) where the organisms produce powerful enterotoxins. Heat-labile enterotoxin (LT) is very similar in structure

and mode of action to cholera toxin produced by *Vibrio cholerae*, and infections with these strains can mimic cholera, particularly in young and malnourished children. Other ETEC strains produce heat-stable enterotoxins (ST) in addition to, or instead of, LT. STs have a similar but distinct mode of action to that of LT. ST_A activates guanylate cyclase activity causing an increase in cyclic guanosine monophosphate, which results in increased fluid secretion. The mechanism of action of ST_B is unknown. Unlike LT, the STs are not immunogenic and therefore cannot be detected by immunological tests (see Fig. 25.6).

Other *E. coli* strains produce a verotoxin (VT), so-called because it is toxic to tissue cultures of 'vero' cells. After attachment to the intestinal mucosa by an 'attaching–effacing' mechanism, the organisms elaborate verotoxin, which has a direct effect on intestinal epithelium resulting in diarrhoea.

Two diseases of previously unknown aetiology, haemorrhagic colitis (HC) and haemolytic uraemic syndrome (HUS), have recently been associated with verotoxin-producing *E. coli* strains. In HC there is destruction of the mucosa and consequent haemorrhage; this may be followed by HUS. Verotoxin receptors have been identified on renal epithelium and may account for the kidney

CHARACTERISTICS OF *ESCHERICHIA COLI* STRAINS CAUSING GASTROINTESTINAL INFECTIONS		
pathogenic group	**epidemiology**	**laboratory diagnosis***
Enterotoxigenic *E. coli* (ETEC)	most important bacterial cause of diarrhoea in children in developing countries most common cause of travellers' diarrhoea water contaminated by human or animal sewage may be important in spread	isolate organisms from faeces test for production of LT (but not ST) by immunological techniques e.g. ELISA *test for production of STs by detecting accumulation of fluid in ligated ileal loops of experimental animals (not in routine use)* *gene probes specific for LT and ST genes available for detection of ETEC in faeces and in food and water samples*
Enteroinvasive *E. coli* (EIEC)	important cause of diarrhoea in areas of poor hygiene infections usually foodborne; no evidence of animal or environmental reservoir	isolate organisms from faeces; *test for enteroinvasive potential in tissue culture cells*
Vero cytoxin-producing *E. coli* (VTEC)	serotype 0157 most important VTEC in human infections outbreaks and sporadic cases occur world-wide food and unpasteurized milk important in spread	isolate organisms from faeces proportion of VTEC in faecal sample may be very low (often <1% of *E. coli* colonies) usually sorbitol non-fermenters *VTEC-producing colonies can be identified with DNA probes in colony hybridisation tests*
Enteropathogenic *E. coli* (EPEC)	EPEC strains belong to particular O serotypes cause sporadic cases and outbreaks of infection in babies and young children importance in adults not known	isolate organisms from faeces determine serotype of several colonies with polyvalent antisera for known EPEC types *adhesion to tissue culture cells can be demonstrated by a fluorescence actin staining test*

Fig. 25.6 *Escherichia coli* is a major cause of gastrointestinal infection, particularly in developing countries and in travellers. There is a range of pathogenic mechanisms within the species which result in more or less invasive disease. *Specialized tests are given in italics.

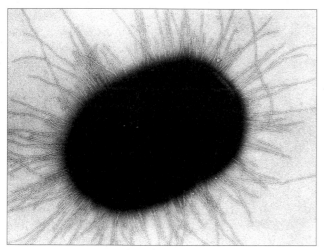

Fig. 25.7 Electron micrograph of enterotoxigenic *E. coli* (ETEC), showing pili necessary for adherence to mucosal epithelial cells. Courtesy of S Knutton.

involvement. The association between haemorrhage and verotoxin-producing *E. coli* has lead to the acronym EHEC – enterohaemorrhagic *E. coli.*

Enteropathogenic *E. coli* (EPEC) were the first group of *E. coli* intestinal pathogens to be described but their mechanism of pathogenicity remains unclear. They do not appear to produce any toxins but have a particular mechanism of adhesion ('attaching–effacing' as with VTEC) to enterocytes which appears to destroy the microvilli (Fig. 25.8).

Enteroinvasive *E. coli* (EIEC) attach specifically to the mucosa of the large intestine and invade the cells by being taken in by endocytosis. Inside the cell they lyse the endocytic vacuole, multiply and spread to adjacent cells, causing tissue destruction and consequently inflammation.

Clinical features. The diarrhoea produced by *E. coli* varies from mild to severe depending on the strain and the

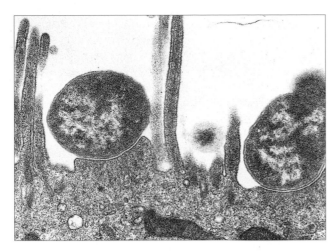

Fig. 25.8 Electron micrograph of enteropathogenic *E. coli* (EPEC) adhering to the brush border of intestinal mucosal cells, with localized destruction of microvilli. Courtesy of S Knutton.

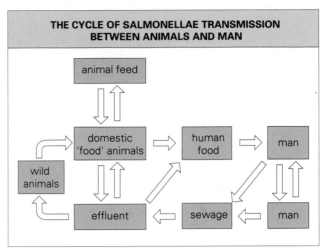

THE CYCLE OF SALMONELLAE TRANSMISSION BETWEEN ANIMALS AND MAN

Fig. 25.10 The recycling of salmonellae. With the exception of *Salmonella typhi*, salmonellae are widely distributed in animals, providing a constant source of infection for man. Excretion of large numbers of salmonellae from infected individuals and carriers allows the organisms to be 'recycled'.

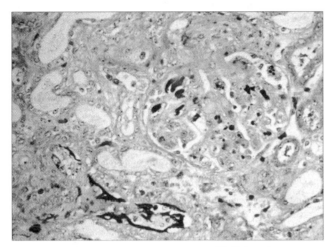

Fig. 25.9 Enterohaemorrhagic *E. coli* (EHEC) infection, showing fibrin 'thrombi' in glomerular capillaries in haemolytic uraemic syndrome. Weigert stain. Courtesy of HR Powell.

Treatment and prevention. Specific antibacterial therapy is not indicated. Fluid replacement may be necessary, especially in young children. Treatment of HUS is urgent and may involve dialysis.

Provision of a pure water supply and adequate systems for sewage disposal are fundamental to the prevention of diarrhoeal disease. Food and unpasteurized milk may be important vehicles of infection, especially for EIEC and EHEC, but there is no evidence of an animal or environmental reservoir.

Salmonella

Until recently salmonellae were the most common cause of food-associated diarrhoea in the western world, but in some countries they have now been beaten into second place by *Campylobacter.* Like *E. coli*, the salmonellae belong to the Enterobacteria and the genus *Salmonella* has been divided into more than 2000 species on the basis of differences in the cell wall (0) and flagellar (H) antigens (Kauffmann–White scheme). However, more recent studies indicate that there is a single species, or at most three species, and that serotypes should not be given species status (see Appendix). Nevertheless it is useful to be able to distinguish between serotypes for epidemiological purposes, for example, when tracing the source of an outbreak.

Epidemiology. All salmonellae except for *S. typhi* and *S. paratyphi* are found in animals as well as humans. There is a large animal reservoir of infection which is transmitted to man via contaminated food (especially poultry and dairy products; Fig. 25.10). Waterborne infection is less frequent. Salmonella infection is also transmitted from person to person and thus secondary spread may occur, for example, within a family after one member has become infected after consuming contaminated food.

underlying health of the host. ETEC is the most important bacterial cause of diarrhoea in children in developing countries and may be clinically indistinguishable from cholera. EIEC and EHEC strains both cause bloody diarrhoea. Following EHEC infection, HUS is characterized by acute renal failure (Fig. 25.9), anaemia and thrombocytopenia and there may be neurological complications. HUS is the most common cause of acute renal failure in children in the UK and USA.

Laboratory diagnosis. Because *E. coli* is a member of the normal gastrointestinal flora, specific tests are required to identify strains that may be responsible for diarrhoeal disease. These are summarized in figure 25.6. Infections are more common in children and are often travel-associated, factors which should be considered when samples are received in the laboratory.

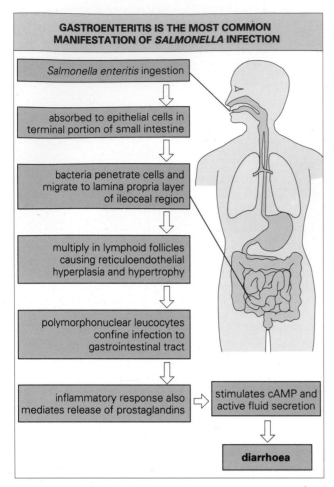

GASTROENTERITIS IS THE MOST COMMON MANIFESTATION OF *SALMONELLA* INFECTION

Salmonella enteritis ingestion

⇩

absorbed to epithelial cells in terminal portion of small intestine

⇩

bacteria penetrate cells and migrate to lamina propria layer of ileoceal region

⇩

multiply in lymphoid follicles causing reticuloendothelial hyperplasia and hypertrophy

⇩

polymorphonuclear leucocytes confine infection to gastrointestinal tract

⇩

inflammatory response also mediates release of prostaglandins ⇨ stimulates cAMP and active fluid secretion

⇩

diarrhoea

Fig. 25.11 The passage of salmonellae through the body to the gut. The vast majority of salmonellae cause infection localized to the gastrointestinal tract and do not invade beyond the gut mucosa. They do not produce enterotoxins.

Pathogenesis of salmonella diarrhoea. Diarrhoeal disease is the most common manifestation of infection caused by *Salmonella* spp. other than *S. typhi* and *S. paratyphi*. These latter species invade the body from the gastrointestinal tract to cause systemic illness and are discussed in a later section.

Diarrhoea is produced as a result of invasion by the salmonellae of epithelial cells in the terminal portion of the small intestine (Fig. 25.11). The bacteria migrate to the lamina propria layer of the ileocaecal region, where their multiplication stimulates an inflammatory response which both confines the infection to the gastrointestinal tract and mediates the release of prostaglandins. These in turn activate cyclic AMP and fluid secretion, resulting in diarrhoea. Salmonella do not appear to produce enterotoxins.

Species of *Salmonella* that normally cause diarrhoea (e.g. *S. enteritidis*, *S. cholerae suis*) may become invasive in patients with particular predispositions (e.g. in children and in patients with cancer or sickle cell anaemia). The organisms are not contained within the gastrointestinal tract but invade the body to cause septicaemia; consequently, many organs become seeded with salmonellae, sometimes leading to osteomyelitis, pneumonia or meningitis.

Clinical features. In the vast majority of cases, *Salmonella* spp. cause an acute but self-limiting diarrhoea, but in the young and the elderly symptoms may be more severe. Vomiting is rare and fever is usually a sign of invasive disease (Fig. 25.12). In the UK there is a reported annual incidence of salmonella bacteraemia of approximately 150, with about 70 deaths. This should be set in context against around 30 000 reported cases of diarrhoea.

Laboratory diagnosis. Diarrhoea caused by salmonellae cannot be distinguished from other causes without culturing faecal specimens on selective media. The methods are summarized in the Appendix. The organisms are not fastidious and can usually be isolated within 24 hours although small numbers may require enrichment in selenite broth prior to culture. Preliminary identification can be made rapidly but the complete result, including serotype, takes at least 48 hours.

Treatment. Diarrhoea is usually self-limiting and resolves without treatment. Fluid and electrolyte replacement may be required particularly in the very young and the elderly. Unless there is evidence of invasion and septicaemia, antibiotics should be positively discouraged because they do not reduce the symptoms or shorten the illness, and may prolong excretion of salmonellae in the faeces. There is some evidence that symptomatic treatment with drugs that reduce diarrhoea has the same adverse effect.

Prevention. Figure 25.10 illustrates the problems associated with prevention of salmonella infections. The large animal reservoir makes it impossible to eliminate the organisms and thus preventative measures must be aimed at 'breaking the chain' between animal and human, and between humans. Such measures include maintaining adequate standards of public health (clean drinking water and proper sewage disposal) and education programmes on hygienic food preparation. Following an episode of salmonella diarrhoea, people may continue to carry and excrete organisms in their faeces for several weeks. Although in the absence of symptoms the organisms will not be dispersed so liberally into the environment, proper hand washing prior to food handling is essential. Persons employed as food handlers are excluded from work until three specimens of faeces have failed to grow salmonella.

Campylobacter

Campylobacter spp. are curved or S-shaped Gram-negative rods (Fig. 25.13). They have long been known to cause diarrhoeal disease in animals, but are also one of the most common causes of diarrhoea in humans. The delay in recognizing the importance of these organisms was due to their cultural requirements which differ from those of the Enterobacteria (they are microaerophilic and thermophilic); thus they do not grow on the media used for isolation of *E. coli* and salmonellae. Several species of the genus *Campylobacter* are associated with human disease but *C. jejuni* is by far the most common. *Campylobacter pylori*, now reclassified as *Helicobacter pylori* is an important cause of gastritis and gastric ulcers (see panel).

			symptoms			
pathogen	**incubation period**	**duration**	**diarrhoea**	**vomiting**	**abdominal cramps**	**fever**
Salmonella	6hrs–2 days	48hrs–7 days	+ +	+	–	+
Campylobacter	2–11 days	3 days–3 wks	+ + +	–	+ +	+ +
Shigella	1–4 days	2–3 days	+ +/+ + +	–	+	+
Vibrio cholerae	2–3 days	up to 7 days	+ + + +	+	–	–
Vibrio parahaemolyticus	8hrs–2 days	3 days	+/+ +	+	+	+
Clostridium perfringens	8hrs–1 day	12hrs–1 day	+ +	–	+ +	–
Bacillus cereus diarrhoeal emetic	8hrs–12hrs 15mins–4hrs	12hrs–1 day 12hrs–2 days	+ + +	– + +	+ +	–
Yersinia enterocolitica	4–7 days	1–2 weeks	+ +	–	+ +	+

CLINICAL FEATURES OF BACTERIAL DIARRHOEAL DISEASE

Fig. 25.12 The clinical features of bacterial diarrhoeal infection. It is difficult, if not impossible, to determine the likely cause of a diarrhoeal illness on the basis of clinical features alone, and laboratory investigations are essential to identify the pathogen.

Epidemiology. As with salmonellae, there is a large animal reservoir of campylobacters in cattle, sheep, rodents, poultry and wild birds. Infections are acquired by consumption of contaminated food especially poultry, milk, or water. Recent studies have shown an association between infection and consumption of milk from bottles with tops that have been pecked by wild birds. Household pets such as dogs and cats may become infected and provide a source for human infection, particularly for young children. Person-to-person spread by the faecal–oral route is rare, as is transmission from food handlers.

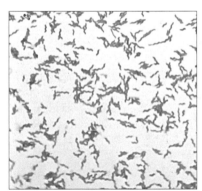

Fig. 25.13 *Campylobacter jejuni* infection. Gram-stain showing Gram-negative, S-shaped bacilli. Courtesy of I Farrell.

Helicobacter pylori

This spiral bacterium is found in the stomach and is strongly associated with gastritis and duodenal ulceration. Whether the organism is truly the cause of these conditions or a consequence of them has been unclear, but self-inoculation studies strongly support a causative role. The mechanism of pathogenicity has still to be identified although production of cytotoxins has been described. The organism also produces large amounts of urease, probably a useful strategy for survival in the acid environment of the gastric mucosa.

Diagnosis is usually made on the basis of histological examination of biopsy specimens. *Helicobacter pylori* can be cultured in the laboratory but is is not an easy organism to grow. Serological diagnosis may in future play a valuable part in investigation of patients thereby avoiding invasive procedures.

Treatment with bismuth salts and antibiotics is successful but relapse is common. At present the epidemiology of *H. pylori* is unknown and it is impossible to distinguish between relapse due to the failure of treatment to eradicate all organisms from the gastrointestinal tract, or due to reinfection from an external source.

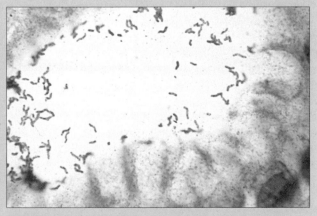

Fig. 25.14 *Helicobacter pylori* gastritis. Silver stain showing numerous spiral-shaped organisms adhering to the mucosal surface. Courtesy of AM Geddes.

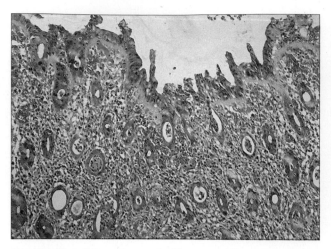

Fig. 25.15 Inflammatory enteritis caused by *Campylobacter jejuni*, involving the entire mucosa with flattened atrophic villi, necrotic debris in the crypts and thickening of the basement membrane. Cresyl-fast violet stain. Courtesy of J Newman.

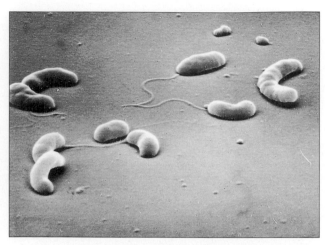

Fig. 25.16 Scanning electronmicrograph *Vibrio cholerae* showing comma-shaped rods and single polar flagellum. x13 000. Courtesy of DK Banerjee.

Pathogenesis. The pathogenesis of campylobacter diarrhoea has not yet been elucidated. The gross pathology and histological appearances of ulceration and inflamed bleeding mucosal surfaces in the jejunum, ileum and colon (Fig 25.15) are compatible with invasion of the bacteria but the production of cytotoxins by *C. jejuni* has also been demonstrated. Invasion and bacteraemia is not uncommon particularly in neonates and debilitated adults.

Clinical features. The clinical presentation is indistinguishable from diarrhoea caused by salmonellae although the disease may have a longer incubation period and a longer duration. The key features are summarized in figure 25.12.

Laboratory diagnosis. Cultures for campylobacter should be set up routinely in every investigation of a diarrhoeal illness. The methods are described in the Appendix but it is important to note that the media and conditions for growth differ from those required for the Enterobacteria. Growth is often somewhat slow compared with the Enterobacteria but a presumptive identification should be available within 48 hours of culture.

Treatment. Erythromycin is the antibiotic of choice for cases of diarrhoeal disease that are severe enough to warrant treatment. Invasive infections may require treatment with an aminoglycoside.

Prevention. The preventative measures for salmonella infections described above are equally applicable to the prevention of campylobacter infection, but there are no requirements for the screening of food handlers because contamination of food by this route is very uncommon.

Cholera

Cholera is an acute infection of the gastrointestinal tract caused by the comma-shaped Gram-negative bacterium *Vibrio cholerae* (Fig. 25.16). The disease has a long history characterized by epidemics and pandemics. The last cases of cholera acquired in the UK were in the last century following the introduction of the bacterium by sailors arriving from Europe and in 1849 Snow published his historic essay *'On the Mode of Communication of Cholera'*.

Epidemiology. Cholera remains endemic in South East Asia and parts of Africa and South America. Unlike salmonellae and campylobacters, *Vibrio cholerae* is a free-living inhabitant of fresh water but causes infection only in humans. Asymptomatic human carriers are believed to be a major reservoir. The disease is spread via contaminated food; shellfish grown in fresh and estuarine waters have also been implicated. Direct person-to-person spread is thought to be uncommon. Thus cholera continues to flourish in communities where the provision of clean drinking water and adequate sewage disposal is absent or unreliable. Cases still occur in developed countries but the standards of hygiene are such that secondary spread does not occur. Over the past 20 years there have been 66 cases reported in the UK and 10 cases in the USA, which amounts to about 1 in 500 000 travellers to areas with endemic cholera.

Vibrio cholerae can be subdivided into serotypes based on somatic (0) antigens. Serotype 01 is the most important and it is further divided into two biotypes: classical and El Tor (Fig. 25.17). The El Tor biotype, named after the quarantine camp where it was first isolated from pilgrims returning from Mecca, differs from classical *V. cholerae* in several ways. In particular it causes only a mild diarrhoea, and has a higher ratio of carriers to cases than with classical cholera; carriage is also more prolonged and survival of the organisms in the environment is better. The El Tor biotype has now spread throughout the world and has largely displaced the classical biotype.

Other species of *Vibrio* also cause a variety of infections in man (see Fig. 25.17). *V. parahaemolyticus* is also a cause of diarrhoeal disease but this is usually much less severe than cholera (see below).

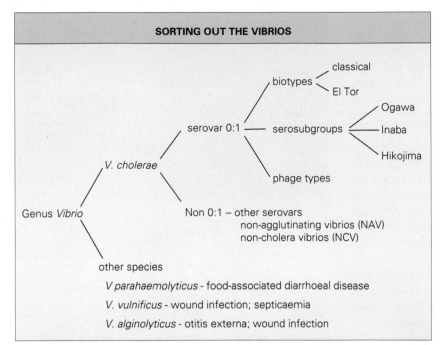

SORTING OUT THE VIBRIOS

Fig. 25.17 *Vibrio cholerae* serovar 0:1, the cause of cholera, can be subdivided into different biotypes which have different epidemiological features, and into serosubgroups and phage types for the purposes of investigating outbreaks of infection. Although *Vibrio cholerae* is the most important pathogen of the genus, other species can also cause infections both of the gastrointestinal tract and other sites.

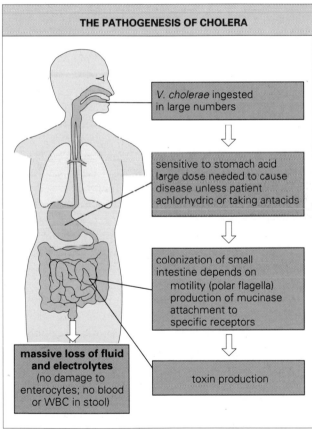

THE PATHOGENESIS OF CHOLERA

Fig. 25.18 The production of an enterotoxin is central to the pathogenesis of cholera, but the organisms must possess other virulence factors to allow them to reach the small intestine and to adhere to the mucosal cells.

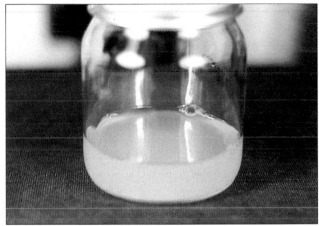

Fig. 25.19 Rice water stool in cholera. Courtesy of AM Geddes.

Clinical features. The clinical features of cholera are summarized in figure 25.12. The severe watery non-bloody diarrhoea (known as rice water stool because of its appearance; Fig. 25.19) can result in the loss of a litre of fluid per hour and it is this fluid loss and the consequent electrolyte imbalance which results in marked dehydration, metabolic acidosis (loss of bicarbonate), hypokalaemia (potassium loss) and hypovolaemic shock resulting in cardiac failure. Untreated, mortality from cholera is 40–60%; fluid and electrolyte replacement, instituted rapidly, reduces mortality to less than 1%.

Laboratory diagnosis. In countries where cholera is prevalent, diagnosis is based on clinical grounds and laboratory confirmation is rarely sought. It is worth remembering that ETEC infection can resemble cholera in its severity but for both diseases, fluid and electrolyte replacement are of paramount important. For diagnosis of sporadic or imported cases and detection of carriers, culture is required to distinguish cholera from other acute diarrhoeas. The methods are given in the Appendix .

Pathogenesis. The symptoms of cholera are entirely due to the production in the gastrointestinal tract of an enterotoxin (see Chapter 16). However, the organism requires additional virulence factors to enable it to survive the host defences and adhere to the intestinal mucosa. These are illustrated in figure 25.18 (see also Chapter 11).

Treatment. Prompt oral or intravenous rehydration with fluids and electrolytes is central to the treatment of cholera. Antibiotics are not necessary, but tetracycline may be given as some evidence indicates that this treatment reduces the time of excretion of *V. cholerae* thereby reducing the risk of transmission. There have, however, been reports of tetracycline-resistant *V. cholerae* in some areas.

Prevention. As with other diarrhoeal disease, a clean drinking-water supply and adequate sewage disposal are fundamental to the prevention of cholera. Because there is no animal reservoir, it should in theory be possible to eliminate the disease. However, carriage in humans, albeit for only a few weeks, occurs in 1–20% of previously infected patients making eradication difficult to achieve.

A killed, whole-cell vaccine is available and is given parenterally, but is only effective in about 50% of vaccinees, with protection lasting only for 3–6 months. It is no longer recommended by WHO for travellers to cholera-endemic areas, although it may be required in certain countries. Field trials of various oral vaccines are in progress.

Shigellosis

Shigellosis is also known as bacillary dysentery (in contrast to amoebic dysentery; see below) because in its more severe form it is characterized by an invasive infection of the mucosa of the large intestine, causing inflammation and resulting in pus and blood in the diarrhoeal stool. However symptoms range from mild to severe depending on the species of *Shigella* involved and on the underlying state of health of the host.

Epidemiology. There are four species, of which *Shigella sonnei* causes most infections at the mild end of the spectrum, *Sh. flexneri* and *Sh. boydii* usually give more severe disease and *S. dysenteriae* is the most serious. Shigellosis is primarily a paediatric disease. When associated with severe malnutrition it may precipitate complications such as the protein deficiency syndrome 'kwashiorkor'. Like *V. cholerae* shigellae are human pathogens without an animal reservoir. But unlike the vibrios, they are not found in the environment, being spread from person-to-person by the faecal–oral route and less frequently by contaminated food and water. Shigellae appear to be able to initiate infection from a small infective dose and thus spread is easy in situations where sanitation or personal hygiene may be poor, e.g. nurseries, day care centres and institutions for the handicapped.

Pathogenesis. The shigellae are effective pathogens in that doses as low as 10–100 organisms may cause disease whereas with salmonellae, campylobacter and *V. cholerae*, higher doses are usually required. The organisms attach to and invade the mucosal epithelium of the distal ileum and colon, causing inflammation and ulceration (Fig. 25.20). However they rarely invade through the gut wall to the bloodstream. Enterotoxin is produced but its role in pathogenesis is uncertain since toxin-negative mutants still produce disease.

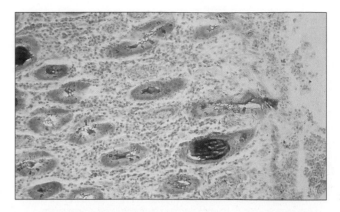

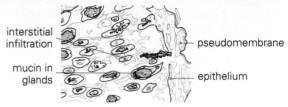

Fig. 25.20 Shigellosis. Histology of the colon showing disrupted epithelium covered by pseudomembrane and interstitial infiltration. Mucin glands have discharged their contents and the goblet cells are empty. Colloidal iron stain. Courtesy of RH Gilman.

Clinical features. The main features of shigella infection are summarized in figure 25.12. Diarrhoea is usually watery at first but later contains mucus and blood. Lower abdominal cramps may be severe. The disease is usually self-limiting but dehydration can occur, especially in the young and elderly. Complications may be associated with malnutrition (see above).

Treatment. Rehydration may be indicated. Antibiotics should not be given except in severe cases. Plasmid-mediated resistance is common and antibiotic susceptibility tests should be performed on shigella isolates if treatment is required.

Prevention. Education in personal hygiene and proper sewage disposal are important. Cases may continue to excrete shigellae for a few weeks but longer term carriage is unusual; thus, with adequate public health measures and no animal reservoir, the disease is potentially eradicable.

Other bacterial causes of diarrhoeal disease

The pathogens described in the previous sections are the major bacterial causes of diarrhoeal disease. *Salmonella* and *Campylobacter* infections and some types of *E. coli* infections are most often food-associated, whereas cholera is more often waterborne and shigellosis is usually spread by direct faecal–oral contact. There are several other bacterial pathogens that cause food-associated infection or food poisoning, as described below.

Gram-negative bacteria. Vibrio parahaemolyticus and *Yersinia enterocolitica* are two Gram-negative organisms which have been associated with food-borne outbreaks of diarrhoeal disease.

Vibrio parahaemolyticus is a halophilic (salt-loving) vibrio which contaminates seafood and fish. If these foods are consumed uncooked, diarrhoeal disease may result. The mechanism of pathogenesis is still unclear. Most strains associated with infection are haemolytic by virtue of production of a heat-stable cytotoxin and have been shown to invade intestinal cells (in contrast to *V. cholerae* which is non-invasive and cholera toxin which is not cytotoxic).

The clinical features of infection are summarized in figure 25.12. The methods used for the laboratory diagnosis of *V. parahaemolyticus* infection are given in the Appendix. Because the special media for cultivation of vibrios are not used routinely, the request form accompanying the specimen must provide adequate information about the patient's history and food consumption to indicate to the laboratory that vibrios should be looked for. Prevention of infection depends on proper cooking of fish and seafood.

Yersinia enterocolitica is a member of the Enterobacteriaceae and is a cause of food-associated infection, particularly in colder parts of the world. The reason for this geographical distribution is unknown, but it has been speculated that it is because the organism prefers to grow at temperatures between 22–25°C. *Yersinia enterocolitica* is found in a variety of animal hosts including rodents, rabbits, pigs, sheep, cattle, horses, and also in domestic pets. Transmission to humans from household dogs has been reported. The organism survives and multiplies, albeit more slowly, at refrigerator temperatures (4°C) and has been implicated in outbreaks of infection associated with contaminated milk as well as other foods.

The mechanism of pathogenesis is unknown but the clinical features of the disease result from invasion of the terminal ileum, necrosis in Peyer's patches and an associated inflammation of the mesenteric lymph nodes (Fig. 25.21). The presentation, with enterocolitis and often mesenteric adenitis, may easily be confused with acute appendicitis, particularly in children. The clinical features are summarized in figure 25.12. The laboratory diagnosis is outlined in the Appendix. As with *V. parahaemolyticus*, an indication of suspicion of *Yersinia* infection is useful to guide the laboratory staff to process the specimen appropriately.

Gram-positive bacteria. The Gram-negative organisms described in the previous sections invade the intestinal mucosa or produce enterotoxins which cause diarrhoea. None of these organisms produces spores. Two Gram-positive species are important causes of diarrhoeal disease particularly in association with spore-contaminated food. These are *Clostridium perfringens* and *Bacillus cereus*.

Clostridium perfringens is associated with diarrhoeal diseases in different circumstances: enterotoxin-producing strains are a common cause of food-associated infection; much more rarely beta-toxin producing strains produce an acute necrotizing disease of the small intestine, accompanied by abdominal pain and diarrhoea. This form occurs

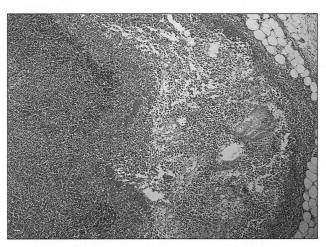

Fig. 25.21 *Yersinia enterocolitica* infection. Hyperplasia and inflammation of a mesenteric lymph node. Courtesy of C Edwards.

after consumption of contaminated meat by people who are unaccustomed to a high protein diet and do not have sufficient intestinal trypsin to destroy the toxin. It is traditionally associated with the orgiastic pig feasts enjoyed by the natives of New Guinea but also occurred in people released from prisoner-of-war camps. The pathogenesis of *Cl. perfringens* food-associated infections are summarized in figure 25.22.

The clinical features of the common type of infection are shown in figure 25.12. The laboratory investigation of suspected *Cl. perfringens* infection is outlined in the Appendix. The organism is an anaerobe which grows readily on routine laboratory media. Enterotoxin production can be demonstrated by a latex agglutination method.

Antibacterial treatment of *Cl. perfringens* diarrhoea is rarely required. Prevention depends on thorough reheating of food before serving, or preferably avoiding cooking food too long in advance of consumption.

Clostridium perfringens is also an important cause of infection of wounds and soft tissue, as described in Chapter 28.

Bacillus cereus. Spores and vegetative cells of *Bacillus cereus* contaminate many foods, and food-associated infection takes one of two forms:
- Diarrhoea resulting from the production of enterotoxin in the gut;
- Vomiting due to the ingestion of enterotoxin in food.

Two different toxins are involved, as illustrated in figure 25.23. The clinical features of the infections are summarized in figure 25.12. Laboratory confirmation of the diagnosis requires specific media as described in the Appendix. The emetic type of disease may be difficult to assign to *B. cereus* unless the incriminated food is cultured.

As with *Clostridium perfringens*, prevention of *Bacillus* food-associated infection depends on proper cooking and rapid consumption of food. Specific antibacterial treatment is not indicated.

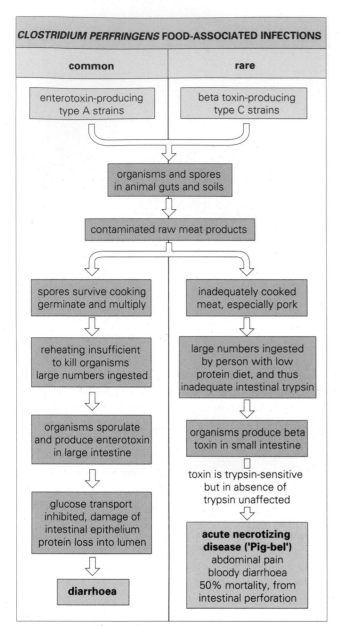

Fig. 25.22 *Clostridium perfringens* is associated with two forms of food-association infection. The common, enterotoxin-mediated infection (left) is usually acquired by eating meat or poultry that has been cooked enough to kill vegetative cells but not spores. As the food cools the spores germinate. If re-heating before consumption is inadequate (as it often is in mass catering outlets), large numbers of organisms are ingested. The rare form associated with beta-toxin producing strains (right) causes a severe necrotizing disease.

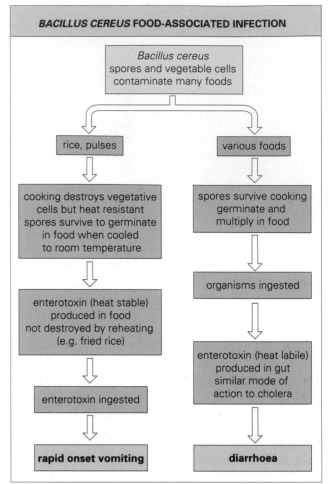

Fig. 25.23 *Bacillus cereus* can also cause two different forms of food-associated infection. Both involve toxins.

Antibiotic-associated diarrhoea

All the infections described so far arise from the ingestion of organisms or their toxins. However, diarrhoea can also arise from disruption of the normal gut flora. Even in the early days of antibiotic use it was recognised that these agents affected the normal flora of the body as well as attacking the pathogens. For example, orally administered tetracycline causes disruption of the normal gut flora and patients sometimes become recolonized not with the usual facultative Gram-negative anaerobes but with *Staph. aureus*, causing enterocolitis, or with yeasts such as *Candida*. Soon after clindamycin was introduced for therapeutic use, it was found to be associated with a severe diarrhoea in which the colonic mucosa became covered with a characteristic fibrinous pseudomembrane (hence pseudomembranous colitis; Fig. 25.24). However, clindamycin is not the cause of the condition; it merely inhibits the normal gut flora and allows the organism *Clostridium difficile* to multiply. This organism is commonly found in the gut of children and sometimes in adults, but it can also be acquired from other patients in hospital by cross infection. In common with other clostridia, *Cl. difficile* produces exotoxins, two of which have been characterized; one is a cytotoxin and the other an enterotoxin, and both appear to play a role in producing diarrhoea.

Although initially associated with clindamycin, *Cl. difficile* diarrhoea has since been shown to follow therapy with many other broad-spectrum antibiotics; hence the term antibiotic-associated diarrhoea or colitis. The infection is often severe and requires treatment with the anti-anaerobic agent, metronidazole, or with oral vancomycin (note that vancomycin is not absorbed from the gut and should not be given orally except for this indication).

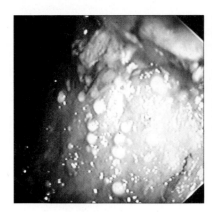

Fig. 25.24
Antibiotic-associated colitis due to *Clostridium difficile*. Sigmoidoscopic view showing multiple pseudomembranous lesions. Courtesy of J Cunningham.

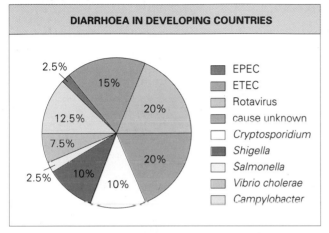

DIARRHOEA IN DEVELOPING COUNTRIES

2.5%
15%
20%
12.5%
7.5%
2.5%
10%
10%

- EPEC
- ETEC
- Rotavirus
- cause unknown
- *Cryptosporidium*
- *Shigella*
- *Salmonella*
- *Vibrio cholerae*
- *Campylobacter*

Fig. 25.25 Diarrhoeal disease is a major cause of illness and death in children in developing countries. This figure shows the proportion of infections caused by different pathogens. Note that in as many as 20% of infections a cause is not identified but many of these are likely to be viral. Data from The World Health Organisation.

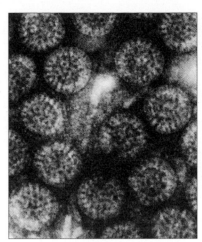

Fig. 25.26
Rotavirus. The virus particles (65 nm in diameter) have a well-defined outer margin, with capsules radiating from an inner core to give the particle a wheel-like (hence 'rota') appearance. Courtesy of JE Banatvala.

Viral diarrhoea

Non-bacterial gastroenteritis and diarrhoea are, for the most part, caused by viruses. Infection is seen in all parts of the world, especially in infants and young children, and in developing countries non-bacterial gastroenteritis is a major cause of death (Fig. 25.25). Its impact is staggering – in parts of Asia, Africa and Latin America 5–10 million infants die of gastroenteritis each year, and children may have a total of 60 days of diarrhoea in each year. It has a major effect on nutritional status and growth. In the USA about 200 000 children of less than 5 years of age are hospitalized each year due to infectious gastroenteritis.

Although viruses appear to be the commonest causes of gastroenteritis in infants and young children, viral gastroenteritis is not distinguishable clinically from other types of gastroenteritis. The viruses are specific to humans and infection follows the general rules for faecal–oral transmission. Oral transmission of non-bacterial gastroenteritis was first demonstrated experimentally in 1945, but it was not until 1972 that viral particles were identified in faeces by electron microscopy. It has been difficult or impossible to cultivate most of these viruses in cell culture.

Rotaviruses

These are morphologically characteristic viruses (Fig 25.26); with a genome consisting of 11 separate segments of double-stranded RNA. Different rotaviruses infect the young of many mammals, including children, kittens, puppies, calves, foals and piglets, but it is thought that viruses from one host species may occasionally cross-infect another. There are at least two human serotypes.

Clinical picture and pathogenesis. The incubation period is 1–4 days. After virus replication in intestinal epithelial cells there is acute onset of vomiting, sometimes projectile, and diarrhoea. The replicating virus damages transport mechanisms in the gut and loss of water, salt and glucose causes diarrhoea (Fig. 25.27). Infected cells are destroyed but there is no inflammation or loss of blood. Exceedingly large numbers of virus particles (1000 million per gram) appear in the faeces. For unknown reasons respiratory symptoms (cough, coryza) are quite common. The disease is more severe in infants in developing countries.

Infection is commonest in those less than two years old, and more frequent in the cooler months of the year. IgA antibodies in colostrum give protection during the first six months of life. Epidemics are sometimes seen in nurseries. Older children are less susceptible, nearly all of them having developed antibodies, but occasional infections occur in adults.

Rotaviruses are well-adapted intestinal parasites. As few as ten ingested particles can cause infection, and by generating a diarrhoea laden with such enormous quantities of infectious particles these organisms have ensured their continued transmission and survival.

Diagnosis. Laboratory methods are generally not available (developing countries) or necessary (developed countries), but during the acute stages the characteristic 65 nm particles can be seen in faecal samples by electron microscopy. They show cubic symmetry and an outer capsid coat arranged like the spokes of a wheel (see Fig. 25.26). Viral antigen can be detected in faeces by ELISA or RIA methods (see Chapter 18).

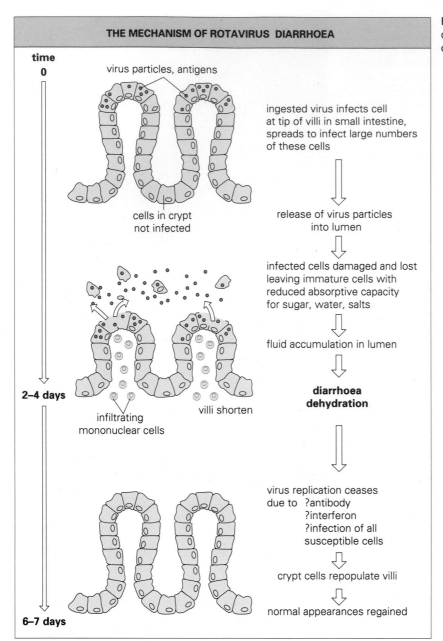

THE MECHANISM OF ROTAVIRUS DIARRHOEA

time 0

virus particles, antigens

ingested virus infects cell at tip of villi in small intestine, spreads to infect large numbers of these cells

cells in crypt not infected

release of virus particles into lumen

infected cells damaged and lost leaving immature cells with reduced absorptive capacity for sugar, water, salts

fluid accumulation in lumen

2–4 days

infiltrating mononuclear cells

villi shorten

diarrhoea dehydration

virus replication ceases due to ?antibody
?interferon
?infection of all susceptible cells

crypt cells repopulate villi

normal appearances regained

6–7 days

Fig. 25.27 The mechanism of rotavirus diarrhoea. Other viruses may have different mechanisms.

Treatment and prevention. Dehydration occurs readily in infants and intravenous fluid replacement can be life-saving. There are no antivirals agents available, but various live, attenuated oral vaccines are undergoing trials.

Other viruses

Other viruses detected in the stools of those with diarrhoea are as follows:

- Caliciviruses, 27nm ssRNA viruses which may cause 'winter vomiting disease'; One representative is the Norwalk virus, which has not yet been cultivated *in vitro* but which causes gastroenteritis when fed to adult volunteers. One of the first identified outbreaks was in a school in Norwalk, Ohio in 1969. Infection is common in older children and adults. In 25–50% cases there may be chills, headache, myalgia or fever as well as nausea, vomiting and diarrhoea, but recovery occurs within about 24 hours and laboratory diagnosis is unnecessary.
- Astroviruses, 28nm ssRNA viruses of which five serotypes are known. Most infections occur in childhood and are mild.

- Adenoviruses (especially types 40,41) most of which cannot be grown in cell culture; second to rotaviruses as causes of acute diarrhoea in young children.
- Small round viruses (SRV), are often implicated in diarrhoea occuring after eating sewage-contaminated shellfish (cockles, mussels, etc.).
- Parvoviruses and coronaviruses. These have an uncertain role.

Although outbreaks of gastroenteritis often have a viral aetiology it may be difficult to be sure about the exact role of a given virus when it is identified in faeces.

Food poisoning

In this chapter the term 'food poisoning' is restricted to the diseases caused by toxins elaborated by contaminating bacteria in food before it is consumed (see above). The emetic toxin of *Bacillus cereus* fits this definition, as do the diseases associated with the consumption of *Staph. aureus* enterotoxin and *Clostridium botulinum* toxin.

STAPHYLOCOCCAL ENTEROTOXINS	
enterotoxin	
A	most commonly associated with food poisoning
B	associated with staphylococcal enterocolitis (rare)
C	rare
D	second most common, alone or in combination with A
	associated with contaminated milk products
E	rare
TSST–1	toxic shock syndrome toxin not food-associated

Fig. 25.28 *Staphylococcus aureus* produces five immunogically distinct enterotoxins. Strains may produce one or more of the toxins simultaneously. Enterotoxin A is by far the most common in food-associated disease. TSST1, the cause of toxic shock syndrome, is not food-associated.

TOXINS OF *CLOSTRIDIUM BOTULINUM*
antigenically distinct polypeptides
types: A B E ⎤ human disease
types: C D ⎤ animal botulism
relative heat labile, destroyed at 80°C for 30 minutes
not destroyed by digestive enzymes

Fig. 25.29 Eight different *Clostridium botulinum* toxins have been identified, but of these only three are associated with human disease and two others with botulism in animals. These protein exotoxins are the most potent biological toxins known to man. They are antigenic and can be inactivated and used to produce antitoxin in animals.

Staphylococcus aureus

Five serologically distinct enterotoxins (A–E) are produced by strains of *Staph. aureus* (Fig. 25.28). All are heat stable and resistant to destruction by enzymes in the stomach and small intestine. Their mechanism of action is not understood but they have an effect on the central nervous system which results in severe vomiting within 3–6 hours of consumption. Diarrhoea is not a feature. Often there are no viable organisms detectable in the food consumed but enterotoxin can be detected by a latex agglutination test.

Botulism

Botulism is a rare but serious disease caused by the exotoxin of *Clostridium botulinum*. The organism is widespread in the environment and spores can be isolated readily from soil samples and from various animals including fish. Eight serologically distinct toxins have been identified, but only three; A, B and E, are associated with human disease (Fig. 25.29). The toxins are ingested in food (often canned or reheated) or produced in the gut after ingestion of the organism; they are absorbed from the gut into the bloodstream and reach their site of action, the peripheral nerve synapses. The action of the toxin is to block neurotransmission (see Chapter 16).

Three forms of botulism have been identified:
- Food-borne botulism
- Infant botulism
- Wound botulism

In food-borne botulism, toxin is elaborated by organisms in food, which is then ingested. In infant and wound, botulism, the organisms are respectively ingested or implanted in a wound, and multiply and elaborate toxin *in*

vivo. Infant botulism is now the most common of the three forms and has been associated with feeding babies with honey contaminated with *Cl. botulinum* spores.

The clinical disease is the same in all three forms and is characterized by flaccid paralysis leading to progressive muscle weakness and respiratory arrest. Intensive supportive treatment is urgently required and complete recovery may take many months. Improvements in supportive care have reduced the mortality from around 70% to about 10% but the disease, although rare, remains life-threatening.

Laboratory diagnosis depends largely on demonstrating the presence of toxin by injecting samples of faeces and food (if available) into mice that have been protected with botulinum antitoxin or left unprotected. There are no *in vitro* tests routinely available at present. Culture of faeces or wound exudate for *Cl. botulinum* should also be performed.

Polyvalent antitoxin is recommended as an adjunct to intensive supportive therapy. Antibacterial agents are not helpful. It is not practicable to prevent food becoming contaminated with botulinum spores so prevention of disease depends on preventing germination of spores in food, by maintaining food at an acid pH or storing at <4°C, or destroying toxin in food by heating for 30 minutes at 80°C.

PARASITES AND THE GASTROINTESTINAL TRACT

Many species of protozoan and worm parasites live in the gastrointestinal tract, but only a few are a frequent cause of serious pathology (Fig. 25.30). These will form the focus of this section.

Transmission of intestinal parasites is maintained by release of life-cycle stages (cysts, eggs, larvae) in faeces. In

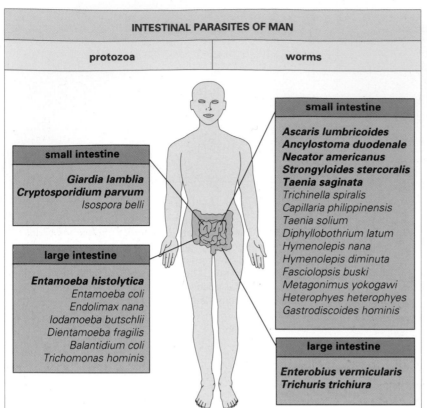

Fig. 25.30 Gastrointestinal parasites of man. The majority of these infections are found in developing countries, but all species also occur in the developed world and some have recently come to prominence because of their association with AIDS. The most important parasite species are highlighted in bold type.

most cases new infections depend, either directly or indirectly, upon contact with faecally derived material, infection rates therefore reflecting standards of hygiene and levels of sanitation. In general, stages of protozoan parasites passed in faeces are either already infective or become infective within a short time. These parasites, therefore, are usually acquired by swallowing infective stages in faecally contaminated food or water. Worm parasites, with two major exceptions (pinworms and tapeworms), produce eggs or larvae that require a period of development outside the host before they become infective. Transmission routes are more complex here. Some species are acquired through food or water contaminated with infective eggs or larvae, or are picked up directly via contaminated fingers; some have larvae which can actively penetrate through the skin, migrating eventually to the intestine; others are acquired by eating animals or animal products that contain infective stages.

The symptoms of intestinal infection range from the very mild, through acute or chronic diarrhoeal conditions associated with parasite-related inflammation, to life-threatening diseases caused by spread of parasites into other organs of the body. Most infections fall into the first of these categories; indeed, in many parts of the world, intestinal parasitism is accepted as a normal condition of life.

Protozoan infections

Three species are of particular importance: *Entamoeba histolytica*, *Giardia lamblia* and *Cryptosporidium parvum*. All three can give rise to diarrhoeal conditions, but the organisms have distinctive features that allow differential diagnosis to be made quite easily (Fig. 25.31).

Entamoeba histolytica

Infections with *Entamoeba histolytica* occur world-wide, but are most often found in subtropical and tropical countries, where prevalence may exceed 50%. The trophozoite stages of the amoebae live in the large intestine, on the mucosal surface, frequently as harmless commensals feeding on bacteria. Reproduction of these stages is by simple binary fission, and there is periodic formation of resistant encysted forms that pass out of the body. These cysts can survive in the external environment and act as the infective stages; asymptomatic individuals are therefore carriers capable of infecting others. Infection occurs when food or drink is contaminated either by infected food-handlers or as a result of inadequate sanitation. Transmission can also take place as a result of anal sexual activity. The cysts pass intact through the stomach when swallowed and excyst in the small intestine, each giving rise to eight progeny. Under certain conditions, still undefined but including variables of both host and parasite origin, *Entamoeba* can become pathogenic, the amoebae invading the mucosa and feeding on host materials including red blood cells, giving rise to amoebic colitis.

Clinical features. Infections with commensal forms of the amoeba are asymptomatic. Invasion of the mucosa may produce small, localized, superficial ulcers or may involve the entire colonic mucosa, with the formation of deep, confluent ulcers (Fig. 25.32). The former causes a mild diarrhoea, whereas more severe invasion leads to 'amoebic dysentery', characterized by mucus, pus and blood in the stools. Dysenteries of amoebic and bacillary origin can be distinguished by a number of features (Fig. 25.33).

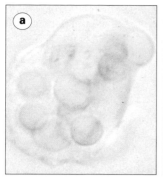

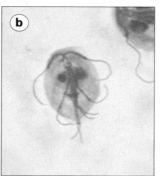

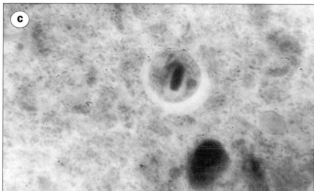

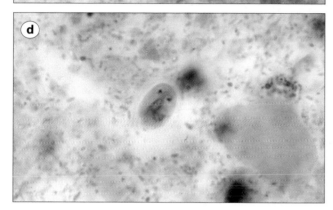

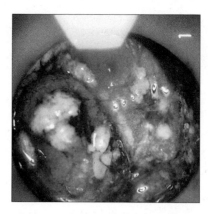

Fig. 25.32 Amoebic colitis. Sigmoidoscopic view showing deep ulcers and overlying purulent exudate. Courtesy of RH Gilman.

FEATURES OF BACILLARY AND AMOEBIC DYSENTERY		
	bacillary	**amoebic**
Organism	shigella	entamoeba
Polymorphs and macrophages in stool	many	few
Eosinophils and Charcot–Leydon crystals in stool	few or absent	often present
Organisms in stool	many	few
Blood and mucus in stool	yes	yes

Fig. 25.33 Features of bacillary and amoebic dysentery.

Fig. 25.31 Protozoan infections of the gastrointestinal tract. (a) *Entamoeba histolytica*. Trophozoite found in the acute stage of the disease, often containing ingested red blood cells. (b) *Giardia lamblia* trophozoite associated with acute infection in man. Courtesy of DK Banerjee. (c) Cyst of *E. histolytica*, with only one of the four nuclei visible. The broad chromatid bar is a semi-crystalline aggregation of ribosomes. H & E stain. (d) Oval cyst of *G. lamblia* showing two of the four nuclei, the remnants of median bodies and flagella, and the rim of an attached disc. Iron haematoxylin stain. Courtesy of R Muller and JR Baker.

Complications include perforation of the intestine, leading to peritonitis, and extraintestinal invasion. Trophozoites can spread via the blood to the liver, with the formation of an abcess, and may secondarily extend to the lung and other organs. Rarely abcesses may spread directly to involve the overlying skin.

Laboratory diagnosis. Infection as such may be diagnosed by the presence of the characteristic 4-nucleate cysts in the stool, although these may be infrequent in light infections and repeated stool examination is necessary. Care must be taken to differentiate *E. histolytica* from other non-

pathogenic species that might be present (Fig. 25.34). Trophozoites can be found in cases of dysentery (when the stools are loose and wet), but they are fragile and deteriorate rapidly; specimens should therefore be preserved prior to examination. Several immunological tests are available. These of course can indicate only that the patient has been exposed to infection at some time in their history, but can be useful in confirming a preliminary diagnosis.

Treatment and prevention. Recovery from infection usually occurs and there is some immunity to reinfection. Acute infections can be treated with metronidazole. Treatment may fail to clear infection completely, and passage of infective cysts can continue. Metronidazole is useful against the extraintestinal sites of infection, but if these become secondarily infected with bacteria, antibiotics and drainage are necessary. Prevention of amoebiasis in the community requires the same approaches to hygiene and sanitation as those adopted for bacterial infections of the intestine.

Giardia lamblia

Giardia was the first intestinal microorganism to be observed under a microscope. It was discovered by Anton van Leeuwenhoek in 1681, using the microscope he had invented to examine specimens of his own stool. At the present time it is the most commonly diagnosed intestinal parasite in the USA.

PROTOZOAN CYSTS				
Entamoeba histolytica	**Entamoeba coli**	**Endolimax nana**	**Iodamoeba bütschlii**	**red blood cell**

Fig. 25.34 Characterisic cysts used to differentiate pathogenic from non-pathogenic protozoa. A red blood cell is shown for comparison.

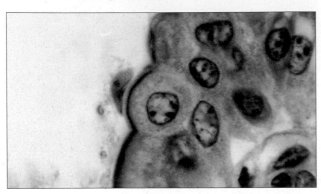

Fig. 25.35 Trophozoite of *Giardia lamblia* attached to the mucosal surface of the small intestine. Iron-haematoxylin stain. Courtesy of R Muller and JR Baker.

Like *Entamoeba*, *Giardia* has only two life-cycle stages, the flagellate (4 pairs of flagella), binucleate trophozoite and the resistant 4-nucleate cyst. The trophozoites live in the upper portion of the small intestine, adhering closely by specialized attachment regions to the brush border of the epithelial cells (Fig. 25.35). They divide by binary fission, and may occur in such numbers that they cover large areas of the mucosal surface. Cyst formation occurs at regular intervals, each cyst being formed as one trophozoite rounds up and produces a resistant wall. Cysts pass out in stools and can survive for several weeks under optimum conditions. Infection occurs when cysts are swallowed, usually as a result of drinking contaminated water. Epidemics of giardiasis have occurred when public drinking supplies have become contaminated, but smaller outbreaks have been traced to drinking from rivers and streams that have been contaminated by wild animals. The genus *Giardia* is widely distributed in mammals and there is suggestive evidence for cross infection between certain animal hosts (e.g. beaver) and humans. Much of this is circumstantial, but case reports provide more direct evidence. Recent data suggest that *Giardia* may also be transmitted sexually.

Clinical features. Light infections are asymptomatic. More severe infections cause a diarrhoea, which can be self-limiting (7 to 10 days being the usual course) or may become chronic, particularly in patients with deficient or compromised immunological defences, developing into a serious condition. The diarrhoea is thought to arise from inflammatory responses triggered by the damaged epithelial cells, and from interference with normal absorptive processes. Characteristically stools are loose, foul-smelling and often

fatty. A link has been suggested between giardiasis and bacterial overgrowth in the intestine, involving *Klebsiella pneumoniae* and *Enterobacter* spp. However, this link, made in 1977, has not been confirmed.

Laboratory diagnosis. Positive diagnosis requires identification of cysts or trophozoites in stool specimens. Repeated examination is necessary in light infections; concentration techniques improve the chances of finding cysts. Duodenal intubation, or the use of recoverable swallowed capsules and threads, may aid in obtaining trophozoites directly from the intestine.

Treatment and prevention. Infections can be treated using a variety of drugs (quinacrine hydrochloride, metronidazole, tinidazole, furazolidone), but none is completely successful. Community measures for prevention include the usual concerns with hygiene and sanitation, but attention has also to be given to improved treatment (largely filtration and chlorination) of drinking supplies where these are suspected as a source. Care in drinking from potentially contaminated natural waters is also indicated.

Cryptosporidium parvum

The implication of *Cryptosporidium parvum* as a cause of diarrhoea in humans is comparatively recent. The parasite is widely distributed in many animals, but is very small and easily overlooked. It has a complex life cycle, going through both asexual and sexual phases of development in the same host. Transmission is by ingestion of the resistant oocyst stage (4–5 μm) in faecally contaminated material (Fig. 25.36). In the small intestine the cyst releases infective sporozoites which invade the epithelial cells, remaining closely-associated with the apical plasma membrane. Here they form schizonts that divide to release merozoites which then reinvade further epithelial cells. Eventually a sexual phase occurs and oocysts are released. Transmission probably most often occurs from drinking water contaminated by oocysts, either from other humans or from animals.

Clinical features. Symptoms of infection range from a moderate diarrhoea to a more severe, profuse diarrhoea that is self-limiting in immunocompetent individuals (lasting up to 20 days), but which can become chronic in immunocompromised patients. Cryptosporidiosis occurs as a common infection in AIDS patients. In these individuals diarrhoea is prolonged, may become irreversible, and can be life-threatening.

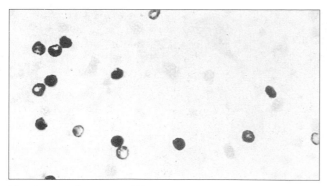

Fig. 25.36 *Cryptosporidium* oocysts in faecal specimen. Courtesy of S Tzipori.

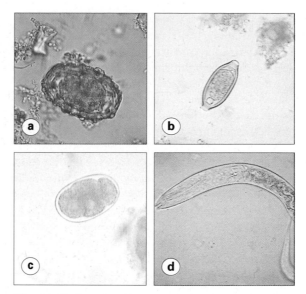

Fig. 25.37 Eggs and larvae of intestinal nematodes passed in faeces. (a) Egg of *Ascaris* (fertile). (b) Egg of *Trichuris*. (c) Egg of hookworm.The ovum continues to divide in the faecal sample and may be at the 16- or 32-cell stage by the time the sample is examined. (d) Larva of *Strongyloides stercoralis*. Courtesy of JH Cross.

Laboratory diagnosis. Routine faecal examinations are inadequate for diagnosis. Concentration techniques and special staining (e.g. modified acid-fast stain) are necessary to recover and identify the oocysts.

Treatment and prevention. Treatment is necessary only in immunocompromised patients; the macrolide spiramycin has been used with limited success.

Public health measures are similar to those outlined for control of giardiasis, although *Cryptosporidium* is even more resistant to chlorination.

Worm infections

The most important intestinal worms are the group of nematodes known collectively as the 'soil-transmitted helminths'. These fall into two distinct groups: first, *Ascaris lumbricoides* (large roundworm) and *Trichuris trichura* (whipworm), in which infection occurs by swallowing the infective eggs; and second, *Ancylostoma duodenale, Necator americanus* (hookworms) and *Strongyloides stercoralis*, which infect by active skin penetration by infective larvae, which then undertake a systemic migration through the lungs to the intestine. With the exception of *Trichuris* (large intestine), all inhabit the small bowel.

Perhaps the commonest intestinal nematode is the least pathogenic, the pinworm or threadworm *Enterobius vermicularis*. The females of this species, which live in the large bowel, release infective eggs onto the perianal skin. Transmission usually occurs directly from contaminated fingers, but the eggs are also light enough to be carried in dust. A number of tapeworms also infect the human intestine, but their pathogenic effects are usually mild, certainly less significant than those of the larval stages.

The soil-transmitted helminths are commonest in the warmer developing countries. About one-quarter of the world's population carry these worms, children being the most heavily infected section of the population. Transmission is favoured where there is inadequate disposal of faeces, contamination of water supplies, use of faeces (night-soil) as fertilizer, and low standards of hygiene (see below).

Life cycle and transmission

Ascaris and Trichuris. The females of these species lay thick-shelled eggs into the intestine, which then pass out with the faeces (Fig. 25.37). The eggs require incubation for several days at optimum conditions (warm temperature, high humidity) for the infective larvae to develop. Once this occurs, the eggs remain infective for many weeks or months, depending on the local microclimate. After being swallowed the eggs hatch in the intestine, releasing the larvae. Those of *Ascaris* penetrate the gut wall and are carried in the blood through the liver to the lungs, climbing up the bronchi and trachea before being swallowed and once again reaching the intestine. The adult worms live freely in the gut lumen, feeding on intestinal contents. In contrast *Trichuris* larvae remain within the large bowel, penetrating into the epithelial cell layer, where they remain as they mature.

Hookworms. Adult female hookworms, *A. duodenale* and *N. americanus* lay thin-shelled eggs that hatch in the faeces shortly after they leave the body of the host (see Fig. 25.37). The larvae feed on bacteria until infective, and then migrate away from the faecal mass. Infection takes place when larvae come into contact with unprotected skin (or additionally, in the case of *Ancylostoma*, are swallowed). They penetrate the skin, migrate via the blood to the lungs, climb the trachea and are swallowed. Adult worms attach by their enlarged mouths to the intestinal mucosa, ingest a plug of tissue, rupture capillaries and suck blood.

Strongyloides. The life cycle of this species is similar to that of hookworms, but shows some important differences. The adult worm exists as a parthenogenetic female that lays eggs into the mucosa. These eggs hatch in the intestine and, usually, the released larvae pass out in faeces (see Fig. 25.37). Development outside the host can follow the hookworm pattern, with the direct production of skin-penetrating larvae, or may be diverted into the production of a complete free-living generation that then produces infective larvae. Under certain conditions, and particularly when the host is immunocompromised, *Strongyloides* larvae can reinvade before they are voided in faeces. This process of autoinfection can give rise to the severe clinical condition known as 'disseminated strongyloidiasis'. All soil-transmitted helminths are relatively long-lived (several months to years), but authenticated cases show that *Strongyloides* infections can persist for more than 30 years, presumably through continuous internal autoinfection.

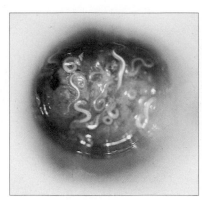

Fig. 25.38
Trichuriasis in a healthy infected child. Proctoscopic view showing numerous adult *T. trichura* secured to the intestinal mucosa. Courtesy of RH Gilman.

Clinical features

In most individuals worm infections produce chronic, mild intestinal discomfort rather than severe diarrhoeal or other conditions. Each infection has a number of characteristic pathological conditions linked with it:

Ascariasis. The migration of *Ascaris* larvae through the lungs can cause severe respiratory distress (pneumonitis) and this stage is often associated with pronounced eosinophilia. Intestinal stages of infection can cause abdominal pain, nausea and digestive disturbances. In children on sub-optimal nutritional intake these disturbances can contribute to clinical malnutrition. Large numbers of adults can cause a physical blockage in the intestine and this may also occur as worms die following chemotherapy. Intestinal worms tend to migrate out of the intestine, often up the bile duct, causing cholangitis. Perforation of the intestinal wall can also occur. Worms have occasionally been reported in unusual locations including the orbit of the eye and the (male) urethra. *Ascaris* is highly allergenic and infections often give rise to symptoms of hypersensitivity, which may persist for many years after infection has been cleared.

Trichuriasis. As with all intestinal worms, children are the members of the community most heavily infected with this parasite. Although usually regarded as of little clinical significance, recent research has shown that moderate to heavy infections in children can cause a chronic diarrhoea (Fig. 25.38), reflected in impaired nutrition and retarded growth. Occasionally heavy infections lead to prolapse of the rectum.

Hookworm disease. Invasion of hookworm larvae through the skin and lungs can cause a dermatitis and pneumonitis respectively. The blood-feeding activities of the intestinal worms can lead to a iron-deficient anaemia if the diet is inadequate. Heavy infections cause a marked debility and growth retardation.

Strongyloidiasis. Heavy intestinal infection causes a persistent and profuse diarrhoea, with dehydration and electrolyte inbalance. Profound mucosal changes can also lead to a malabsorption syndrome, sometimes confused with tropical sprue. Patients suffering from diseases that suppress immune function, such as AIDS and cancer, or being treated with immunosuppressant drugs, are susceptible to the development of disseminated strongyloidiasis. Invasion of the body by many thousands of autoinfective larvae can be fatal.

Pinworm (threadworm). The commonest signs of infection by these worms are anal pruritis, only occasionally accompanied by mild diarrhoea. Migrating worms sometimes invade the appendix and have been linked with appendicitis. In female children invasion of the vagina has been reported.

Laboratory diagnosis

All five of the soil-transmitted species can be diagnosed by finding eggs or larvae in the fresh stool; direct smears or concentration techniques can be used. Immunodiagnosis of intestinal parasites is still at an early stage.

Ascaris, Trichuris and hookworms. The eggs of each are characteristic (see Fig. 25.37) and easily recognized. Identification of the species of hookworm present requires culture of the stool to allow the eggs to hatch and the larvae to mature into the infective third stage. The presence of adult *Ascaris* can sometimes be confirmed directly by carrying out x-ray examination (Fig. 25.39).

Strongyloides. Infection is diagnosed by finding larvae in fresh stools.

Pinworm. Although adult pinworms sometimes appear in stools, the eggs seldom do so because they are laid directly onto the perianal skin (Fig. 25.40). They can be found by wiping this area with a piece of clear adhesive tape (the 'Scotch tape' test) and examining the tape under the microscope.

Infections with *Ascaris*, hookworms and *Strongyloides* are often accompanied by a marked blood eosinophilia. Although this is not diagnostic, it is a very strong indicator of worm infection.

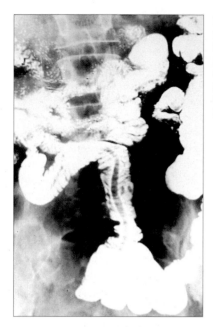

Fig. 25.39 Filling defect in the small intestine due to the presence of *Ascaris*, shown up by x-ray after barium meal. Courtesy of W Peters.

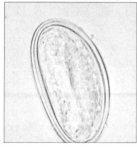

Fig. 25.40 Egg of *Enterobius* on perianal skin. Courtesy of JH Cross.

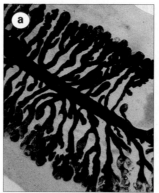
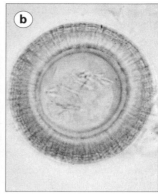

Fig. 25.41 *Taenia saginata*. (a) Gravid proglottids, stained with India ink to show numerous side branches. (b) Egg containing six-hooked hexacanth larva. Courtesy of R Muller and JR Baker.

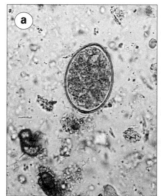
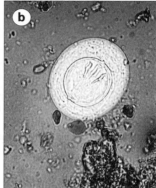

Fig. 25.42 Eggs of (a) *Diphyllobothrium latum* and (b) *Hymenolepis nana*. Courtesy of R Muller and JR Baker.

Treatment and prevention

A variety of antihelminthic drugs are available for treatment of intestinal nematodes. Piperazine has been used with great success against *Ascaris*, hookworms and pinworm; many more recent drugs (albendazole, mebendazole, levamisole, pyrantel) can also be used, and these are effective also against trichuriasis and strongyloidiasis (especially albendazole, levamisole). At the community level prevention can be achieved through improved hygiene and sanitation, making sure that faecal material is disposed of properly.

Other intestinal worms

Although many other species of helminth can occur in the intestine the majority are unlikely to be found in developed countries. Of the human tapeworms the beef tapeworm *Taenia saginata,* transmitted through infected beef, is the most widely distributed. However, infection is usually asymptomatic, apart from the nausea felt on passing the large segments! Diagnosis involves finding these segments or the characteristic eggs in the stool (Fig. 25.41). *Diphyllobothrium latum,* the broadfish tapeworm, is widely distributed geographically, but infection is restricted to individuals eating raw or undercooked fish carrying the

infective larvae. The eggs of this species have a terminal 'lid' and are the diagnostic stage in the stool (Fig. 25.42). *Hymenolepis nana*, the dwarf tapeworm, occurs primarily in children, infection occuring directly by swallowing eggs (see Fig. 25.42). This worm has the ability to undergo autoinfection within the host's intestine, so that large numbers of worms can build up rapidly, leading to diarrhoea and some abdominal discomfort. All of the tapeworms described can be removed by praziquantel or niclosamide.

Intestinal symptoms (predominantly diarrhoea and abdominal pain) are also associated with infections by the nematode *Trichinella spiralis*, better known clinically for the pathology caused by the parenteral muscle phase (see Chapters 28 and 31). Infection with the two species of schistosome associated with mesenteric blood vessels (*S. japonicum* and *S. mansoni*) may also cause symptoms of intestinal disease. As the eggs pass through the intestinal wall they cause marked inflammatory responses; granulomatous lesions form, and diarrhoea may occur in the early, acute phase. Inflammatory polyps in the colon are associated with heavy, chronic *S. mansoni* infection; severe involvement of the small bowel is more common with *S. japonicum.*

SYSTEMIC INFECTION INITIATED IN THE GASTROINTESTINAL TRACT

We opened this chapter by noting that infections acquired by ingestion of pathogens could remain localized in the gastrointestinal tract or could disseminate to other organs and systems. Important examples of the latter are the enteric fevers and viral hepatitis type A and E. Listeriosis also appears to be acquired via the gastrointestinal tract. For the sake of clarity and convenience, other types of viral hepatitis will also be discussed in this chapter.

Enteric fevers: typhoid and paratyphoid

The term 'enteric fever' was introduced in the last century in an attempt to clarify the distinction between typhus (see Chapter 30) and typhoid. For many years these two diseases had been confused, as the common root of their names suggests (typhus – a fever with delirium, and typhoid – resembling typhus). But even before the causative agents were isolated (typhoid caused by *Salmonella typhi* and typhus caused by *Rickettsia* spp.) it was pointed out that it was "just as impossible to confuse the intestinal lesions of typhoid with the pathological findings of typhus as it was to confuse the eruptions of measles with the pustules of smallpox". In fact, enteric fevers can be caused by *S. paratyphi* as well as *S. typhi*, but the name 'typhoid' has stuck.

Aetiology and transmission

Salmonella typhi and *S. paratyphi* types A, B, and C all cause enteric fevers. These species of *Salmonella* are restricted to humans and do not have a reservoir in animals. Thus, spread of the infection is from person to person, usually through contaminated food or water. After infection, people can carry the organism for months or years providing a continuing source from which others may become infected. Typhoid Mary, a cook in New York City in the early 1900s, is one such example. She was a long-term carrier who succeeded in initiating at least 10 outbreaks of the disease.

Pathogenesis

After ingestion, the salmonellae that survive the antibacterial defences of the stomach and small intestine penetrate the gut mucosa through the Peyer's patches, probably in the jejunum or the distal ileum (Fig. 25.43). Once through the mucosal barrier, the bacteria reach the intestinal lymph nodes where they survive and multiply within macrophages (see Fig. 13.5). They are transported in these cells to the mesenteric lymph nodes, thence to the thoracic duct and are eventually discharged into the bloodstream. Circulating in the blood, the organisms can seed many organs, most importantly in areas where cells of the reticuloendothelial system are concentrated (i.e. the spleen, bone marrow, liver and Peyer's patches) and contribute to the multisystem disease characteristic of enteric fever. In the liver they multiply in Kupffer cells. From the reticuloendothelial system there is reinvasion of the blood, to reach other organs (e.g. kidney). The gall bladder is infected either from the blood or from the liver via the biliary tract, the bacterium being particularly resistant to bile. As a result *S. typhi* enter the intestine for the second time, in much larger numbers than in the primary encounter, and in Peyer's patches cause a strong inflammatory response leading to ulceration, with the danger of intestinal perforation.

Clinical features

After an incubation period of 10–14 days (which may range from 7–21 days), the disease has an insidious onset, with non-specific symptoms of fever and malaise accompanied by aches and respiratory symptoms which may resemble a flu-like illness (see Chapter 13). Diarrhoea may be present but constipation is just as likely. At this stage the patient often presents as a PUO (pyrexia of unknown origin; see Chapter 32). In the absence of treatment the fever increases and the patient becomes acutely ill. Rose spots (erythematous maculopapular lesions which blanch on pressure; Fig. 24.44) are characteristic on the upper abdomen but may be absent in up to 50% of patients. These spots are transient and disappear within hours to days. Without treatment, an uncomplicated infection lasts 4–6 weeks.

Complications

These can be classified into: (1) those secondary to the local gastrointestinal lesions, e.g. haemorrhage and perforation (Fig. 25.45); (2) those associated with toxaemia, e.g.

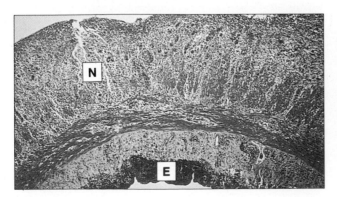

Fig. 25.43 Typhoid. Section of ileum showing a typhoid ulcer, with transmural inflammatory reaction, focal areas of necrosis (N) and a fibrinous exudate (E) on the serosal surface. H & E stain. Courtesy of MSR Hutt.

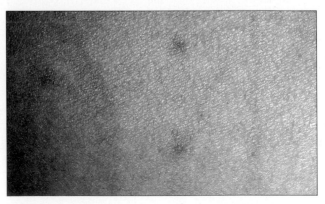

Fig. 25.44 Rose spots on the skin in typhoid fever. Courtesy of WE Farrar.

myocarditis, hepatic and bone marrow damage; (3) those secondary to the prolonged serious illness; and (4) those resulting from multiplication of the organisms in other sites, causing meningitis, osteomyelitis, or endocarditis. Before antibiotics became available, 12–16% of patients died, usually of complications occuring in the third or fourth week of the disease. Relapse after an initial recovery was also common.

Carriage

Patients usually continue to excrete *S. typhi* in the faeces for several weeks after recovery and 1–3% become chronic carriers (defined as excretion in faeces or urine for a year after infection). Chronic carriage is more common in women and in older patients, and in those with underlying disease of the gallbladder (e.g. stones) or urinary bladder (e.g. schistosomiasis).

Laboratory diagnosis

This cannot be made on clinical grounds alone, although the presence of rose spots in a febrile patient is highly suggestive. A positive diagnosis depends on the isolation of *S. typhi or S. paratyphi* from the patient. Blood during the first two weeks, or faeces and urine at 2–4 weeks should be cultured on selective media (see Chapter 18). An antibody response to infection can be detected by an agglutination test (Widal test) but interpretation of the results depends on a knowledge of the normal antibody titres in the population and whether the patient has been vaccinated. Demonstration of a rising titre between acute- and convalescent-phase sera is more useful than examination of a single sample. At best the results confirm the microbiological diagnosis; at worst they are misleading.

Treatment

Treatment with chloramphenicol, ampicillin, cotrimoxazole, or ciprofloxacin should be commenced as soon as the diagnosis is made and should continue for at least a week after the temperature has returned to normal. Isolates of *S. typhi* resistant to one or more of the above agents have been reported. Many other agents are active *in vitro* but do not achieve a clinical cure, presumably because they do not reach the bacteria in their intracellular location.

Prevention

Breaking the chain of spread of infection from person to person depends on good personal hygiene, adequate sewage disposal and a clean water supply. In general these conditions exist in the developed world and outbreaks of enteric fever are rare, but still occur.

Typhoid carriers are a public health concern and should be excluded from employment which involves food handling. Every effort should be made to eradicate carriage by antibiotic treatment and if this is unsuccessful, removal of the gall bladder (the most common site of carriage) should be considered.

A killed vaccine against *S. typhi* and one which includes *S. paratyphi* is available and is recommended for travellers to developing countries; protection, however, is incomplete. Side effects of vaccination include pain at the site of injection, fever and headache. Live oral vaccines are currently being tested in the anticipation that they will produce better immunity and fewer side effects.

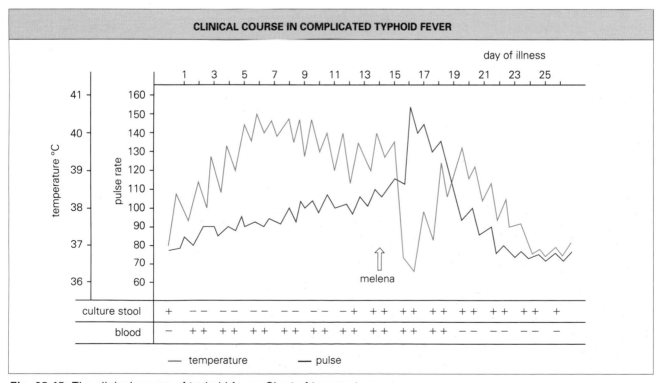

Fig. 25.45 The clinical course of typhoid fever. Chart of temperature, pulse rate and bacteriological findings in a patient whose illness was complicated by massive haemorrhage. Courtesy of HL DuPont.

VIRAL HEPATITIS								
virus	virus group	type of virus	mode of infection	incubation period	frequency of infection in UK/USA	severity of hepatitis	persistent carriage of virus	other comments
Hepatitis A (HAV)	enterovirus 72	ssRNA	faecal–oral	2–4 weeks	++	±	–	common in UK and USA
Hepatitis B (HBV)	hepadnavirus	dsDNA	from blood (also sexual)	1–3 months	±	++	+	carriage associated with liver cancer
Hepatitis C (HCV)	togavirus	ssRNA	from blood (?also sexual)	2 months	±	+	±	uncommon in UK, USA
Hepatitis D (HDV)	very small	ssRNA	from blood	2–12 weeks	±	+	+	needs concurrent hepatitis B virus infection
Hepatitis E (HEV)	calicivirus	ssRNA	faecal–oral	6–8 weeks	–	±	–	common in Far East
Yellow fever	togavirus	ssRNA	mosquito	3–6 days	–	++	–	no person-to-person spread

Fig. 25.46 The main viruses causing hepatitis in humans. Other viruses include Epstein-Barr virus (mild hepatitis in 15% of infected adults and adolescents), herpes simplex virus (rarely) and hepatitis in the newborn due to intra-uterine infection with rubella or cytomegalovirus.

Listeriosis

Listeria monocytogenes is a Gram-positive coccobaccillus which is widespread in animals and in the environment. It is becoming increasingly recognized as a food-borne pathogen, associated particularly with uncooked foods such as paté, contaminated milk, soft cheeses and coleslaw. It is likely that large numbers of organisms must be ingested to cause disease, but the ability of the organism to multiply, albeit slowly, at refrigeration temperatures allows an infective dose to accumulate in goods stored in this way. Even then, the population at risk appears to be limited to pregnant women, with the possibility of infection of the baby in the uterus or during birth, and immunocompromised patients. The disease usually presents as meningitis (see Chapters 27 and 33).

Hepatitis

Hepatitis means inflammation and damage to the liver, and can be caused by viruses and, less commonly bacteria (e.g. *Leptospira* spp.) or other microorganisms. The disease picture varies from malaise, anorexia and nausea, to (rarely) acute life-threatening liver failure. More than half the liver must be damaged or destroyed before liver function fails. Regeneration of liver cells is rapid but fibrous repair, especially when infection persists, can lead to cirrhosis.

At least five different viruses are referred to as hepatitis viruses (Fig. 25.46), and they generally cannot be distinguished clinically. Other viruses cause hepatitis as part of a disease syndrome and are dealt with elsewhere. Dramatic elevations of serum aminotransferases (alanine amino transferase, ALT; aspartate aminotransferase, AST) are characteristic of acute viral hepatitis. Specific laboratory tests for hepatitis A and B viruses have been available for some years and tests for others, originally referred to as

'nonA-nonB' viruses are now becoming available. Except in the cases of hepatitis A and B, there are no licensed vaccines, and except for interferons (hepatitis B and C) there are no specific treatments.

Hepatitis A

This disease is caused by a typical enterovirus (ssRNA) referred to as hepatitis A virus (HAV) or enterovirus 72. There is only one serotype.

Transmission. This occurs by the faecal–oral route. Virus is excreted in large amounts in faeces (one-hundred million infectious doses per gram), and spreads from person to person by contact (hands) or by contamination of food or water. The incubation period between infection and illness is 2–4 weeks; virus is present in faeces for a week or two before symptoms appear and during the first week (sometimes also the second and third week) of the illness. Person-to-person transmission can lead to outbreaks in schools, camps, etc. and viral contamination of water or food is a common source of infection (see panel). In developed countries 20–50% of adults have been infected and have antibody, whereas in developing countries infection is more common and >90% of adults have been infected.

Clinical picture and pathogenesis. After infection the virus enters the blood from unknown sites in the gastrointestinal tract, where it may replicate. It then infects liver cells, passing into the biliary tract to reach the intestine and appear in faeces (Fig. 25.48). Relatively small amounts of virus enter the blood at this stage. Events during the rather lengthy incubation period are poorly understood, but liver cells are damaged, possibly by direct viral action. Common clinical manifestations are fever, anorexia,

Hepatitis A

In August 1988 the Florida Department of Health and Rehabilitation Services traced 61 persons who had suffered serologically confirmed infection with hepatitis A virus. These individuals resided in 5 different states but 59 of them had eaten raw oysters from the same growing areas in Bay County coastal waters. The oysters had been gathered illegally from outside the approved harvesting areas and were contaminated with hepatitis A virus. The mean incubation period of the disease was 29 days (range 16–48 days). Probable sources of faecal contamination near the oyster beds included boats with inappropriate sewage disposal systems and discharge from a local sewage treatment plant that contained high levels of faecal coliforms.

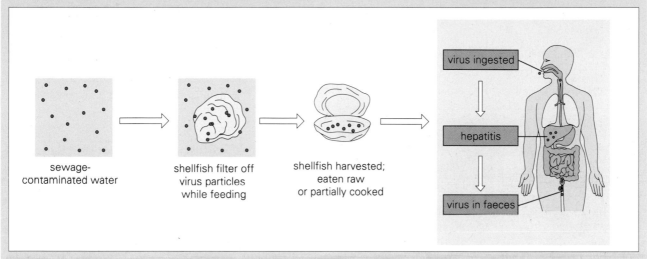

Fig. 25.47 Contamination of shellfish by hepatitis A virus can lead to human infection.

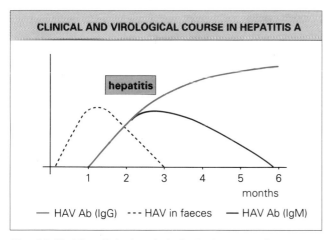

Fig. 25.48 The clinical and virological course of hepatitis A.

nausea, vomiting, and sometimes jaundice. The illness generally has a more sudden onset than hepatitis B, and is milder in young children than in older children and adults.

Laboratory diagnosis. The best laboratory method is by detecting hepatitis A-specific IgM antibody in serum, or the demonstration of antigen (using an ELISA method; see Chapter 18) in faeces.

Treatment and prevention. Pooled normal immunoglobulin contains antibody to hepatitis A virus, and gives a month or two of protection when injected into travellers to developing countries. There is no antiviral therapy, but a formaldehyde-inactivated vaccine is now available.

Hepatitis B

This disease is caused by hepatitis B virus (HBV), a hepadna (hepatitis DNA) virus (see Appendix and overleaf), containing a partially double-stranded circular DNA genome and three important antigens – HBsAg, HBcAg, and HBeAg (Figs 25.49 and 25.50). There is only one serotype in the sense that infection with a given strain of virus confers resistance to all strains, but antigenic variation in HBsAg gives four subtypes (adw, adr, ayn and ayr). These do not differ in virulence or chronicity, but are useful in epidemiological studies.

Transmission. The virus is present in blood and can spread between intravenous drug abusers or male homosexuals, between mother and child (intrauterine, peri- and postnatal infection; see Chapter 27) and also in association with tattooing, earpiercing and acupuncture. Heterosexual transmission probably occurs, perhaps when there are genital ulcers. Bloodsucking arthropods do not appear to be important. Because blood contains up to a million infectious doses per microlitre, invisible amounts of blood can transmit the infection. Virus carriers, of which there are about 200 million world-wide, play a major role in transmission.

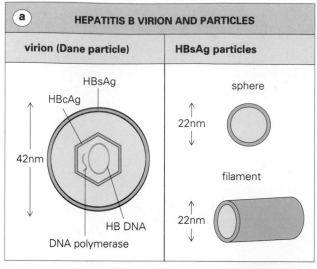

a   HEPATITIS B VIRION AND PARTICLES

virion (Dane particle)	HBsAg particles

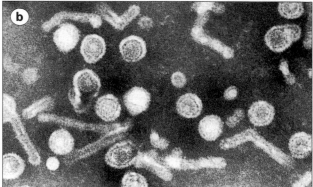

Fig. 25.49 During acute infection and in some carriers. 10^6–10^7 infectious (Dane) particles are present per microlitre of serum, and as many as 10^{12} HBsAg particles per microlitre. Electronmicrograph courtesy of JD Almeida.

HEPATITIS B ANTIGENS AND ANTIBODIES	
HBsAg	envelope (surface) antigen of HBV particle also occurs as free particle (spheres and filaments) in blood; indicates infectivity of blood
HBsAb	antibody to HBsAg; provides immunity; appears late (not in carriers)
HBcAg	antigen in core of HBV
HBcAb	antibody to HBcAg; appears early
HBeAg	antigen derived from core; indicates transmissibility
HBeAb	antibody to HBcAg; indicates low transmissibility

Fig. 25.50 Characteristics of hepatitis B antigens (Ag) and antibodies (Ab).

About 10% of infected individuals fail to eliminate the virus from the body and become virus carriers. The blood remains infectious, often for life, and although continuing liver damage can cause chronic hepatitis, the damage is often so slight that the carrier remains in good health.

Those with a more vigorous immune response to the infection clear the virus more rapidly, but tend to suffer a more severe illness. Immunodeficient patients develop a milder disease but are more likely to become carriers. There is also a marked age-related effect. In Taiwan, for instance, 90–95% of perinatally infected infants became carriers compared with 23% of those infected at 1-3 years of age and only 3% of those infected as university students.

In countries where infection in infancy and childhood is common (possibly because there is a high carrier rate in mothers), overall carrier rates are higher. Thus in West Africa where more than 70% of the population have antibodies, 12-20% are carriers, compared with western Europe and North America where up to 5% have antibodies and 0.9% are carriers. Sex is another factor, with males being more likely to become carriers than females.

Complications. These include:
• Cirrhosis, as a result of chronic active hepatitis
• Hepatocellular carcinoma. Hepatitis B carriers are 200-times more likely to get liver cancer than non-carriers. This is not seen until 20-30 years after infection. The

Clinical features and pathogenesis. After entering the body there is probably a preliminary period of virus replication in lymphoid tissue, following which the virus reaches the blood, and then the liver. This results in inflammation and necrosis. The virus is not directly cytopathic for liver cells, and much of the pathology is immune-mediated, for instance attack on infected liver cells by virus-specific cytotoxic T cells. It is not known why the incubation period is so lengthy (1–3 months). As the first virus-specific antibodies are formed there may be a brief, prodromal illness with rash and arthralgia. This is seen in 10–20% of icteric (jaundiced) patients and is due to the formation in the circulation of immune complexes between HBs and anti-HBs antibody, in antigen excess. (free antibody then being undetectable) These are deposited in the skin, joints, etc. (see Chapter 16).

As liver damage increases clinical signs of hepatitis appear (Fig. 25.51); the disease is generally more severe than in the case of hepatitis A. The immune response slowly becomes effective, virus replication is curtailed, and eventually, although sometimes not for many months, the blood becomes non-infectious. It is interesting to note that the host's alpha and beta interferon responses to the infection are specifically suppressed by the gene products of this resourceful viral parasite.

Hepadnaviruses

Other hepadnaviruses are found in woodchucks, ground squirrels and Pekin ducks. In each case the infection persists in the body, with HBs-like particles present in the blood, and chronic hepatitis and liver cancer as sequelae. These viruses often infect non-hepatic cells. In north-east USA for instance, 30% of woodchucks carry their own type of hepadnavirus and most develop liver cancer by later life. The virus replicates not only in liver cells but also in lymphoid cells in spleen, peripheral blood and thymus, a well as in pancreatic acinar cells and bile duct epithelium.

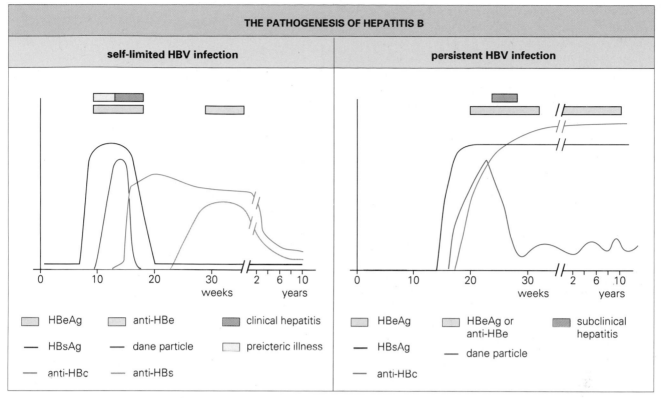

Fig.25.51 Hepatitis B. (a) Clinical and virological course of hepatitis B, with recovery. (b) Clinical and virological course in a carrier of hepatitis B. Results for hepatitis B virus DNA polymerase and DNA are not routinely available, but parallel those for HBeAg. Redrawn from WE Farrar *et al.*, 1992

cancer cells contain multiple integrated copies of hepatitis B viral DNA (integration takes place in infected liver cells after about two years or carriage) and this could be the carcinogenic factor. Alternatives would be the constant regenerative mitosis of liver cells in response to chronic infection, or the presence of an unknown cocarcinogen.

Laboratory diagnosis. HBsAg appears in serum during the incubation period and as the amount increases it signifies that infectious ('Dane') particles are also present (see Fig. 25.51). HBsAg levels generally fall and finally disappear during recovery and convalescence, but remain present in carriers. As HBsAg disappears, anti-HBs antibody becomes detectable and can be used for diagnosis. Anti-HBs is demonstrable in previously infected non-carriers.

Detection of HBeAg means that there are large amounts of virus in the blood, and after it has disappeared anti-HBe antibody becomes detectable.

Treatment and prevention. There is no standard antiviral therapy. However, large doses of alpha/beta interferon have been used to clear the virus, sometimes permanently, from carriers.

A safe, effective vaccine is available. It consists either of purified HBsAg prepared from the serum of carriers and chemically treated to kill any contaminating viruses, or genetically engineered HBsAg produced in yeasts. Two to three injections of vaccine generally give good protection, and vaccination is recommended, especially for those frequently exposed to blood or blood products (surgeons, dentists, multiply-transfused or dialysed patients, intravenous drug abusers, etc.). One problem is that up to 10% of normal individuals fail to produce the protective anti-HBs antibody, even when revaccinated. This could be because of genetically determined defects in the immune repertoire or because of induction of immune suppressor cells.

After accidental exposure to infection, hepatitis B immunoglobulin (HBIg) can be used to provide immediate passive protection. This is prepared from serum of haemophiliacs or others with high titres of antibody to HBs.

Hepatitis C

Hepatitis C virus (HCV) was discovered in 1989 as a cause of 90–95% of cases of transfusion-associated nonA-nonB hepatitis. It is a single-stranded RNA virus that is related to the flaviviruses and pestiviruses. The viral RNA was extracted from blood, a cDNA clone was made, and viral protein produced. Antibody to viral protein could then be tested for in sera. The discovery of hepatitis C virus was a *tour de force* in molecular virology; although it has been cloned it has still not been visualized or grown in the laboratory.

Transmission. The virus is present in blood (about 10^4–10^5 infectious doses per μl), and spreads in the same way as hepatitis B, by blood transfusion, intravenous drug abuse, and probably by both homosexual and heterosexual contact. There may be other methods of transfer, because infection also occurs in the general community with no evidence for parenteral exposure.

Clinical picture and pathogenesis. The incubation period is 2–4 months and the disease can be mild, but nothing is known of its pathogenesis. Virus is often detectable in the blood after recovery from illness, and carriers are a source of infection. In Europe and the USA up to 1% of apparently normal individuals have antibody and may be infectious.

Complications. About 50% patients develop chronic active hepatitis and 20% progress to cirrhosis. Infection also appears to be associated with liver cancer.

Laboratory diagnosis. If antibody is present it is possible that the virus is also present and the patient is infectious, but this is not necessarily the case. As tests for different viral antigens or for virus-specific cDNA by the polymerase chain reaction become routinely available, a clearer answer will be provided.

Treatment and prevention. Results of treatment with alpha interferon and ribavirin have been encouraging. There is no vaccine. Because hepatitis C virus is now the commonest cause of transfusion-associated hepatitis, blood donors are routinely tested for antibody to hepatitis C.

Hepatitis D

This is caused by hepatitis D virus (HDV or delta virus). It has a very small circular ssRNA genome and is a defective virus, so named because it can successfully multiply in a cell only when the cell is at the same time infected with hepatitis B virus (see Appendix). When it buds from the surface of a hepatic cell it acquires an envelope consisting of HBs (Fig 25.52). The HBs envelope makes the 35–37nm virus particle infectious by attaching it to hepatic cells.

Transmission. Infected blood contains very large amounts of virus (up to 10^{10} infectious doses per μl in experimentally infected chimpanzees), and transmission, which includes heterosexual transmission, is similar to HBV and HCV.

Clinical effects and pathogenesis. When HDV infection accompanies or is added to HBV infection the resulting disease is more severe than with HBV alone. Infection is uncommon in the UK and USA but common in parts of South America and Africa. World-wide it is present in about 5% of HBV carriers.

Diagnosis. The laboratory test is for HD antigen ('delta' antigen) or antibody to HD antigen. Hepatitis B surface antigen will be present although not necessarily at detectable levels.

Prevention. There is no vaccine, but vaccination against hepatitis B prevents infection with hepatitis D.

Hepatitis E

This disease, also known as enteric nonA-nonB hepatitis, is caused by a small ssRNA virus, probably a calicivirus. The virus is excreted in faeces, and spreads by the faecal–oral route. Although uncommon in developed countries, it occurs as a waterborne infection in India, and may be responsible for 50% of sporadic hepatitis in developing countries. The incubation period is 6–8 weeks. The disease

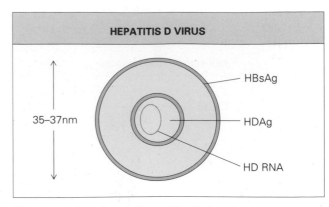

HEPATITIS D VIRUS

35–37nm

HBsAg

HDAg

HD RNA

Fig. 25.52 Structure of hepatitis D virus in serum.

is generally mild but is severe in pregnant women, with high mortality (up to 20%) involving disseminated intravascular coagulation, during the third trimester. The virus is eliminated from the body on recovery, and there are no carriers. The possible protective value of passively administered normal immunoglobulin is being investigated. Serological tests are also under development.

Hepatitis F

Around 5–10% of hepatitis cases known to be transmitted by blood transfusion cannot be attributed to a known virus. Perhaps there are even more human hepatitis virus waiting to be discovered.

Parasitic infections affecting the liver

Liver pathology in parasitic infections is most severe in patients suffering from infection with *Schistosoma mansoni*. Although the worms spend only a relatively short time in the liver itself before moving to the mesenteric vessels, eggs released by the females can be swept by the bloodstream into the hepatic circulation, becoming filtered out in the sinusoids. The inflammatory response to these trapped eggs is the primary cause of the complex changes that result in hepatomegaly, fibrosis and formation of varices (Fig. 25.53).

Whereas schistosomiasis is widespread in tropical and subtropical regions, other parasitic infections affecting the liver are much more restricted in their distribution. In Asia infections with the human liver fluke *Clonorchis sinensis* are acquired by eating fish infected with the metacercarial stage. Juvenile flukes, released in the intestine, move up the bile duct and attach to the duct epithelium, feeding on the cells and blood and tissue fluids. In heavy infections there is a pronounced inflammatory response, with proliferation and hyperplasia of the biliary epithelium, cholangitis, jaundice and liver enlargement as possible consequences. There may be an association with cholangiocarcinoma, but the evidence for this in humans is not strong.

A number of animal liver flukes can also establish in humans. These include species of *Opisthorchis* (in Asia and Eastern Europe) and the common liver fluke *Fasciola hepatica*. In general the symptoms associated with these infections are similar to those described for *C. sinensis*. Other parasitic infections associated with liver pathology are malaria, leishmaniasis, extra-intestinal amoebiasis, hydatid disease and ascariasis.

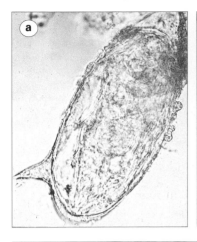

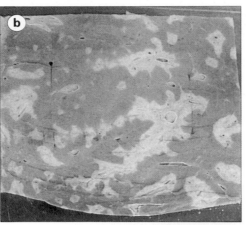

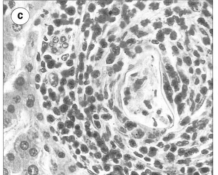

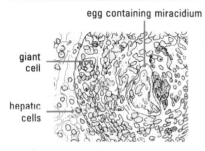

egg containing miracidium

giant cell

hepatic cells

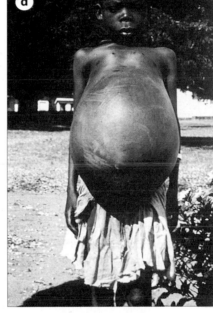

Fig. 25.53 The portal cirrhosis of *Schistoma mansoni* infection is the end result of huge numbers of granulomas formed around worm eggs deposited in the liver. In the related *S. haematobium* infection, a similar process occurs in the wall of the bladder. (a) Egg of *S. mansoni*. x400. (b) 'Pipe-stem cirrhosis in the liver as a result of coalescent calcified granulomata. (c) Cellular reaction around egg in liver. (a)-(c) Courtesy of R Muller. (d) Clinical schistosomiasis with massive hepatosplenomegaly and ascites due to portal obstruction. Courtesy of G Webbe.

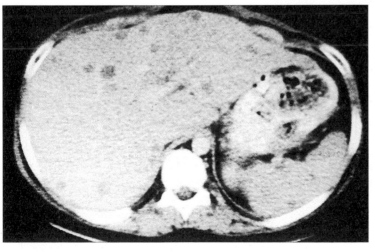

Fig. 25.54 Multiple pyogenic liver abscesses due to *Pseudomonas aeruginosa*. Courtesy of N Holland.

Liver abscesses

Entamoeba histolytica can escape from the gastrointestinal tract and cause disease in other sites, including the liver (see above). However the term 'amoebic liver abscess' is not strictly accurate because the lesions formed in the liver consists of necrotic liver tissue rather than pus. True liver abscesses, i.e. walled-off lesions containing organisms and dead or dying polymorphs (pus), are frequently polymicrobial containing a mixed flora of aerobic and anaerobic bacteria (Fig. 25.54). Lesions caused by *Echinococcus granulosus* in hydatid disease may become secondarily infected with bacteria The source of infection may be local to the lesion or at another body site, but is most often undiagnosed. Broad-spectrum antimicrobial therapy is required to cover both aerobes and anaerobes.

Biliary tract infections

Although infection is not often the primary cause of disease in the biliary tract, it is a very common complication. Many patients with gallstones obstructing the biliary system develop infective complications caused by organisms from the normal gastrointestinal flora, such as enterobacteria and anaerobes. Local infection may result in cholangitis and subsequently liver abscesses, or invade the bloodstream to cause septicaemia and generalized infection. Removing the underlying obstruction in the biliary tree is a prerequisite to successful therapy. Antibacterial therapy is usually broad-spectrum, covering both aerobes and anaerobes.

Peritonitis and intra-abdominal sepsis

The peritoneal cavity is normally sterile but is in constant danger of becoming contaminated by bacteria discharged through perforations in the gut wall arising from trauma (accidental or surgical) or infection. The outcome of peritoneal contamination depends on the volume of the inoculum (a millilitre of gut contents contains many millions of organisms), and the ability of the local defences to wall off and destroy the organisms.

Although the gut contains an enormous range of different bacterial species, peritonitis and intra-abdominal abscesses are usually caused by only a few, primarily strict anaerobes of the *Bacteroides fragilis* group mixed with facultative anaerobes such as *E. coli*. It is unusual to find a single species causing the infection. *Mycobacterium tuberculosis* and *Actinomyces* may also cause intra-peritoneal infection (Fig. 25.55).

Peritonitis usually begins as an acute inflammation in the abdomen and progresses to the formation of localized intra-abdominal abscesses. In the absence of appropriate antibiotic therapy the infection is frequently fatal and even with proper treatment, mortality remains at 1–5%. Antibiotic therapy must be chosen to cover both aerobic and anaerobic pathogens. Suitable regimens include a combination of gentamicin (for the aerobic Gram-negative rods), ampicillin (for enterococci) and metronidazole (to cover the anaerobes). Mycobacterial infection requires

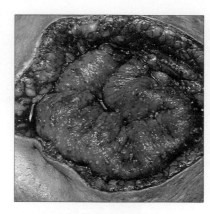

Fig. 25.55 Tuberculous peritonitis. Oedematous bowel with multiple white lesions on the peritoneal surface. Courtesy of M Goldman.

specific anti-tuberculous therapy (see Chapter 35); actinomycosis responds well to prolonged treatment with penicillin.

SUMMARY

The length and complexity of the gastrointestinal tract is matched by the variety of microorganisms that can be acquired by this route, causing damage locally or invading to cause disseminated disease. Diarrhoeal disease is a major cause of morbidity and death in malnourished populations in the developing world, and will only be combatted successfully when adequate public health measures are in place. Meanwhile in the developed world, diarrhoeal disease is still common, and causes severe illness in the very young and the very old.

Certain infections (e.g. typhoid) are initiated in the gastrointestinal tract but cause systemic disease, and hepatitis A is acquired and excreted by the intestinal route. The remaining members of the hepatitis 'alphabet' are also dealt with in this chapter. Infections can arise not only by the ingestion of pathogens from an external source but also from the normal flora of the gastrointestinal tract, if it escapes through accidental or man-made breaches of the mucosa, to cause intra-abdominal sepsis.

Further Reading

Farrar WE *et al. Infectious Diseases.* 2nd edn. London: Gower Medical Publishing, 1992.

Field M, Rao MC, Chang FB. Intestinal electrolyte transport and diarrhoeal disease. *N Engl J Med* 1989; **321:** 800–806.

Gross RJ. The pathogenesis of *Escherichia coli* diarrhoea. *Rev Med Microbiol* 1991; **2:** 37–44.

Howe GM. *Man, environment and disease in Britain.* London: Penguin Books, 1976.

Kapikian AZ, *et al.* Prospects for development of a rotavirus vaccine against rotavirus diarrhoea in infants and young children. *Rev Infect Dis* 1989; **II (Suppl 3):** S539.

Lemon SM. Type A viral hepatitis: new developments in an old disease. *N Engl J Med* 1985; **313:** 1059–1067.

McMahon BL, *et al.* Acute hepatitis B infection: relation of age to the clinical expression of disease and subsequent development of the carrier state. *J Infect Dis* 1985; **151:** 599–603.

World Health Organization. *Readings on Diarrhoea.* Student Manual. (WHO/CDD/SER/90,13) Geneva, 1990.

26 OBSTETRIC AND PERINATAL INFECTIONS

Contents

INTRODUCTION

During pregnancy certain infections in the mother can be more severe or can reactivate. In addition a novel set of potentially susceptible tissues appear, including the foetus, the placenta and the lactating mammary glands. On the other hand, the placenta acts as an effective barrier, protecting the foetus from most circulating microorganisms, along with the fetal membranes, which serve to shield the foetus from microorganisms in the genital tract. Perforation of the amniotic sac, for instance, at a late stage of pregnancy, often results in fetal infection.

A few infections occur at around the time of birth. The infant may be directly exposed during passage down a birth canal that is infected with gonococci, chlamydia or herpes simplex virus, or is contaminated with faecal bacteria from the mother. In the immediate post-natal period, the mother's blood (hepatitis B virus) or milk (HTLV1) can also be a source of infection. Here we describe infections that occur during pregnancy and around the time of birth, and discuss their effects on the mother, the foetus, and the neonate.

INFECTIONS OCCURRING IN PREGNANCY

The foetus may be considered as an immunologically incompatible transplant which must not be rejected by the mother. Reasons for the failure to reject the foetus include absence or low density of MHC antigens on placental cells, covering of antigens with blocking antibody, and subtle defects in maternal immune responses. A severe or generalized immunosuppression in the mother would be undesirable because it would mean potentially disastrous susceptibility to infectious disease. Certain infections, however, are known to be more severe (Fig. 26.1) and certain persistent infections reactivate (Fig. 26.2) during pregnancy. The hormonal changes that accompany pregnancy can also increase susceptibility. The picture is further complicated when there is malnutrition, which in itself impairs

INFECTIONS THAT ARE MORE SEVERE DURING PREGNANCY	
infection	**comments**
Malaria	?depressed cell-mediated immunity
Viral hepatitis	?additional metabolic burden of pregnancy
Influenza	higher mortality during pandemics
Poliomyelitis	paralysis more common
Urinary tract infections	cystitis, pyelonephritis more common; atony of bladder and ureter leads to less effective flushing, emptying
Candida	vulvovaginitis
Listeriosis	influenza-like illness
Coccidiomycosis	leading cause of maternal mortality in endemic areas in SW USA and Latin America

Fig. 26.1 The effect of pregnancy on the severity of infectious disease.

INFECTIONS THAT CAN REACTIVATE DURING PREGNANCY	
infection	**phenomenon**
Polyomavirus (JC, BK)	viruses appear in urine
Cytomegalovirus	increased shedding from cervix virus in milk of nursing mother
Herpes simplex virus	increased replication in cervical region
Epstein–Barr virus	increased antibody titres increased shedding of virus in oropharynx

Fig. 26.2 Reactivation of persistent infections during pregnancy.

CONGENITAL (*IN UTERO*) INFECTIONS	
microorganism	**effects**
Rubella virus	congenital rubella
Cytomegalovirus	congenital CMV – deafness, mental retardation
Human immuno-deficiency virus	congenital infection – childhood AIDS; about 1 in 5 infants born to infected mothers are infected *in utero*
Varicella-zoster virus	skin lesions; musculo-skeletal, CNS abnormalities severe disease in newborn if mother infected too late in pregnancy to have provided transplacental IgG for foetus*
Herpes simplex virus	neonatal herpes simplex, often disseminated – infection *in utero* is rare
Hepatitis B virus	congenital hepatitis B – persistent infection*†
Treponema pallidum	congenital syphilis – classical syndrome
Toxoplasma gondii	congenital toxoplasmosis
Listeria monocytogenes	congenital listeriosis – pneumonia septicaemia, meningitis*
Mycobacterium leprae	congenital infection common in mothers with lepromatous leprosy

* infection also occurs during and immediately after birth
† protection of newborn by hepatitis B vaccine plus specific immunoglobulin is probably less effective after *in utero* infection

Fig. 26.3 Maternal infections that are transmitted to the foetus. Congenitally infected babies may be symptomless, especially in CMV infection. They are often small, or fail to thrive or show detectable abnormalities later in childhood. In all cases the baby remains infected, often for long periods, and may infect others.

COMPARISON BETWEEN TERATOGENIC VIRUSES AND OTHER TERATOGENS		
	viral teratogens (e.g. rubella)	**other teratogens (e.g. drugs, radiation)**
Critical stages of susceptibility during pregnancy (organogenesis)	+	+
Foetal death a possible outcome	+	+
Maternal effects minimal or absent	+	+
Cause retarded foetal growth	+	+
Increase in frequency of naturally occurring abnormalities	–	+
Influence of genetic factors in mother/foetus	–	+

Fig. 26.4 Teratogenic viruses show many similarities to other types of teratogen.

isms generally have more subtle, non-lethal effects, interfering with fetal development or causing lesions, so that a live but damaged baby is born.

CONGENITAL INFECTIONS

After primary infection during pregnancy, certain microorganisms enter the blood, establish infection in the placenta, and then invade the foetus. The foetus sometimes dies, leading to abortion, but when the infection is less severe, as in the case of a relatively non-cytopathic virus, or when it is partially controlled by the maternal IgG response, the foetus survives. It may then be born with a congenital infection, often showing malformations or other pathological changes. The infant is generally small and fails to thrive. It produces specific antibodies, but often, for instance with cytomegalovirus (CMV), fails to generate an adequate virus-specific cell-mediated immune response, remaining infected for a long period. Hence, the lesions may progress after birth. It is a striking feature of these infections that they are generally mild or unnoticed in the mother.

Important causes of congenital infections are shown in figure 26.3. Viruses that induce fetal malformations (i.e. act as teratogens) share certain characteristics with other teratogens, such as drugs or radiation (Fig. 26.4). The foetus tends to show similar responses to different infectious agents (hepatosplenomegaly, encephalitis, eye lesions, low birth weight), and the diagnosis is difficult on purely clinical grounds. Most of these infections (rubella, CMV, syphilis) can also, at times, kill the foetus. They generally follow primary infection of the mother during pregnancy, so that their incidence depends on the proportion of non-immune females of child-bearing age. Routine

host defences by weakening immune responses, decreasing metabolic reserves and interfering with the integrity of epithelial surfaces.

Once the foetus in infected it is exquisitely susceptible. Its immune defences are poor; indeed if it were able to generate a vigorous response to maternal antigens, a troublesome graft-versus-host reaction could be unleashed. IgM and IgA antibodies are not produced in significant amounts until the second half of pregnancy, there is no IgG antibody synthesis, and cell-mediated immune responses are poorly developed or absent, with inadequate production of the necessary cytokines.

Most microorganisms have sufficient destructive activity to kill the foetus, leading to spontaneous abortion, or stillbirth. Here, our interests focus on the few microorganisms that can overcome the placental barrier by infecting it, so that the infection then spreads to the foetus. These organ-

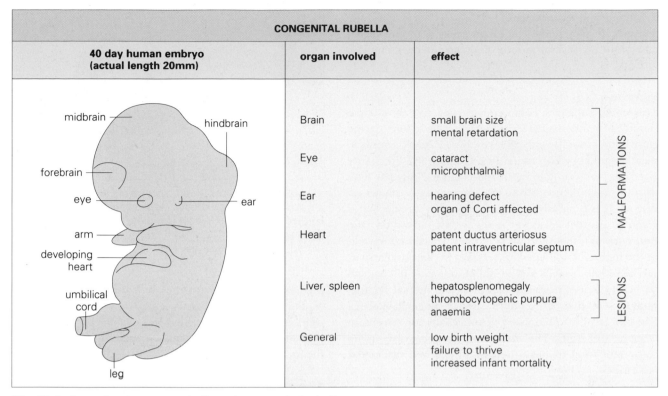

CONGENITAL RUBELLA		
40 day human embryo (actual length 20mm)	**organ involved**	**effect**
	Brain	small brain size mental retardation
	Eye	cataract microphthalmia
	Ear	hearing defect organ of Corti affected
	Heart	patent ductus arteriosus patent intraventricular septum
	Liver, spleen	hepatosplenomegaly thrombocytopenic purpura anaemia
	General	low birth weight failure to thrive increased infant mortality

(MALFORMATIONS: Brain, Eye, Ear, Heart; LESIONS: Liver, spleen)

Fig. 26.5 Organ involvement and effects in congenital rubella.

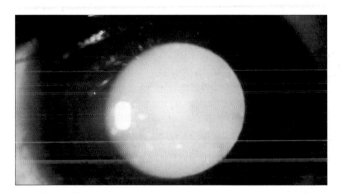

Fig. 26.6 Cataract in congenital rubella. Courtesy of RJ Marsh and S Ford.

antenatal screening for antibodies to rubella, syphilis and HIV identifies susceptible (rubella) and infected (syphilis, HIV) mothers. In the case of CMV, reactivation of an earlier infection can occur during pregnancy and lead to fetal infection. Better control of the infection by maternal antibody under these circumstances means that the baby is generally born normal. Congenital syphilis can also result from earlier, untreated infection of the mother.

There is no good evidence to suggest that maternal mumps, influenza or poliovirus infection during pregnancy leads to harmful effects in the foetus. The human parvovirus (see Chapter 28), however, occasionally causes foetal damage or death (in about 10% of cases) following maternal infection in early pregnancy. The infected foetus develops severe anaemia with pallor, ascites and hepatosplenomegaly (hydrops foetalis), following extensive growth of virus in the liver and elsewhere.

Congenital rubella

The foetus is particularly susceptible when maternal infection occurs during the first three months of pregnancy. At this time the heart, brain, eyes and ears are being formed and the infecting virus interferes with their development. If the foetus survives it may show certain abnormalities (Fig. 26.5). About 25% of congenitally infected children eventually develop insulin-dependent diabetes mellitus, but rubella is a very uncommon cause of this disease. The virus replicates in the pancreas.

The classical features of congenital rubella infection were first described by Gregg in Australia in 1941, long before the virus had been isolated and characterized. Not all foetuses are affected; in one study detectable congenital defects were seen in 15.3% of cases when maternal rubella occurred in the first month of pregnancy, 24.6% when in the second month, 17.5% in the third month and 6.5% in the fourth month. The figure for the first month is low because foetal death is a common sequel at this stage. Rubella causes malformations by a primary effect on blood vessels in the developing organs, and also a virus-mediated inhibition of mitosis which contributes to the reduced number of cells and the small size of rubella babies.

Diagnosis

Clinical appearances include low birth weight, eye (Fig. 26.6) and heart lesions. Effects on the brain and ears may not become detectable until later in childhood in the form of mental retardation and deafness. There is a 15% mortality in infants showing signs of infection at birth, often associated with hypogammaglobulinaemia.

Infected foetuses produce their own IgM molecules to rubella virus, which can be detected in cord blood. Maternal IgG antibodies are also present and, together with interferons, help to control the spread of infection in the foetus. Virus can be isolated from the infant's throat or urine.

Treatment and management

There is no treatment. The infant sheds virus into throat and urine for several months and can infect susceptible individuals.

Prevention

Congenital rubella is completely preventable by vaccination with live attenuated virus vaccine. This is done during childhood, usually with the combined MMR (mumps, measles and rubella) vaccine (see Chapter 36). Pregnancy is a contra-indication to vaccination, and the only safe time during reproductive life is the immediate post-partum period. This is an interesting example of a vaccine that is given to protect an as yet non-existent individual (the future foetus), the infection being only subclinical or mild in the mother. Until effective vaccines became available in the late 1960s, rubella was an important cause of congenital heart disease, deafness, blindness and mental retardation. In 1990 there were only 5 cases of congenital rubella and less than 30 pregnancy terminations for rubella in England and Wales. The virus continues to circulate in the community and damage foetuses in less well vaccinated countries.

Congenital cytomegalovirus infection

Clinical features of congenital CMV (see also Chapter 29) include mental retardation, spasticity, eye abnormalities, hearing defects, hepatosplenomegaly, thrombocytopenic purpura and anaemia (Fig. 26.7). Mothers that develop a poor T cell proliferative response to CMV antigens are more likely to infect their foetus.

After primary maternal infection during pregnancy about 40% of foetuses are infected and 5% of these show signs at birth. It is not known whether the foetus is especially vulnerable at certain stages of pregnancy. The foetus is also infected following pregnancy reactivation of CMV in immune (sero-positive) mothers, but fetal damage is then uncommon. As many as 1–2% of infants born in the USA are infected (less in the UK) and up to about 10% of these are symptomatic with up to a million infectious doses of virus present per ml of urine. Deafness and mental retardation may not be detectable until later in childhood.

Diagnosis and prevention

Diagnosis is by detecting CMV-specific IgM antibodies in cord blood, and more reliably by virus isolation from throat or urine. Live attenuated vaccines are presently being developed (AD169 and Towne strains); in preliminary studies, none of those who became pregnant after vaccination transmitted the virus to the infant.

Congenital syphilis

As a result of routine serological screening for syphilis in antenatal clinics and treatment with penicillin (see Chapter 24), this condition is now rare but is more common in developing countries. Treatment of the mother before the fourth month of pregnancy prevents foetal infection.

Clinical features in the infant include rhinitis (snuffles), skin and mucosal lesions, hepatosplenomegaly, lym-

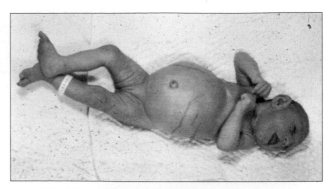

Fig. 26.7 Microcephaly with associated severe psychomotor retardation and hepatosplenomegaly in congenital cytomegalovirus infection. Courtesy of WE Farrar.

phadenopathy, abnormalities of bones, teeth, cartilage (saddle shaped nose), etc. Pregnancy often masks the early signs of syphilis, but antibodies will be present in the mother, and *Treponema pallidum*-specific IgM antibodies in the foetus.

Congenital toxoplasmosis

This results from acute, asymptomatic infection by *Toxoplasma gondii* during pregnancy. About one-third of normal adults are seropositive. Clinical features in the infant include convulsions, microcephaly, chorioretinitis, hepatosplenomegaly, jaundice, with later hydrocephaly, mental retardation and defective vision (see Chapter 21). There are often no detectable abnormalities at birth but signs (e.g. chorioretinitis) generally appear within a few years. The incidence of foetal infection and damage (leading to abortion, stillbirth or disease in the newborn) increases from 14% when maternal infection is in the first trimester to 59% when in the third trimester.

Diagnosis, treatment and prevention

Toxoplasma-specific IgM antibodies may be detected in cord blood. Treatment of a pregnant woman or an infected infant is with spiramycin, or (with care) sulphonamide or pyrimethamine.

There is no vaccine. Prevention is by avoidance of primary infection (via cysts from cat faeces or in lightly cooked meat) during pregnancy.

Congenital HIV infection

At least 1 in 5 of infants born to HIV infected mothers are infected *in utero*. They show poor weight gain, susceptibility to sepsis, developmental delays, lymphocytic pneumonitis, oral thrush, enlarged lymph nodes, hepatosplenomegaly, diarrhoea, pneumonia, and some develop AIDS within the first year. Infection may also take place during or shortly after birth.

Laboratory diagnosis is at present difficult (see Chapter 24). If IgG antibodies are present they will be of maternal origin and can persist for at least a year; there is no satisfactory test for HIV-specific IgM antibodies, which would signify *in utero* infection. Reliable blood tests for viral antigens or nucleic acid sequences would solve this problem.

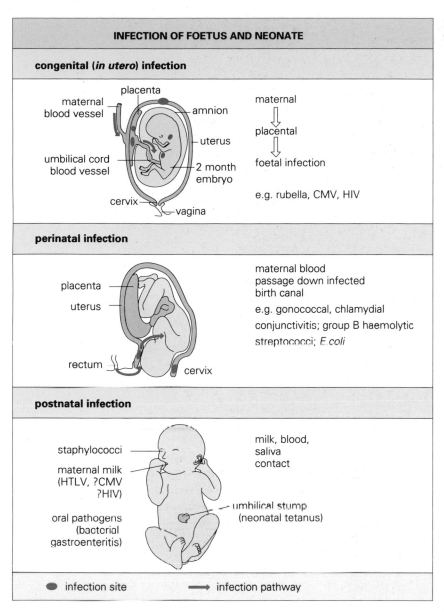

INFECTION OF FOETUS AND NEONATE

congenital (*in utero*) infection

maternal blood vessel
placenta
amnion
umbilical cord blood vessel
uterus
2 month embryo
cervix
vagina

maternal
⇩
placental
⇩
foetal infection

e.g. rubella, CMV, HIV

perinatal infection

placenta
uterus
rectum
cervix

maternal blood passage down infected birth canal

e.g. gonococcal, chlamydial conjunctivitis; group B haemolytic streptococci; *E. coli*

postnatal infection

staphylococci
maternal milk (HTLV, ?CMV ?HIV)
oral pathogens (bacterial gastroenteritis)
umbilical stump (neonatal tetanus)

milk, blood, saliva contact

● infection site   → infection pathway

Fig. 26.8 Routes of infection in the foetus and neonate.

Congenital and neonatal listeriosis

Aetiology and transmission
Listeria monocytogenes is a small Gram-positive rod, which is motile and beta-haemolytic. It is distributed world-wide in a great variety of animals including cattle, pigs, rodents and birds. Transmission to man is by contact with infected animals and their faeces, or by consuming unpasteurized milk or soft cheeses. Up to 70% of people may carry listeria in the gut for short periods, without disease. Unlike most bacteria, *Listeria* can grow at regular refrigeration temperatures (e.g. 6°C). The bacteria also occur in plants and in soil, and infection can be due to eating contaminated vegetables. *Listeria* are not a common cause of disease; in England and Wales in 1989 there were 67 reported cases of listeriosis, 36 of them materno-foetal or neonatal, and in 1990 this fell to 24 cases, with only 5 materno-foetal or neonatal.

Clinical features and pathogenesis
Listeria monocytogenes in the pregnant woman causes a mild, influenza-like illness or is asymptomatic. But there is a bac-

teraemia, which leads to infection of the placenta and then the foetus. This may cause abortion, premature delivery, neonatal septicemia, pneumonia, with abscesses or granulomas. The infant can also be infected shortly after birth, for instance from other babies or from hospital staff, and this may lead to a meningitic illness.

Diagnosis, treatment and prevention
Listeria monocytogenes is isolated from blood cultures, CSF or skin lesions. Treatment is with penicillin or ampicillin. There are no vaccines. Although pregnant women should not be exposed to infected material, the exact source of infection is generally unknown.

INFECTIONS OCCURRING AROUND THE TIME OF BIRTH

Effects on the foetus and neonate
The routes of infection of the foetus and neonate are shown in figure 26.8. Viral infections (rubella, CMV) are generally less damaging to the foetus when maternal infection takes place late in pregnancy, but primary infection

NEONATAL INFECTIONS ACQUIRED DURING PASSAGE DOWN INFECTED BIRTH CANAL		
infectious agent	**site of infection**	**phenomenon**
Neisseria gonorrhoeae	conjunctiva	neonatal conjunctivitis (ophthalmia neonatorum)
Chlamydia trachomatis	conjunctiva, respiratory tract	neonatal conjunctivitis (ophthalmia neonatorum) neonatal pneumonia
Herpes simplex virus	?	neonatal herpetic infection*
Genital papillomavirus	respiratory tract	laryngeal warts in young children
Group B streptococci** Gram-negative bacilli (*E. coli* etc.)	respiratory tract	septicaemia; death if not treated
Candida albicans	?	neonatal oral thrush

* although preventable by caesarean section, it is often difficult to detect maternal genital infection; infants can be treated prophylactically with acyclovir

** up to 30% of women carry these bacteria in vagina or rectum

Fig. 26.9 Neonatal infections acquired during passage down an infected birth canal.

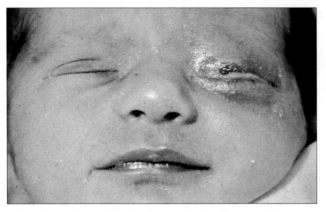

Fig. 26.10 Gonococcal ophthalmic neonatorum. Signs appear 2–5 days after birth. The inflammation and oedema is more severe than with chlamydia infection. Courtesy of JS Bingham.

with varicella-zoster virus at this time can lead to limb deformities and other severe lesions in the newborn. Bacterial infections originating from the vagina and perineum are more important, occurring especially when foetal membranes have been ruptured for more than 1–2 days, and resulting in chorioamnionitis, maternal fever, premature delivery and stillbirth. Infants of low birth weight (less than 1500g) tend to be more severely effected. Bacteria involved include group B haemolytic streptococci, *E. coli, Klebsiella, Proteus, Bacteroides,* staphylococci, *Mycoplasma hominis.* These infections may also be acquired after delivery, to give later onset disease. Neonatal septicaemia often progresses to meningitis (see Chapter 27)

and this is frequently fatal unless treated. Clinical diagnosis is difficult because the infant shows generalized signs such as respiratory distress, poor feeding, diarrhoea and vomiting, but early diagnosis is essential and requires emergency treatment. 'Blind' antibiotic treatment should be started as soon as cerebrospinal fluid (Gram-stain and culture) and blood samples have been taken.

The foetus can also be infected during labour by direct contact as it passes down an infected birth canal (Fig. 26.9). For instance, cutaneous lesions of herpes simplex may develop a week after delivery, with generalized infection and severe CNS involvement, and both gonococci (Fig. 26.10), chlamydia or staphylococci (see Chapter 21) can wipe the eye to cause ophthalmia neonatorum. Maternal blood can be a source of hepatitis B virus infection during or shortly after birth and 80–90% infants from HBV carrier mothers become infected and then carry the virus. This is preventable by giving the vaccine plus specific immunoglobulin to the newborn.

Human milk may contain rubella virus, CMV, HTLV1, and (probably) HIV. Virus titres are generally low, and, except in the case of HTLV1, milk is not thought to be an important source of infection. But it makes sense to pasteurize milk in human milk banks, just as we pasteurize cow's milk.

Effects on the mother

After delivery (or abortion) a large area of damaged, vulnerable uterine tissue is exposed to infection. Puerpural sepsis (childbed fever) was a major cause of maternal death in Europe in the 19th Century. In 1843 Oliver Wendell Holmes made the unpopular suggestion that it

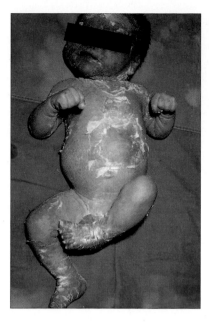

Fig. 26.11 Staphylococcal scalded skin syndrome. There are large areas of epidermal loss where bullae have burst. Courtesy of L Brown.

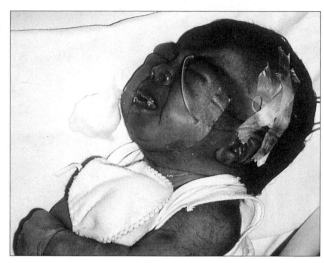

Fig. 26.12 Tetanus. Risus sardonicus in a newborn infant. Courtesy of WE Farrar.

was carried on the hands of doctors, and four years later Ignaz Semmelweiss in Vienna showed how it could be prevented if doctors and midwives washed their hands before attending a woman in labour and practised aseptic techniques. Group A beta-haemolytic streptococci were major culprits. Other possible organisms include anaerobes such as *Clostridium perfringens* or *Bacteroides*, and *E. coli*. The streptococci came from the nose, throat or skin of hospital attendants whereas the others were derived from the mother's own faecal flora. Puerpural sepsis, which carried up to 10% mortality until the 1930s, is now, like septic abortion, less common in developed countries. Predisposing factors include premature rupture of the membranes, instrumentation and retained fragments of membrane or placenta. Where there is postnatal pyrexia or offensive discharge, high vaginal swabs and blood cultures should be taken.

Miscellaneous neonatal infections

Infection may reach the newborn infant during the first week or two after birth, rather than during delivery. Group B beta-haemolytic streptococci and Gram-negative bacilli (see above) can still cause serious infection at this time, often with meningitis. Herpes simplex may come from cold sores or herpetic witlows of attending adults. Staphylococcal infection from noses and fingers of adult carriers may cause staphylococcal conjunctivitis or 'sticky eye' (see Chapter 21), skin sepsis in the neonate, and sometimes the staphylococcal 'scalded skin' syndrome (Fig. 26.11) due to a specific 'epidermolytic' staphylococcal toxin. During the first week or two of life the nose of the neonate becomes colonized with *Staphylococcus aureus*

which can enter the nipple during feeding to cause a breast abscess. These infections are preventable when hospital staff pay vigorous attention to hand washing, aseptic techniques, and so on.

The umbilical stump, especially in developing countries, may by infected with *Clostridium tetani*, resulting in neonatal tetanus (Fig. 26.12). It can be prevented by immunizing mothers with tetanus toxoid. In developing countries gastroenteritis is an important problem during the neonatal period as well as during infancy. Diarrhoea leading to water and electrolyte depletion is particularly serious in low birth weight infants. Causative agents include strains of *E. coli*, salmonella etc., rather than rotaviruses. Breast feeding gives some protection by supplying specific antibodies and other less well-characterized protective factors.

SUMMARY

A small number of infections can be more severe when they occur during pregnancy, and there can be reactivation of certain persistent infection. The few infections that are able to pass to the foetus and cause damage are generally (rubella, CMV, toxoplasmosis) but not always (syphilis) mild or subclinical in the mother. The foetus may die, but more importantly may survive and be born infected, showing characteristic malformations. Rubella is the only congenital infection that can at present be prevented by vaccination.

Infection during birth or shortly afterwards can cause local disease (conjunctivitis due to gonococci or chlamydia), or occasionally severe life-threatening illness (*E. coli* meningitis, herpes simplex virus infection).

Further Reading ──

Preece P, Pearl K, Peckham C. Congenital cytomegalovirus. *Arch Dis Child* 1984; **59:** 1120–1126.

Scott. GB, Hutto. C, Makuch RW *et al.* Survival in children with perinatally acquired human immunodeficiency virus type I infection. *N Engl J Med* 1989; **311:** 1791–1796.

Kovar IZ. Neonatal and pediatric infections. *Curr Opin Infect Dis* 1990; **3:** 479–500.

27 CENTRAL NERVOUS SYSTEM INFECTIONS

Contents

INTRODUCTION

The brain and spinal cord are protected from mechanical pressures or deformations by enclosure in rigid containers (skull and vertebral column), which also act as barriers to the spread of infection. The blood vessels and nerves that traverse the walls of the skull and vertebral column are the main routes of invasion. Blood-borne invasion is the commonest (e.g. poliovirus, meningococcus), while invasion via peripheral nerves is less common (e.g. herpes simplex, varicella-zoster, rabies viruses). Local invasion from infected ears or sinuses, or from local injury or congenital defects, such as spina bifida, also occurs; invasion from the olfactory tract (amoebic meningitis) is rare. Here we discuss the main routes of CNS invasion by microorganisms (see also Chapter 10) and the body's response, followed by a more detailed discussion of the diseases that result.

INVASION OF THE CENTRAL NERVOUS SYSTEM

Blood-borne invasion

Blood-borne invasion takes place across the blood–brain barrier to give encephalitis, or the blood–cerebrospinal fluid (CSF) barrier to given meningitis (Fig. 27.1). The blood–brain barrier consists of tightly joined endothelial cells surrounded by glial processes, while the brain–CSF barrier, at the choroid plexus, consists of endothelium, with fenestrations, and tightly joined choroid plexus epithelial cells. Microbes can traverse these barriers by: 1) growing across, infecting the cells that comprise the barrier; 2) being passively transported across in intracellular vacuoles; or 3) carried across by infected white blood cells.

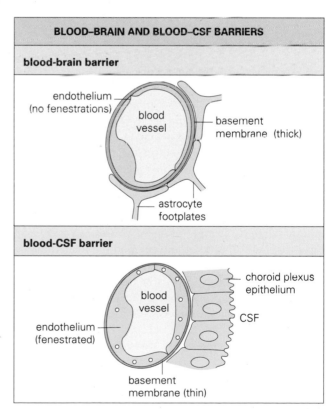

Fig. 27.1 Structures of the blood–brain and blood–CSF barriers.

In the case of viruses examples of each mechanism are known. Poliovirus, for instance, invades the CNS across the blood–brain barrier. After oral ingestion of virus, a complex stepwise series of events provides the mechanism for CNS invasion (Fig. 27.2). Poliovirus also invades the

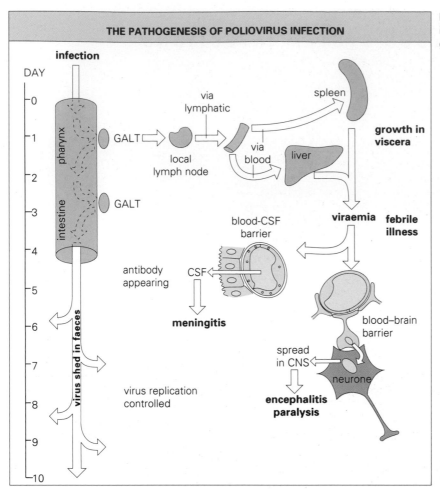

Fig. 27.2 The mechanism of CNS invasion by poliovirus. GALT, gut-associated lymphoid tissue

meninges after localizing in vascular endothelial cells, and can cross the blood–CSF barrier. Mumps virus behaves in the same way, as do circulating *Haemophilus influenzae*, meningococci or pneumococci. Once infection has reached the meninges and CSF, the brain substance can in turn be invaded if passage across the pia takes place. In poliomyelitis, for instance, a meningitic phase often precedes encephalitis and paralysis.

CNS invasion, however, is a rare event because most microorganisms fail to pass from blood to CNS across the natural barriers. A large variety of viruses can grow and cause disease if introduced directly into the brain, but circulating viruses generally fail to invade, and CNS involvement by polio, mumps, rubella or measles viruses is seen only in a very small proportion of infected individuals. The factors which determine such CNS invasion are unknown.

Invasion via peripheral nerves

Invasion of the CNS via peripheral nerves takes place in several viral infections. Herpes simplex and varicella-zoster viruses present in skin or mucosal lesions (see Chapter 28) travel up axons using the normal retrograde transport mechanisms that can move virus particles (as well as foreign molecules such as tetanus toxin) at the rate of about 200mm per day, to reach dorsal root ganglia. Rabies virus introduced into muscle or subcutaneous tissues by the bite of a rabid animal, infects muscle fibres and muscle spindles after binding of the virus to the nicotinic acetylcholine receptor. It then enters peripheral nerves and

travels up to the CNS, to reach glial cells and neurones, where it multiplies.

THE RESPONSE TO INVASION

The response to invading viruses is reflected by an increase in lymphocytes (mostly T cells) and monocytes in the CSF (Fig. 27.3). A slight increase in protein also occurs, the CSF remaining clear. This is termed 'aseptic' meningitis. The response to pyogenic bacteria shows a more spectacular and more rapid increase in polymorphonuclear leucocytes and proteins (Fig. 27.4), so that the CSF becomes visibly turbid. This is termed 'septic' meningitis. Certain slower growing or less pyogenic microorganisms induce less dramatic changes, such as in tuberculous or listerial meningitis.

In the CNS itself viruses can infect neural cells, sometimes showing a marked preference. Polio and rabies viruses, for instance, invade neurones whereas JC virus invades oligodendrocytes. Because there is very little extracellular space, spread is mostly direct from cell to cell, along established nervous pathways. Invading bacteria and protozoa generally induce more dramatic inflammatory events which limit local spread, so that infection is soon localized to form abscesses.

The pathological consequences of CNS infection depend on the microorganism. Viruses induce perivascular infiltration of lymphocytes and monocytes, sometimes, as in the case of polio, with direct damage to infected cells.

Fig. 27.3 Changes in cerebrospinal fluid in response to invading microbes.

CEREBROSPINAL FLUID CHANGES DURING CNS INFECTION				
	cells per μL	protein mg/dl	glucose mg/dl	causes
Normal	0–5	15–45	45–85	—
Septic (purulent) meningitis	200–20 000 (mainly neutrophils)	high (>100)	<45	bacteria amoebae brain abscess
Aseptic* meningitis or meningo-encephalitis	100–1000 (mainly mononuclear)	moderately high (50–100)	normal**	viruses tuberculosis leptospira fungi brain abscess partly treated bacterial meningitis

* Aseptic because the CSF is sterile on regular bacteriological culture

** low (<45) in the case of tuberculosis, fungi, leptospira

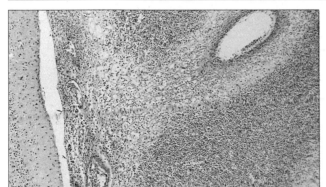

Fig. 27.4 Bacterial meningitis. Exudate of acute inflammatory cells in the subarachnoid space. H & E stain. Courtesy of P Garen.

The pathogenesis of viral encephalomyelitis is illustrated on page 27.10. Associated immune responses not only to viral but often to host CNS components play a part (see 'post vaccinial encephalitis', below). Infiltrating B cells produce antibody to the invading microorganism and T cells react with microbial antigens to release cytokines that attract and activate other T cells and macrophages. The pathological condition evolves over the course of several days, and occasionally, when partly controlled by host defences, (e.g. subacute sclerosing panencephalitis) over the course of years. Bacteria cause more rapidly evolving pathological changes, with local responses to bacterial antigens and toxins playing an important part.

In all cases, a degree of inflammation and oedema that would be trivial in striated muscle, skin or liver may be life threatening when it occurs in the vulnerable 'closed box' containing the lepto-meninges, brain and spinal cord. It may be several weeks after clinical recovery that cellular infiltrations are removed and histological appearances are restored to normal.

From the point of view of a parasitic microorganism that needs to be transmitted to a fresh host, invasion of the CNS is generally foolish, or at least unnecessary. The only occasions on which it makes sense are:

- When dorsal root ganglion neurones are invaded, as an essential step in establishing latency (herpes simplex and varicella-zoster viruses). This gives a mechanism for reactivation and further episodes of shedding from mucosal or skin lesions;

- In the case of rabies (see below), where CNS invasion in the animal host is necessary for two reasons. First, it enables the virus to spread from the CNS, down peripheral nerves to the salivary glands, from which transmission takes place. Second, invasion of the limbic system of the brain causes a change in behaviour of the infected animal, so that it becomes less retiring, more aggressive and more likely to bite, thus transmitting the infection. Invasion of the limbic system can be regarded as a fiendish strategy on the part of rabies virus to promote its own transmission and survival.

BACTERIAL MENINGITIS

Acute bacterial meningitis is a life-threatening infection, needing urgent specific treatment. It is more severe, but fortunately less common, than viral meningitis (see below). The important causative agents are shown in figure 27.5. *Neisseria meningitidis*, *Haemophilus influenzae*, and *Streptococcus pneumoniae* invade the meninges in healthy individuals and account for more than three-quarters of all bacterial meningitis. These three pathogens have several virulence factors in common (Fig. 27.6), including possession of a polysaccharide capsule (Fig. 27.7).

Meningococcal meningitis

Neisseria meningitidis is a Gram-negative diplococcus which closely resembles *N. gonorrhoeae* in structure (see Chapter 23), but with an additional polysaccharide capsule that is antigenic and by which the serotype of *N. meningitidis* can be recognized. The bacteria are carried asymptomatically in up to 20% of the population, attached by their pili to the epithelial cells in the nasopharynx. Invasion of the blood and meninges is a rare and poorly understood event. The known virulence factors are summarized in

NON-VIRAL MENINGITIS - CAUSES, TREATMENT AND PREVENTION		
pathogen	**treatment**	**prevention**
Neisseria meningitidis	penicillin (or chloramphenicol)	rifampicin prophylaxis for close contacts

polysaccharide vaccine (poor protection against group B) |
| *Haemophilus influenzae* | ampicillin* or chloramphenicol or cefotaxime | rifampicin prophylaxis for close contacts

vaccine |
| *Streptococcus pneumoniae* | penicillin (or chloramphenicol) | prompt treatment of otitis media & respiratory infections

polyvalent (23 serotypes) polysaccharide vaccine |
E. coli (& other coliforms) Group B streptococci *Listeria monocytogenes Staph. epidermidis*	gentamicin & penicillin or chloramphenicol**	no vaccines available
Mycobacterium tuberculosis	isoniazid & rifampicin & pyrazinamide ± streptomycin	BCG vaccination isoniazid prophylaxis for contacts recommended in USA
Cryptococcus neoformans	amphotericin B & flucytosine	no vaccines available
* if strain shown to be susceptible (10–20% of isolates are resistant because they produce a plasmid coded b-lactamase)

** until antibiotic susceptibles are availanle | | |

Fig. 27.5 The important causative agents of non-viral meningitis, their treatment and prevention.

BACTERIAL MENINGITIS-VIRULENCE FACTORS FOR MAJOR PATHOGENS			
virulence factor	**bacterial pathogen**		
	N. meningitidis	***H. influenzae***	***S. pneumoniae***
Capsule	+	+	+
IgA protease	+	+	+
Pili	+	+	–
Endotoxin	+	+	–
OMPs*	?	+	–
* outer membrane proteins			

Fig. 27.6 Virulence factors in bacterial meningitis.

figure 27.6. People possessing specific, complement-dependent bacterial antibodies to capsular antigens are protected against invasion. Those with C5–C9 complement deficiencies show increased susceptibility to bacteraemia (as they do to *N. gonorrhoeae* bacteraemia; see Chapter 24). Those most often infected are young children, who have lost the antibodies acquired from their mother, and adoles-

cents who have not previously encountered the infecting serotype and therefore have no type-specific immunity. Person-to-person spread takes place by droplet infection, and is facilitated by other (viral) respiratory infections which cause increased respiratory secretions, and by overcrowding. During outbreaks of meningococcal meningitis the carrier rate may reach 70%. In the UK and USA serotype B infections are the commonest, but in Africa, China and South America there have been repeated epidemics due to serotypes A and C.

Clinical features
After an incubation period of 1–3 days, the onset is sudden with sore throat, headache, development of drowsiness and signs of meningitis (fever, irritability, neck stiffness). There is often a haemorrhagic skin rash, with petechiae, reflecting the associated septicaemia (Fig. 27.8). In about one-third of patients this is fulminating, with complications due to disseminated intravascular coagulation (DIC), endotoxaemia and shock, and renal failure. In the most severe cases there is an acute addisonian crisis, with bleeding into the brain and adrenal glands (Waterhouse–Friederichsen syndrome). Mortality from meningococcal meningitis reaches 100% if untreated but remains around 10% even if treated. However, serious sequelae are uncommon in survivors compared with the outcome of *H. influenzae* or *Strep. pneumoniae* meningitis (Fig. 27.9).

CAPSULES - IMPORTANT VIRULENCE FACTORS			
pathogen	**capsule**	**important type**	**vaccine**
Neisseria meningitidis	polysaccharide	A,B,C,Y,W-135	good for A & C; poor for B
Haemophilus influenzae	polysaccharide	b	new vaccine available for <1 year old
Streptococcus pneumoniae	polysaccharide	many	pneumovax:23-valent most common types
Group B streptococcus	polysaccharide rich in sialic acid	(Ia,Ib, II) III in meningitis	- ? future
E. coli		KI in meningitis	- ? future

Fig. 27.7 Polysaccharide capsules are important virulence factors in the pathogenesis of bacterial meningitis.

Diagnosis

The diagnosis of acute meningitis is usually suspected on clinical examination. Laboratory identification of the bacterial cause is essential, however, so that appropriate antibiotic therapy can be given and prophylaxis of contacts initiated. Preliminary results should be available within an hour of receipt of the CSF sample in the laboratory. Results of culture of CSF and blood should follow after 24 hours (see Chapter 18). Serology is not helpful in the diagnosis of bacterial meningitis because the infection is too acute for an antibody response to be detectable.

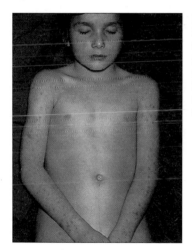

Fig. 27.8 Meningococcal septicaemia showing a mixed petechial and maculopapular rash on the extremities and exterior surfaces. Courtesy of W E Farrar.

Treatment

Bacterial meningitis is a medical emergency and antibiotic therapy (usually penicillin or ampicillin) should be instigated if the diagnosis is suspected (see Fig. 27.5). Early treatment saves lives, although it may make recovery of viable organisms from specimens more difficult.

Prevention

Close contacts in the family ('kissing contacts') should be given rifampicin chemoprophylaxis for 2–3 days. Note that penicillin is not used for prophylaxis because it does not eliminate nasopharyngeal carriage of meningococci. Patients should be given a course of rifampicin to clear carriage after the acute phase of the infection is passed. Sulphonamides can no longer be relied upon for prophylaxis because resistance in meningococci is common.

Haemophilus meningitis

Haemophilus influenzae is a Gram-negative coccobacillus. 'Haemophilus' means 'blood-loving', and the name 'influenzae' was given because it was originally thought to be the cause of influenza, but is now known to be a common secondary invader in the lower respiratory tract. There are six types (a–f) of *H. influenzae*, distinguishable serologically by their capsular polysaccharides. Unencapsulated strains are common and are present in the throat of most healthy people. It is the capsulated type b, a

BACTERIAL MENINGITIS - CLINICAL FEATURES				
pathogen	**host (patient)**	**important clinical features**	**mortality (as % of treated cases)**	**sequelae (as % of treated cases)***
Neisseria meningitidis	children & adolescents	acute onset (6–24h) skin rash	7–10	<1
Haemophilus influenzae	children <5yrs	onset often less acute (1–2 days)	5	9
Streptococcus pneumoniae	all ages but especially children <2yrs and elderly	acute onset may follow pneumonia &/or septicaemia in elderly	20–30	15–20
* Major CNS deficit. In addition up to 10% of patients develop deafness				

Fig. 27.9 Clinical features of bacterial meningitis.

common inhabitant of the respiratory tract of infants and young children (where it may cause infection: see Chapter 21), that very occasionally invades the blood and reaches the meninges. Maternal antibody protects the infant up to 3–4 months of age but as it wanes there is a 'window of susceptibility' until the child produces its own antibody. Anticapsular antibodies are good opsonins (see Chapter 13), which allow the bacteria to be phagocytosed and killed, but children do not generally produce them until 2–3 years of age, possibly because these antibodies are T independent. In addition to the capsule, *H. influenzae* has several other virulence factors, as shown in figure 26.6.

Clinical features

The incubation period is 5–6 days and the onset often more insidious than meningococcal or pneumococcal meningitis (see fig. 27.9). The condition is less frequently fatal but there is a higher incidence of serious sequelae (hearing loss, delayed language development, mental retardation and seizures) than with meningococcal infection.

Diagnosis

General diagnostic features are the same as for meningococcal meningitis, as explained above. For laboratory diagnosis see Chapter 18. It is important to note than the organisms may be difficult to see in Gram-stained smears of CSF, particularly if they are present in small numbers.

Treatment and prevention

General features of treatment are referred to above, under meningococcal meningitis; details are summarized in figure 27.5. There is a vaccine containing the capsular polysaccharide of *H. influenzae* type b, but unfortunately this is ineffective in those less than 2 years old, who are most vulnerable. More effective vaccines are, however, becoming available. Close contacts of patients are sometimes given rifampicin prophylaxis.

Pneumococcal meningitis

Streptococcus pneumoniae was first isolated more than 100 years ago and has since received intensive study both as a pathogen and as the subject of early work on bacterial transformation. Despite this, relatively little is known about its virulence attributes apart from its polysaccharide capsule (see Figs 27.6 and 27.7) and the pneumococcus remains a major cause of morbidity and mortality. (Pneumococcal respiratory tract infections are reviewed in Chapter 21.) *Strep. pneumoniae* is also of major importance as a cause of bacterial meningitis. It is a capsulate Gram-positive coccus carried in the throats of many healthy individuals. Invasion of the blood and meninges is a rare event, but is more common in the very young (less than 2 years of age), in the elderly, in those with sickle cell disease, in debilitated or splenectomized patients and following head trauma. Susceptibility to infection is associated with low levels of antibodies to capsular polysaccharide antigens: antibody opsonizes the organism and promotes phagocytosis, thereby protecting the host from invasion. However, this protection is type-specific and there are more than 85 different capsular types of *Strep. pneumoniae*.

Clinical features

Clinical features of pneumococcal meningitis are summarized in figure 27.9.

Diagnosis

General features are the same as for meningococcal meningitis, as described above. Details are referred to in Chapter 18.

Treatment and prevention

Treatment and prevention of pneumococcal meningitis is summarized in figure 27.5. The role of the 23-valent polysaccharide vaccine in prevention of meningitis is uncertain.

Listeria monocytogenes meningitis

This gram-positive coccobacillus is an important cause of meningitis in immunocompromised adults, especially in renal transplant and cancer patients. It also causes intra-uterine infections and infections of the newborn, as summarized in Chapter 25. *L. monocytogenes* is less susceptible than *Strep. pneumoniae* to penicillin and the recommended treatment is a combination of penicillin or ampicillin with gentamicin.

Neonatal meningitis

This can be caused by a wide range of bacteria but the most frequent are *E. coli* and group B haemolytic streptococci (Fig. 27.10; see also Chapter 25). Infection is fatal in about one-third of cases and in others often leads to permanent sequelae such as cerebral or cranial nerve palsy, epilepsy, mental retardation or hydrocephalus. This is partly because the clinical diagnosis of meningitis in the neonate is difficult, perhaps with no more specific signs than fever, poor feeding, vomiting, respiratory distress or diarrhoea. Because the possible range or organisms is wide, 'blind' antibiotic therapy, in the absence of susceptibility tests, may not be optimal and many antibiotics penetrate inadequately into the CSF. Host defences are poor, especially in low birth weight (less than 1000g) babies.

Tuberculous meningitis

Patients with tuberculous meningitis always have a focus of infection elsewhere, but one in four have no clinical or historical evidence of such an infection. In more than half the cases, meningitis is associated with acute miliary tuberculosis (Fig. 27.11). There is a gradual onset of generalized illness beginning with malaise, apathy and anorexia and proceeding within a few weeks to photophobia, neck stiffness and impairment of consciousness. Occasionally the onset is much more rapid and may be mistaken for a sub-arachnoid haemorrhage. The variability of presentation means that the clinician needs to maintain an awareness of possible tuberculous meningitis to make the diagnosis. A delay in making the diagnosis and in starting appropriate antimicrobial therapy (see Fig. 27.5) results in serious complications and sequelae.

In spinal tuberculosis, uncommon now except in developing countries, bacteria in the vertebrae destroy the intervertebral discs to form epidural abscesses, which compress the spinal cord and lead to paraplegia.

FUNGAL MENINGITIS

Cryptococcus neoformans and *Coccidioides immitis* can invade the blood from a primary site of infection in the lungs and thence to the brain to cause meningitis. *Cryptococcus neoformans* meningitis is seen in those with depressed cell-mediated immunity and is a problem in AIDS patients. The onset is usually slow, over days or weeks. The capsulate yeasts can be seen in India ink stained preparations of CSF (Fig. 27.12) and can be cultured (see Chapter 18). Antigen detection is also a useful diagnostic tool and evidence of a decline in antigen and an increase in antibody levels in the CSF can be used as a measure of successful therapy. Treatment with the antifungal drugs amphotericin B and flucytosine in combination is recommended.

Exposure to *Coccidioides immitis* infection is very common in particular geographical locations, notably south-west USA, Mexico and South America. CNS infection may be part of the generalized disease or may represent the only extrapulmonary site. It occurs in fewer than 1% of infected individuals but is fatal unless treated. The organisms are rarely visible in the CSF and cultures are positive in less than half of cases, but the diagnosis can be made by demonstrating complement-fixing antibodies in the serum. Treatment with amphotericin B or miconazole is recommended.

NEONATAL MENINGITIS		
group B streptococci and neonatal meningitis		
Group B streptococci (*Streptococcus agalactiae*) are normal inhabitants of the female genital tract and may be acquired by the neonate		
	at or soon after birth	in the nursery
	early onset disease	**late onset disease**
Age	<7 days	1 week – 3 months
Risk factors	Heavily colonized mother lacking specific antibody Premature rupture of membranes Pre-term delivery Prolonged labour, obstetric complications	Lack of maternal antibody Exposure to cross-infection from heavily colonized babies Poor hygiene in nursery
Type of disease	Generalized infection including bacteraemia, pneumonia and meningitis	Predominantly meningitis
Type of group B streptococcus	All serotypes but meningitis mostly due to type III	90% type III
Outcome	~60% fatal; serious sequelae in many survivors	~20% fatal
Treatment	Take blood & CSF, for culture Treat on suspicion Gentamicin and ampicillin or cefotaxime/ceftazidime	Treat on suspicion Take blood & CSF for culture Gentamicin and ampicillin or cefotaxime/ceftazidime
Prevention	Antibiotic treatment does not reliably abolish carriage in mother; not recommended 'Blind' treatment of sick baby who has risk factors Future: ?? immunize antibody-negative females of child-bearing age.	Good hygienic practices in nursery Do not allow mothers to handle other babies

Fig. 27.10 Group B streptococci as a major cause of neonatal meningitis.

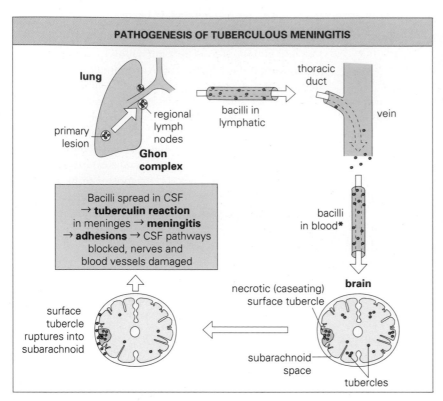

PATHOGENESIS OF TUBERCULOUS MENINGITIS

Bacilli spread in CSF
→ **tuberculin reaction**
in meninges → **meningitis**
→ **adhesions** → CSF pathways
blocked, nerves and
blood vessels damaged

Fig. 27.11 The association between acute miliary tuberculosis and meningitis. *This leads to miliary tuberculosis (Latin *milium* millet seed, each tubercle resembling a millet seed). Miliary tuberculosis also occurs in lungs and elsewhere.

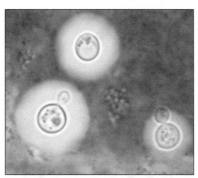

Fig. 27.12 *Cryptococcus neoformans* in India ink stained preparation of CSF sediment. Courtesy of A E Prevost.

VIRAL MENINGITIS		
virus	**virus group**	**comments**
Herpes simplex	alpha herpes virus	uncommon
Mumps	paramyxovirus	a quite common complication
Lymphocytic choriomeningitis	arenavirus	uncommon infection from urine etc. of mice, hamsters carrying the virus
Polio, Coxsackie, Echo etc.	picornaviruses (enterovirus group)	commonly seen (especially due to echoviruses) although an uncommon complication of infection
Japanese encephalitis	togavirus	India, S.E. Asia, Japan
E and W equine encephalitis	togavirus	E and W USA
Louping ill	togavirus	Scotland

Fig. 27.13 Causes of viral meningitis.

PROTOZOAL MENINGITIS

Free-living amoebae (*Naegleria* or *Hartmanella* sp.) can multiply in stagnant fresh water in warm countries, especially in the sludge at the bottom of lakes and swimming pools. They reach the meninges via the olfactory tract and cribriform plate, and cause an acute or subacute meningitis. These slowly motile amoebae can be seen on careful examination of a fresh wet sample of CSF. The mortality rate from such infection is high.

VIRAL MENINGITIS

This is the commonest type of meningitis. It is a milder disease than bacterial meningitis, with headache, fever and general illness but less neck stiffness. The CSF is clear, bacteria-free, and the cells are mainly lymphocytes, although polymorphs may be present in the early stages (see Fig. 27.3). The causes of viral meningitis are listed in figure 27.13, but viruses are isolated from the CSF in less than 50% of cases. Because there are many types of enteroviruses (32 echoviruses, 29 coxsackie viruses, 3 polioviruses) and because infection is commonly asymptomatic, a virus isolated from throat or stool of a child with mild meningi-

tis may be of no aetiological significance. In contrast to bacterial meningitis, and in spite of the fact that there are no antiviral drugs (except for herpes simplex), complete recovery generally takes place.

VIRAL ENCEPHALITIS

Nearly all encephalitis is caused by viruses (Figs 27.14 and 27.15). Characteristically, there are signs of cerebral

CAUSES OF ENCEPHALITIS		
Cause	**Infectious agent**	**comment**
Viruses (sporadic occurrence)	Herpes simplex	infant and adult forms distinguished
	Mumps	much less common than meningitis
	Varicella-zoster	a rare complication of ophthalmic zoster
	CMV	*in utero* and in immunosuppressed (e.g. AIDS)
	Rabies	in India 15–20 000 deaths/yr, in USA less than 10
	Louping ill	one of tick-borne encephalitis virus complex (others cause Russian spring–summer encephalitis etc.)
	Retroviruses HTLV1	tropical spastic paraparesis in small proportion of those infected
	HIV	subacute encephalitis (often together with other CNS infections)
Viruses (may be outbreaks)	Polio and other enteroviruses	uncommon; may be spastic paralysis
	Eastern and Western equine encephalitis	⎤
	St. Louis encephalitis virus	⎥ mosquito-borne togaviruses
	Japanese encephalitis virus	⎦
	California encephalitis virus	mosquito-borne bunyavirus
Slow viruses	Rubella	infection *in utero* (microcephaly etc.) or SSPE-type disease
	Measles	SSPE following uncomplicated measles after interval of up to 10 years
	PML (JC virus)	usually in immunocompromised
Atypical agents of scrapie group (non-viral)	?	Creutzfeld–Jacob disease and Kuru in humans Incubation period up to 20 years 'spongiform' encephalopathy
Post-vaccinial or post-infectious	?	occurs as a rare complication 2–3 weeks after exposure to certain viruses (e.g. measles) or vaccines; strong autoimmune component
Protozoa and fungi	*Toxoplasma gondii*	encephalitis a rare complication
	Cryptococcus neoformans	meningoencephalitis
	Plasmodium falciparum	cerebral malaria
	Trypanosoma sp.	sleeping sickness in Africa
Bacteria	*Treponema pallidum*	rare
	Mycoplasma pneumoniae	rare
	Borrelia borgdorferi	uncommon

Fig. 27.14 Infectious agents in encephalitis.

dysfunction such as abnormal behaviour, seizures and altered consciousness, often with nausea, vomiting and fever. However, *Toxoplasma gondii* and *C. neoformans* can also cause life-threatening encephalitis or meningoencephalitis, especially in those with defective cell-mediated immunity, and cerebral malaria as a complication of *P. falciparum* infection is frequently fatal. In Lyme disease (*Borrelia burgdorferi*) and Legionnaires' disease (*Legionella pneumophila*) encephalitis may occur, but the relative importance of bacterial invasion, bacterial toxins and immunopathology, is unknown.

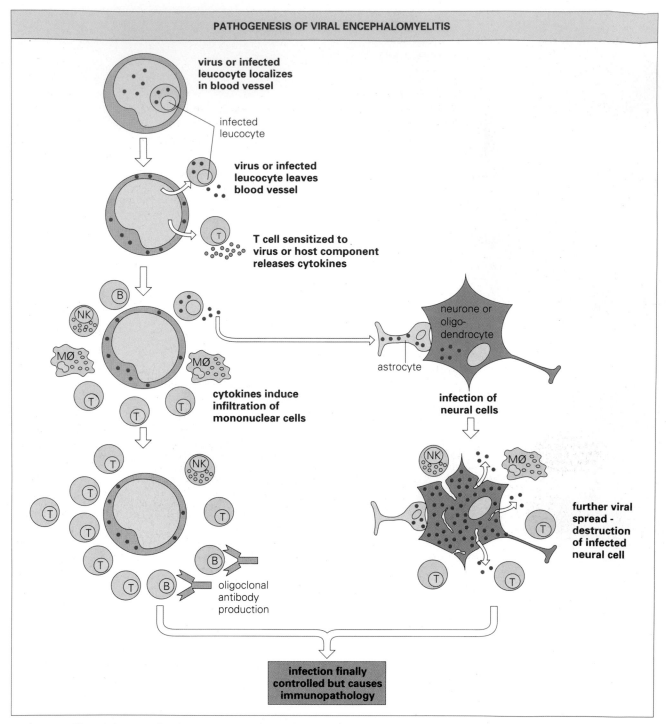

Fig. 27.15 The pathogenesis of viral encephalomyelitis

Herpes simplex

This is the commonest cause of severe sporadic encephalitis. One form occurs following primary and generalized infection in infancy, and another, seen in adults, is probably due to virus reactivation in the trigeminal ganglia (see Chapters 15), the infection then passing back to the temporal lobe of the brain. Herpetic skin or mucosal lesions may be present. Diagnosis is indicated by clinical signs of a space-occupying lesion in the temporal lobe, and a CT or radioactive (Technetium-99) brain scan (Fig. 27.16). Brain biopsy is sometimes justified. The 70% mortality rate in untreated patients is greatly reduced by early treatment with acyclovir.

Other herpes viruses less commonly cause encephalitis. With V-2 virus, encephalitis generally occurs following reactivation, and with cytomegalovirus either during primary infection *in utero* (see Chapter 26) or reactivation as a complication of immunodeficiency (e.g. in AIDS).

Poliovirus

Poliovirus was once a common cause of encephalitis; 9000 cases of paralysis, nearly all in children less than 5 years old, were reported in the great 1916 epidemic in New York City. CNS disease occurs in less than 1% of those infected. After an initial 1–4 days of fever, sore throat, malaise, meningeal signs and symptoms appear, followed by

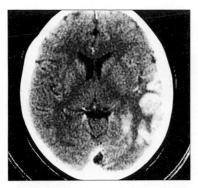

Fig 27.16 Herpes simplex encephalitis. CT scan showing enhancement of gyral structures in left temporal lobe and associated cerebral oedema. Courtesy of Dr J Curé.

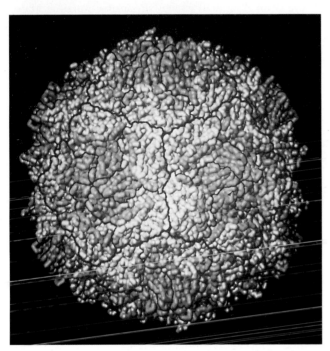

Fig. 27.17 Computer graphic model of the surface of poliovirus, based on x-ray diffraction studies. The capsid protein subunits visible on the surface of the virus particle are viral protein 1 (VP_1) in blue, VP_2 in green, and VP_3 in grey. Courtesy of A J Olson, Research Institute of Scripps Clinic, La Jolla, California.

involvement of motor neurones and paralysis (see Fig. 27.2). In spite of the fact that there are successful vaccines and we now have sophisticated information about the structure (Fig. 27.17) and replication of the virus, the disease poliomyelitis is still common in developing countries (there were 200 000 cases in India in 1989). The disease is completely preventable by vaccination (see Chapter 34) and has been disappearing in developed countries since vaccination programmes were first carried out in the 1950s (Fig. 27.18). There are three serologic (antigenic) types of poliovirus, with little cross-reaction between them, so that antibody to each type is necessary for protection. At least three-quarters of paralytic cases are due to type 1 polioviruses.

Other enteroviruses (coxsackie, echoviruses) also occasionally cause encephalitis.

Mumps virus

The mumps virus is a common cause of mild encephalitis. Asymptomatic CNS invasion may be common, because there are increased numbers of cells in the CSF in about half those patients with parotitis; on the other hand meningitis and encephalitis is often seen without parotitis.

Rabies

The causative agent of rabies is a rhabdovirus, a bullet-shaped single-stranded (ss)RNA virus. The virus is excreted in the saliva of infected dogs, foxes, jackals, wolves, skunks, raccoons, vampire bats, etc., and transmission to man follows a bite or salivary contamination of other types of skin abrasions or wounds. Some species of animal, e.g. foxes, are more infectious because larger amounts of virus (up to 10^6 infectious doses per ml) are present in the saliva. The infection is eventually fatal, although the course of the disease varies considerably among species. If an apparently healthy dog is still healthy 10 days after biting a human, rabies is extremely unlikely. However, the virus may be excreted in the dog's saliva before the animal shows any clinical signs of disease.

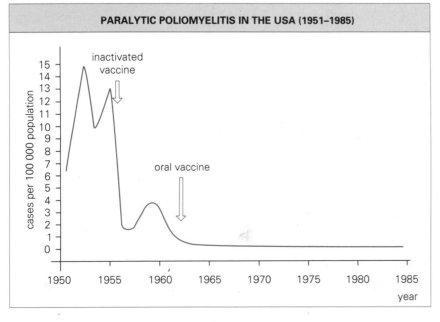

PARALYTIC POLIOMYELITIS IN THE USA (1951–1985)

inactivated vaccine

oral vaccine

cases per 100 000 population

year

Fig. 27.18 The incidence of paralytic poliomyelitis in the USA from 1951–1985.

The virus can infect all warm-blooded animals. Rabies from vampire bats causes more than one million deaths per year in cattle in Central and South America. Dogs transmit most of the estimated 75 000 cases of human rabies that occur in the world each year. In all the mainland masses the infection maintains itself in non-human mammalian hosts; islands such as Australia, Great Britain, Japan, Hawaii, most of the Caribbean islands, and also Scandinavia, are free of rabies because of strict controls over the importation of dogs, cats etc. In the USA, human rabies has been falling since the 1940s and 1950s, when most cases followed exposure to infected dogs. Since then the source has more often been non-domesticated animals such as skunks, raccoons and bats, or exposure to dogs in other countries. Raccoon rabies spread slowly northwards from Florida in the 1950s, and in the 1980s caused an explosive epidemic in Virginia, Maryland and Colombia. This outbreak was due to the importation of raccoons from infected areas, for sporting purposes.

The incubation period in humans is generally 4–13 weeks, although it may occasionally be as long as 6 months, possibly due to a delay in virus entry into peripheral nerves. The virus travels up peripheral nerves (see above) and in general the further the bite is from the CNS, the longer the incubation period. For instance, a bite on the foot gives a longer incubation period than a bite on the face.

Diagnosis

After developing a sore throat, headache, fever and discomfort at the site of the bite, the patient becomes excited, with muscle spasms and convulsions. Involvement of the muscles of swallowing when attempting to drink water gave the old name for rabies – hydrophobia, the symptoms sometimes being precipitated by the mere sight of water. Once the disease has developed it is fatal, death occurring following cardiac or respiratory arrest. One or two patients treated in intensive care units have recovered, but with serious neurological sequelae.

Laboratory diagnosis can be made by detection of viral antigen by immunofluorescence observations on skin biopsies, corneal impression smears, or brain biopsy. Characteristic intracytoplasmic inclusions (Negri bodies) are seen in neurones (Fig. 27.19).

Pathogenesis

While the virus is travelling up the axons of motor or sensory neurones, there is no detectable antibody or cell-mediated immune response, possibly because antigen remains sequestered in infected muscle cells. Hence, passively administered immunoglobulin may be given during the incubation period to initiate active immunization, rabies virus antigens being highly immunogenic.

Once in the brain, the virus spreads from cell to cell until a large proportion of neurones are infected but there is little cytopathic effect, even when viewed by electron microscopy, and almost no cellular infiltration. Presumably the striking symptoms of this disease are largely due to dysfunction rather than visible damage to infected cells. The change in behaviour of infected animals as a result of virus invasion of the limbic system has been discussed above.

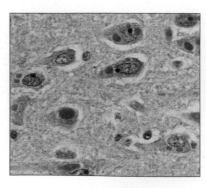

Fig. 27.19 Multiple cytoplasmic negri bodies in pyramidal neurones of the hippocampus in rabies. Courtesy of P Garen.

Treatment and prevention

There is no treatment except supportive nursing. Many countries have developed vaccination programmes for domestic dogs (e.g. France) and in Canada there have been efforts to vaccinate wild foxes by dropping food baited with live virus vaccine from the air. For the rabies-free countries, constant vigilance at borders and strict quarantine regulations are necessary to prevent the introduction of infected animals. As recently as 1906, when rabies was endemic in England, there were deaths due to rabies in the deer in Hampton Court Park, London.

After exposure to a possibly infected animal the following steps should be taken:
- Prompt cleaning of the wound (alcoholic iodine, debridement);
- Confirmation of whether or not the animal is rabid (clinical observation of suspected dogs, histological observation on the brain of other suspected species);
- Administration of human rabies immunoglobulin, to ensure prompt passive immunization. Half the dose is given into the wound and half intramuscularly;
- If the risk is definite, active immunization with killed diploid cell-derived rabies virus (see Chapter 36). The chances of preventing the disease are greater when vaccination is begun as early as possible after infection.

Togaviruses

Numerous arthropod-borne togaviruses can cause meningitis or encephalitis (see Figs 27.13 and 27.14), sometimes in outbreaks. In different parts of the world different mammals, birds or even reptiles act as reservoirs and there are a variety of arthropod (mosquito and tick) vectors. Usually less than 1% of humans infected develop neurological disease (see Chapter 30). There may be a febrile illness, but asymptomatic infection is common. In California, for instance, WEE (western equine encephalomyelitis) virus and SLE (St. Louis encephalitis) virus are prevalent and transmitted by the mosquito *Culex tarsalis;* a WEE vaccine is available, but only for horses. Japanese encephalitis virus infection is common in India and may cause a mortality of more than 50% in older age groups; a vaccine for humans has been developed.

Retroviruses

HIV (see Chapter 24) often invades the CNS shortly after initial infection, with an increase in cells in CSF and a mild meningitic illness. At a later stage, and quite independently of the disease picture that results from immune deficiency (ARC, AIDS), a subacute encephalitis may develop,

INFECTIOUS DISEASES WHICH MAY BE MANIFEST AS CHRONIC MENINGITIS OR BRAIN ABCESS	
bacterial	
Tuberculosis	Mycobacterium tuberculosis
Syphilis	Treponema pallidum
Brucellosis	Brucella abortus
Lyme disease	Borrelia burgdorferi
Nocardiosis*	Nocardia asteroides
Actinomycosis*	Actinomyces fumigatus
fungal	
Cryptococcosis	Cryptococcus neoformans
Coccidioidomycosis	Coccidioides immitis
Histoplasmosis	Histoplasma capsulatum
Candidiasis	Candida albicans
Blastomycosis*	Blastomyces dermatitidis
parasitic	
Toxoplasmosis*	Toxoplasma gondii
Cysticercosis*	Taenia solium
* disease manifest as brain abscess	

Fig. 27.20 Infections causing chronic meningitis or brain abscess.

often with dementia (AIDS-dementia complex). This is sometimes difficult to distinguish from the neurological disease caused by *Toxoplasma gondii, Cryptococcus neoformans,* cytomegalovirus, JC virus, etc. The brain is shrunken with enlarged ventricles and vacuolation of myelin tracts. HIV mainly infects macrophages and microglia in the CNS, and because the clinical disease is more severe than might be expected from the pathological changes, additional pathogenic mechanisms have been proposed. For instance, there are amino acid sequence similarities between the HIV envelope protein gp 120 and certain transmitter molecules, so that HIV-derived molecules could block the action of natural neurotransmitters.

Some of those infected with HTLV1 develop the disease 'tropical spastic paraparesis'. The spinal cord is involved but little is known of the pathogenesis.

NEUROLOGICAL DISEASES OF POSSIBLE VIRAL AETIOLOGY

It has often been suggested that certain neurological diseases of unknown origin, including multiple sclerosis, amyotrophic lateral sclerosis, Parkinson's disease, schizophrenia and senile dementia, have a viral origin. Although so far there is no acceptable evidence for this, it is possible that viruses may, at times, trigger off dangerous autoimmune-type responses in the CNS.

SLOW VIRUSES

In these rare infections a regular virus (rubella, measles or JC virus) invades the CNS, but virus growth is slow, often incomplete, and partially controlled by host defences (see Chapter 15); clinical disease appears after an incubation period of up to 10 years. For instance in otherwise uncomplicated measles, CNS invasion can take place and eventually result in SSPE (subacute sclerosing panencephalitis). Rubella very occasionally causes a similar disease, but more commonly, like cytomegalovirus it invades the brain of the foetus, interfering with development to cause mental retardation. JC virus (a polyomavirus) occasionally invades oligodendrocytes in immunodeficient people and eventually gives rise to PML (progressive multifocal leucoencephalopathy).

BRAIN ABSCESSES

Since the development of antibiotics brain abscesses have become rare and usually follow surgery or trauma, chronic osteomyelitis of neighbouring bones, septic embolism or chronic cerebral anoxia. They are also seen in children with congenital cyanotic heart disease, where the lungs fail to filter off circulating bacteria. They are diagnosed clinically and by scans. When an abscess is suspected, lumbar puncture is contraindicated, but if performed shows CSF cells and proteins generally raised (see Fig. 27.3). Treatment is by surgical drainage if the abscess is well-encapuslated, and antibiotics should be given for at least a month. Acute abscesses are caused by various bacteria, generally of oropharyngeal origin, including anaerobes. There is usually a mixed bacterial flora. Chronic abscesses are often due to *M. tuberculosis* or *C. neoformans*.

Other infections which may be manifest as chronic meningitis or brain abscess are summarized in figure 27.20.

ENCEPHALOPATHY DUE TO SCRAPIE-TYPE AGENTS

These agents form a closely related group, infect a variety of mammals, including humans, and are all transmissable to laboratory rodents or primates. They show a number of remarkable features:
- They replicate extremely slowly, taking more than a week to double in number. Hence the incubation period is long, usually a large fraction of the life span;
- They are of virus size but are not true viruses. Their exact nature (DNA or RNA genome) and method of replication is unknown. A prion protein, closely associated with the infectious agent, is host-coded but slightly altered in the infected brain;
- They show amazing resistance to heat, chemical agents and irradiation, and are not completely killed by boiling or immersion for years in formalin;
- They cannot be cultivated in test tubes, and since there is no antibody or other immune response to infection, diagnosis is by clinical appearances and characteristic pathological changes in the brain. Microscopic vacuoles

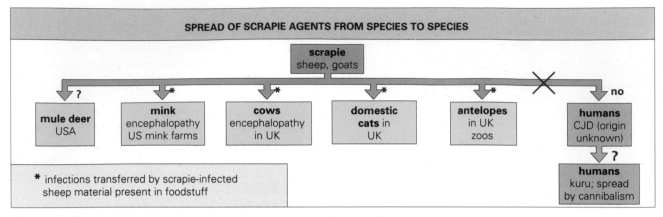

Fig. 27.21 The spread of scrapie agents between species. Nearly all have been transmitted to laboratory rodents and primates.

are seen, giving a spongiform appearance with little or no inflammatory response. The infectious agent is restricted to the CNS and lymphoid tissues;

- There is no treatment and no vaccine.

In animals, infection seems to have originated from sheep and goats with scrapie (Fig. 27.21), present in Europe for two to three hundred years. Affected animals itch, and scrape themselves against posts for relief.

Creutzfeld–Jakob Disease (CJD)

This is a rare chronic encephalopathy of humans, with associated dementia. Its natural mode of transmission is unknown, and it does not appear to be acquired from sheep. It has been occasionally transmitted by:

- Stereotactic electrodes used by neurosurgeons, with incomplete sterilization between patients;
- Corneal grafts;
- Injections of growth hormone preparations extracted from pooled 'normal' human pituitary glands, before genetically engineered growth hormone became available. A total of 15–20 cases have been reported, with incubation periods of up to 19 years.
- About 10% of CJD occurs in certain families, affected individuals having mutations in the gene coding for the prion protein (see above). It is possible that mere posession of the abnormal gene is enough to initiate the disease, the abnormal prion protein being more easily converted into pathogenic form. In this case CJD would be vertically rather than horizontally transmitted (see Chapter 11) and the role of a replicating agent not clear.

Kuru

This was a fatal neurological disease, with cerebellar signs, exclusive to the Fore tribes in Papua, New Guinea. A total of 3700 cases occurred in a population of 35 000, and transmission from human to human was associated with ritual cannibalism, involving the consumption of the body of a dead member of the family. The disease occurred equally in boys and girls but was most common in adult females, so that in some villages the men outnumbered the women by 3 to 1. Adult males rarely participated in the ritual and were less commonly affected. Although transmission was clearly associated with cannibalism, infection may have taken place via abrasions on fingers and mouth rather than in the gastrointestinal tract. There was a remarkable absence of communicability from person to person, and none of the hundreds of children born and suckled by mothers with Kuru developed the disease.

The incubation period of this disease was 4–20 years. No cases have been seen in those born since 1957, when cannibalism ceased. In some villages it was the commonest cause of death, and because deaths were attributed to sorcery, the second commonest cause of death was reprisal murder! A suggested origin of Kuru was from the cannibalistic consumption of a missionary who was dying from CJD.

POST-VACCINIAL AND POST-INFECTIOUS ENCEPHALITIS

Encephalitis very occasionally occurs a week or two after apparently normal measles, and even less commonly after varicella. It is also seen after vaccination with live vaccinia virus (against smallpox), after *Mycoplasma* infection, and after various influenza-like illnesses. Virus is generally not recoverable from the CNS and the perivascular infiltration, sometimes with demyelination, suggests an autoimmune pathogenesis. A similar condition occurs after administration of brain-derived inactivated rabies vaccines (now obsolete), and after other immunizations with non-infectious materials. The clinical picture resembles experimental allergic encephalitis, and is probably due to autoimmune responses triggered by the infection or by the injected material.

An analogous inflammatory demyelinating condition of the peripheral nervous system (the Guillain–Barré syndrome) has been associated with a variety of viral infections, as well as with immunization with non-infectious material. In 1976, most adults in the USA were given inactivated influenza virus vaccine, which resulted in a small but highly significant number of cases of Guillain–Barré syndrome.

CNS DISEASE DUE TO HELMINTH PARASITES

Toxocariasis

The cat and dog roundworms *Toxocara cati* and *Toxocara canis* infect humans, usually children, when toxocara eggs derived from kitten or puppy faeces are ingested (see

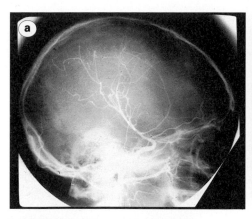

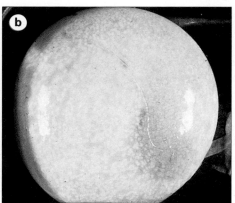

Fig. 27.22 Echinococcosis (a). Cerebral angiography showing displacement of vessels by a large frontal mass. (b) Cyst removed from patient in (a). Courtesy of H Whitwell.

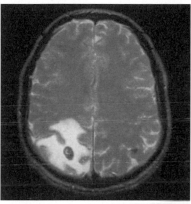

Fig. 27.23 Cerebral cysticerosis. MRI scan showing a cyst containing a developing larva. Courtesy of J Curé.

Chapter 3). Although transmission can be direct in cats and dogs, it is thought that these parasites originally required rodents as intermediate hosts, the life cycle being completed when these animals were eaten by cats or dogs. After ingestion by humans, the eggs hatch and the larvae migrate from the gut to the liver, lung, eye (see Chapter 21), brain and so on, the same as in the rodent. Granulomas form around the larvae, which in the brain may cause epilepsy, and in the retina a tumour-like mass can cause detachment and eventually blindness. There is usually a marked eosinophilia. However, infection is often asymptomatic.

Serum can be tested for fluorescent antibody to toxocara antigen. The disease is prevented by de-worming puppies and kittens, and by reduction of the pollution of children's play areas by dog excreta.

Hydatid disease

Hydatid disease is caused by the tapeworm *Echinococcus granulosus* (see Chapter 3) which has a world-wide distribution, especially in sheep-rearing areas. When humans ingest eggs from infected dogs, the embryos emerge, migrate through the gut to the portal blood vessels, and subsequently develop into hydatid cysts, especially in the liver, but also in the lungs, brain and kidney. Disease is caused by local pressure from the cyst, and sometimes hypersensitivity reactions to hydatid antigens. Neurological symptoms include nausea and vomiting, seizures and altered mental status,

Diagnosis is by detecting antibody to hydatid antigens, and by CT scanning, radiography or ultrasound examination to demonstrate cysts (Fig. 27.22). The disease is prevented by interrupting the natural dog–sheep, dog–goat, etc. transmission cycle.

Cysticercosis

Cysticercosis is due to *Taenia solium,* a human tapeworm. The eggs present in human faeces infect pigs, where they develop cysts in muscle tissue ('measly pork') and are a source of further human infection. Occasionally the eggs produced in the human intestine re-infect the same individual, perhaps as a result of ingestion of faecal material. After passing through the gut wall, the parasite develops into cysts in the brain (Fig. 27.23), eye and elsewhere, causing epilepsy or encephalopathy. Diagnosis is by detecting specific antibody in serum or CSF, and visualizing cysts by CT scans, MRI or x-rays.

TETANUS AND BOTULISM

Several bacteria release toxins that act on the nervous system (see Chapter 16) but do not themselves invade the central nervous system. In the case of *Clostridium tetani* and *Clostridium botulinum,* the major clinical impact is neurological.

Tetanus

Pathogenesis
Tetanus spores are widespread in soil, and originate from the faeces of domestic animals. The spores enter a wound, and when necrotic tissue or the presence of a foreign body permits local and anaerobic growth of bacteria, the toxin tetanospasmin (see Chapter 16) is produced. All strains of *C. tetani* produce the same toxin. The wound can be anything from a small gardener's scratch or cut, to a large automobile or battlefield injury. However, in as many as 20% of cases there is no history of injury. Infection of the umbilical stump can cause neonatal tetanus, and kills about 10^6 infants per year in developing countries (see Chapter 26).

The toxin is carried in peripheral nerve axons and probably in the blood to the central nervous system, where it binds to neurones and blocks the release of inhibitory mediators in spinal synapses, causing over-activity of motor neurones. It can also pass up sympathetic nerve axons and lead to over-activity of the sympathetic nervous system.

Clinical features and diagnosis
After a period of 3–21 days, but sometimes longer, there are exaggerated reflexes, muscle rigidity and uncontrolled muscle spasms. Lockjaw (trismus) is due to contraction of

jaw muscles, and dysphagia, 'risus sardonicus' (a sneering appearance), neck stiffness and opisthotonus (especially in neonatal tetanus; see Chapter 26) are also seen. Muscle spasms may lead to injury and eventually there is respiratory failure. Tachycardia and sweating can result from effects on the sympathetic nervous system. Mortality is up to 50%, depending on severity and the quality of treatment.

The diagnosis is clinical. Organisms are rarely isolated from the wound, and only a small number of bacteria are needed to form enough toxin to cause disease.

Treatment
Human anti-tetanus immunoglobulin should be given as soon as the clinical diagnosis is suspected. The wound should be excised if necessary and penicillin given to inhibit bacterial replication. Muscle relaxants are used and, if necessary, respiratory support in an intensive care unit.

Prevention
Immunization with toxoid prevents tetanus, the effects of the vaccine lasting for 5 years after the last dose. Wounds should be cleansed, necrotic tissue and foreign bodies removed, and a tetanus toxoid booster given. Those with badly contaminated wounds should also be given tetanus immunoglobulin and penicillin.

Botulism
Spores of *Clostridium botulinum* are widespread in soil and contaminate vegetables, meat, fish and so on. When foods are canned or preserved without adequate sterilization (often at home), contaminating spores survive and can germinate in the anaerobic environment, leading to the formation of toxin.

Pathogenesis
Pre-formed botulinus toxin is ingested, then absorbed from the gut into the blood. It acts on peripheral nerve synapses by blocking the release of acetylcholine (see Chapter 16). It is, therefore, a type of food poisoning that effects the motor and autonomic nervous systems. Sometimes spores contaminate a wound and the toxin is then absorbed from this site. If the organism is ingested by infants, in the honey smeared on pacifiers for instance, it can multiply in the gut and produce the toxin, causing infant botulism.

Clinical features and diagnosis
After an incubation period of 2–72 hours, there is descending weakness and paralysis, with dysphagia, diplop-

ia, vomiting, vertigo, and respiratory muscle failure. There is no abdominal pain, diarrhoea or fever. Infants develop generalized weakness ('floppy babies'), but usually recover.

Diagnosis is mainly clinical. The toxin can be demonstrated in contaminated food and occasionally in the patient's serum.

Treatment
Antibodies (preferably human) specific for types A, B and E toxins are given (types C and D cause botulism in birds) plus respiratory support. The mortality is less than 20%, depending on the success of respiratory support.

Prevention
Prevention is by avoidance of imperfectly sterilized canned or preserved food. Contaminated cans are often swollen due to the release of gas by clostridial enzymes. Home preserved foods are often incriminated, but fruit, with its acidic pH, usually prevents the development of the spores. The toxin is heat labile and is destroyed by adequate cooking (80°C for 4 minutes). The spores, however, can survive for up to 2 hours at boiling point (100°C).

SUMMARY

Fortunately, microbial invasion of the CNS is uncommon, due to the presence of the blood–brain or blood–CSF barriers, which limit the spread of infection. Once infectious agents have traversed these barriers, however, they generally cause neurological disease by involving the meninges (meningitis) or the brain substance (encephalitis). Viral meningitis is the commonest condition, bacterial meningitis the next commonest, with cerebral abscesses and viral encephalitis as rarities. The spinal cord (in myelitis) or peripheral nerves (in neuritis) are occasionally affected. Disease results from interference with the function of infected nerve cells (e.g. rabies), from direct damage to infected nerve cells (e.g. poliomyelitis), or from the inflammatory sequel to CNS invasion (e.g. bacterial meningitis, viral encephalitis). Because the anatomically defined compartments of the nervous system are adjacent or interconnected, however, more than one of them can be involved in a given infectious disease. CNS disease is sometimes seen in the helminth infections toxocariasis, hydatid disease and cysticercosis. CNS disease can also result when bacterial neurotoxins reach the CNS either from extraneural sites of growth (tetanus) or from contaminated food (botulism).

Further Reading

Johnson RT. The pathogenesis of acute viral encephalitis and post infectious encephalomyelitis. *J Inf Dis* 1987; **155:** 359.

Prusiner SB. Molecular biology of prion diseases. *Science* 1991; **252:** 1515–1522.

Warrell DA. Warrell MJ. Human rabies and its prevention: An overview. *Rev Inf Dis* 1988; **10:** (Suppl) S726.

Weinstein L. Tetanus. *New Eng J Med* 1973; **289:** 1293.

28 INFECTIONS OF THE SKIN, MUSCLE, JOINTS, BONE AND HAEMOPOIETIC SYSTEM

Contents

INTRODUCTION

Normal healthy intact skin protects the underlying tissues and provides the host with an excellent defence against invading microbes. In addition to the structural barrier, the skin is colonized by an array of organisms which forms its normal flora. The numbers and identity of the flora varies somewhat between different skin sites; the relatively arid areas of the forearm or back are colonized with fewer organisms, predominantly Gram-positive bacteria and yeasts. In the moister areas such as the groin and the armpit the organisms are more numerous and more varied and include Gram-negative bacteria. The normal flora of the skin plays an important role, as does the normal flora in other body sites, in defending the surface from 'foreign invaders'. The microbial load of normal skin is kept in check by various factors, as shown in figure 28.1. Alterations in these factors (e.g. prolonged exposure to moisture) upsets the ecological balance of the commensal flora, and predisposes to infection.

FACTORS CONTROLLING THE SKIN'S MICROBIAL LOAD
the limited amount of moisture present
acid pH of normal skin
surface temperature < optimum for many pathogens
salty sweat
excreted chemicals such as sebum, fatty acids and urea
competition between different species of the normal flora

Fig. 28.1 The numbers of bacteria on the skin vary from a few hundred per cm^2 on the arid surfaces of the forearm and back, to tens of thousands per cm^2 on the moist areas such as the axilla and groin. This normal flora plays an important role in preventing 'foreign' organisms from colonizing the skin but it too needs to be kept in check.

28.1

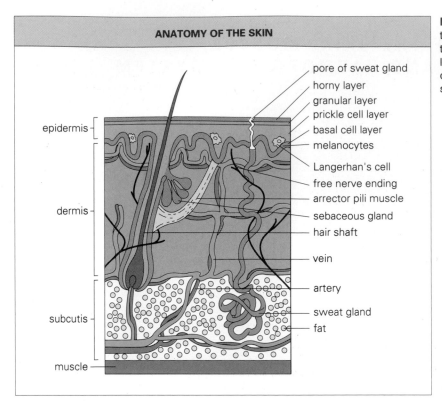

ANATOMY OF THE SKIN

Fig. 28.2 Infection of the skin and soft tissue can be related to the anatomy of the skin. Pathogens usually enter the lower layers of the epidermidis and dermis only after the skin surface has suffered some degree of trauma.

A small number of microbes cause diseases of muscle, joints or the haemopoietic system and are also considered here. Invasion of these sites is generally from the blood, but the reason for localization to particular tissues is often obscure. Circulating microbes tend to localize in growing or damaged bones (acute osteomyelitis) and in damaged joints, but we do not know why Coxsackieviruses or *Trichinella spiralis* invade muscle. On the other hand *Plasmodia* invade erythrocytes and some viruses infect a given target cell because they have specific attachment sites for these cells.

INFECTIONS OF THE SKIN

An appreciation of the structure of the skin helps in the understanding of the different sorts of infection to which the skin and its underlying tissues are prone (Fig. 28.2). If organisms breach the stratum corneum the host defences are mobilized, the epidermal Langerhans' cells elaborate cytokines, neutrophils are attracted to the site of invasion and complement is activated via the alternative pathway.

Modes of infection
Microbial disease of the skin may result from any of three lines of attack:
- breach of intact skin, allowing infection from the outside;
- skin manifestations of systemic infections; these may arise as a result of blood-borne spread from the infected focus to the skin, or by direct extension as in draining sinuses from actinomycotic lesions or necrotizing anaerobic infection from intra-abdominal sepsis;
- toxin-mediated skin damage due to production of a microbial toxin at another site in the body (e.g. scarlet fever, toxic shock syndrome).

The sequence of events in the pathogenesis of muco-cutaneous lesions caused by bacterial, fungal and virus infections is outlined in figure 28.3. Breaches in the skin range from the microscopic to major trauma which may be accidental (e.g. lacerations or burns) or intentional (e.g. surgery). Hospitalized patients are liable to other skin breaches arising from, for example, pressure sores and intravenous catheter insertions, which may become infected (see Chapter 39). Infections in compromised individuals such as burn patients will be discussed in Chapter 33. Here we will consider primary infections of the skin and underlying soft tissues, together with mucocutaneous lesions resulting from certain systemic virus infections. Systemic bacterial and fungal infections that cause mucocutaneous lesions are summarized in figure 28.4.

BACTERIAL INFECTIONS OF SKIN, SOFT TISSUE AND MUSCLE

These can be classified on an anatomic basis depending on the layers of skin and soft tissue involved, although some infections may involve several components of the soft tissues:
- Abscess formation. Boils and carbuncles are the result of infection and inflammation of the hair follicles in the skin (folliculitis).
- Spreading infections. Impetigo is limited to the epidermis and presents as a bullous, crusted or pustular eruption of the skin. Erysipelas involves the dermal lymphatics and presents as a well-defined, spreading erythematous inflammation, often accompanied by pain and fever. If the focus of infection is in the subcutaneous fat, cellulitis, a diffuse form of acute inflammation, is the usual presentation.

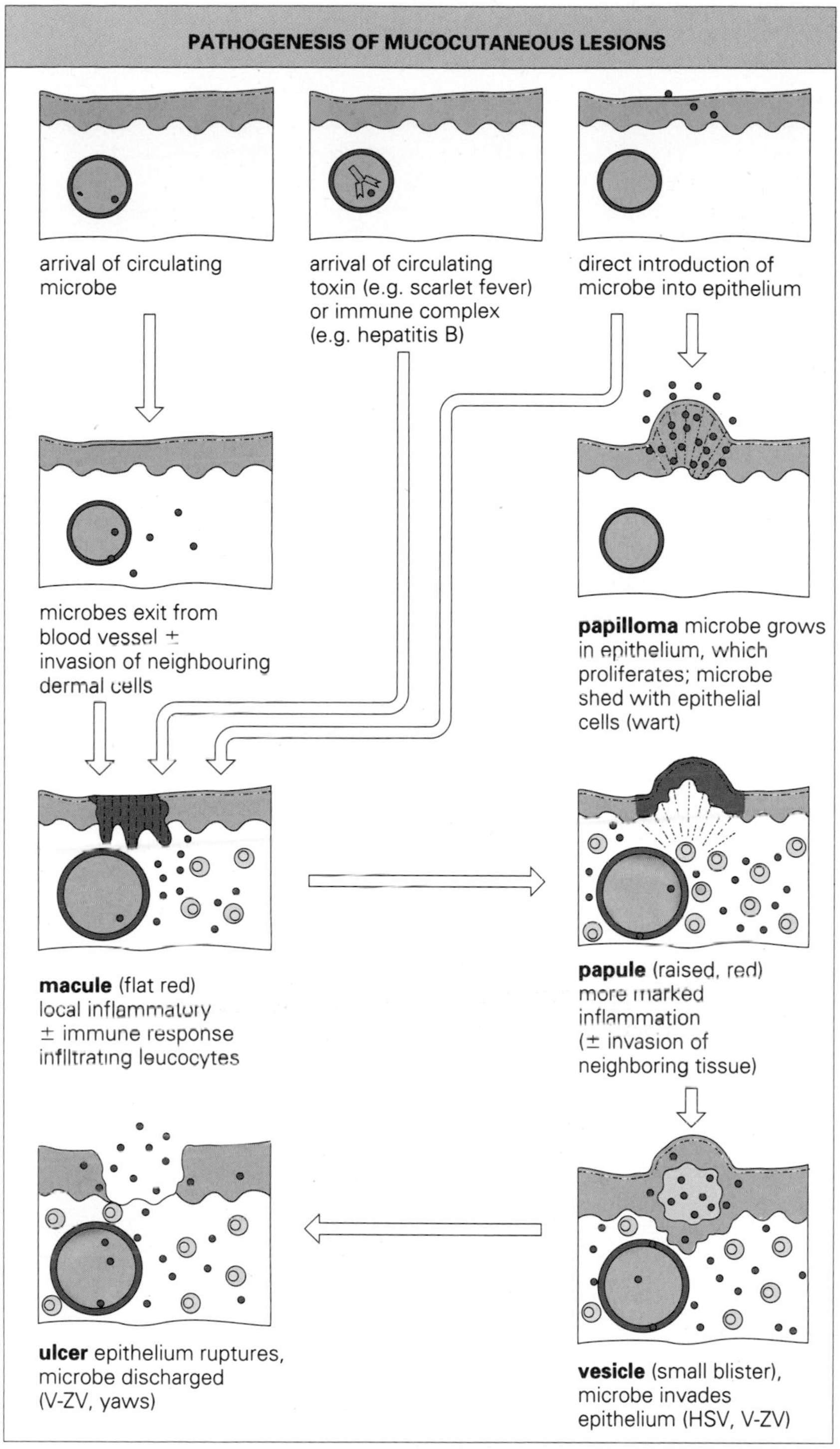

PATHOGENESIS OF MUCOCUTANEOUS LESIONS

arrival of circulating microbe

arrival of circulating toxin (e.g. scarlet fever) or immune complex (e.g. hepatitis B)

direct introduction of microbe into epithelium

microbes exit from blood vessel ± invasion of neighbouring dermal cells

papilloma microbe grows in epithelium, which proliferates; microbe shed with epithelial cells (wart)

macule (flat red) local inflammatory ± immune response infiltrating leucocytes

papule (raised, red) more marked inflammation (± invasion of neighboring tissue)

ulcer epithelium ruptures, microbe discharged (V-ZV, yaws)

vesicle (small blister), microbe invades epithelium (HSV, V-ZV)

Fig. 28.3 The pathogenesis of mucocutaneous lesions. In different infections the starting point (arrival of microbe or toxin or immune complex) and the final picture (e.g. maculo-papular rash, vesicle) will be different.

- Necrotizing infections. Fasciitis describes the inflammatory response to infection of the soft tissue below the dermis. Infection spreads, often with alarming rapidity, along the fascial planes causing disruption of the blood supply. Gangrene or myonecrosis may follow infection associated with ischaemia of the muscle layer. Gas resulting from the fermentative metabolism of anaerobic organisms may be palpable in the tissues (gas gangrene).

The common causative organisms are shown in figure 28.5. Note that the same pathogen e.g. *Streptococcus pyogenes* can cause different infections in different layers of the skin and soft tissue.

Staphylococcal skin infections

Aetiology and transmission

Staphylococcus aureus is the most common cause of minor skin infections such as boils or abscesses, as well as more serious post-operative wound infection. Infection may be acquired by 'self-inoculation' from a carrier site, e.g. the nose, or acquired by contact with an exogenous source, usually another person. People who are nasal carriers of virulent *Staphylococcus aureus* may suffer from recurrent boils but an inoculum of about 100 000 organisms is thought to be required in the absence of a wound or foreign body.

SKIN MANIFESTATIONS OF SYSTEMIC INFECTIONS CAUSED BY BACTERIA AND FUNGI

organisim	disease	skin manifestation
Salmonella typhi *Salmonella paratyphi* B	enteric fever	'rose spots' containing bacteria
Neisseria meningitidis	septicaemia, meningitis	petechial or maculopapular lesions containing bacteria
Pseudomonas aeruginosa	septicaemia	ecthyma gangrenosum, skin lesion pathognomic if infected with this organism
Treponema pallidum *Treponema pertenue*	syphilis yaws	disseminated infectious rash seen in secondary stage of disease, 2–3 months after infection
Rickettsia prowazeki *Rickettsia rickettsiae* *Rickettsia conori*	typhus spotted fevers	macular or haemorrhagic rash
Streptococcus pyogenes	scarlet fever	erythematous rash caused by erythrogenic toxin
Staphylococcus aureus	toxic shock syndrome	rash and desquamation due to toxin
Blastomyces dermatitidis	blastomycosis	papule or pustule develops into granuloma lesions containing organisms
Cryptococcus neoformans	cryptococcosis	papule or pustule, usually on face or neck

Fig. 28.4 Skin lesions are often associated with systemic infection with particular bacteria and fungi. The lesions may provide useful diagnostic aids. Sometimes they are a site from which organisms are shed.

COMMON BACTERIAL AND FUNGAL CAUSES OF SKIN INFECTIONS

structure involved	infection	common cause
Keratinized epithelium	ringworm	dermatophyte fungi (*Trichophyton, Epidermophyton* and *Microsporum*)
Epidermis	impetigo	*Strep. pygenes* and/or *Staph. aureus*
Dermis	erysipelas	*Strep. pyogenes*
Hair follicles	folliculitis boils (furuncles) carbuncles	*Staph. aureus*
Subcutaneous fat	cellulitis	*Strep. pyogenes*
Fascia	necrotizing fasciitis	anaerobes and microaerophiles, usually mixed infections
Muscle	myonecrosis gangrene	*Clostridium perfringens* (and other clostridia)

Fig. 28.5 Direct introduction of bacteria or fungi into the skin is the most common route of skin infection. Infections range from mild, often chronic, conditions such as ringworm to acute and life-threatening fasciitis and gangrene. Relatively few species are involved in the common infections.

Staphylococcus aureus can also cause serious and potentially fatal skin disease due to toxin production (scalded skin syndrome; see below).

Pathogenesis, clinical features and complications
A boil begins, within 2–4 days of inoculation, as a superficial infection in and around a hair follicle (folliculitis; Fig. 28.6). In this site the organisms are relatively protected from the host defences, multiply rapidly and spread locally. This provokes the host to produce an intense inflammatory response with an influx of neutrophils; fibrin is deposited, and the site is walled off. Abscesses typically contain abundant yellow creamy pus formed by the massive number of organisms and necrotic white cells. They

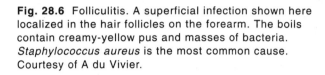

Fig. 28.6 Folliculitis. A superficial infection shown here localized in the hair follicles on the forearm. The boils contain creamy-yellow pus and masses of bacteria. *Staphylococcus aureus* is the most common cause. Courtesy of A du Vivier.

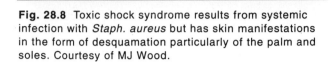

Fig. 28.8 Toxic shock syndrome results from systemic infection with *Staph. aureus* but has skin manifestations in the form of desquamation particularly of the palm and soles. Courtesy of MJ Wood.

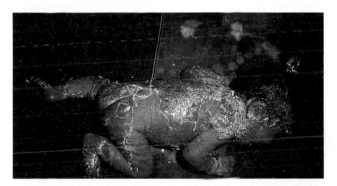

Fig. 28.7 Scalded skin syndrome results from infection of the skin with strains of *Staph. aureus* producing a specific toxin which destroys the intercellular connections in the skin resulting in large areas of desquamation. The appearance may be confused with a burn. Courtesy of A du Vivier.

continue to expand slowly, eventually erode the overlying skin, 'come to a head' and drain. Drainage inwards can result in seeding of the staphylococci to underlying body sites to cause serious infections such as peritonitis, empyema or meningitis.

Diagnosis and treatment

Staphylococcus aureus is the most common cause of boils and diagnosis is made on clinical grounds. Isolation and further identification of the infecting staphylococcus in hospital patients and staff is important in the investigation of hospital infections (see Chapter 39).

Treatment involves drainage and this is usually sufficient for minor lesions but antibiotics may be given in addition when the infection is severe and the patient has a fever. Most *Staph. aureus* are beta-lactamase producers and therefore enzyme-stable penicillins such as cloxacillin or flu-

cloxacillin are indicated. Treatment with these agents does not necessarily eradicate carriage of the staphylococci.

Prevention

Recurrent infections may be prevented by treating nasal carriers of *Staph. aureus* with nasal creams containing antibiotics such as bacitracin or neomycin; mupirocin has been used to advantage for carriers of methicillin-resistant staphylococci (see Chapter 39). Good skin care and personal hygiene should be encouraged.

Staphylococcal scalded skin syndrome

This condition, also known as 'Ritter's disease' in infants and 'Lyell's disease' or 'toxic epidermal necrolysis' in older children, occurs sporadically and in outbreaks. It is caused by strains of *Staph. aureus* producing a toxin known as 'exfoliatin' or 'scalded skin syndrome toxin'. The initial skin lesion may be minor but the toxin causes destruction of the intercellular connections and separates layers within the epidermis so that within one or two days large areas of skin are lost (Fig. 28.7) leaving normal skin underneath. The baby is irritable and uncomfortable but rarely severely ill. However, treatment should take into account the risk of increased loss of fluid from the damaged surface and fluid replacement may be needed. A beta-lactamase stable penicillin (e.g. cloxacillin) should be administered parenterally.

Toxic shock syndrome

This systemic infection is caused by *Staph. aureus* strains which produce toxic shock syndrome toxin (TSST). The disease came to prominence through its association with tampon use by healthy women, but it is not confined to women and can occur as a result of *Staph. aureus* infection at non-genital sites. There is septicaemia and toxaemia and skin manifestations include a rash followed by desquamation of the skin, particularly on the soles and palms (Fig. 28.8).

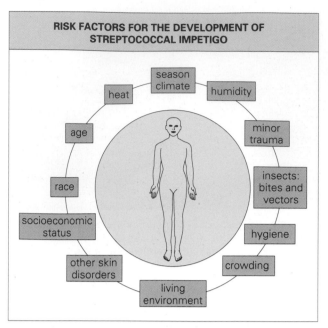

RISK FACTORS FOR THE DEVELOPMENT OF STREPTOCOCCAL IMPETIGO

- heat
- season climate
- humidity
- age
- minor trauma
- race
- insects: bites and vectors
- socioeconomic status
- hygiene
- other skin disorders
- crowding
- living environment

Fig. 28.9 Various factors relate to the development of streptococcal skin infections. Particular M types of *Strep. pyogenes* have a prediliction for skin but various factors predispose the host (usually a child) to infection. Mixed infections with *Staph. aureus* are also common.

Streptococcal skin infections

Aetiology and transmission

These infections are caused by *Streptococcus pyogenes* (Group A streptococci). Streptococcal impetigo develops independently of streptococcal upper respiratory tract infection, and although up to a third of patients carry the same strain in their nose or throat, colonization may well occur after the skin has become infected. The organisms are acquired through contact with other people with infected skin lesions and may first colonize and multiply on normal skin prior to invasion through minor breaks in the epithelium and the development of lesions. The various risk factors relating to the development of streptococcal impetigo are illustrated in figure 28.9. *Streptococcus pyogenes* may also infect deeper in the dermis causing erysipelas.

Streptococcus pyogenes possesses certain surface proteins (M and T) which are antigenic. The species can be subdivided (typed) on the basis of these antigens, and it has been recognized that certain M and T types are associated with skin infection (and these differ from the types associated with sore throats). T proteins play no known role in virulence and their function is unknown. M proteins are important virulence factors because they inhibit opsonization and confer on the bacterium resistance to phagocytosis.

Clinical features

The infections are typically acute (Figs 28.10 and 28.11), developing within 24–48 hours of skin invasion, and they trigger a marked inflammatory response as the host attempts to localize the infection. *Strep. pyogenes* elaborates a number of toxic products and enzymes, such as hyaluronidase, which help the organism to spread in

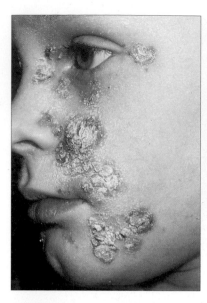

Fig. 28.10 Impetigo is a condition limited to the epidermis, with typically yellow, crusted lesions. It is commonly caused by *Strep. pyogenes* either alone or together with *Staph. aureus*. Courtesy of MJ Wood.

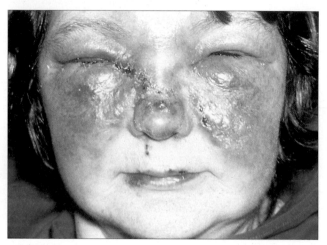

Fig. 28.11 Erysipelas. Infection with *Streptococcus pyogenes* involving the dermal lymphatics and giving rise to a clearly demarcated area of erythema and induration. When the face in involved there is often a typical 'butterfly-wing' rash, as shown here. Courtesy of MJ Wood.

tissue. Lymphatic involvement is common, with lymphadenitis and lymphangitis being manifest.

Complications

Certain M types (e.g. M49) of *Strep. pyogenes* are associated with the development of acute glomerulonephritis (AGN) and this complication occurs more often after skin infections than after infections of the throat (see Chapter 20). AGN is characterized by deposition of immune complexes on the basement membrane of the glomerulus but the precise role of the streptococcus in the causation is still unclear (see Chapter 16); 10–15% of individuals infected with a nephritogenic strain will develop AGN about 2–3 weeks after the primary infection. Most people recover completely and recurrence, after a subsequent streptococcal infection, is rare. Rheumatic fever rarely follows skin infections with *Strep. pyogenes*.

About 5% of patients with erysipelas go on to develop bacteraemia and this infection carries a high mortality if untreated.

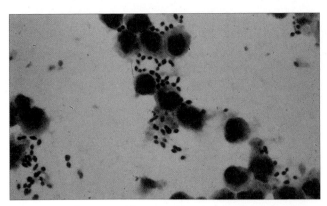

Fig. 28.12 Gram-positive cocci in pus.

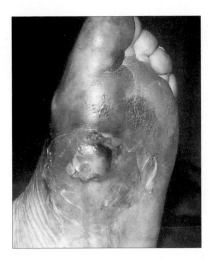

Fig. 28.14 Severe progressive cellulitis of the foot. Usually caused by anaerobic bacteria or a mixture of aerobes and anaerobes, is a particular problem in diabetic patients who suffer from peripheral vascular and neuropathic damage. Courtesy of JD Ward.

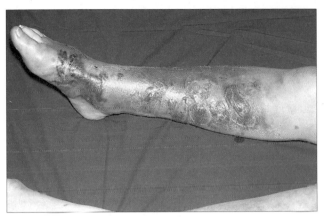

Fig. 28.13 When the focus of infection is in the sub-dermal fat cellulitis, a severe and rapidly progressive infection, is the typical presentation. Large blisters and scabs may also be present on the skin surface. Courtesy of MJ Wood.

Diagnosis

The diagnosis is usually made on clinical findings. Gram stains of pus from vesicles in impetigo show Gram-positive cocci and culture reveals *Strep. pyogenes* sometimes mixed with *Staph. aureus* (Fig. 28.12). In erysipelas, skin cultures are often negative although culture of fluid from the advancing edge of the lesion may be successful.

Treatment

Penicillin is the drug of choice, administered orally or intramuscularly in the long-acting benzathine formulation. Erythromycin should be used for penicillin-allergic patients. Severe infections may require hospitalization.

Prevention

Prevention of impetigo requires improvement in the host factors associated with acquisition of the disease, as illustrated in figure 28.9. Since AGN rarely recurs on subsequent streptococcal infection, long-term prophylaxis with penicillin is not indicated (in contrast to patients who suffer from rheumatic fever; see Chapter 20) .

Cellulitis and gangrene

Cellulitis is an acute spreading infection of the skin, extending deeper than erysipelas to involve subcutaneous tissues. Infection usually originates either from superficial skin lesions such as boils or ulcers, or following trauma. It is rarely blood-borne but, conversely, cellulitis made lead to invasion of bacteria into the bloodstream. Infection develops within a few hours or days of trauma and quickly produces a hot, red swollen lesion (Fig. 28.13). Regional lymph nodes are enlarged and the patient suffers malaise, chills and fever.

The great majority of cases of cellulitis are caused by *Strep. pyogenes* and *Staph. aureus*. Occasionally, in patients who have had particular environmental exposure, other organisms may be implicated. For example, *Erysipelothrix rhusiopathiae* is associated with cellulitis in butchers and fishmongers, while *Vibrio vulnificus* and *Vibrio alginolyticus* may complicate traumatic wounds acquired in salt water environments (see Chapter 25).

Attempts can be made to confirm the clinical diagnosis by culture of aspirates from the advancing edge of the cellulitis, the site of trauma (if present), skin biopsies and blood cultures, but a pathogen is isolated in only about a quarter to a third of cases. Treatment should be initiated on the basis of the clinical diagnosis because of the rapid progression of the disease, particularly when caused by *Strep. pyogenes*. Initial therapy should cover both streptococci and staphylococci and a combination of benzyl penicillin and a beta-lactamase stable penicillin such as cloxacillin should be given.

Anaerobic cellulitis may develop in areas of traumatized or devitalized tissue such as that associated with surgical or traumatic wounds and in ischaemic extremities. Diabetic patients are particularly prone to anaerobic cellulitis of their feet (Fig. 28.14). The causative organisms depend on the circumstances of the trauma; infections in the lower parts of the body are most often caused by organisms from the faecal flora whereas wounds from human bites are infected with oral organisms. Foul-smelling discharge, marked swelling and gas in the tissues are characteristic of anaerobic cellulitis and a mixture of organisms is usually cultured from the wound. Treatment needs to be aggressive to halt the spread of infection; both antibiotics and surgical debridement are required. Osteomyelitis (see below) is a common sequela.

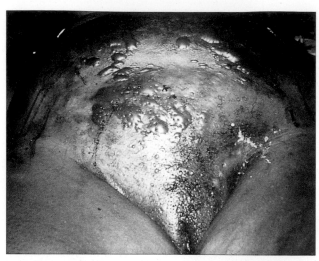

Fig. 28.15 Necrotizing fasciitis of the abdominal wall. In patients such as this, infection can be seen rapidly spreading from its origin and causing deep and widespread necrosis. Complete debridement and intensive antimicrobial therapy is required, but the condition is often fatal. Courtesy of WM Rambo.

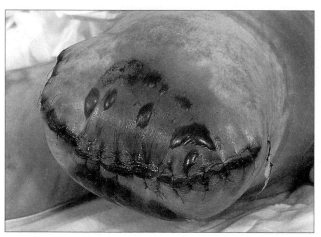

Fig. 28.16 Gas gangrene caused by *Clostridium perfringens*. Organisms from the faecal flora may contaminate the wound and grow and multiply in poorly perfused (anaerobic) tissue. Infection spreads rapidly and gas can be felt in the tissue and seen on on x-rays. Courtesy of J Newman.

Synergistic bacterial gangrene is a rare but relentlessly destructive infection caused by a mixture of organisms, typically microaerophilic streptococci and *Staph. aureus*. Meleney, who first described the condition (hence the alternative name 'Meleney's gangrene') could not reproduce the infection in an animal model unless both bacterial species were inoculated together. The gangrene most commonly follows surgery in the groin or genital area, starting at the site of a drain or suture. Cellulitis develops in the surrounding skin and extends rapidly (within hours), leaving a black necrotic centre. The full skin thickness is affected but subcutaneous tissues are spared. The patient suffers intense pain and the condition is often fatal. Treatment requires radical excision of the necrotic area and systemic antibiotic therapy.

Necrotizing fasciitis, myonecrosis and gangrene

Necrotizing fasciitis, a mixed infection of anaerobes and facultative anaerobes, although apparently resembling synergistic bacterial gangrene it is a much more acute and highly toxic infection which causes widespread necrosis and undermining of the surrounding tissues, such that the underlying destruction is more widespread than the skin lesion (Fig. 28.15). Patients deteriorate rapidly and frequently die. Radical excision of all necrotic fascia is the essential part of therapy, along with antibiotics given both locally to the wound and systemically.

Wounds resulting from trauma or surgery can become infected with various species of the genus *Clostridium*. *Clostridium tetani* gains access to the tissues through trauma to the skin but the disease it produces is entirely due to the production of a powerful exotoxin (see Chapter 16). Gas gangrene or clostridial myonecrosis can be caused by several species of clostridia, but *Clostridium perfringens* is the most common. The organism and its spores are found in soil and in faeces of humans and animals, and thus can gain access to traumatized tissues by contamination from these sources. Infection develops in areas of the body with poor blood supply (anaerobic) and the buttocks and perineum are common sites particularly in patients with ischaemic vascular disease or peripheral arteriosclerosis. The organisms multiply in the subcutaneous tissues producing gas and an anaerobic cellulitis. But a characteristic of clostridial infection is that the organisms invade deeper into the muscle where they cause necrosis and produce bubbles of gas which can be felt in the tissue and sometimes seen in the wound (Fig. 28.16). The infection proceeds very rapidly and causes the patient acute pain.

Much of the damage is due to the production by *Clostridium perfringens* of a lecithinase (also known as alpha toxin) which hydrolyses the lipids in cell membranes resulting in cell lysis and death (Fig. 28.17). The presence of dead and dying tissue further compromises the blood supply and the organisms multiply and produce more toxin and more damage. Other extracellular enzymes may also play a role in helping the clostridia to spread. If the toxin escapes from the affected area and enters the bloodstream, there is massive haemolysis, renal failure and death.

Because of the rapid progression and fatal outcome gangrenous areas require immediate surgery to excise all the affected tissue and amputation may be necessary to prevent further spread of the disease. Anti-alpha toxin may help if given early enough and treatment in a hyperbaric oxygen chamber has also been recommended to improve the oxygenation of the tissues. Antibiotics (penicillin or metronidazole) should be considered only as adjuncts to, not in place of, surgical debridement.

Prevention of infection is of foremost importance. Wounds should be cleaned and debrided early to remove the dead and poorly perfused tissue which the anaerobes favour. Prophylactic antibiotics (penicillin or metronidazole) should be given pre-operatively to patients having elective surgery of body sites liable to contamination with faecal flora (see Chapters 35 and 39).

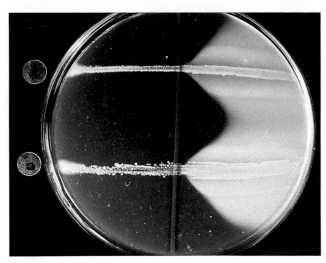

Fig. 28.17 The Nagler reaction. *Clostridium perfringens* produces alphatoxin, which is a lecithinase. If the organism is grown on a medium containing egg yolk (lecithin) enzyme activity can be detected as opacity around the line of growth (right). If anti-alpha toxin is applied to the surface of the plate before inoculation of the organism, the action of the toxin is inhibited (left). This test can be used to confirm the identity of a clostridial isolate.

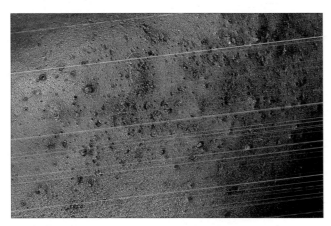

Fig. 28.18 Typical lesions of acne. 'Blackheads' are seen when plugs of keratin block the pilosebaceous canal. Courtesy of A du Vivier.

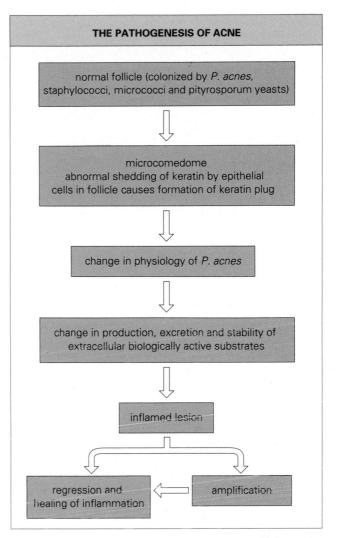

Fig. 28.19 The proposed mechanism of pathogenesis of acne. Host factors probably initiate the formation of comedomes from normal follicles and thereby change the environment of *Propionibacterium acnes* and its physiological properties. The organism, (which used to be called *Corynebacterium parvum*) is known to be an immunostimulator.

Does *Propionibacterium acnes* cause acne?

The Gram-positive anaerobic rod *Propionibacterium acnes* has not been shown to fulfil Koch's postulates as the causative agent of acne, but there is considerable evidence that the skin microflora in general, and *P. acnes* in particular, play an important role in the development of acne (Fig. 28.18). Lesions develop in the pilosebaceous follicles whose normal flora is composed of propionibacteria (especially *P. acnes*), staphylococci, micrococci and *Pityrosporum ovale* (a yeast). Two stages can be identified: the formation of comedomes, and inflammation. Comedomes are greasy plugs composed of a mixture of keratin, sebum and bacteria and capped by a layer of melanin (blackheads in popular terminology). The bacterial flora in comedomes is essentially the same as in normal follicles but it is postulated that in this environment *P. acnes* secretes extracellular products which cause direct damage and/or act as mediators of inflammation (Fig. 28.19).

Treatment of acne includes long-term administration of oral antibiotics (usually tetracycline but also erythromycin) combined with topical antibiotic or antiseptic therapy. Orally administered antibiotics reduce the surface numbers of *P. acnes* only 10-fold but are also thought to influence metabolic activity. Acne can be a problem for teenagers but often disappears in older age groups as the sebaceous follicles become less active.

Other Gram-positive rods related to *P. acnes* such as corynebacteria and brevibacteria, can also cause skin infections.

MYCOBACTERIAL DISEASES OF THE SKIN

Leprosy

Leprosy has been recognized since biblical times, but in the past the word was a generic term applied to several different diseases and also implying 'moral uncleanliness'.

THE PATHOGENESIS OF ACNE

normal follicle (colonized by *P. acnes*, staphylococci, micrococci and pityrosporum yeasts)

⬇

microcomedome
abnormal shedding of keratin by epithelial cells in follicle causes formation of keratin plug

⬇

change in physiology of *P. acnes*

⬇

change in production, excretion and stability of extracellular biologically active substrates

⬇

inflamed lesion

⬇

regression and healing of inflammation ⬅ amplification

Leprosy is thought to have spread to Europe in the sixth century, and by the thirteenth century there were some 200 leper hospitals in England. Over the centuries that followed leprosy declined in incidence and by the fifteenth century was no longer endemic in the UK; in contrast tuberculosis was on the increase. Nowadays, leprosy is rare in UK and USA but world-wide the disease affects 12–15 million people.

Aetiology and transmission

Leprosy is caused by *Mycobacterium leprae*. The organism appears to be confined to humans and no animal reservoir has been defined, although it is possible that one exists unrecognized. Transmission of infection is directly related to overcrowding and poor hygiene. Relatively few organisms are shed from skin lesions, but nasal secretions of patients with lepromatous leprosy are laden with *M. leprae*. Arthropod vectors may play a role in transmission. Leprosy is not highly contagious and prolonged exposure to an infected source is necessary; it seems that children living under the same roof as an open case of leprosy are most at risk. Ironically, because the lesions of leprosy are more obvious, patients were in the past excluded from the community and gathered in leper colonies, whereas

tuberculosis is much more contagious but sufferers were not shunned.

Pathogenesis

Mycobacterium leprae cannot be grown in artificial culture media and little is known about its mechanism of pathogenicity. Two animal models have been used: infection in the armadillo and in the footpads of mice. The organism grows better at temperatures below 37°C, hence its concentration in the skin, and it grows extremely slowly; in the mouse footpad the generation time is 11–13 days. Likewise in man the incubation period may be many years.

    Mycobacterium leprae grows intracellularly, typically within skin histiocytes and endothelial cells and the Schwann cells of peripheral nerves.

Clinical features

The organism shares many pathobiological features with *M. tuberculosis* but the clinical manifestations of the diseases are quite different. After an incubation period of several years the onset of leprosy is gradual and the spectrum of disease activity is very broad. This spectrum has been classified into a five group system (Fig. 28.20). The two extremes are characterized by the presence or absence

CLASSIFICATION OF LEPROSY			
	group	**skin lesions**	**nerve involvement**
limited disease low infectivity	full tuberculoid (TT)	few erythematous or hyperpigmented plaques granulomas containing giant cells very few acid-fast fods	one or two peripheral nerves infiltrated and damaged loss of sensation nerve involvement dominates clinical picture
	borderline tuberculoid (BT)		
	borderline (BB)	more numerous than in (TT)	more nerves involved but degree of damage less than in TT
	borderline lepromatous (BL)		
generalized disease high infectivity	full lepromatous (LL)	many erythematous nodules extensive tissue damage with nasal ulceration and septal destruction foamy histiocytes rather than granulomas many acid-fast rods	diffuse, with patchy loss of sensation

Fig. 28.20 Classification of leprosy. Humans respond in a variety of ways to infection with *Mycobacterium leprae*. Their immunological response is all-important in deciding the type of disease. Leprosy is classified into five groups. The two extremes are immunologically stable conditions whereas patients in the borderline groups tend to gravitate to one extreme or the other.

of cell-mediated immunity (CMI) to *M. leprae* (Fig. 28.21). At one end of the spectrum is tuberculoid leprosy, characterized by blotchy red lesions with anaesthetic areas on the face, trunk and extremities (Fig. 28.22). There is palpable thickening of the peripheral nerves because the organisms multiply in the nerve sheaths. The local anaesthesia renders the patient prone to repeated trauma and secondary bacterial infection. This disease state is equivalent to secondary tuberculosis (see Chapter 22), with a vigorous CMI response and exaggerated allergic responses. Tuberculoid leprosy carries a better prognosis than lepromatous leprosy and in some cases is self-limiting but in others may progress across the spectrum to lepromatous leprosy.

In lepromatous leprosy there is extensive skin involvement with large numbers of bacteria in affected areas. As the disease progresses there is loss of eyebrows, thickening and enlargement of the nostrils, ears and cheeks, resulting in the typical leonine (lion-like) facial appearance (Fig. 28.23). There is progressive destruction of the nasal septum and the nasal mucosa is loaded with organisms (Fig. 28.24). This form of the disease is equivalent to mil-

iary tuberculosis (see Chapter 22) with many organisms visible in the lesions and a weak CMI response. The gross deformities characteristic of late disease result primarily from infectious destruction of the nasomaxillary facial structures, and secondarily from pathological changes in the peripheral nerves predisposing to repeated trauma of the hands and feet and subsequent superinfection with other organisms.

Whether a patient develops tuberculoid or lepromatous leprosy may in part be genetically determined. Patients with intermediate forms of the disease may progress to either extreme.

Diagnosis

An alertness to the possibility of leprosy when confronted with a patient with dermatologic, neurologic or multi-system complaints is of fundamental importance. Although the majority of cases are in people who are not native to Europe or USA the diagnosis should also be considered in those who have worked in endemic areas.

Nasal scrapings and biopsies of skin lesions should be stained by Ziehl-Neelsen or auramine stain (see Appendix) to demonstrate acid-fast rods. In lepromatous leprosy these are numerous but in the tuberculoid form of the disease few if any organisms are seen. However, the appearance of granulomas are sufficiently typical to allow the diagnosis to be made (Fig. 28.25). Remember that, in contrast to *M. tuberculosis*, the organism cannot be grown *in vitro*.

Treatment

If the disease is diagnosed early and treatment initiated promptly the patient has a much better prognosis. Dapsone (see Chapter 35) has long been the mainstay of

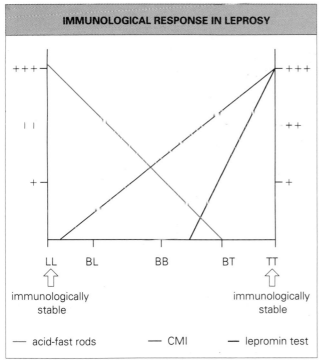

IMMUNOLOGICAL RESPONSE IN LEPROSY

LL   BL   BB   BT   TT

immunologically stable   immunologically stable

— acid-fast rods   — CMI   — lepromin test

Fig. 28.21 Immunological responses in leprosy. In tuberculoid leprosy (TT) the patient is capable of mounting an effective cell-mediated response which makes it possible for macrophages to destroy the organisms and contain the infection. At the other extreme in lepromatous leprosy (LL) the patient is incapable of producing a cell-mediated response and the organisms multiply unhindered. These patients have many acid-fast rods in their skin and nasal secretions, and are much more infectious than TT patients. The lepromin test, in which the patient is challenged with a crude preparation of *M. leprae* antigens, is a non-specific skin test and useless for diagnostic purposes, but it is of value in classifying a case of leprosy. The reaction (an erythematous papule) is strongly positive in TT patients, weakly positive in borderline tuberculoid (BT) and negative in borderline (BB), borderline lepromatous (BL) and full lepromatous (LL) disease.

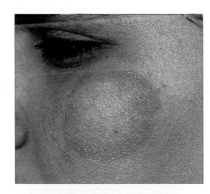

Fig. 28.22 Tuberculoid leprosy. Characteristic dry blotchy lesion on face but the diagnosis needs to be confirmed by microscopic examination of skin biopsy (see Fig. 28.25). Courtesy of the Institute of Dermatology.

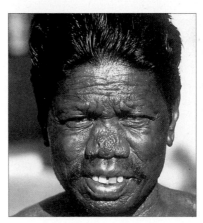

Fig. 28.23 Extensive skin involvement in lepromatous leprosy results in a characteristic leonine appearance. Courtesy of DA Lewis.

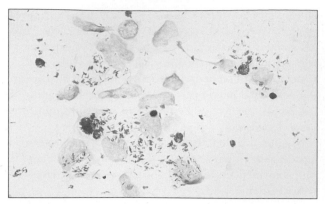

Fig. 28.24 In lepromatous leprosy the nasal mucosa is packed with *Mycobacterium leprae* seen here in an acid-fast stain (Ziehl-Neelson) of nasal scrapings. Courtesy of I Farrell.

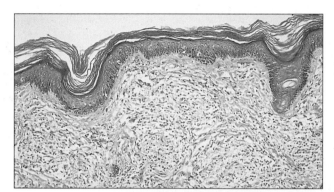

Fig. 28.25 In tuberculoid leprosy the organisms are much more sparse but characteristic granulomata form in the dermis as shown in this histological preparation. Courtesy of CJ Edwards.

therapy, but the current World Health Organisation recommendations are for multidrug therapy aimed both to slow the increase in incidence of dapsone resistance and to reduce the duration of treatment. For lepromatous and borderline leprosy, triple therapy with dapsone and clofazamine (daily) and rifampicin (once monthly) is the preferred choice but ethionamide can replace clofazamine if side effects (gastrointestinal intolerance and skin pigmentation) make this drug unacceptable. Combined therapy should be given for a minimum of two years and may be life-long, or until all skin scrapings and biopsies are negative for acid-fast rods. For tuberculoid leprosy, a combination of dapsone taken daily and rifampicin monthly for 6 months is recommended, the rationale being that in this form of disease there are many fewer organisms and thus less chance of emergence of resistant mutants.

Destruction of the organisms by effective antimicrobial therapy may result in an inflammatory response, erythema nodosum leprosum, which may be severe, and occasionally fatal. Treatment with corticosteroids or thalidomide may be indicated.

Prevention

As stated above, leprosy is not highly contagious but prophylaxis with dapsone is advised for household contacts (particularly children) of lepromatous leprosy cases. Contacts of tuberculoid cases do not require prophylaxis

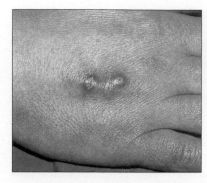

Fig. 28.26 Fish tank granuloma caused by *Mycobacterium marinum* infection of a lesion acquired while cleaning out a fish tank. Courtesy of MJ Wood.

but should be examined regularly and any suspicious lesions should be biopsied.

Trials aimed to determine the role of BCG immunization for the prevention of leprosy have shown conflicting results. A vaccine of heat-killed *M. leprae* is being tested but it will be some time before the long-term follow-up, necessary for such a slowly developing disease, will be complete.

Other mycobacterial skin infections

Two other slow-growing mycobacterial species cause skin lesions: *M. marinum* and *M. ulcerans*. As its name suggests, *M. marinum is* associated with water and marine organisms. Human infections follow trauma, often minor such as a graze acquired while climbing out of a swimming pool or while cleaning out an aquarium, which becomes contaminated with mycobacteria from the wet environment. After an incubation period of 2–8 weeks, initial lesions appear as small papules which enlarge, suppurate and may ulcerate. Histologically the lesions are granulomas and hence the name 'swimming pool granuloma' or 'fish-tank granuloma' (Fig. 28.26). Sometimes the nodules follow the course of the draining lymphatic and produce an appearance which may be mistaken for sporotrichosis (see below). The species is resistant to some of the first-line antituberculous drugs but rifampicin and ethambutol are active *in vitro*. Some strains are susceptible to tetracyclines and trimethoprim-sulphamethoxazole (cotrimoxazole).

Mycobacterium ulcerans causes chronic, relatively painless cutaneous ulcers known as 'Buruli' ulcers. This disease is prevalent in Africa and Australia but is rarely seen elsewhere. Experience with treatment is limited but combination therapy with streptomycin and isoniazid may be effective; excision and skin grafting may also be required.

Tuberculosis of the skin is exceedingly uncommon. Infection can occur by direct implantation of *M. tuberculosis* during trauma to the skin (lupus vulgaris) or may extend to the skin from an infected lymph node (scrofuloderma). In both forms the disease is very slow in its progression but responds, albeit slowly, to treatment with isoniazid.

FUNGAL INFECTIONS OF THE SKIN

Fungal infections of the skin may be confined to the very outermost layer (superficial mycoses) or penetrate into the epidermal or dermal layers (subcutaneous mycoses). In addition, some systemic fungal infections acquired by the airborne route have skin manifestations (see Fig. 28.4).

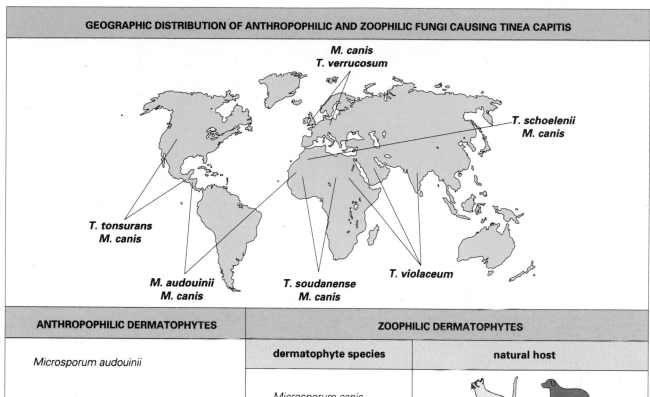

GEOGRAPHIC DISTRIBUTION OF ANTHROPOPHILIC AND ZOOPHILIC FUNGI CAUSING TINEA CAPITIS

ANTHROPOPHILIC DERMATOPHYTES	ZOOPHILIC DERMATOPHYTES	
	dermatophyte species	natural host
Microsporum audouinii	Microsporum canis	
Trichophyton mentagrophytes var. mentagrophytes		
T. rubrum	M. gallinae	
T. tonsurans		
T. violaceum	Trichophyton verrucosum	
T. soudanense	T. equinum	
T. schoenleinii T. concentricum	T. mentagrophytes var. mentagrophytes	
Epidermophyton floccosum	T. erinacei	

Fig. 28.27 Three genera of dermatophytes are important causes of disease: *Microsporum*, *Trichophyton* and *Epidermophyton*. Within each genus there are anthropophilic, zoophilic and geophilic species. Anthropophilic species vary in their natural host and thus also their distribution. *Microsporum gypseum* is the geophilic species of importance.

Superficial mycoses

Superficial fungal infections are among the most common infections in humans. The important causative agents are the dermatophyte fungi of the genera *Epidermophyton*, *Trichophyton* and *Microsporum*, and the yeast *Malassezia furfur.*

Dermatophyte infections

Aetiology and transmission

The dermatophytes are known as zoophilic, anthropophilic or geophilic depending on their primary source (animal, human or soil). Their geographical distribution and routes of transmission to man therefore depend on their normal habitat (Fig. 28.27). In temperate countries, *Trichophyton verrucosum*, the cause of cattle ringworm, and *Microsporum canis* , which causes infections in cats and dogs, are the most common zoophilic causes of human infection. Geophilic species such as *Microsporum gypseum* are uncommon causes of human disease but are seen in people who have appropriate exposure, such as gardeners and agricultural workers. The anthropophilic dermatophytes are the most common causes of dermatophyte

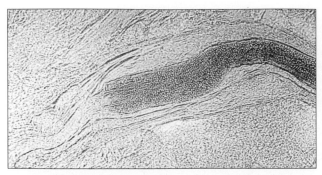

Fig. 28.28 Arthrospores of *Trichophyton tonsurans* in an infected hair shaft. These thick-walled spores are the form in which infection is spread. They can survive in the environment for weeks or months before infecting a new host. Courtesy of AE Prevost.

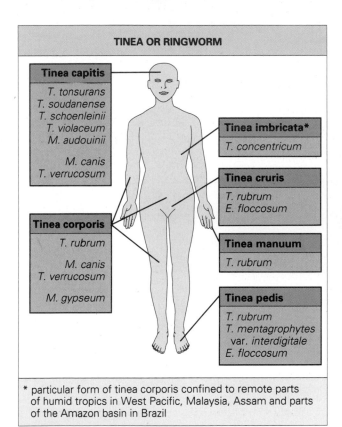

TINEA OR RINGWORM

Tinea capitis
T. tonsurans
T. soudanense
T. schoenleinii
T. violaceum
M. audouinii
M. canis
T. verrucosum

Tinea imbricata*
T. concentricum

Tinea cruris
T. rubrum
E. floccosum

Tinea corporis
T. rubrum
M. canis
T. verrucosum
M. gypseum

Tinea manuum
T. rubrum

Tinea pedis
T. rubrum
T. mentagrophytes
var. interdigitale
E. floccosum

* particular form of tinea corporis confined to remote parts of humid tropics in West Pacific, Malaysia, Assam and parts of the Amazon basin in Brazil

Fig. 28.29 Tinea (or ringworm) is the disease of skin, hair and nails caused by dermatophyte fungi. Different species have predelictions for different body sites.

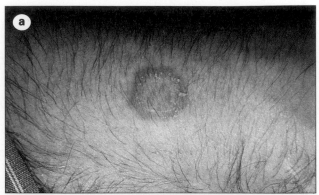

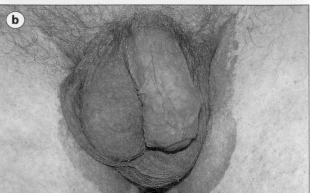

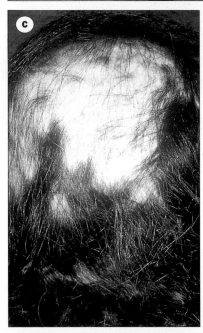

Fig. 28.30 (a) Classic annular lesion of tinea corporis, caused here by infection with a *Microsporum* species. Courtesy of AE Prevost. (b) Tinea cruris or 'jock itch' produced a scaly rash on the thighs but the scrotum is usually spared. Courtesy of MJ Wood. (c) Tinea capitis causes scaling on the scalp and hair loss. Some dermatophytes fluoresce under UV light and this can be an aid to diagnosis. Courtesy of MH Winterborn.

infections. The species differ in their geographical distribution and in their predelection for different body sites (see below).

Infections are spread by contact with arthrospores, the thick-walled vegetative cells formed by dermatophyte hyphae (Fig. 28.28), which are shed from the primary host probably in skin scales and hair and can survive for months.

Pathogenesis and clinical features
The dermatophytes are keratin-loving organisms and invade the keratinized structures of the body, i.e. skin, hair and nails. The arthrospores adhere to keratinocytes, germinate and invade. The latin word *tinea* (meaning a

maggot or grub) or ringworm is used for dermatophyte infections because they were originally thought to be caused by a worm-like parasite. Thus tinea capitis affects the hair and skin of the scalp, tinea corporis the body, and tinea pedis the feet (Fig. 28.29).

The typical lesion of dermatophyte infection is an annular scaling patch with a raised margin. The main symptom is itching but this is variable in degree. The skin is often dry and scaly and sometimes cracks, e.g. between the toes in tinea pedis, and infections of hair cause hair loss (Fig. 28.30). The degree of associated inflammation varies with the infecting species, usually being greater with zoophilic than anthropophilic species. Individuals also differ in their susceptibility to infection but the factors determining

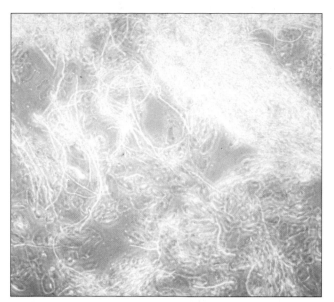

Fig. 28.31 Dermatophytes. Samples of skin, hair and nails need to be 'cleared' by treatment with potassium hydroxide before examining under the microscope for the presence of fungal hyphae. Courtesy of RY Cartwright.

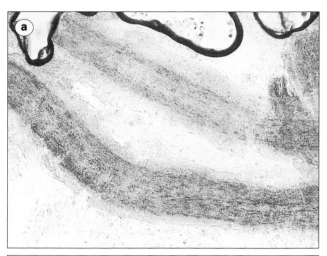

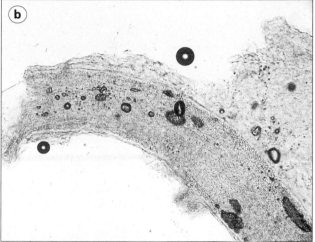

Fig. 28.32 Dermatophytes may form arthrospores on the outside of hair shafts (ectothrix infections) as shown in (a) but more commonly are formed within the shaft (endothrix infection) as shown in (b). Courtesy of Y Clayton and G Midgley.

these differences are not clearly understood. Likewise dermatophyte species differ in their ability to elicit an immune response; some such as *Trichophyton rubrum* cause chronic or relapsing conditions, whereas other species induce long-term resistance to reinfection. In some patients circulating fungal antigens give rise to immuno logically mediated hypersensitivity phenomena in the skin (e.g. erythema or vesicles) known as dermatophytid reactions. When the skin becomes cracked and macerated as a result of infection, it is liable to superinfection with other organisms such as Gram-negative bacteria in moist sites.

Very rarely, dermatophytes invade the subcutaneous tissues via the lymphatics causing granulomas, lymphoedema and draining sinuses. Further extension to sites such as the liver and brain may be fatal.

Diagnosis

Some, but not all dermatophyte species fluoresce under ultraviolet light and this can be used as a diagnostic aid, particularly for tinea capitis, in the clinic. Laboratory diagnosis depends on microscopic examination for fungal hyphae and culture on Sabouraud agar of scrapings or clippings from lesions (Fig. 28.31; see Chapter 18 and Appendix). Dermatophytes infecting hair show characteristic distribution which may be helpful for identification. Some, such as most *Microsporum* species form arthrospores on the outside of the hair shaft (ectothrix infections) whereas the majority of *Trichophyton* infections form arthrospores within the hair shaft (endothrix infection; Fig. 28.32). Confirmation of identity depends on the colonial and microscopic characteristics of the fungi cultured on Sabouraud agar (Fig. 28.33). Growth may take up to two weeks but identification is not difficult and is useful for determining the source of infection.

Treatment

Topical therapy is used where possible, but infections of nails and hair are better treated by oral administration of antifungal drugs. A range of agents is available for topical treatment, both antifungals and keratolytic agents such as Whitfield's ointment (a mixture of salicylic and benzoic acids). The orally administered agent most commonly used is griseofulvin. Scalp infections take 6–12 weeks to respond, fingernail infections up to 6 months and toenail infections may take a year or longer. The relapse rate of treated nail infections is high and many physicians advise against treatment unless there is pain or more widespread skin involvement.

The azole antifungals (see Chapter 35) are also active against the common dermatophyte fungi and some are available in topical formulations. Oral ketoconazole is useful for patients who cannot tolerate griseofulvin or who have failed to respond. However the risk of hepatitis associated with ketoconazole administration makes it the second choice to griseofulvin and liver function should be monitored regularly throughout treatment.

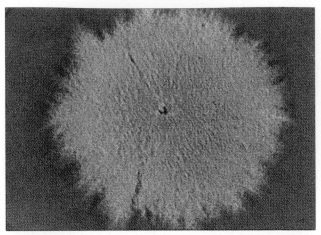

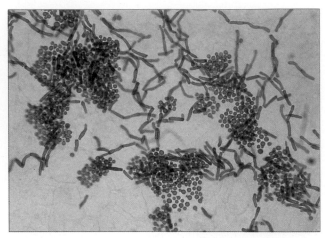

Fig. 28.34 Infected skin scales stained to show the thick-walled yeast forms of *Malassezia furfur* and the short angular hyphae. Courtesy of Y Clayton and G Midgley.

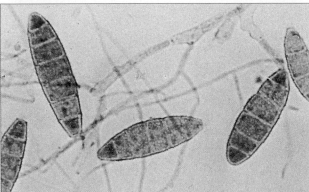

Fig. 28.33 Macroscopic growth (colony) and microscopic preparation showing the macroconidia of *Microsporum gypseum*.

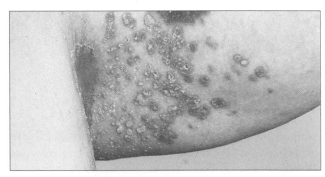

Fig. 28.35 *Candida* infection of the skin. Here, infection has occurred between two apposing skin surfaces which provide a suitably moist environment for this yeast to multiply. Courtesy of A du Vivier and St Mary's Hospital.

Pityriasis versicolor

The yeast *Malassezia (Pityrosporum) furfur* is a common skin inhabitant which produces the infection pityriasis or tinea versicolor. The change from commensalism to pathogenicity appears to be associated with the phase change from yeast to hyphal forms of the fungus, but the stimulus for this is unknown. Infections are usually confined to the trunk or proximal parts of the limbs and are associated with hypo- or hyperpigmented macules that coalesce to form scaling plaques. The lesions are not usually itchy and in some patients they resolve spontaneously. Treatment with a topical azole antifungal (see above) or with selenium sulphide (2%) lotion is appropriate. Diagnosis can be confirmed by direct microscopy of scrapings showing characteristic round yeast forms (Fig. 28.34). *Pityrosporum* yeasts are also thought to be involved in the pathogenesis of seborrheic dermatitis.

Candida and the skin

The relative dryness of most areas of skin limits the growth of fungi such as *Candida* that require moisture. *Candida* is found in low numbers on healthy intact skin but rapidly colonizes damaged skin and intertriginous sites (apposed skin sites which are often moist and become chafed; Fig. 28.35). *Candida* also colonizes the oral and vaginal mucosa and overgrowth may result in disease in these sites (thrush; see Chapter 24). However a substantial lowering of host resistance is necessary for *Candida* to invade deeper subcu-

taneous tissue, and disseminated candidiasis does not often originate from skin infection unless there is instrumentation through infected areas (see Chapter 33). Chronic mucocutaneous candidiasis is associated with a specific immune defect and is discussed in Chapter 33.

Subcutaneous mycoses

Subcutaneous fungal infections can be caused by a number of different species. Lesions usually develop at sites of trauma where the fungus becomes implanted. With the exception of sporotrichosis, subcutaneous fungal infections are rare but similar diseases can be caused by certain bacteria such as *Actinomyces* and atypical mycobacteria, and thus it is important to establish the aetiology in order to select optimal therapy. The fungi involved are difficult to eradicate with antifungal agents, and surgical intervention, in the form of excision or amputation, is often required.

Sporotrichosis

Sporothrix schenckii is a saprophytic fungus widespread in nature in soil, on rose and *Berberis* bushes, tree bark and sphagnum moss. Infection is acquired through trauma (e.g. a thorn) and is an occupational hazard for people such as farmers, gardeners and florists. A small papule or

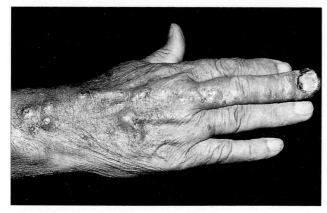

Fig. 28.36 Sporotrichosis spreading up the draining lymphatics of the hand following a primary infection in the nail bed of the third finger. Courtesy of TF Sellers, Jr.

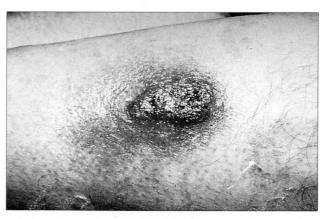

Fig. 28.37 Typical skin lesion of blastomycosis. Infection is acquired by the respiratory route and the primary site of infection is the lung. However, in chronic blastomycosis the skin is the most common extra-pulmonary site of infection. Courtesy of KA Riley.

subcutaneous nodule develops at the site of trauma one week to six months after inoculation and infection spreads, producing a series of secondary nodules along the lymphatics that drain the site (Fig. 28.36). Diagnosis is made by culture of draining or aspirated material on to Sabouraud agar. Treatment with oral potassium iodide is effective for cutaneous lymphatic disease.

Disseminated disease can occur following cutaneous or pulmonary infection with *Sporothrix schenckii*. It is more common in compromised patients such as those with carcinoma or sarcoidosis but many cases occur in people in whom no underlying disease is recognized. Treatment with amphotericin B is indicated and the prognosis is often poor.

Systemic fungal infections with skin manifestations

Skin lesions are the most common presenting symptom of blastomycosis. This disease, caused by *Blastomyces dermatitidis,* is acquired by aspiration of the fungal spores and invasion and blood-borne spread of infection from the primary site in the lung. Blastomycosis is one of the endemic fungal diseases of Central and North America and Africa which cause systemic infections in apparently immunologically normal hosts (Fig. 28.37).

Cryptococcus neoformans is a yeast which causes infection of the lungs. Blood-borne dissemination occurs and the organism has a particular predeliction for the central nervous system, but skin and bones are also common sites of infection. Many of the patients with disseminated infection have no demonstrable underlying disease, but immunocompromised patients are more prone to rapidly progressive disease (see Chapter 33).

PARASITIC INFECTIONS OF THE SKIN

The skin is a major route of entry for parasites, whether these penetrate directly (e.g. schistosomes, nematodes) or whether they are injected by blood-feeding vectors. Many of these parasites leave the skin almost immediately, but some remain there and others may become trapped. A few parasites actually exit from the body through the skin. Pathological responses to parasites associated with the skin range from mild to disablingly severe. Some of the species causing severe conditions are described briefly below.

Leishmaniasis

Two major disease complexes caused by these protozoans affect the skin. Both are transmitted by the bite of sandfly vectors. The cutaneous leishmaniases, which occur in both the Old and New Worlds, include conditions ranging from localized, self-healing ulcers to non-curing, disseminated lesions akin to leprosy in appearance. In the New World there are mucocutaneous leishmaniases, conditions where the parasite is localized in the skin or invades skin – mucous surfaces (nose, mouth) giving rise to chronic, disfiguring conditions. Leishmaniasis is discussed in detail in Chapter 30.

Schistosomiasis

Transmission of these parasites from the snail vector is achieved by active skin penetration of larvae (see Chapter 30). With those species adapted to man, this stage of infection can give rise to a dermatitis. A similar, though more pronounced, skin reaction is seen when bird schistosomes invade. This condition, known as 'swimmer's itch', is relatively common where bodies of natural water used for recreation are populated with aquatic birds. Topical anti-inflammatory treatments are effective in control.

Cutaneous larval migrans

Human hookworms (the nematodes *Ancylostoma* and *Necator*) invade the body through the skin, the infective larvae burrowing into the dermis and then migrating via the blood to eventually reach the intestine. Invasion may cause dermatitis, and this becomes more severe upon repeated infection. Humans, however, can also be invaded by the larvae of the cat and dog species of hookworm. Infection is acquired when exposed skin comes into contact with soil that has been contaminated by animals carrying the adult worms in their intestines. Eggs in the

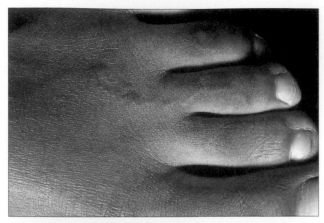

Fig. 28.38 Cutaneous larva migrans (creeping eruption), showing the raised inflammatory track left by the invading hookworm larvae. Courtesy of A du Vivier.

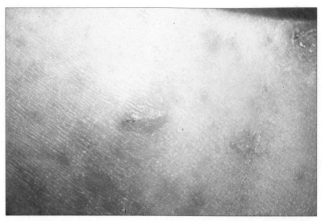

Fig. 28.39 A characteristic cutaneous burrow in scabies. Courtesy of MJ Wood.

faeces hatch to produce the infective larvae, which remain viable for prolonged periods. Because the human host is foreign for these species the larvae fail to escape from the dermis after invasion, and may live for some time migrating parallel to the skin, leaving intensely itchy, sinuous inflammatory trails, easily visible at the surface (Fig. 28.38). Topical treatment to control inflammation, together with the use of an anthelmintic such as thiabendazole, can be used.

Onchocerciasis (river blindness)

The adult stages of *Onchocerca volvulus* live for many years in subcutaneous nodules. Female worms release live microfilaria larvae, which migrate away from the nodules, remaining largely in the dermal layers. The slow build-up of parasite numbers, and the development of hypersensitivity response to the antigens released by living and dying larvae, give rise to inflammatory skin conditions. In the early stages these appear as erythematous papular rashes, accompanied by intense itching. Later on there is skin thickening, elasticity is lost and excessive wrinkling occurs; depigmentation is also common. The microfilarial larvae can be killed by ivermectin treatment, but the skin conditions, once advanced, are irreversible. Dermal inflammatory conditions are not uncommon during infections with other filarial nematodes.

Arthropod infections

Myiasis is a condition associated with invasion of the body by the larvae of dipteran flies. Many species of fly have a cycle in which the larvae feed and grow just below the skin of a mammal, escaping before or after pupation to release the aerial adult forms. Female flies may lay eggs or larvae directly onto the skin, and larvae may then invade wounds or natural orifices. The activities and feeding of the larvae cause intense, painful reactions, and large lesions may develop. A number of species have been found in humans, and infections have been recorded in many countries, although primarily in tropical and subtropical regions. Treatment involves removal of the larvae, alleviation of symptoms and prevention of secondary infection.

Several species of arthropod live by obtaining meals of blood or tissue fluids from the bodies of humans. Some feed non-selectively on humans and other species, others are host specific. The feeding processes, and the inevitable release of saliva, give rise to skin irritation, which becomes more intense as the body responds immunologically to the proteins present in the saliva. Prolonged feeding, as practised by ticks, may leave painful lesions in the skin which can became secondarily infected. Those species, like lice and scabies mites, which spend the greater part, or the whole of their lives on the human body, can cause severe skin conditions when populations accumulate. These conditions arise from the activity of the insects themselves, their production of excreta and the oozing of blood and tissue fluids from the feeding sites, as well as from the host's inflammatory reaction. Pediculosis, infection with head and body lice of the genus *Pediculus*, can, when severe, give rise to encrusting inflammatory masses in which fungal infections may establish. Good personal hygiene prevents infestation; use of insecticidal creams, lotions, shampoos and powders containing malathion or carboryl helps to clear the insects directly.

The scabies mite has a more intimate contact with the human host than do lice, living its whole life in burrows within the skin. The female lays eggs into these burrows, and so the area of infection can spread to cover large areas of the body from the original site, which is usually on the hands or wrists (Fig. 28.39; but see also Chapter 24). Infection causes a characteristic rash, with itching, and secondary infections may follow scratching. Very heavy infections may develop in immunocompromised individuals or in people who are unable to care adequately for themselves. Under these conditions there is extensive thickening and crusting of the skin (Norwegian scabies). Treatment with malathion, gamma-benzene hexachloride or lindane is recommended; benzyl benzoate can also be used on unbroken skin.

MUCOCUTANEOUS LESIONS CAUSED BY VIRUSES

Mucocutaneous lesions caused by viruses can be divided into those in which the virus remains restricted to the body

MUCOCUTANEOUS LESIONS CAUSED BY VIRUSES			
	virus	**lesion**	**virus shedding from lesion**
no systemic spread	Papilloma (wart)	common wart plantar wart genital wart	+
	Molluscum contagiosum (poxvirus)	fleshy papule	+
	Orf (poxvirus from sheep, goats)	papulovesicular	+
systemic spread	Herpes simplex Varicella-zoster	vesicular (neural spread and latency)	+
	Coxsackie virus A (9, 16, 23)	vesicular, in mouth (herpangina)	+
	Coxsackie virus A16	vesicular (hand, foot and mouth disease)	+
	Human parvovirus (B19)	facial maculopapular (erythema infectiosum)	–
	Human herpes virus 6	exanthem subitum (roseola infantum)	–
	Measles	maculopapular skin rash	–
	Rubella Echoviruses (4, 6, 9,16)	maculopapular not distinguishable clinically	–
	Dengue and other arthropod transmitted viruses	maculopapular	–

Fig. 28.40 Mucocutaneous lesions caused by viruses. The pathogenesis of these diseases is illustrated in figure 28.3. Papillomas and vesicular lesions are generally sites of virus shedding. The distribution as well as the nature of the lesion can be important in diagnosis (e.g. varicella), but many maculopapular rashes are in themselves clinically indistinguishable.

surface at the site of initial infection, and those in which the virus causes mucocutaneous lesions after spreading systemically through the body (Fig. 28.40). The infections that spread systemically can in turn be divided into those in which the skin lesions (vesicular) are sites of virus growth and are infectious, and those in which the skin lesions (maculopapular) are non-infectious and immunologically mediated. The skin rash has a characteristic distribution in many infectious diseases but, with the exception of zoster, the reason for this is unknown.

Rashes are particular features of human infection and are rare in animals. This is because human skin is naked and is a turbulent, highly reactive tissue, in which immune and inflammatory events are clearly visible. Rashes are not often in themselves a source of suffering but they may be a godsend to the clinician, who needs to make a diagnosis. The veterinarian is less privileged because the skin of most other mammals is largely covered with fur, and skin lesions generally involve hairless areas such as udders, scrotums, ears, prepuces, teats, noses or paws, which have the human properties of thickness, sensitivity and vascular reactivity.

Papillomavirus infection

Aetiology and transmission

These small (55nm) icosahedral dsDNA viruses cause skin papillomas (warts). There are more than 60 different types (showing less than 50% cross-hybridization of DNA) that infect humans, although not all types are common. Human papillomaviruses (HPV) are species-specific and distinct from animal papillomaviruses. Evidently they are highly adapted to human skin and mucosa, ancient associates of our species that most of the time cause little or no disease. They show some adaptation to definite sites on the body. At least five types (HPV 6, 11, 16, 18, 32) regularly infect the genital areas and are sexually transmitted, while HPV 1 and 4 tend to cause plantar warts and HPV 2, 3 and 10 warts on knees and fingers. Papillomaviruses are generally transmitted by direct contact but they are stable and can also be spread indirectly. For instance, plantar warts can be acquired from contaminated floors or from the non-slip surfaces at the edges of swimming pools, and in a given individual warts can be spread from one site to another by shaving.

Clinical features and pathogenesis

After entering via surface abrasions the virus infects cells in the basal layers of the skin or mucosa (see Fig. 28.3). There is no spread to deeper tissues. Virus replication is slow and is critically dependent on the differentiation of host cells. Viral DNA is present in basal cells , but viral antigen and infectious virus is produced only when the cells begin to become squamified and keratinized as they approach the surface (see Chapter 14). The infected cells are stimulated to divide and the mass of infected cells finally, 1–6 months after initial infection, protrudes from the body surface to form a visible papilloma or wart (Fig. 28.41). There is marked proliferation of prickle cells and vacuolated cells are present in the more superficial layers. Warts can be filiform with finger-like projections, flat topped, or flat because they grow inwards due to external pressure (plantar warts). Genital warts can blossom into cauliflower-like protuberances, but in the cervix the lesion is a flat area of dysplasia. Immune responses eventually bring virus replication under control and, several months after infection, the wart regresses. Antibodies are demonstrable but CMI responses are more important in recovery. It seems likely that viral DNA remains in a latent state in the basal cell layer, infecting an occasional stem cell and therefore is retained within the layer as epidermal cells differentiate and are shed from the surface. Hence, when patients are subsequently immunocompromised (e.g. post-transplant) there may be crops of warts as a result of reactivation of latent virus in the skin.

Complications

The association between genital warts and cancer of the cervix, vulva, penis and rectum is referred to in Chapter 16. It is not clear whether this association is causal or merely casual. There is no evidence that regular skin warts are involved in the development of skin cancer. There is, however, a rare autosomal recessive disease, epidermodysplasia verruciformis, characterized by multiple warts containing many different types of wart virus, and poorly understood immunological defects. Warts may undergo malignant change in these patients.

Diagnosis

The diagnosis is clinical. Wart viruses cannot be cultivated in the laboratory, and at present serological tests are neither useful nor available.

Treatment and prevention

An astounding variety of treatments have been used for warts, some of them doubtless seeming effective because warts eventually disappear without treatment. Post-hypnotic suggestion has at times been successful. Current treatments include the application of karyolytic agents such as salicylic acid, and destruction of wart tissue by freezing with dry ice (solid CO_2) or with liquid nitrogen. The latter is the most commonly used and the most effective treatment.

Molluscum contagiosum

Molluscum contagiosum is caused by a poxvirus which infects epidermal cells to form a fleshy lesion, often with an umbilicated centre (Fig. 28.42). It only infects humans and is spread by contact, or in the case of genital lesions, by sexual intercourse. There are two antigenically distinct types. Poxvirus particles can be seen by electron microscopy (see Chapter 3).

Orf (contagious pustular dermatitis)

This uncommon infection of the epidermis is caused by a poxvirus and is acquired by direct contact with infected sheep or goats. There is a papulovesicular lesion, generally on the hands, which may ulcerate.

Herpes simplex virus infection

Aetiology and transmission

Herpes simplex virus (HSV) is a medium sized (120 nm) dsDNA virus of the herpes virus group. Two types, HSV1 and HSV2, are distinguishable antigenically. They cause a wide variety of clinical syndromes, the basic lesion being an intraepithelial vesicle, from which the virus is shed. Infection is universal and occurs in early childhood, usually transmitted from the saliva or cold sores of other individuals and frequently by kissing.

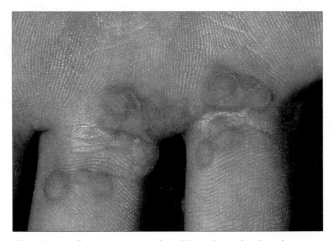

Fig. 28.41 Common warts (papilloma) on the hand. Courtesy of MJ Wood.

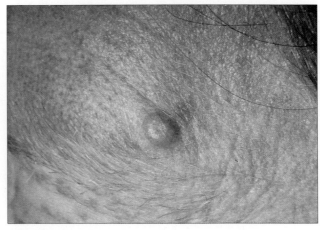

Fig. 28.42 Single umbilicated lesion in molluscum contagiosum. Courtesy of MJ Wood.

Clinical features and pathogenesis

After infection the virus replicates in cells in the oral mucosa and forms virus-rich vesicles. The patient suffers at most a mild febrile illness. The vesicles ulcerate and become coated with a whitish-grey slough (Fig. 28.43).

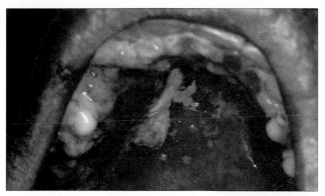

Fig. 28.43 Primary herpes simplex. Shallow ulcers with white exudate on the palate and gums. Courtesy of JA Innes.

During the primary infection virus particles enter sensory nerve endings in the lesion and are transported to the dorsal root (trigeminal) ganglion, where they initiate latent infection in sensory neurones (see Chapter 15). The lesion resolves as antibody and CMI responses develop. The latent virus remains in the sensory ganglion for life, and under certain circumstances can reactivate and spread down sensory nerves to give cold sores at the site of the original infection (Fig. 28.44).

Primary infection can also occur in:
- The conjunctiva, to cause conjunctivitis and keratitis, often w... vesicles on the eyelids (see Chapter 21);
- The finger, to cause herpetic whitlow;
- Other skin sites following direct contact with infected individuals where there is rubbing or trauma. This is seen for instance in rugby football ('scrum pox') or in wrestlers ('herpes gladiatorum');
- The genital tract (see Chapter 24). Although HSV2 arose as a sexually transmitted variant of HSV1, the sites infected by the two types are now less clearly distinct.

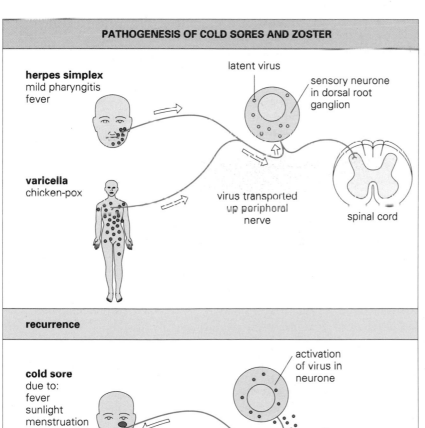

PATHOGENESIS OF COLD SORES AND ZOSTER

herpes simplex
mild pharyngitis
fever

latent virus

sensory neurone
in dorsal root
ganglion

varicella
chicken-pox

virus transported
up peripheral
nerve

spinal cord

recurrence

cold sore
due to:
fever
sunlight
menstruation
nerve section
at *

activation
of virus in
neurone

*

zoster (shingles)
due to:
age
immunocompromise
local injury

virus transported
down peripheral
nerve

spinal cord

Fig. 28.44 Pathogenesis of cold sores and zoster. In both HSV and V-ZV infections the virus in mucocutaneous nerve endings travels up the axon to reach the sensory neurones, where it becomes latent. Recurrences are due to reactivation of the virus within the neurone to become infectious followed by passage of virus down the axon to mucocutaneous site(s) and local spread and replication to form clinical lesion(s).

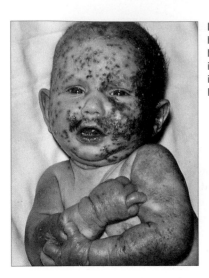

Fig. 28.45 Eczema herpeticum due to herpes simplex infection in an infant. Courtesy of MJ Wood.

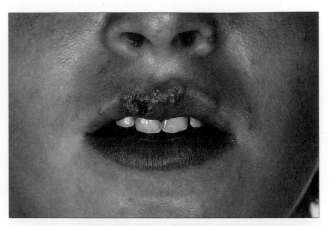

Fig. 28.46 Recurrent herpes simplex vesicles on the mucocutaneous margin of the lip. Courtesy of A du Vivier.

Complications

Serious complications associated with herpes simplex infection include:

- Herpetic infection of eczematous skin areas, leading to severe disease in young children (Fig. 28.45);
- Acute necrotizing encephalitis following either primary infection or reactivation (see Chapter 27);
- Neonatal infection acquired from the genital tract of the mother (see Chapter 26);
- Primary or reactivating HSV infection in immunocompromised individuals, causing very severe disease (see Chapter 33).

Recurrent HSV

In healthy individuals virus reactivation is provoked by certain febrile illnesses (e.g. common cold, pneumonia), by direct sunlight, by stress, and in association with menstruation (see Chapter 14). Reactivation also occurs and is more severe in immunocompromised patients (see Chapter 33). A sensory prodrome (pain, burning, itching) precedes the appearance of the lesion and is due to virus activity in sensory neurones. The lesion, a so-called 'cold sore', generally occurs around the mucocutaneous junctions in the nose or mouth (Fig. 28.46). Less commonly, when the ophthalmic branch of the trigeminal ganglion is involved, the lesion is a dendritic ulcer in the cornea. Large amounts of virus are shed in the cold sore, which scabs over and heals over the course of about a week. Occasionally the sensory prodrome occurs without proceeding to a cold sore (see also V-ZV recurrence).

Diagnosis

The virus is readily isolated from vesicle fluid, saliva or conjunctival fluid, and causes a well-marked cytopathic effect in human embryo lung and other cells. Significant rises in complement-fixing (CF) antibodies may be useful in diagnosing primary infection but recurrent infection rarely leads to a rise in titre.

Treatment and prevention

Acyclovir has revolutionized the treatment of HSV infection (see Chapter 35), and can be used either topically or systemically. It is relatively non-toxic and acts specifically in virus-infected cells. Recurrent herpetic eruptions have been successfully treated with low doses of acyclovir twice daily for up to three years.

Other topical treatments include 0.1% idoxuridine for herpes keratitis, or 5–40% idoxuridine in dimethylsulphoxide for herpetic skin lesions.

Varicella-zoster virus infection

Aetiology and transmission

Varicella-zoster virus (V-ZV) is a medium-sized (100-200 nm diameter) dsDNA virus of the herpesvirus group and is morphologically indistinguishable from HSV. There is only one serological type. The virus grows more slowly than HSV and is not released from the infected cell. Infection is by inhalation of droplets from respiratory secretions and saliva, or by direct contact from skin lesions. Primary infection with V-ZV causes varicella (chicken-pox). Immunity develops and prevents reinfection (a second attack of varicella) but the virus persists in the body and later in life, after reactivation, causes zoster (shingles). Varicella is highly contagious and nearly all humans, world-wide, are infected during childhood. The vesicles of zoster are slightly less infectious but are an important source of varicella in the community (see Chapter 15).

Clinical features and pathogenesis

After primary infection the virus passes across surface epithelium in the respiratory tract to infect mononuclear cells, and is then carried to lymphoid tissues. There are no symptoms and no detectable lesions at the site of entry into the body. The virus slowly replicates in lymphoreticular tissues for about a week, and then enters the blood in association with mononuclear cells and is seeded out to epithelial sites. These are mainly the respiratory tract and the skin, but also include the mouth, often the conjunctiva, and probably also the alimentary and urinogenital tracts. In the skin, for unknown reasons, the trunk, face and scalp are especially involved. At these epithelial sites the virus exits from small blood vessels, infecting subepi-

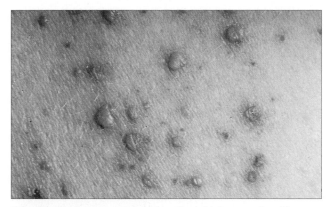

Fig. 28.47 Early rash in varicella (chicken-pox), with macules, papules and vesicles. Courtesy of MJ Wood.

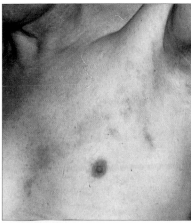

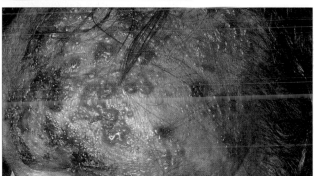

Fig. 28.48 Zoster rash. (a) A band of faint erythema, an early sign of shingles, along an intercostal nerve. (b) Rash effecting the ophthalmic division of the trigeminal nerve. Courtesy of MJ Wood.

thelial and finally epithelial cells. Multinucleated giant cells with intranuclear inclusions are present in the lesions. In the oropharynx and respiratory tract the virus reaches the surface and is shed to the exterior to infect other individuals about two weeks after initial infection. In the skin it takes a day or two longer, and it is at this stage, when the characteristic varicella vesicles appear, that a clinical diagnosis can be made (Fig. 28.47) The mean incubation period is 14 days (range 10–23 days).

The patient remains well until a day or two before the rash, when there may be slight fever and, malaise, but the illness is usually mild and often unnoticed. The vesicles appear first on the trunk, then on the face and scalp, and less commonly on arms and legs. They often come in 'crops', over the course of several days, then develop into pustules, break down, and scab over. The lesions are deeper than with HSV, and scarring is more common. Lesions in the mouth may be painful.

Complications

Skin lesions can become infected with staphylococci or streptococci to produce secondary impetigo, but varicella in a child is characteristically a very mild illness. It is generally more severe and complications are commoner in adults. The main complications are:

- Interstitial pneumonia; this can be detected radiologically, although it is often subclinical, in up to 20% of adults with varicella. Secondary bacterial pneumonia can also occur;
- CNS involvement, which may consist of a lymphocytic meningitis or an encephalomyelitis (see Chapter 27).

Thrombocytopenia can occur but it is usually symptomless. In immunocompromised patients, particularly children with leukaemia, varicella can be a life-threatening disease. After primary infection during pregnancy the virus may infect the foetus (see Chapter 26), but maternal antibody is present by then and the infection is generally without serious consequences. However, when the mother is infected a few days after delivery the infant is exposed without the protection of maternal antibody and can suffer a serious disease.

Recurrent V-ZV infection

During primary infection V-ZV in mucocutaneous lesions enters sensory nerve endings and establishes latent infection in sensory neurones in dorsal root ganglia (see Fig. 28.44). Later in life reactivation can occur to cause zoster (shingles) in the dermatome at the site of the reactivation. Thoracic dermatomes are most commonly involved because the original varicella lesions are commonest here. Zoster is unilateral because the reactivation is a localized event in a single dorsal root ganglion. Zoster thus originates from inside the body and is not directly acquired from either varicella or zoster in other individuals. During reactivation in sensory neurones (see Fig. 28.44), there is paraesthesia and pain. Pain may be severe and preceeds by several days the development of the erythematous rash in which virus-rich vesicles appear (Fig. 28.48). Fever and malaise may accompany the rash. Sometimes the immune response controls the reactivating virus before skin lesions have had time to form, and in this case the sensory phenomena occur without the skin eruption.

The following conditions predispose to zoster:

- Increasing age. Although zoster is very occasionally seen in childhood, its incidence increases with increasing age, rising from three cases per thousand per year in 50–59 year olds to ten per thousand per year in 80–89 year olds;
- Immunocompromise due to leukaemia, lymphoma, AIDS, renal transplant or other drug-induced immunosuppression. For instance zoster occurs in about 20% of patients with Hodgkin's disease;
- Fractures or tumours affecting the brain or spinal cord.

The skin areas affected by zoster reflect the distribution of the original varicella rash, as might be expected from its pathogenesis (see Fig. 28.44). Hence the trunk is most commonly involved. Ophthalmic zoster, with the upper eyelid, forehead and scalp also affected, is a particularly unpleasant manifestation.

Complications of zoster. In the normal host post-herpetic (post-zoster) neuralgia is a common complication, especially in the elderly. Pain, which can also be severe early in the illness, continues to cause suffering for up to several months after the lesions have resolved. It is difficult to treat.

In the immunocompromised patients zoster may be very severe. A few days after the localized eruption, the virus, with inadequate control by CMI, spreads via the blood to cause skin and visceral lesions throughout the body. Haemorrhagic complications and pneumonia may occur.

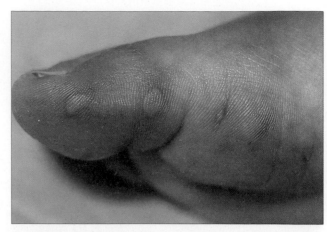

Fig. 28.49 Vesicular lesions on the foot in hand, foot and mouth disease. Courtesy of M J Wood.

Diagnosis

Isolation of the virus is difficult and is not routinely attempted in laboratories. Herpesvirus particles can be seen by electron microscopy in vesicle fluid but they are indistinguishable from HSV particles. In varicella and usually in zoster a rise in CF antibody titre between acute and convalescent sera is detectable. Past immunity is determined from the presence of antibodies by ELISA or other tests.

Treatment and prevention

Varicella skin lesions are treated with baths and soothing applications to relieve itching and to prevent scratching and secondary infection. V-ZV is much less sensitive than HSV to acyclovir, but severe infections can be treated with intravenous acyclovir. V-ZV immune globulin contains a high titre of human antibody to the virus, and is used to prevent varicella in vulnerable individuals after exposure. A live attenuated vaccine is available for the protection of immunocompromised children, but is not yet approved for general use.

Rashes caused by coxsackieviruses and echoviruses

Coxsackieviruses and echoviruses cause a variety of exanthems (skin rashes), sometimes with an enanthem (lesions on internal epithelial surfaces such as the oral cavity). These infections are generally seen in young children, are not usually distinguishable on clinical examination, and are not severe. These viruses are also responsible for illnesses affecting the central nervous system (see Chapter 27), the upper respiratory tract (see Chapter 20), and striated and heart muscle (see below). Coxsackievirus A lesions are usually vesicular and occur mostly on the buccal mucosa and the tongue. Most children complain of sore mouth or tongue and there is slight fever. When vesicular lesions are also seen on the skin, principally on the hands, feet, buttocks, the condition is called 'hand-foot-and-mouth disease' (Fig. 28.49). The virus is present in the lesions and coxsackievirus A16 is the commonest cause.

Maculopapular rashes resembling rubella are common manifestations of echovirus infection; a number of different serotypes may be involved.

Rashes caused by human parvovirus

Parvoviruses are very small (22 nm diameter) ssDNA viruses. The defective parvoviruses (see Appendix) require a helper (adeno-) virus to replicate, and are called 'adeno-associated viruses'; there are four serotypes and infection is common but they have not been implicated in any human disease. There is a non-defective parvovirus (B19) that causes a febrile illness in children with a characteristic maculopapular rash on the face ('slapped cheek syndrome'). The condition is referred to as 'erythema infectiosum', and sometimes 'fifth disease', it being the fifth of the six common exanthematous infections recognized by nineteenth century physicians. Symptomless infection is common and nearly half the population have antibodies. The virus grows in haemopoietic cells in the bone marrow and although this normally causes no more than a temporary and barely detectable fall in haemoglobin levels, it can lead to serious consequences in those with chronic anaemias. In children with sickle cell anaemia for instance, the effect on erythopoiesis may cause an aplastic crisis. The virus can also cause arthralgia when it infects adults. It was first discovered by electron microscopy, and cannot be isolated in cell culture. Virus-specific IgM antibody tests are available.

Other maculopapular rashes

Maculopapular rashes are seen in a number of other virus infections. They appear to be immune-mediated, there being little or no viral invasion of the skin and no shedding of virus from the skin.

Human herpes virus 6 (HHV6) infects nearly all humans during the first five years of life (see Chapter 29). Although it grows in T and B cells its main clinical manifestation is a maculopapular rash known as exanthem subitum or roseola infantum. After an incubation period of about two weeks there is fever for a few days with cervical lymphadenopathy, the rash appearing 1–2 days after disappearance of the fever.

The maculopapular rashes caused by measles and rubella viruses, and the maculopapular rashes seen in certain arthropod–borne virus infections (e.g. dengue) and in zoonotic virus infections (e.g. Marburg disease) are referred to in Chapters 29, 30 and 31. A maculopapular rash is often seen in the prodromal stage of hepatitis B virus infection (see Chapter 24), and is immune complex-mediated.

There are a variety of rashes or other skin lesions produced in other bacterial and fungal infections. Most of these are referred to elsewhere in this book, and they are listed in figure 28.4. Rashes in rickettsial infections are often striking, as in the case of Rocky Mountain spotted fever or typhus (see Chapter 30). Most rickettsia invade vascular endothelial cells, from whence they are shed into the blood to infect blood-sucking arthropod vectors. Invasion of vascular endothelial cells in the skin provides the basis for the skin rash but is not a source of direct shedding to the exterior.

VIRAL INFECTIONS OF MUSCLE

Viral myositis, myocarditis and pericarditis

Aetiology and transmission

Group B , and to a lesser extent group A, coxsackieviruses and certain enteroviruses, are the main viral causes of myocarditis and pericarditis. Both conditions are seen principally in adult males and are important because they can be mistaken for myocardial infarction, yet the prognosis is good and complete recovery is the rule. These infections are spread by the faecal–oral route and occasionally from pharyngeal secretions. Mumps and influenza are less common causes of myocarditis or pericarditis. Rubella (see Chapter 26) can cause myocarditis and associated congenital lesions in the foetus.

Group B coxsackieviruses also cause pleurodynia or epidemic myalgia. This condition is sometimes called 'Bornholm disease', after the Danish island where there was an extensive outbreak in 1930. There is pain and inflammation involving intercostal or abdominal muscles. Influenza (especially influenza B in children) can cause pain and tenderness in muscles, but it is not known whether this is associated with viral invasion of muscle. Myalgias are also seen in dengue and in certain rickettsial infections but here too the mechanism is unknown.

Clinical features and pathogenesis

Ingested coxsackieviruses spread from the pharynx or gut wall to the lymphatics and then to the blood. Invasion of striated muscles, heart or pericardium takes place across small blood vessels and results in acute inflammation. In the heart and pericardium this gives rise to dyspnoea, pain in the chest, and sometimes mimics a myocardial infarction.

Diagnosis, treatment and prevention

Coxsackievirus may be isolated from throat swabs, faecal specimens or pericardial fluid. Rising titres of neutralizing antibody may be demonstrable, or the presence of IgM antibodies in ELISA tests.

There are no specific treatments and no vaccines for coxsackievirus infections.

Postviral fatigue syndrome

The postviral fatigue syndrome is sometimes referred to as myalgic encephalomyelitis, but this is inappropriate because there is no evidence for CNS pathology. The condition has been difficult to establish as a clinical entity. It consists of:
* Chronic and severe muscle weakness, lasting at least six months, often as a sequel to an acute febrile illness;
* Severe tiredness;
* Less regularly associated symptoms such as depression, headache and anxiety.

It is more reliably identified when the first two symptoms appear in a previously healthy individual with no history of psychosomatic illness. Several viruses have been suggested as causes. A small proportion of cases appear to be due to chronic infection with Epstein–Barr virus. There have been repeated claims for the role of coxsackie B viruses, based on antibody tests and on the detection of a virus-specific protein in the serum of patients. But these results have not been widely confirmed and the picture remains unclear. Occasional reports have associated the condition with HHV6 and with other viruses. It has also been suggested that it is due to 'allergic reactions' triggered by virus infection.

KAWASAKI DISEASE

Kawasaki disease is a childhood illness of unknown aetiology. Patients, who are less than eight years old, develop fever, congested conjunctiva, and a rash. There is dryness and redness of the lips, red palms and soles with some oedema, desquamation of fingertips, often together with arthralgia, and a carditis that gives a case mortality of about 2%. Epidemics have occurred in the USA, and the disease is commoner in those of Japanese ancestry. Although there is no evidence for person-to-person transmission and no microbe has been regularly isolated, it is quite possibly of infectious origin.

PARASITIC INFECTIONS OF MUSCLE

Relatively few parasites commonly invade muscle tissues or cause serious disease. Three are described here to illustrate the variety of organisms and the range of pathology.

Trypanosoma cruzi infection

This protozoan causes Chagas' disease or American trypanosomiasis (see Chapter 30). This disease, is restricted to Central and South America, where it affects an estimated 10 to 12 million people. The parasite is carried by blood-sucking bugs, which deposit infective trypomastigote stages on to the skin as they defecate whilst feeding. If these are rubbed into mucous membranes or wounds, the parasites penetrate cells, transform into amastigotes and proliferate. The infected cells then burst, liberating trypomastigotes that disperse around the body to reinvade other cells. Major sites of infection include the CNS, intestinal myenteric plexus, reticuloendothelial system and cardiac muscle. Disease occurs as an acute febrile phase, with intense inflammatory changes, and as a chronic phase, lasting many years, where there is gradual tissue destruction, autoimmune damage playing an important role. In the heart, where the parasite invades the myofibrils (see Fig. 30.19), muscle fibrils and Purkinje fibres may be replaced by fibrous tissue. As a result of the conduction defects this causes, the heart enlarges, there are cardiac arrhythmias and heart failure can occur. No satisfactory prophylaxis is available, and the chronic disease is irreversible. Prevention of infection is the most important measure.

Taenia solium infection

Although tapeworms are usually thought of as intestinal parasites the larval stages of a number of species may invade deeper tissues of the body. The most important of these are the larvae of *Echinococcus granulosus* (which cause hydatid disease; see Chapter 31) and of the pork tapeworm *Taenia solium*. Humans acquire the latter infection by eating undercooked infected pig meat in which the cysticercus larvae are found as small, bladder-like structures in the muscle tissue. These larvae are digested out in the intestine and mature into the adult tapeworm, which may reach a length of several metres. *Taenia solium* is unusual in that its eggs can hatch directly in the human intestine. This may result from accidental swallowing of water contaminated with eggs, but can occur directly from the eggs released by adult worms. If hatching occurs, the larvae cross the intestinal wall and are carried via the blood to internal organs. Sites of development include the CNS and body muscles. In the latter the cysts eventually become calcified and can be seen on x-ray (Fig. 28.50). Muscle infection is not serious, being largely asymptomatic. Infections are common in many parts of the world, particularly South and Central America and Asia. Avoidance of undercooked pork products is the safest precaution; infections can be treated with praziquantel.

Trichinella spiralis infection

The life cycle of this nematode has many unique features. The parasite is able to infect almost any warm-blooded animal, and has a life cycle in which a complete generation (infective stage to infective stage) develops within the body of a single host. Transmission depends upon the ingestion of muscle tissue containing viable infective larvae. As far as humans are concerned, the commonest route of transmission is via infected pig meat, but many other meat sources have been known to transmit infection (e.g. bear, boar, horse). Infections occur world-wide. When infected undercooked meat is eaten, the larvae are digested out in the small intestine and develop rapidly into the adult worms. These live in the mucosa, the females releasing newborn larvae directly into the intestinal tissues. From there the larvae are carried in blood or lymph around the body, eventually penetrating into striated muscles where they mature into the infective stage, transforming muscle cells into a parasite-sustaining nurse cell (see Fig. 31.14).

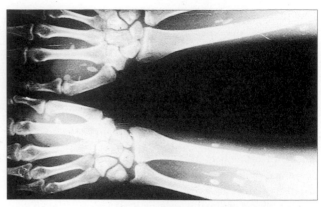

Fig. 28.50 X-ray showing numerous calcified cysts of *T. solium* in the forearms. Courtesy of R Muller and JR Baker.

Although light infections are asymptomatic, the migration and penetration of the larvae is associated with inflammatory reactions, which can be severe and life-threatening when a person is heavily infected. A variety of symptoms are associated with this phase, of which fever, muscle pains, weakness and eosinophilia are characteristic. Myocarditis may also occur, although the parasite does not develop in the heart. The muscle stage of infection can be treated with mebendazole; steroids may also be required.

JOINT AND BONE INFECTIONS

Joints and bones will be considered separately for convenience, but joint lesions often spread to involve neighbouring bone, and vice versa (e.g. in tuberculosis).

Reactive arthritis, arthralgia and septic arthritis

Aetiology, pathogenesis, diagnosis and treatment

Arthralgia and arthritis occur in a variety of infections, as outlined in figure 28.51. Joints can become infected by the haematogenous route or directly following trauma or surgery, but in many cases the condition is immunologically mediated rather than due to microbial invasion of the joint. The microbe responsible is at a distant site in the body, and it is a 'reactive arthritis'. Reactive arthritis and arthralgia occur after certain enteric bacterial infections, and the arthralgia in rubella and hepatitis B infections is of similar origin. In this type of arthritis more than one joint is usually affected. Ankylosing spondylitis is associated with *Klebsiella* infection, and it has been suggested that the antigenic similarity between *Klebsiella* and HLA B27 antigens provokes a cross-reactive immune response that causes the disease. So far there is no evidence that rheumatoid arthritis is caused by either viruses or other microbes. Circulating bacteria sometimes localize in joints, especially following trauma, and can then cause a suppurative (septic) arthritis. Generally a single joint is involved.

Joints are very susceptible, particularly if they are already damaged for instance by rheumatoid arthritis, or if a pros-

ARTHRALGIA AND ARTHRITIS IN INFECTIOUS DISEASES		
	infectious agent	**comments**
viral arthritis	Hepatitis B	occurs in prodromal period; due to circulating immune complexes
	Rubella	especially in young women, often follows live virus vaccine
	Mumps	unusual, mostly in men
	Ross River and other togaviruses	mosquito-transmitted infections in Australia (Ross River) and Africa
	Parvovirus	may follow adult infection
reactive arthritis	*Campylobacter. Yersinia, Salmonella, Shigella, Chlamydia trachomatis* (Reiter's syndrome*)	'post-infectious' arthritis, HLA B27-associated, no bacterial invasion of joint, immune mediated
septic arthritis	*Staphylococcus aureus*	commonest cause of suppurative arthritis
	Salmonella	occurs in children
	Haemophilus influenzae	occurs in children
	Neisseria gonorrhoeae	may affect multiple joints
	Mycobacterium tuberculosis	often together with bone lesions, especially weight bearing joints and bones
	Borrelia burgdorferi	arthritis a late feature of Lyme disease
	Streptococci, *Pseudomonas aeruginosa*	uncommon
	Mycoplasma hominis	bacteria can enter maternal blood during delivery and invade joints. Uncommon
	Sporothrix schenckii	most common fungal infection of joints

* Urethritis, arthritis, uveitis ± mucocutaneous lesions; complicates 1–2% of cases of chlamydial urethritis

Fig. 28.51 Arthralgia and arthritis in infectious diseases.

thesis has been inserted. Knees are most commonly affected, followed by hips, ankles (see Fig. 24.9) and elbows. Patients show fever, joint pain, limitation of movement, swelling, and usually a joint effusion. Bacteria can be isolated from the joint fluid or seen in the centrifuged deposit, and the commonest organism is *Staphylococcus aureus*. Sometimes the source of the circulating bacteria is obvious (e.g. a septic skin lesion) but often no source is apparent.

Osteomyelitis

Aetiology and pathogenesis

As with joints, infection can be by the direct route (e.g. from a nearby focus of infection, after fractures, after orthopaedic surgery) or from circulating microbes. The commonest cause of haematogenous osteomyelitis is *Staphylococcus aureus*, but when infection is from a neighbouring site it is generally mixed, with Gram-negative rods

and occasionally anaerobes also present. There seems to be no equivalent to reactive arthritis, in which inflammation is due to infection at a distant site.

Acute osteomyelitis typically involves the growing end of a long bone, where sprouting capillary loops adjacent to epiphysial growth plates promote the localization of circulating bacteria. It therefore tends to be a disease of children and adolescents, and may follow non-penetrating injury to the bone.

Clinical features, diagnosis and treatment

There is a painful tender bone lesion and a general febrile illness. Diagnosis is from blood cultures taken before the start of antimicrobial therapy or, when there is an open lesion, from a bone biopsy. Periosteal reaction and bone loss may be visible radiologically (Fig. 28.52). Treatment is begun on a 'most likely' basis (cloxacillin, for penicillinase-producing *Staph. aureus*) as soon as microbiological samples have been taken.

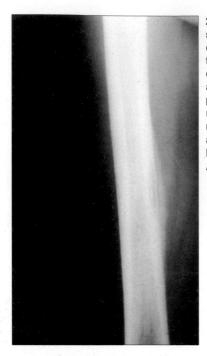

28.52 Acute staphylococcal osteomyelitis in the femur of a 24-year-old woman. There is a well defined periosteal reaction in relation to the midshaft of the femur and an underlying lucency. Courtesy of AM Davies.

Osteomyelitis becomes chronic, especially when there are necrotic bone fragments to act as a continued source of infection. Surgical intervention for debridement and drainage, as well as prolonged courses of antibiotics, may be necessary.

Tuberculosis may affect the spine, the hip, the knee, or the bones of the hands and feet, and in the west is seen especially in immigrants from the Indian subcontinent. Constitutional disturbances are often absent, but the site is generally painful and pressure from a tuberculous abscess in the spine can cause paraplegia.

INFECTIONS OF THE HAEMOPOIETIC SYSTEM

A great variety of infectious agents cause alterations in circulating blood cells. For instance, *Bordetella pertussis* causes lymphocytosis, Epstein–Barr and cytomegaloviruses cause mononucleosis, while the *Plasmodia* cause anaemia and thrombocytopenia. A smaller number of infectious agents act directly on cells in the bone marrow (human parvovirus) or cause malignant transformation of lympho-cytes (HTLV1 and HTLV2). The range of possibilities is summarized in figure 28.53. HTLV1 and 2 are mentioned in Chapters 24 and 27, but are described more fully below.

MICROBES AFFECTING BLOOD CELLS OR HAEMOPOIESIS			
microbe	**disease**	**effect**	**mechanism**
Plasmodium spp	malaria	anaemia	replication in erythrocytes
Babesia spp	babesiosis (uncommon, tick–borne)	anaemia	replication in erythrocytes
Bartonella brucelliformis	oroya fever* (rare, sandfly-transmitted, occurs in Peru)	anaemia	replication in erythrocytes
Human parvovirus	erythema infectiosum	temporary fall in haemoglobin levels (adult) aplastic crisis (child with chronic anaemia)	replication in erythropoietic cells
Colorado tick fever virus	colorado tick fever	no effect on survival of infected erythrocytes	replication in erythropoietic cells
HTLV1,HTLV2	T cell leukaemia, lymphoma	malignant transformation of infected T cells	replication in T cells
HIV **	AIDS	immunosuppression	infection of CD4 positive T cells
EB virus	infectious mononucleosis	thrombocytopenia (common) anaemia (complication)	autoantibody to platelets, erythrocytes
Cytomegalovirus	congenital CMV, complication of adult infection	anaemia, thrombocytopenia	infection of, or autoantibody to, erythrocytes, platelets

* a cutaneous form (Verrugas) also occurs. In 1885 a peruvian medical student, Daniel Carrion, demonstrated the common bacterial origin by inoculating himself with infected blood from the cutaneous form of the disease and developing oroya fever.

** many other viruses infect immune cells and depress immune responses less dramatically (e.g. CMV, measles).

Fig. 28.53 Microbes affecting blood cells or haemopoiesis.

HTLV1 infection

Aetiology and transmission

HTLV1 (human T cell lymphotropic virus type 1) was first isolated in 1980 from a patient with adult T cell leukaemia. Infection is widespread, especially in certain islands in the West Indies and Japan, where 5–15% of the population are seropositive, and also in S. America and parts of Africa. Transmission is primarily via maternal milk, and in addition via homosexual and heterosexual routes, and by blood in intravenous drug abusers.

Clinical features and pathogenesis

The virus infects T cells so that blood is infectious, and the infection is persistent. The tax protein (coded by the pxV region of the viral genome) stimulates transcription of host genes controlling production of IL-2, IL-2 receptor and other molecules. Infected T cells proliferate, and if in addition there are certain chromosomal abnormalities, then malignant transformation takes place. The patient develops a mild febrile disease, with lymphadenopathy. The skin is often involved (nodules, plaques) and pleural effusion or aseptic meningitis can occur. There is also increased susceptibility to opportunist infections (*Pneumocystis carinii*, CMV), associated with depressed delayed hypersensitivity responses to tuberculin. Polymyositis has been described. Up to 5% of infected individuals eventually develop T cell leukaemia, and others (about the same proportion) progress to 'tropical' spastic paraparesis, a myelopathy in which there is primary demyelination (see Chapter 27). Neural cells do not appear to be infected and it is not known how the virus causes a neurological disease.

Diagnosis, treatment and prevention

HTLV1-specific antibodies are demonstrable, but false positive results can occur. Retrovir inhibits viral replication but is not known to influence the leukaemia or the myelopathy once they have appeared. Seropositive individuals are assumed to be infectious and should not donate blood or organs.

HTLV2 infection

HTLV2 (human T cell lymphotropic virus type 2) was first isolated in 1982 from a patient with T cell hairy leukaemia, although it is not the usual cause of this condition. HTLV2 is closely related to HTLV1, and is not distinguishable by routine laboratory tests. Almost nothing is known of its distribution, transmission, or natural history.

SUMMARY

The intact skin provides an invaluable barrier that defends the body against invasion. Bacteria, fungi and viruses usually gain access through breaches of the barrier caused by trauma. Some parasites on the other hand are capable of initiating their own penetration into the skin. Arthropod vectors are important in transmission of several microbial species which then set up local infections or disseminate through the body to distant sites. Conversely, pathogens may be acquired by other routes, disseminate in the body and localize in the skin or cause toxic or immunopathologic manifestations in the skin. Thus a very wide range of organisms is associated with skin infection and disease.

Superficial infections of the skin are among the commonest human infections and usually cause little more than cosmetic distress. Invasion of pathogens deeper into dermal and subdermal tissues, however, may produce severe infections that can be rapidly fatal, as in gangrene, or slow but progressive deformation and destruction, as in leprosy.

Infections of muscle usually arise from invasion from the outside whereas infections of joints is more often blood-borne. Bone infections may arise either by local spread from an infected joint or as a result of haematogenous seeding. Bone marrow cells are occasionally invaded by viruses which interfere with haemopoiesis (parvovirus) or cause malignant transformation (HTLV1 and 2).

Further Reading

Corey L, Spear PG. Infections with herpes simplex viruses. *N Engl J Med* 1986; **314:** 686; 749.

Demeter LM, Reichman RC. Human papillomavirus. *Curr Opin Infect Dis* 1990; **3:** 796–804.

Jones HE, Reinhardt JH, Renaldi MG. Acquired immunity to dematophytes. *Arch dermatol* 1974; **109:** 840.

Miller AE. Selective decline in cellular immune response to varicella-zoster in the elderly. *Neurology* 1980; **30:** 582–587.

Roth RR, James WD. Microbial ecology of the skin. *Ann Rev Microbiol* 1988; **42:** 411–464.

Spodick DK (1986) Infection and infarction. Acute viral (and other) infection in the onset, pathogenesis and mimicry of acute myocardial infarction. *Am J Med* 1986; **81:** 661–668.

Spruance SL, Overall JC, Jr, Kern ER, Krueger GC, Pliam V, Miller W. The natural history of recurrent herpes simplex labialis: Implications for antiviral therapy. *N Engl J Med* 1977; **297:** 69–75.

Stevens JG. Human herpes viruses; a consideration of the latent state. *Microbiol Rev* 1989; **53:** 318–332.

Straus SE., Ostrove JM, Inchauspé G. Varicella-zoster virus infections: Biology, natural history, treatment and prevention. *Ann Int Med* 1988; **108:** 221–237.

Swartz MN. The chronic fatigue syndrome – one entity or many? *N.Engl J Med* 1988; **319:** 1726–1727.

Weller TH. Varicella and herpes zoster. Changing concepts of the natural history, control, and importance of a not-so-benign virus. *N. Engl J Med* 1983; **309:** 1362–1368; 1434–1440.

DIAGNOSIS AND CLINICAL MANIFESTATIONS

part 3 **Multisystem and other Infections**

29 WORLD-WIDE VIRUS INFECTIONS

Contents

INTRODUCTION

The infectious agents described in the previous chapters characteristically cause diseases in which damage and symptoms predominate in a particular part of the body, even though spread to other systems may occur. Thus, tuberculosis, typhoid and syphilis are considered in chapters on the respiratory tract, intestine and urogenital tract, respectively, these being the main sites involved in infection and/or transmission. Many other microbes cannot be so easily pigeon-holed. These include a number of important and common virus infections which cause diseases that are not obviously localized to any one system of the body. These multisystem infections are discussed in this chapter.

The viruses described occur in all parts of the world, and are exclusively human infections. Some of them, like the viruses included in Chapter 28 (HSV, V-ZV, HPV, etc.), cause skin rashes (exanthems), but differ because they are not primarily dermatotrophic. Most of them involve young children, but some (mumps, Epstein–Barr virus) cause more severe illness when primary infection takes place during adolescence or adult life. This is more common in developed countries, especially with EB virus, where individuals often escape infection during childhood. Some (measles, mumps, rubella) are readily controllable by vaccines, but so far this has been achieved only in developed countries.

MEASLES

Measles has several special features:
- Nearly all infected individuals become unwell and develop disease. This is in contrast to most other virus infections, in which a significant proportion of individuals undergo an asymptomatic or subclinical infection;
- The disease is so characteristic that a clinical diagnosis can nearly always be made without the need for laboratory help. We can recognize measles as described a thousand years ago by the Arabian physician Rhazes;
- There is only one antigenic type of measles virus;
- After infection there is complete resistance to reinfection which is probably life-long. Second attacks are almost unknown;
- Measles is highly infectious, and nearly all susceptible children contract the disease on exposure. Until recently measles was regarded as a routine, inescapable part of childhood, and more than 99% of individuals were infected;
- There is a striking contrast between measles in well-nourished children with good access to medical care (i.e. in developed countries) and measles under conditions of malnutrition or starvation or with poor medical services (developing countries). The seed (virus) is the same in each case but differences in the soil (human host) lead to a different outcome (Fig. 29.1).

Aetiology and transmission

The basic virology of this paramyxovirus is described in Chapter 3 and in the Appendix. Transmission takes place readily via respiratory droplets. Although the virus is soon inactivated as it dries on surfaces, it is more stable in droplets suspended in the air. In unvaccinated populations, outbreaks tend to occur every few years when the number of susceptible children reaches a high enough level.

Clinical features and pathogenesis

The pathogenesis of measles is illustrated in Chapter 13. The inhaled virus enters the body at unknown sites in the upper or lower respiratory tract and spreads to subepithelial and local lymphatic tissues, without causing detectable lesions or symptoms. During the next few days the virus slowly spreads and multiplies in lymphoid tissues elsewhere in the body, including the spleen. The virus then enters the blood in larger amounts and, about a week after infection, is seeded out to a variety of epithelial sites. In the respiratory tract, where there are only one or two layers of epithelial cells, clinical signs soon appear. Nine to ten days after infection, the patient, until now perfectly well, develops an acute respiratory illness with running nose, fever and cough. Conjunctivitis is also present and, as a result of the large amounts of virus being shed in respiratory secretions, the patient is highly infectious. The diagnosis may be suspected during this prodromal illness, especially after known exposure to measles. It takes a day or two longer for the foci of infection at mucosal and skin surfaces to cause lesions. Koplik's spots appear inside the cheek

(Fig. 29.2), and shortly afterwards the unmistakable maculopapular rash (Fig. 29.3) is seen, first on the face, then spreading down the body to the extremities. The diagnosis is now clear.

Antibodies are formed, but a cell mediated immune (CMI) response is needed to control the growth of virus in the lungs and elsewhere. Without it the virus continues to grow and gives rise to giant cell pneumonia (see Chapter 21).The CMI response is also responsible for the skin lesions, which are not seen in patients with serious defects in this type of immunity. Children with agammaglobulin-aemia, on the other hand, have a normal course of disease, develop normal immunity, and can be protected by vaccination. In uncomplicated cases recovery is rapid.

During measles, as in a variety of other acute infections, there are temporary defects in immune responses to unrelated antigens. For instance, at about the time the rash appears, individuals who are known to be tuberculin-positive give negative skin-test responses to tuberculin. This returns to normal in about a month. During the 'Virgin-soil' epidemic, when measles reappeared after a long absence in Southern Greenland in 1953 and adults as well as children were infected, there was increased mortality in those previously infected with tuberculosis.

Complications

Complications can occur for the following reasons:
- As a result of virus damage to respiratory surfaces, opportunistic bacterial superinfections are quite common, especially otitis media and pneumonia;

THE CLINICAL IMPACT OF MEASLES		
site of virus growth	well nourished child good medical care	malnourished child poor medical care
Lung	temporary respiratory illness	life threatening pneumonia
Ear	otitis media quite common	otitis media commoner more severe
Oral mucosa	Koplik's spots	severe ulcerating lesions
Conjunctiva	conjunctivitis	severe corneal lesions secondary bacterial infection blindness may result
Skin	maculopapular rash	haemorrhagic rashes may occur ('black–measles')
Intestinal tract	no lesions	diarrhoea – exacerbates malnutrition, halts growth, impairs recovery
Urinary tract	virus detectable in urine	no known complications
Overall impact	serious disease in a small proportion of those infected	major cause of death in childhood (estimated 1.5 million deaths/yr worldwide)

Fig. 29.1 The clinical impact of measles depends on the host. Measles is a much more serious disease in malnourished children with poor access to medical care. The same epithelial surfaces are infected, but more extensively and with more serious sequelae.

- A primary measles virus pneumonia (giant-cell pneumonia) is seen in patients with serious cell-mediated immune defects;
- Encephalitis occurs in about 1 in a 1000 cases (see Chapter 27);
- Very rarely sub-acute sclerosing panencephalitis (SSPE) occurs. This develops one to ten years after apparent recovery from acute infection;
- Children in countries where there is poor medical care and malnutrition develop a more serious disease (see Fig. 29.1). This is especially the case during famine. It is attributable to:
    1) Poor local mucosal defences, which can be improved by vitamin A administration;
    2) Impaired immune defences due to protein–calorie malnutrition, with the added impact of measles virus-induced immunosuppression;
    3) Poor medical services, with antibiotics to control secondary infection less readily available;
    4) High levels of bacterial contamination of the environment;
    5) Exposure to a larger virus dose, a possible factor if others with severe measles shed larger amounts of virus from the respiratory tract.

Diagnosis, treatment and prevention

The diagnosis is nearly always obvious clinically. Greater than four-fold rises in antibody titre can be detected in difficult cases. Virus isolation in cell culture is rarely necessary. No antiviral therapy is available, but a live attenuated vaccine is effective, safe and long lasting. It is combined with mumps and rubella vaccines (MMR vaccine; see Chapter 36).

MUMPS

Aetiology and transmission

There is only one serotype of this (ssRNA) paramyxovirus. It spreads by airborne droplets, salivary secretions and possibly urine. Intimate contact is necessary, either at school (peak incidence is at 5 to 14 years) or in crowded adult communities (e.g. prisons, garrisons, ships).

Clinical features, pathogenesis and complications

After entry into the body at unknown sites, probably in the upper respiratory tract, the virus spreads systemically, undergoing a lengthy period of growth in lymphoid tissues (lymphocytes and monocytes) and reticuloendothelial cells. After about 7 to 10 days the virus re-enters the blood and localizes in salivary and other glands (Fig. 29.4). Infected cells lining ducts degenerate and finally, after an incubation period of 18–21 days, the inflammation, with lymphocyte infiltration and often oedema, results in disease. After a prodromal period of malaise and anorexia lasting 1 to 2 days, the parotid gland becomes painful, tender and swollen. This is the classical sign of mumps (Fig. 29.5) although it is present only in 30–40% of infections. Cell-mediated as well as antibody responses appear, and the patient normally recovers within a week. There is life-long resistance to re-infection. However, other tissues in the body may be invaded, with clinical consequences as outlined in figure 29.4.

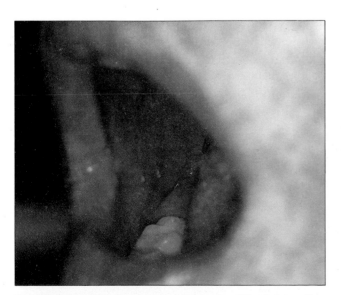

Fig. 29.2 Koplik's spots seen as minute white dots on the inflamed buccal mucosa of a patient with measles. Courtesy of MJ Wood.

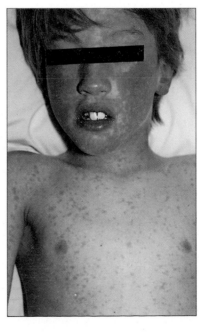

Fig. 29.3 Maculopapular rash on the face and trunk of a patient with measles. Courtesy of MJ Wood.

Diagnosis

Clinical diagnosis is made on the basis of parotitis. Laboratory diagnosis is:
- By isolating virus in cell culture from saliva, CSF or urine;
- By detecting:
  1) A greater than four-fold rise in antibody;
  2) Mumps-specific IgM antibody;
  3) CF (complement fixing) antibody to the S (soluble, nucleocapsid) mumps antigen. These antibodies disap-

pear within months and suggest recent infection. CF antibody to the V (viral envelope) antigen persists for years.

Treatment and prevention

There is no specific treatment. Mumps is prevented by a single injection of attenuated live virus vaccine which is safe and effective. This is usually given in combination with measles and rubella vaccines (MMR vaccine).

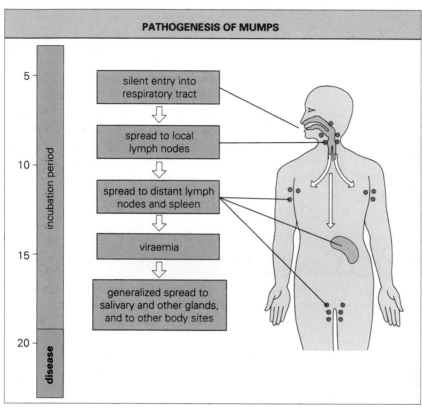

PATHOGENESIS OF MUMPS

Fig. 29.4 The pathogenesis of mumps. Understanding the pathogenesis of this infection helps to explain the disease picture, sites of shedding and the complications that can arise. Unfortunately, little is known about the events that occur during the first week of infection.

site of growth	result	comment
Salivary glands	inflammation, parotitis virus shed in saliva (from 3 days before to 6 days after symptoms)	often absent; can be unilateral
Meninges Brain	meningitis ⎤ ⎟ up to 7 days after parotitis encephalitis ⎦	common (in about 10% cases) less common; complete recovery is the rule; nerve deafness is a rare complication
Kidney	virus present in urine	no clinical consequences
Testis, ovary	epididymo-orchitis; rigid tunica albuginea around testis makes orchitis more painful, more damaging, in male	common in adults (20% in adult males); often unilateral; not a significant cause of sterility
Pancreas	pancreatitis	rare complication (possible role in juvenile diabetes)
Mammary gland	virus detectable in milk; mastitis in 10% post-pubertal females	–
Thyroid	thyroiditis	rare
Myocardium	myocarditis	rare
Joints	arthritis	rare

RUBELLA

Aetiology and transmission

There is only one serotype of this (ssRNA) togavirus. Although it causes a multisystem infection its principal impact is on the foetus (see Chapter 26). It is transmitted by droplet infection, and is less contagious than measles, but more so than mumps.

Clinical features and pathogenesis

After entering the body silently at unknown sites in the respiratory tract, the virus grows for a period in local lymphoid tissues, followed by spread to the spleen and to lymph nodes elsewhere in the body. A week after infection further multiplication in these tissues leads to viraemia and localization of virus in the respiratory tract, skin, and sometimes the placenta, joints, and kidney. The pathogenesis of rubella is outlined in figure 29.6. After an incubation period of 14–21 days there is a mild disease, with fever, malaise and an irregular maculopapular rash lasting 3 days. Enlarged lymph nodes are often seen behind the ear but the infection is often subclinical.

Diagnosis

Clinical diagnosis is sometimes possible. Laboratory diagnosis is made by demonstrating rubella-specific IgM antibodies or a four-fold or greater rise in HI or ELISA antibodies (see Chapter 18). Virus isolation from the throat is rarely indicated – the virus fails to damage cells in culture and indirect methods are needed to demonstrate its growth.

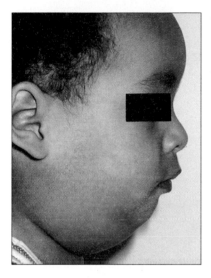

Fig. 29.5 Enlarged submandibular glands in a child with mumps. Courtesy of JA Innes.

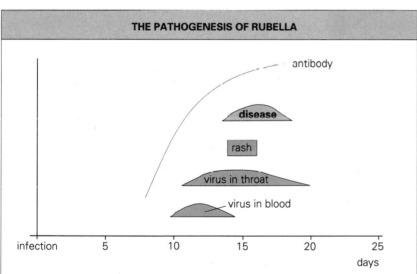

Fig. 29.6 The pathogenesis of rubella. Rubella is generally a very mild, often subclinical infection, but it can cause arthritis and has a major impact when it infects the foetus.

THE PATHOGENESIS OF RUBELLA

site of virus growth	result	comment
Respiratory tract	virus shedding but symptoms minimal (mild sore throat, coryza, cough)	patient infectious 5 days before to 3 days after symptoms
Skin	Rash	often fleeting, atypical; immunopathology involved (Ag–Ab complexes)
Lymph nodes	lymphadenopathy	commoner in posterior triangle of neck or behind ear
Joints	mild arthralgia, arthritis	immunopathology involved (circulating immune complexes)
Placenta/foetus	placentitis foetal damage	congenital rubella

Treatment and prevention

There is no antiviral treatment. A live attenuated rubella vaccine that is safe and effective is given by injection, generally in combination with measles and mumps vaccines (MMR vaccine). Prevention of congenital rubella is referred to in Chapter 26.

CYTOMEGALOVIRUS INFECTION

Aetiology and transmission

Cytomegalovirus (CMV) is the largest human herpesvirus (Fig. 29.7), and there is only one serotype. As with animal cytomegaloviruses it is species specific; humans are the natural hosts and animal cytomegaloviruses do not infect humans. The name refers to the multinucleated cells which, together with the intranuclear inclusions, are characteristic responses to infection with this virus. Transmission is via saliva, and cytomegaloviruses were originally called 'salivary gland' viruses.

Urine is an additional source of infection in children, and in infected pregnant women the virus can spread via the blood to the placenta and foetus. Also, semen and cervical secretions may contain virus so that it can be spread via sexual contact. It is often present in milk in small quantities but this is of doubtful significance in transmission. In hospitals it can be transmitted by blood transfusions and organ transplants.

Clinical features and pathogenesis

After clinically silent infection of unknown cells in the upper respiratory tract the virus spreads locally to lymphoid tissues and then systemically in circulating lymphocytes and monocytes to involve lymph nodes and the spleen. The infection then localizes in epithelial cells in salivary glands and kidney tubules, and in cervix, testes and epididymis, from whence the virus is shed to the outside world (Fig. 29.8). Infected cells may be multinucleated or bear intranuclear inclusions, but pathologic changes are minor, and infection is generally asymptomatic. In young adults a glandular fever type illness can occur, but without heterophile antibodies (see below). There is fever, lethargy, and abnormal lymphocytes and mononucleosis in blood smears. The virus inhibits T cell responses and there is a temporary reduction in their immune reactivity to other antigens.

Although specific antibodies and CMI responses are generated, these fail to clear the virus (see Chapter 15), which often continues to be shed in saliva and urine for many months. The infection is, however, eventually controlled by CMI mechanisms, although infected cells remain in the body throughout life and can be a source of reactivation and disease when CMI defences are impaired.

Complications

In the natural host, the human infant or child, CMV causes no illness and at most a mild illness in adults. Two circumstances, however, interfere with this harmonious host–parasite balance:
- Primary infection during pregnancy allows spread of virus from blood to placenta and then to the foetus, with

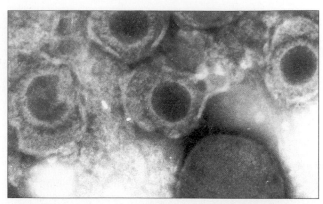

Fig. 29.7 Electron micrograph of cytomegalovirus particles. This is the largest human herpesvirus, with a diameter of approximately 100nm and a dense DNA core. Courtesy of DK Banerjee.

production of congenital abnormalities as described in Chapter 26. Reactivation of infection during pregnancy also occurs and leads to foetal infection but rarely to congenital abnormalities;
- In immunodeficient patients (bone marrow or kidney transplant recipients, AIDS patients, etc.; see Chapter 33) an interstitial pneumonia is seen with infiltrating infected mononuclear cells. Also focal cerebral 'micronodular' lesions, again with infected mononuclear cells, occur together with a variety of other complications, including retinitis.

Diagnosis

Clinical diagnosis of primary infection is rarely possible, because it is so commonly asymptomatic. The virus can be isolated in cell culture from the throat or urine. This generally takes a few days, the viral antigens being identified in cells by fluorescent antibody staining. In lung biopsies multinucleated cells or cells with prominent intranuclear inclusions may be seen. Antibody tests (four-fold or greater rise) can also be used.

Treatment and prevention

Dihydroxypropoxymethylguanine (DHPG; ganciclovir) is often effective in treatment of CMV retinitis and pneumonia. Acyclovir however is ineffective.

There is no vaccine, but trials of live and inactivated vaccines have been carried out. Contact between congenitally infected children and susceptible pregnant women should be avoided. Blood for transfusion of newborns, and kidneys and bone marrow for transplantation should preferably come from CMV antibody-negative donors.

EPSTEIN–BARR VIRUS INFECTION

Aetiology and transmission

Epstein-Barr virus (EBV), like CMV, is species specific. EBV is structurally and morphologically identical to other herpesviruses (see Chapter 3) but is antigenically distinct.

CYTOMEGALOVIRUS INFECTION		
site of infection	result	comment
Salivary glands	salivary transmission	importance of kissing and contaminated hands
Tubular epithelium of kidney	virus in urine	probable role in transmission
Cervix Testis/epididymis	sexual transmission	up to 10^7 infectious doses per ml of semen in an acutely infected male
Lymphocytes Macrophages	virus spread through body via infected cells mononucleosis may occur immunosuppressive effect	probable site of persistent infection
Placenta Foetus	congenital abnormalities	greatest damage in foetus after primary maternal infection rather than reactivation

Fig. 29.8 The effects of cytomegalovirus infection. CMV is a well-behaved parasite, causing little or no damage to the host unless it infects the foetus or placenta to cause congenital abnormalities, or it reactivates following depressed cell-mediated immunity (post-transplant, AIDS) to cause viraemia, fever, hepatitis or pneumonia.

A major antigen is the viral capsid antigen (VCA) used in diagnostic tests. Other useful antigens diagnostically are the early antigens (EA) which are produced prior to viral DNA synthesis, and the viral nuclear antigens (EBNA) which are located in the nucleus of the infected cells. Humans are the natural hosts.

EBV is transmitted by the exchange of saliva, for instance during kissing. It is a world-wide infection. In developing countries infection takes place, probably via fingers etc., in early childhood and is subclinical. In developed countries infection is generally delayed until adolescence or early adult life (peak incidence 15–25 years), and in most cases causes illness.

Clinical features and pathogenesis

Clinical and immunological events in EBV infection are illustrated in figure 29.9. EBV replicates in B lymphocytes, after making a specific attachment to the C3d receptor on these cells, and also in certain epithelial cells. The pathogenesis of the disease and the clinical features can be accounted for on this basis. Virus is shed in saliva from infected epithelial cells and possibly lymphocytes in salivary glands, and from the oropharynx, with clinically silent spread to B lymphocytes in local lymphoid tissues and elsewhere in the body (lymph nodes, spleen).

T lymphocytes respond immunologically to the infected B cells (outnumbering the latter by about 50 to 1) and appear in peripheral blood as 'atypical lymphocytes' (Fig. 29.10). Much of the disease is attributable to an immunological civil war, as specifically activated T cells respond to the infected B cells. In the naturally infected infant or small child these immune responses are weak and there is generally no clinical disease. Older children, however, become unwell, and young adults especially develop infectious mononucleosis or glandular fever 4 to 7 weeks after initial infection. This is characterized by fever, sore throat (see Chapter 20), often with petechiae on the hard palate,

lymphadenopathy, splenomegaly, with anorexia and lethargy as prominent features. Hepatitis may occur, with mild elevations of hepatocellular enzymes in 90% of cases and jaundice in 9%. Rarely there is encephalitis.

The symptoms are presumably due to the action of cytokines released during the intense immunological activity. The infected B cells are stimulated to differentiate and produce antibodies; this polyclonal activation of B cells is responsible for the production of heterophile antibodies (reacting with erythrocytes of sheep or horses) and a variety of autoantibodies. Spontaneous recovery usually occurs in 2–3 weeks but the symptoms may persist for a few months. The virus stays in the body in spite of antibody and CMI responses, and saliva often remains infectious for months after clinical recovery.

EBV remains latent in a small proportion of B lymphocytes, with EBV DNA present in episomal form and a few copies integrated into the cell genome. Later in life, immunodeficiency can lead to reactivation of infection so that EB virus reappears in the saliva, usually with no clinical symptoms; this occurs in more than half of renal transplant patients.

Complications

The autoantibodies include IgM antibodies to erythrocytes (cold agglutinins), which are present in most cases. About 1% of cases develop an autoimmune haemolytic anaemia, which subsides within a month or two.

Less than 1% of cases suffer neurological complications (aseptic meningitis, encephalitis) nearly always with complete recovery. A 'hairy tongue' condition caused by EBV replication in squamous epithelial cells in the tongue occurs in immunodeficient patients.

Diagnosis, treatment and prevention

Infectious mononucleosis is diagnosed clinically by the characteristic syndrome and the appearance of the throat.

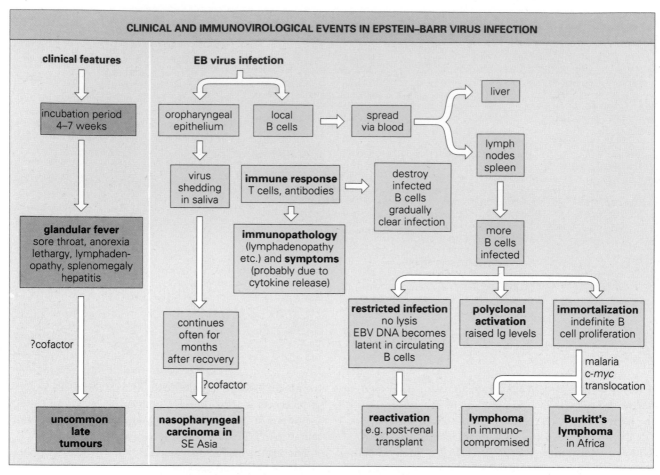

CLINICAL AND IMMUNOVIROLOGICAL EVENTS IN EPSTEIN–BARR VIRUS INFECTION

Fig. 29.9 Clinical and immunovirological events in Epstein–Barr virus infection in adolescents or adults. A milder, often subclinical infection occurs in children.

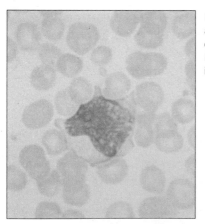

Fig. 29.10 An atypical lymphocyte characteristic of Epstein–Barr virus infection.

Laboratory diagnosis is by:
- Demonstrating atypical lymphocytes, comprising up to 30% of nucleated cells, in a blood smear;
- Demonstrating heterophil antibodies to horse (or sheep) erythrocytes in the 'Monospot' test (see Chapter 8). These are present in 90% of cases, but less commonly in infected children. Titres fall during recovery and disappear by 6 months, so that previous infection is not detected;

- Demonstrating EBV specific antibody. IgM antibody to the viral capsid antigen (VCA) indicates current infection, and IgG antibody past infection. Antibody to the various forms of EBNA persist for life;
- Demonstrating EBV itself, by cultivation of cells from clinical samples with cord blood lymphocytes and testing for transformation of the lymphocyte. This is difficult and rarely undertaken;
- Demonstrating EBV DNA by DNA hybridization or polymerase chain reaction (PCR; see Chapter 8). These methods are being developed and refined;

At present there is no reliable antiviral agent, although high doses of acyclovir are sometimes useful. There is no vaccine, but trials are in progress using various viral envelope glycoproteins.

Burkitt's lymphoma

EB virus is closely associated with Burkitt's lymphoma in African children (Fig. 29.11). It is also associated with other B cell lymphomas in immunodeficient patients, occuring, for instance, in 1–10% of renal and heart transplant patients surviving up to 15 years, especially when primary infection took place during immunosuppression. EBV DNA and EBNA is found in the tumour cells, which also show a translocation of the *c-myc* oncogene on chromosome 8 to the immunoglobulin heavy chain locus on

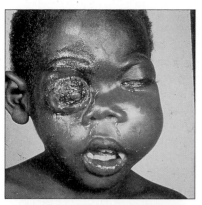

Fig. 29.11 Burkitt's lymphoma affecting the maxilla in an African child. Courtesy of DH Wright.

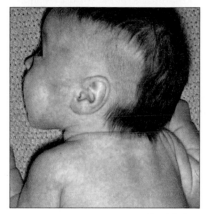

Fig. 29.12 Maculopapular rash in roseola infantum. Courtesy of MJ Wood.

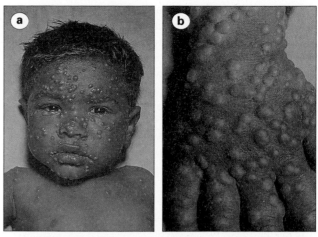

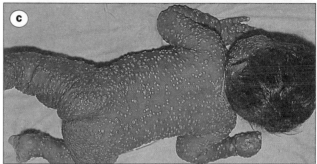

Fig. 29.13 Smallpox. These pictures were used as smallpox recognition cards by the World Health Organisation during its smallpox elimination campaign. After upper respiratory tract infection the virus reached the skin where it replicated to cause a widespread vesiculo-pustular rash, with later scarring, especially on the face. The fatality rate was up to 40%, depending on the age of the host and the strain of the virus. Courtesy of the World Health Organisation.

chromosome 14 (see Chapter 16). Because Burkitt's lymphoma is virtually restricted to parts of Africa and Papua-New Guinea it is clear that EBV alone is not enough to cause the lymphoma. The most likely co-carcinogen is malaria, which acts by weakening T cell control of EBV infection and perhaps by causing polyclonal activation of B cells, whose increased turnover renders them more susceptible to neoplastic transformation.

Nasopharyngeal carcinoma

EBV is also closely associated with nasopharyngeal carcinoma (NPC), a very common cancer in China and SE Asia. Here too, EBV DNA (100 episomal copies per cell) and EBNA is detectable in the tumour cells, and a co-carcinogen (possibly ingested nitrosamines from preserved fish) is likely. Host genetic factors controlling HLA antigens and immune responses also attract susceptibility to NPC.

HUMAN HERPES VIRUS 6 INFECTION

Human herpes virus 6 (HHV6), the latest human herpesvirus (preceding ones HSV1, HSV2, V-ZV, CMV, EBV), was discovered in 1988, and its behaviour and natural history is still being studied. Infection, which occurs in the first 3 years of life, is world-wide. The virus replicates in T and B cells and also in the oropharynx, from whence it is shed into saliva. The virus persists in the body after initial infection and can be demonstrated in the saliva of more than 85% of healthy adults.

Clinical features

HHV6 is the cause of exanthem subitum (or roseola infantum), a very common acute febrile illness in infants and young children. After an incubation period of about two weeks there is onset of fever which lasts for several days. The disease is mild and within two days of the fever subsiding a maculopapular rash is seen (Fig. 29.12).

HUMAN HERPES VIRUS 7 INFECTION

Yet another human herpesvirus, HHV7, has recently been isolated, from CD4–positive T cells. Infection, as determined by seroconversion, occurs in most children but later than is the case of HHV6.

The virus persists, and is present in 75% of normal adult saliva samples. It is not yet known whether it is a significant cause of disease.

SMALLPOX

Smallpox (variola) was, for at least 3000 years, a major scourge of humankind. It was caused by a poxvirus and spread from person to person by contact with skin lesions and via the respiratory tract. The disease was severe, with a generalized rash (Fig. 29.13), and was fatal in up to 20% of cases, depending on the strain of virus. During the first part of the 20th Century it was largely eradicated from Oceania, N. America and Europe by widespread vaccination as originally developed by Edward Jenner (see

Chapter 36), using a live attenuated strain of virus (vaccinia virus), together with strict controls at frontiers. In 1967 the WHO started a campaign to eliminate smallpox from the world, focusing on S. America, Africa, India and Indonesia, making use of vaccination, surveillance and containment of cases. Despite the daunting difficulties of cultural barriers, warfare, transport to remote areas etc., the campaign was successful. Occasional cases had continued to occur in the USA until the 1940s, and in 1974 there were 218 000 cases world-wide, mostly in Asia, but the last case as recorded in Somalia in October 1977. Global eradication of this major human pestilence was officially certified in December 1979. The total cost to the WHO was about $US 150 million. Global eradication of smallpox was possible because:

- There were no subclinical infections, so that cases were readily identified;
- The virus was eliminated from the body on recovery, with no carriers;
- Humans were the only host (no animal reservoir);
- An effective vaccine was available.

For a few years there were concerns about monkeypox, a simian disease caused by a similar virus and acquired by contact with infected monkeys in Africa. It is, however, poorly transmitted from human to human. It has been agreed that stocks of smallpox virus held in certain laboratories in the USA and CIS will be destroyed by 21st December 1993, giving sufficient time for the complete sequencing of the viral DNA.

SUMMARY

Measles, mumps, rubella, CMV, EBV and human herpesviruses 6 and 7 infect almost everyone throughout the world. Measles always gives rise to a detectable, clinically characteristic illness, whereas mumps may be subclinical, and laboratory tests are often needed for diagnosis of rubella, CMV and EBV infections.

These are essentially childhood infections which have more serious consequences when infection is delayed until adolescence or adult life. In the adult, the CNS (mumps), the conceptus (CMV, rubella) or the liver (EBV) are frequently infected, and in certain parts of the world EBV infection can result in lymphoma or nasopharyngeal carcinoma.

It should be noted that patterns of disease are not fixed. Smallpox, once a major world-wide virus infection, often with fatal consequences, was eradicated from the world 20 years ago. Thanks to improved health care and the development of safe, effective vaccines (measles, mumps, rubella polio), many other infections are fast disappearing from developed countries. However, as long as a reservoir of disease remains elsewhere in the world they could reappear in force if barriers break down or immunity in the population is allowed to wane. Conversely, the world-wide increase in travel and the effects of immunosuppression as a result of HIV infection, has meant that almost forgotten diseases are beginning to reappear in developed countries (e.g. malaria).

Further Reading

Behbehani AM. The smallpox story: life and death of an old disease. *Microbial Res* 1983; **47**: 455–509.

Koster FT, Curlin GC, Aziz KMA, Hague A. Synergistic impact of measles and diarrhoea on nutrition and mortality in Bangladesh. *Bull WHO* 1981; **59**: 901-908.

Latchmann DS. Molecular biology of herpes simplex virus latency. *Int J Exp Pathol* 1990; **71**: 133–142.

Miller AE. Selective decline in cellular immune response to varicella zoster in the elderly. *Neurology* 1980; **30**: 582–587.

Mach M, Stamminger T, Jahn G. Human cytomegalovirus: recent aspects from molecular biology. *J Gen Virol* 1989; **70**: 3117–3146.

Neiderman JC, Miller G, Pearson HA, Pagano JS, Dowaliby JM. Infectious mononucleosis: EB virus shedding in saliva and oropharynx. *New Engl J Med* 1976; **294**: 1355–1359.

30 VECTOR–BORNE INFECTIONS

Contents

INTRODUCTION

At least 85% of all known animal species are arthropods, and among them two classes make a major contribution to disease by transmitting parasites from one individual to another. These are the six-legged 'Insects' and the eight-legged 'Acarine Arachnids'. Their habit of feeding on human blood allows them to both ingest parasites from and inject them into the bloodstream. The most important diseases transmitted in this way are discussed in this chapter.

This form of spread has major implications for the host, the vector, and the parasite. To consider the parasite first, it requires the organism to be present in the right place (in the blood) and at the right time (some insects, for example, bite only at night). Blood is an inhospitable environment and this may require quite subtle evasion mechanisms for parasite survival. Moreover the conditions found in the vector are likely to be extremely different from those in the human host, and the parasite may have to make a remarkably complex transition in a short time; with the larger protozoal and helminth parasites this often involves clearly visible changes in appearance and is responsible for much of the complicated nomenclature of parasite 'life cycles'. Since some insect vectors have lifespans hardly longer than those of their parasites, there is considerable wastage due to death of the vector before the parasite has matured to the infective stage for man. A difference of a few days in mosquito lifespan can make an enormous difference in the effectiveness of malaria transmission, and indeed this simple factor is believed to underlie much of the difference between the African pattern of endemic infection and the Indian pattern of sporadic epidemics. But what may be lost from wastage is more than compensated for by the enormously increased distance over which dissemination of the parasite can occur, and in thinly-populated areas this makes transmission by insects a most effective means of spread.

On the host side, there is the advantage that the disease may be controllable merely by controlling the vector – although this is much easier said than done, as was discovered during the attempts to eradicate malaria by DDT spraying of the mosquito breeding areas. In the event the mosquitoes developed resistance and more damage was done to the environment than to the insects. Nevertheless, vector control remains a highly desirable goal in relation to the diseases discussed in this chapter and is, for instance, the only reason malaria is not endemic in northern Europe. Another potential advantage for the host is the perhaps surprising fact that it is sometimes possible to immunize specifically against the transmission stage. Again malaria can serve as an example, vaccines against the gametocytes and gametes having been clearly shown, in animal models, to completely block transmission. Once transmission is blocked there is a mathematically calculable possibility that the disease will die out.

ARBOVIRUS INFECTIONS

A wide range of about 500 different viruses is transmitted by arthropods such as ticks, mosquitoes and sandflies. These 'arboviruses' (arthropod-borne viruses) multiply in the arthropod vector, and for each virus there is a natural cycle involving vertebrates (various birds or mammals) and arthropods. The virus enters the arthropod when it takes a blood meal from the infected vertebrate, and passes through the gut wall to reach the salivary gland where replication takes place. Once this has occurred, 1–2 weeks

30.1

after ingesting the virus, the arthropod becomes infectious, and can transmit virus to another vertebrate during a blood meal. Certain arboviruses that infect ticks are also transmitted directly from adult tick to egg (vertical transmission), so that future generations of ticks are infected without the need for a vertebrate host.

Arboviruses tend to replicate in vascular endothelium, CNS, skin, muscle etc., and are therefore multisystem infections. They are generally named after the clinical disease (yellow fever) or the place where they were first discovered (Rift Valley fever, Japanese encephalitis). Only a small number are important causes of human disease, but they provide endless fascination for virologists, zoologists and ecologists.

The human stage of the virus cycle may be essential (urban yellow fever, dengue), there being no other vertebrate host, or it may be 'accidental' from the virus's point of view, with humans acting as 'dead end' hosts who do not form a necessary part of the natural cycle (e.g. equine encephalitides).

Yellow fever

Aetiology and transmission

Yellow fever is a flavivirus and there is only one antigenic type. It is restricted to Africa, Central and South America and the Caribbean. It was brought to the Americas by the early slave traders and the first recorded case was in Yucatan in 1640. Yellow fever virus is transmitted by two different cycles: 1) From human to human by the mosquito *Aedes aegypti*. The infection can be maintained in this way as 'urban' yellow fever; 2) from infected monkeys to humans by mosquitoes such as *Haemagogus*. This is 'jungle' yellow fever and is seen in Africa and South America. Yellow fever is not transmitted directly from human to human.

Clinical features and pathogenesis

The virus enters dermal tissues or blood vessels at the site of a mosquito bite and spreads through the body, infecting vascular endothelium and liver. After an incubation period of 3–6 days there is sudden onset of fever, headache and muscular aches. Although mild cases occur, prostration and shock are not uncommon, and severe liver damage may result in death. Coagulation defects (largely due to prothrombin deficiency) cause haemorrhage into the gastrointestinal tract (haematemesis) and elsewhere. Renal damage is also seen, with proteinuria and occasionally tubular necrosis.

Diagnosis, treatment and prevention

The diagnosis is usually clinical. Virus can be isolated from blood during the acute stage and a post-mortem diagnosis can be made from the severe mid-zonal changes and acidophilic inclusion bodies seen in the liver.

No specific antiviral therapy is available. By far the best prevention is to give the live attenuated '17D' yellow fever vaccine to those who may be exposed. Protection lasts at least 10 years and vaccination is necessary for entry into and travel through endemic areas. Vaccination is also a legal requirement for travellers from endemic areas to other countries where the disease does not occur (e.g. from tropical Africa to India). As with all arthropod-borne infections, control of arthropod vectors (insecticides, attention to breeding sites) and reduced exposure (insect repellants, mosquito nets) is also important.

Dengue fever

Aetiology and transmission

Dengue virus is a flavivirus with four antigenic subtypes. Dengue fever occurs in S.E. Asia, the Pacific area, India and the Caribbean. The mosquito *Aedes aegypti* is the principal human vector. The virus also circulates in monkeys and can be transmitted by mosquitoes to cause 'jungle' dengue in humans, a disease analagous to jungle yellow fever.

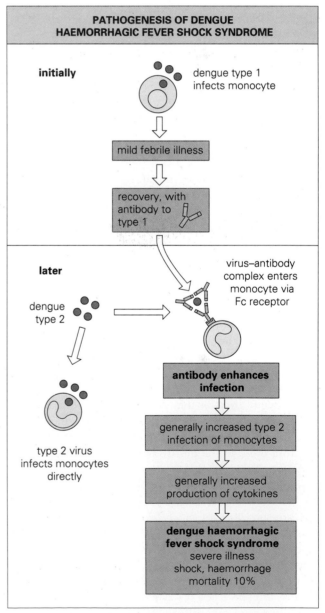

Fig. 30.1 The pathogenesis of dengue haemorrhagic fever shock syndrome. There are four serotypes of dengue virus. Types 1 and 2 are illustrated as an example. Antibody to type 1 binds to type 2 without preventing infection with type 2.

Clinical features

The virus replicates in monocytes and possibly in vascular endothelium. After an incubation period of 4–8 days there is malaise, fever, headache, arthalgia, nausea and vomiting, and sometimes a maculopapular rash. On recovery, prostration and depression are quite common.

Complications

A particularly severe form of disease, the 'dengue haemorrhagic fever shock syndrome', occurs in children in endemic areas, with mortality of up to 10%. The pathogenesis of this syndrome (Fig. 30.1) is as follows. After an earlier attack of dengue, antibodies are formed that are specific for that serotype. On subsequent infection with a different serotype the antibodies bind to the virus and not only fail to neutralize it (as might be expected for a different subtype), but actually enhance its ability to infect monocytes. The Fc portion of the virus-bound immunoglobulin molecule attaches to Fc receptors on monocytes and entry into the cell by this route increases the efficiency of infection. Infection of increased numbers of monocytes results in increased release of cytokines into the circulation (see Chapter 16) and this leads to vascular damage, shock, and haemorrhage, especially into the gastrointestinal tract and skin. Similar 'enhancing' antibodies are formed in many other virus infections, but it is only in dengue haemorrhagic fever that they are known to play a pathogenic role.

Treatment and prevention

No antiviral therapy or vaccine is available, and there is the obvious danger that a vaccine could induce a dangerous type of antibody.

Arbovirus encephalitis

Five of the nine encephalitic arboviruses listed in figure 30.2 cause disease in the USA, and although most infections are subclinical or mild, encephalitis can occur. Vaccines against WEE, EEE and VEE, each of which may cause disease in horses, have been used for laboratory workers and a Japanese encephalitis vaccine is available in Japan and India. Laboratory diagnosis is carried out in special centres, occasionally by virus isolation, but more commonly by demonstrating a rise in specific antibody.

Arboviruses and haemorrhagic fevers

Arboviruses are major causes of fever in endemic areas of the world. Infection is often subclinical or mild but unlucky individuals develop a severe haemorrhagic illness. Some of the best known of these infections are listed in figure 30.3. Laboratory diagnosis by isolation of virus or by demonstration of a rise in antibody is possible in special centres.

ARBOVIRUSES THAT CAN CAUSE ENCEPHALITIS				
virus and disease	geographical distribution	vector for human infection	vertebrate resevoir	severity of infection
Eastern equine encephalitis (EEE) (alphavirus)	USA (Atlantic Gulf states)	*Aedes* sp. mosquitoes	wild birds horses (dead–end hosts)	50% case fatality
Western equine encephalitis (WEE) (alphavirus)	USA (west of Mississippi)	*Culex* sp. mosquitoes	wild birds horses (dead–end hosts)	2% case fatality
St. Louis encephalitis (SLE) (flavivirus)	USA (S, Central and W States)	*Culex* sp. mosquitoes	wild birds	10% case fatality
California encephalitis (CE) (bunyavirus)	USA (N and Central States)	*Aedes* sp. mosquitoes	small mammals	fatalities rare
Japanese encephalitis (JE) (flavivirus)	Far East, SE Asia	*Culex* sp. mosquitoes	birds, pigs	8% case fatality
Murray valley encephalitis (MVE) (flavivirus)	Australia	*Culex* sp. mosquitoes	birds	up to 70% case fatality (variable)
Tick-borne encephalitis (flavivirus)	Eastern Europe	tick	mammals, birds	up to 10% case fatality (variable)
Venezuelan encephalitis (VEE) (alphavirus)	Southern USA Central and South America	mosquitoes	rodents	70% case fatality (cases rare)
Powassan (flavivirus)	USA, Canada	tick	rodents	cases rare

Fig. 30.2 Arboviruses causing encephalitis. The great majority of infections are either subclinical or are associated with non-specific febrile illness, e.g. 70% case fatality in encephalitis due to VEE virus, but only 3% develop encephalitis.

RICKETTSIAL INFECTIONS

General features

Rickettsia are small bacteria (see Chapter 3 and Appendix) that multiply by binary fission, but which are obligate intracellular parasites (with the exception of *R. quintana*, the causative agent of 'trench fever'). Howard T Ricketts identified 'Rocky Mountain spotted fever' in 1906 and showed that it was transmitted transovarially in ticks. All the rickettsia except *Coxiella burnetii* (which causes Q fever; see Chapter 31) are transmitted to humans by arthropods (Fig. 30.4) and all except epidemic typhus have a vertebrate reservoir. They multiply in vascular endothelium to cause pathology (vasculitis) in skin, CNS and liver, and hence are multisystem infections (Fig. 30.5). In spite of immune responses there is a tendency for rickettsial infections to persist in the body for long periods or become latent.

Rickettsia probably arose as parasites of blood-sucking or other arthropods in which they were maintained by vertical transmission, transfer to the arthropod's vertebrate host being initially 'accidental' and not necessary for rickettsial survival. The infected arthropod does not appear to be adversely affected. *Rickettsia prowazeki* is perhaps a more recent parasite of the human body-louse, because the louse dies 1–3 weeks after infection. As with most arthropod-borne infections, transmission from person to person does not occur.

Diagnosis

Typical clinical symptoms (except for Q fever) are fever, headache and rash. A history suggesting contact with rickettsial vectors or reservoir animals may suggest a diagnosis, e.g. camping, working, or engaging in military activities in endemic areas.

Laboratory diagnosis is based on serological tests. Complement fixation (CF) tests are specific for different rickettsia, and a 40-fold or greater rise in titre can be demonstrated. Microimmunofluorescence tests (IgG and IgM) are also used. Infected patients also make antibody to the rickettsiae that cross-react with the O antigen polysaccharide of various stains of *Proteus vulgaris*, as detected by agglutination in the Weil–Felix test. The agglutination pattern with three strains of *Proteus* can be used to identify the rickettsia. Although the phenomenon is of interest, the test is not of great value because of false positive and false negative results. Earlier diagnosis can often be made by fluorescent-antibody staining of skin biopsy material. Isolation of rickettsia is difficult and dangerous and laboratory infections have occurred.

Treatment and prevention

All rickettsiae are susceptible to tetracycline, with chloramphenicol as an alternative. Prevention is based on reducing exposure to ticks. A killed *R. prowazeki* vaccine is available for the military, and a killed *C. burnetii* vaccine for those at risk (veterinarians, shepherds, etc.).

Rocky Mountain spotted fever

The rickettsiae causing this disease are carried by the dog tick (*Dermacentor andersoni*) and in this host are transmitted vertically from adult tick to egg. Human infection occurs in the warm months of the year as ticks become active. Children are most commonly infected but their disease is milder.

ARBOVIRUSES THAT CAN CAUSE FEVERS AND HAEMORRHAGIC DISEASES				
viruses	**disease**	**geographical distribution**	**vector**	**animal reservoir**
Yellow fever (alphavirus)	fever, hepatitis	Africa, Central and South America	mosquito *Aedes* sp.	nil (monkeys for jungle type)
Dengue (4 serotypes) (flavivirus)	fever, rash (haemorrhagic shock syndrome)	India, SE Asia Pacific, South America, Caribbean	mosquito	nil
Kyasanur forest (flavivirus)	haemorrhagic fever	India	tick	monkeys, rodents
Ross river (alphavirus)	fever, arthralgia arthritis	Australia	mosquito	birds
Rift-valley fever (bunyavirus)	fever sometimes haemorrhage	Africa	mosquito	sheep, cattle camels
Sandfly fever (phlebovirus)	fever (mild disease)	Asia, South America, Mediterranean	sandflies	gerbils
Congo-Crimean haemorrhagic fever (bunyavirus)	fever, haemorrhage	Asia, Africa	tick	rodents
Colorado tick fever (reovirus)	fever, myalgia	USA (Rocky Mountains)	tick	rodents

Fig. 30.3 Arboviruses causing fevers and haemorrhagic diseases. There are many other less important arboviruses. For example, there are almost 200 in the bunyavirus family, most of which are anthropod-borne, with about 40 occasionally causing human disease.

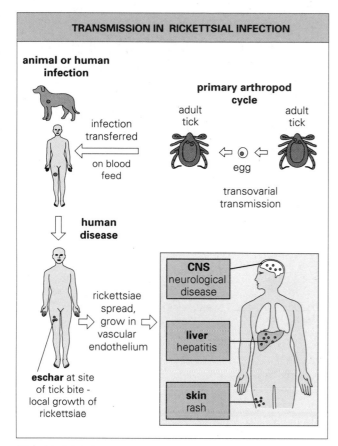

TRANSMISSION IN RICKETTSIAL INFECTION

Fig. 30.4 Typical events in rickettsial infection. There is no direct person-to-person spread. Q fever is atypical (see text). Typhus is unusual because the infected arthropod transmits from person-to-person, eventually dies and there is no eschar.

Clinical features and pathogenesis

The rickettsiae multiply in the skin at the site of the tick bite, then spread to blood and infect vascular endothelium in lung, spleen, brain and skin. After an incubation period of about a week there is onset of fever, severe headache, myalgia, and often respiratory symptoms. A generalized maculopapular rash appears a few days later, often becoming petechial or purpuric (Fig. 30.6). Splenomegaly is seen, and neurological involvement is frequent, with later onset of clotting defects (disseminated intravascular coagulation), shock and death. Fatal cases are usually those with delayed diagnosis. Peak mortality (10%) is seen in 40–60 year olds.

Mediterranean spotted fever

This disease is caused by *Rickettsia conorii*, carried by the dog tick *Rhipicephalus sanguineus*. Human infection, which occurs mainly in October, is known in all Mediterranean countries and can occur in urban as well as rural areas. After an incubation period of about a week, half of cases develop fever, headache, myalgia, and 2–4 days later a rash, especially on the palms and soles. The bite usually goes unnoticed as it is caused by immature ticks and is painless; a local lesion is not usually seen. Mortality in hospitalized cases is similar to Rocky Mountain spotted fever.

Rickettsialpox

About five days after the bite of an infected mite a local eschar develops, followed a week later by fever and headache. After a few days a generalized papulovesicular rash then appears. The disease is, however, mild.

PRINCIPAL RICKETTSIAL DISEASE OF HUMANS

	organism	disease	arthropod vector	vertebrate resevoir	clinical severity	geographical distribution
Spotted fevers***	R. rickettsia	Rocky Mountain spotted fever	tick*	dogs, rodents	+	Rocky Mountain states, Eastern USA
	R. akari	rickettsial pox	mite*	mice	–	Asia, Far East Africa, USA
	R. conorii	Mediterranean spotted fever	tick	dogs	+	Mediterranean
Typhus	R. prowezeki	epidemic typhus	louse	human**	++	Africa, South America
	R. typhi	endemic typhus	flea	rodents	–	world-wide
	R. tsutsugamushi	scrub typhus	mite*	rodents	++	Far East
Others	Coxiella burnetii	Q fever	none	sheep, goats cattle	+	world-wide
	R. quintana	trench fever	louse	human	+	Asia, Africa Central and South America †

* vertically transmitted in arthropod
** non-human vertebrates are possibly also involved
*** other rickettsiae cause similar tick-borne fevers in Africa, India, Australia
† multiply extracellularly; 1 million soldiers infected in World War 1

Fig. 30.5 The principal rickettsial diseases in humans.

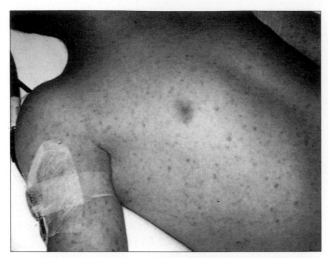

Fig. 30.6 Generalized maculopapular rash with petechia in Rocky Mountain spotted fever. Courtesy of TF Sellers, Jr.

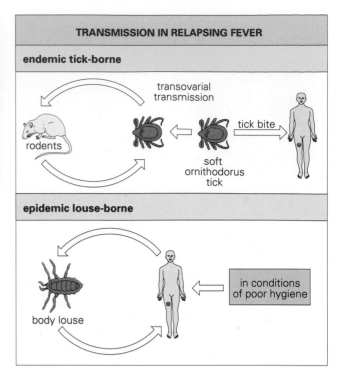

Fig. 30.7 Transmission in relapsing fever.

Epidemic typhus

Epidemic typhus is transmitted from person to person by the human body louse (*Pediculus corporis*). The rickettsia (*R. prowazeki*) multiply in the gut epithelium of the louse and are excreted in faeces during the act of biting. The rickettsia enter the skin when the bite is scratched. The disease cannot maintain itself unless enough people are infested with lice. Epidemic typhus is therefore classically associated with poverty and war, when clothes and bodies are washed less frequently. Thirty million cases occurred in Eastern Europe and the Soviet Union during 1918–1922. The disease is seen in Africa and South America, but the last case in the USA was in 1922. Because there is no direct person-to-person spread outbreaks can be terminated by de-lousing campaigns.

Clinical features and pathogenesis

Rickettsia proliferate at the site of the bite and then spread in the blood to infect vascular endothelium in skin, heart, CNS, muscle and kidney. About a week after the louse bite (there is no eschar) the infected person develops fever, headache and flu-like symptoms. The generalized maculopapular rash appears 5–9 days later and sometimes severe meningoencephalitis with delirium and coma. In untreated cases mortality can be as high as 40%, due to peripheral vascular collapse or secondary bacterial pneumonia.

Convalescence may take months. In some individuals the rickettsia are not eliminated from the body on clinical recovery and remain in the lymph nodes. As long as 50 years later the infection can reactivate to cause Brill-Zinsser disease, and the patient once again acts as a source of infection for any lice that may be present.

Endemic typhus

Endemic typhus is caused by *R. typhi* and is transmitted to humans by the rat flea. The disease is similar to epidemic typhus but is less severe.

Scrub typhus

Scrub typhus is caused by *R. tsutsugamushi* and is transmitted to humans by trombiculid mites (chiggers). It occurs only in the Far East; cases were seen in US soldiers in Vietnam. The rickettsia are maintained in the mites by transovarial transfer and are transmitted to humans or to rodents during feeding. There is an eschar, and a macular rash appears after about five days of illness.

BORRELIA INFECTIONS

Relapsing fever

Aetiology and transmission

Relapsing fever (Fig. 30.7) is caused by *Borrelia recurrentis*. This spirochaete consists of an irregular spiral, 10–30μm long, and is highly flexible, moving by rotation and twisting. Infection is endemic in rodents in many parts of the world, including western USA, and it is transmitted by soft ticks of the genus *Ornithodorus*. Human infection results from tick bites. In the tick the bacteria are transmitted transovarially from generation to generation. Also, ticks survive months or years between feeds, which helps maintain the endemic cycle of tick-borne relapsing fever.

In humans, epidemics of relapsing fever are due to transmission of infection by the human body louse. Bacteria multiply in the louse, and when louse bites are rubbed the lice are crushed and the bacteria are introduced into the bite wound. Lice are essential for person-to-person transmission of louse-borne relapsing fever. As with other louse-borne infections (e.g. typhus), spread of the disease in humans is favoured when people rarely wash and when clothes are not changed (i.e. in wars, natural disasters, etc.).

Clinical features and pathogenesis

The bacteria multiply locally and enter the blood. After an incubation period of 3–10 days there is sudden onset of illness with chills and fever, lasting for 3–5 days (Fig. 30.8).

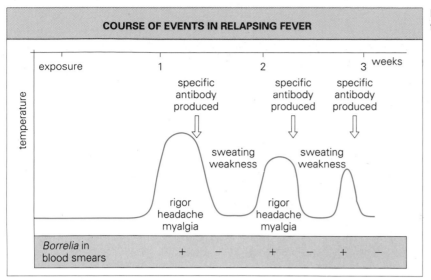

COURSE OF EVENTS IN RELAPSING FEVER

Fig. 30.8 Course of events in relapsing fever.

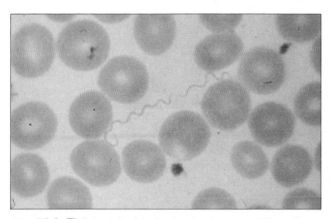

Fig. 30.9 Tightly coiled helical spirochaetes of *Borellia recurrentis* in the blood of a patient with relapsing fever. Courtesy of TF Sellers.

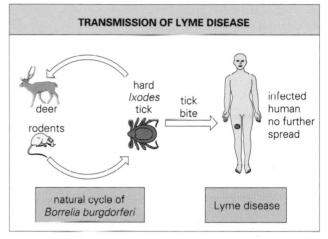

TRANSMISSION OF LYME DISEASE

Fig. 30.10 Transmission of Lyme disease.

The afebrile period lasts about a week before there is a second attack of fever, which is followed by another afebrile period. Generally there are from 3–10 such episodes, of diminishing severity. More serious illness can occur when there is extensive growth of bacteria in spleen, liver and kidneys.

The repeated febrile episodes are due to antigenic variation in the spirochaetes. Agglutinating and lytic antibodies are formed against the infecting bacteria, which are cleared from the blood. Under the 'pressure' of this immune response a new antigenic type emerges and is free to multiply and cause a fresh febrile episode. Antigenic variation involves switching of the variable major protein (VMP) on the bacterial surface. The borrelia have arrays of VMP genes that are activated by gene conversion. A single cloned bacterium can give rise spontaneously to more than 20 serotypes and switching occurs at a rate of 1 in 1000 to 1 in 10 000 per cell generation. Similar phenomena are seen in trypanosomes. Direct person–to–person transmission does not occur. Mortality with endemic (tick-borne) relapsing fever is <5% but may be up to 40% in epidemic (louse-borne) relapsing fever.

Diagnosis
The bacteria can be cultivated in the laboratory and can

be seen in Giemsa-stained smears of blood taken during the febrile period (Fig. 30.9). CF antibody tests are available but are rarely useful because of the problem of antigenic variation.

Treatment and prevention
Tetracycline is used in treatment and to prevent relapses. The best preventative measure is avoidance of arthropod vectors.

Lyme disease

Aetiology and transmission
Lyme disease occurs in Europe, USA, and in most continents of the world, and is named after the town in Connecticut, USA where the first cases were recognized in 1975. It is caused by *Borrelia burgdorferi*. The natural cycle of infection takes place in mice and deer in whom it is transmitted by hard ticks of the genus *Ixodes* (Fig. 30.10). Human infection follows the bite of an infected tick (larval, nymph or adult form). In Europe and USA infection is commoner in summer months when recreational exposure to infected ticks is more likely. Person–to–person transmission does not occur.

Clinical features and pathogenesis

The bacteria multiply locally, and after an incubation period of about one week there is fever, headache, myalgia, lymphadenopathy, and a characteristic lesion develops at the site of the tick bite. This skin lesion is called 'erythema chronicum migrans' (Fig. 30.11), its name describing its main features. It begins as a macule and enlarges over the next few weeks, remaining red and flat but with the centre clearing, until it is several inches in diameter. In 50% of patients fresh, transient lesions appear on the skin elsewhere in the body. Immunological findings include circulating immune complexes and sometimes elevated serum IgM levels and cryoglobulins that contain IgM.

In 75% of untreated patients, in spite of antibody and T cell responses to the *Borrelia* , there are additional later manifestations of disease. These are seen from one week to more than two years after onset of illness. The first are neurological (meningitis, encephalitis, peripheral neuropathy) and cardiological (heart block, myopericarditis). The second are arthralgia and arthritis, which may persist for months or years. Immune conplexes are found in affected joints. These late manifestations are immunological in origin, and are probably due to antigenic cross-reactivity between *Borrelia* and host tissues. The *Borrelia* themselves are rarely detectable at this stage.

Diagnosis

The *Borrelia* are rarely seen in skin biopsies but can sometimes be isolated from biopsies obtained at an early stage, although this may take weeks. Serological tests (e.g. ELISA) are more useful. Specific IgM antibodies are detected 3–6 weeks after infection and IgG antibodies at a later stage. Antigenic cross reactivity may result in false positive results.

Treatment and prevention

Penicillin or tetracycline are effective and penicillin can be used to treat the late arthritis. Prevention is by avoidance of tick bites.

PROTOZOAL INFECTIONS

Malaria

Egyptian papyruses from the 16th century BC chronicle the association between fever, shivering, and enlargement of the spleen. Since the Middle Ages, Europe knew this condition as malaria, although the causative organism was not identified until 1880. Four species of *Plasmodium* cause malaria in man, of which *P. falciparum* is the most virulent (Fig. 30.12). In addition, occasional infections may occur with the simian parasites *P. knowlesi*, *P. cynomolgi* and *P. simium*.

Epidemiology

The human disease is initiated by the bite of an infected female anopheline mosquito, and so is restricted to areas where these can breed. At present this includes most of

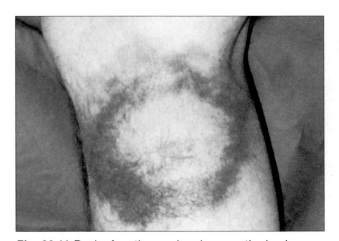

Fig. 30.11 Rash of erythema chronicum on the leg in Lyme disease. Courtesy of E Sahn.

HUMAN MALARIA PARASITES				
species	**P. falciparum**	**P. vivax**	**P. malariae**	**P. ovale**
Major distribution	West, East and Central Africa, Middle East Far East, South America	India, N and E Africa South America Far East	tropical Africa India Far East	tropical Africa
Common name	malignant tertian	benign tertian	quartan	ovale tertian
Duration of liver stage (incubation period)	6–14 days	12–17 days (with relapses up to 3 years)	13–40 days (with relapses up to 20 years)	9–18 days (with rare relapses)
Duration of asexual blood cycle (fever cycle)	48 hrs	48 hrs	72 hrs	50 hrs
Major complications	cerebral malaria anaemia hypoglycaemia jaundice pulmonary oedema shock	–	nephrotic syndrome	–

Fig. 30.12 Human malaria parasites. The most important and life-threatening complications occur with *P. falciparum*, hence its old name 'malignant tertian malaria'.

the tropics between 60°N and 40°S (except areas more than about 2000 metres above sea level), with a major impact in Africa, India, the Far East and S. America. Early hopes of eradication via mosquito control and chemotherapy have been dashed by the emergence of drug resistance and, globally, malaria is now on the increase. About one-third of the world's population is estimated to be infected, with some 10 million new cases annually and perhaps 2 million deaths. As a result of increased air travel, new cases are regularly seen in the developed world, and unless the diagnosis is constantly borne in mind, vital treatment may be withheld, with fatal results. Malaria can also be transmitted by blood transfusion or needle accidents, and, very rarely, from mother to foetus.

Aetiology and transmission

The malaria parasite has the most complex life cycle of any human infection, comprising three quite distinct stages and characterized by alternating extracellular and intracellular forms, as described in detail in figures 30.13 and 30.14.

The symptoms of malaria, which range from fever to fatal cerebral or renal disease, are associated exclusively with the asexual blood stage (see Fig. 30.13). Invasion of red cells requires at least two separate receptor–receptor interactions, and the lack of one red cell surface molecule, the 'Duffy' antigen, explains the resistance to *P. vivax* of most West Africans. Other genetic traits that appear to have been selected because they contribute to resistance to malaria include haemoglobin S (sickle-cell), ß-thalassaemia, and glucose-6-phosphate dehydrogenase deficiency.

The genetic recombination allowed by the sexual stage of the process is one element in the remarkable antigenic diversity seen within malaria parasite populations. It is interesting to note that the successful transmission of malaria depends crucially on the mosquito surviving long enough for sporozoites to develop, and that quite small species differences in mosquito lifespan can drastically affect transmission; this may be an important cause of regional differences in malaria incidence.

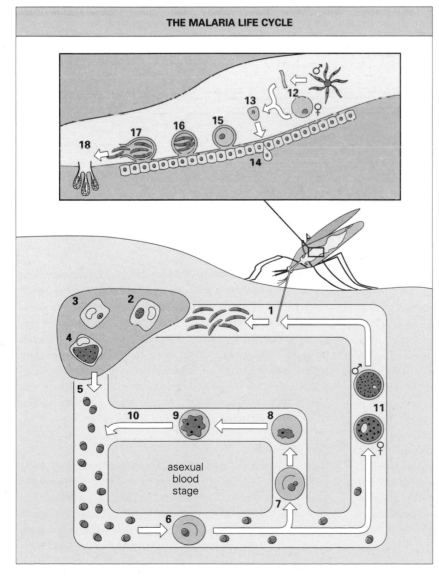

THE MALARIA LIFE CYCLE

asexual blood stage

Fig. 30.13 The life cycle of malaria in man and mosquito. In the symptomless pre-erythrocytic stage, sporozoites from the saliva of an infected *Anopheles* mosquito are injected into the human bloodstream when the mosquito bites(1). They then enter the parenchymal cells of the liver (2), where they mature in approximately 2 weeks into tissue schizonts (4), finally rupturing to produce 10 000 to 40 000 merozoites (5). These circulate in the blood for a few minutes before entering the red blood cells (6) to initiate the asexual blood stage. Some parasites, however, remain within the liver to lie dormant as hypnozoites (3), which are the cause of relapses. Once in the red blood cells, the merozoites mature into the ring form (7), trophozoite (8) and schizont (9), which complete the cycle by maturing to release merozoites back into the circulation (10). This cycle may last for months or even years. Some merozoites, however, go on to initiate the sexual stage, maturing within the red blood cells to form male and female gametocytes (11), which can be taken up by the *Anopheles* mosquito on feeding. On entering the gut of the insect, the male gametocyte exflagellates (12) to form male microgametes, which fertilize the female gamete to form the zygote (13). This then invades the gut mucosa (14), where it develops into an oocyst (15). This develops to produce thousands of sporozoites (16), which are released into the gut (17), finally migrating to the salivary glands of the insect (18), whence the cycle begins again.

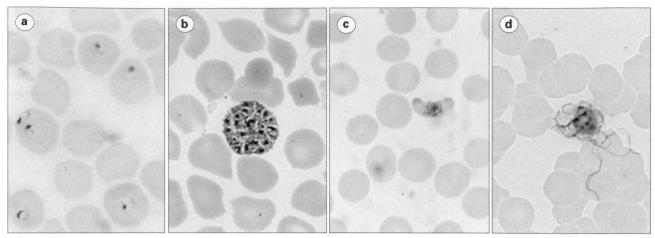

Fig. 30.14 Different stages of the malaria parasites.(a) *P. falciparum ring* forms in red blood cells. (b) *P. vivax* erythrocytic schizont. (c) *P. falciparum* female gametocyte. (d) *P. vivax* male gametocytes exflaggelating to form microgametes 20–25 μm long.

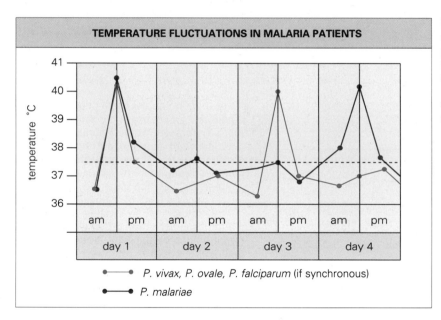

Fig. 30.15 Malaria fever charts showing cyclical fluctuations in temperature. The peaks coincide with the maturation and rupture of the intraerythrocytic schizonts, occuring every 48 hours (*P. falciparum, P. vivax* and *P. ovale*) or every 72 hours (*P. malariae*), when the cycles are synchronized.

Clinical features and pathogenesis

The clinical picture of malaria depends on the age and immune status of the patient, as well as the species of parasite. The most characteristic feature is fever, which follows closely upon rupture of erythrocytic schizonts and is thought to be mainly due to the induction of cytokines such as IL-1 and tumour necrosis factor (TNF). Because of their regular and synchronous cycle times, the different species of malaria give characteristic patterns of fever, with either a 48 hour (tertian, i.e. days 1 and 3) or 72 hour (quartan, i.e. days 1 and 4) periodicity (Fig. 30.15). A typical paroxysm of fever starts with a feeling of intense cold with shivering followed by a hot dry stage and finally a period of drenching sweats. Headache, muscle pains and vomiting frequently occur. *Plasmodium falciparum* infections do not always display the typical periodicity, causing a daily evening fever due to superimposed nonsynchronous parasite cycles. It is in such cases that the diagnosis is likely to be missed and the symptoms attributed to influenza or some other pyrexial disease. Enlargement of the spleen and liver is common and anaemia almost invariable. In the absence of treatment or reinfection, *P. vivax*, *P. ovale* and *P. malariae* malaria is normally self-limiting. though relapses may occur. *Plasmodium falciparum* malaria, however, is frequently fatal during the first 2–3 weeks, due to the development of a variety of complications (Fig. 30.12). Relapses may occur after months or even years, especially in *P. vivax* malaria, where they are due to parasites that lie dormant in the liver ('hypnozoites').

Complications

In areas where malaria is endemic, complicated *P. falciparum* malaria is most common in children between the ages of 6 months and 5 years and in pregnant women, particularly primagravidae. However, it can occur at any age in the non-immune (e.g. tourists). The most dangerous complication is 'cerebral malaria', with progressive headache, neck stiffness, convulsions and coma. There is much

IMMUNITY TO MALARIA	
stage	**mechanism**
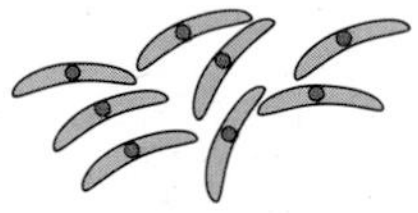 sporozoites	antibody
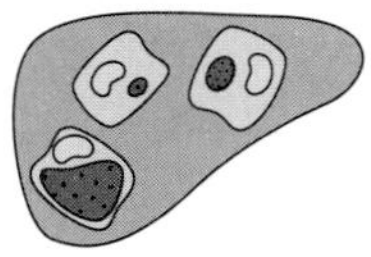 liver stage	cytotoxic T cells TNF IFN–α IL–1
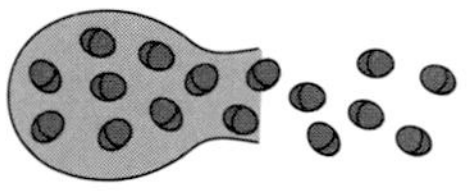 merozoites	antibody
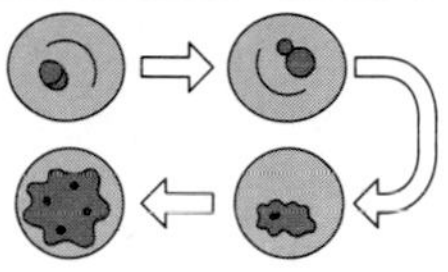 asexual erythrocyte stage	antibody ROI, RNI ECP TNF
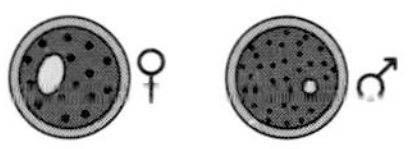 gametocytes	antibody ?cytokines
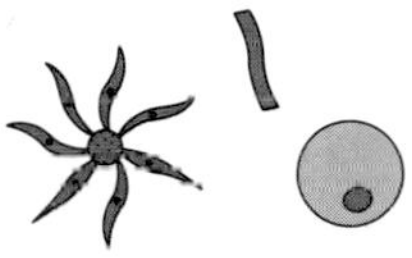 gametes	antibody

ROI, reactive oxygen intermediates
RNI, reactive nitrogen intermediates
ECP, eosinophil cationic proteins

Fig. 30.16 Immunity to malaria. The principal mechanisms thought to be responsible for immunity at each stage of the cycle.

debate as to whether this is caused by sludging or binding of parasitized red cells in cerebral capillaries, by increased permeability of the blood–brain barrier, or by the excessive induction of cytokines such as TNF. If successfully treated, however, it usually leaves behind little or no impairment of cerebral function, though neurological and psychiatric sequelae may occur in 5–10% of childhood cases.

Severe anaemia is also common, due partly to red cell destruction and partly to dyserythropoiesis in the bone marrow; the spleen appears to be the major site of red cell removal. Of the other complications, hypoglycaemia and lactic acidosis are thought to be important contributors to mortality. Reduced food intake, impaired liver gluconeogenesis and possible glucose consumption by the large number of parasites may all be involved and a role for TNF has been proposed, as it has for many of the complications. Immune complex glomerulonephritis is common, and there is a particular tendency to progressive nephrotic disease in *P. malariae* (quartan) malariae.

Immunity

Immunity develops gradually and in stages. In endemic areas, children who survive early attacks become resistant to severe disease by about the age of five. Parasite levels fall progressively until adulthood when they are low or absent most of the time. A period of a year spent away from exposure is sufficient for most of this immunity to wane, suggesting that repeated boosting is needed to maintain it. The actual mechanisms are controversial and seem to involve both antibody and cell-mediated immunity (Fig. 30.16).

Diagnosis

Diagnosis is by finding parasitized red cells in a blood film (thick if necessary) or the bone marrow. Because the later (schizont) stages may be sequestered in deep tissues, parasites may be deceptively scarce in, or even absent from, the blood. Any case of fever, especially with anaemia, splenomegaly or cerebral signs, in a patient who conceivably could have malaria is therefore best treated as such. However, the presence of parasites in the blood of an ill patient from an endemic area does not mean malaria is the cause of the illness, since parasitaemia may be asymptomatic. The demonstration of antibody by immunofluorescence or ELISA confirms previous exposure and a predominance of IgM would suggest a recent attack.

Treatment and prevention

The effect of cinchona bark on malaria has been known for 400 years and the active principle, quinine, remains the drug of choice in life-threatening malaria. Complications of quinine treatment include massive intravascular haemolysis ('blackwater fever'). Other major drugs are chloroquine (to which *P. falciparum* is increasingly resistant), and the new Chinese drug quinghaosu, with primaquine for preventing relapses. The most promising form of prevention is bednets impregnated with mosquito repellents, but drugs such as proguanil or chloroquine are also used. The prospects for a malaria vaccine are discussed in Chapter 36.

Trypanosomiasis

Three species of the flagellated protozoan *Trypanosoma* cause human disease: *T. brucei gambiense* and *T. b. rhodesiense* (the cause of African trypanosomiasis or sleeping sickness) and *T. cruzi* (the cause of South American trypanosomiasis or Chagas' disease). The diseases differ quite markedly in the nature of the insect vector, the habitat of the parasite, and the effects on the immune system.

African trypanosomiasis

The vector, *Glossina* (the tsetse fly), restricts this disease to equatorial Africa, with a reservoir of infection in several domestic and wild animals (cattle, pigs, deer). In man, *T. brucei* remains extracellular, first in the tissues near the insect bite and then in the blood, where it divides rapidly and continuously.

Clinical features and pathogenesis

Following an infected bite a swollen chancre develops at the site, with widespread lymph node enlargement,

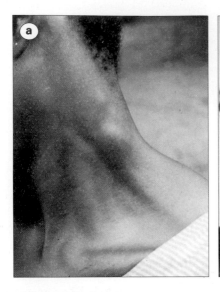
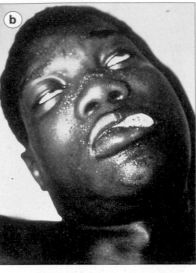

Fig. 30.17 African trypanosomiasis. (a) Enlargement of the lymph nodes in the neck (Winterbottom's sign). Courtesy of PG Janssens. (b) Coma (sleeping sickness) due to generalized encephalitis. Courtesy of ME Krampitz and P de Raadt.

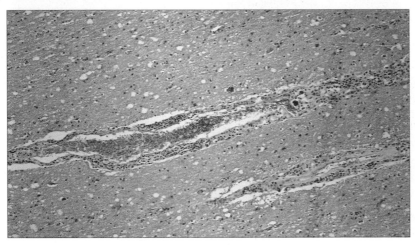

Fig. 30.18 Lymphocytic infiltration around a blood vessel in the brain in *T. brucei* infection. H & E stain. Courtesy of R Muller and JR Baker.

especially in the back of the neck (Winterbottom's sign; Fig. 30.17). The parasite becomes established in the blood where it multiplies rapidly, with fever, splenomegaly, and often signs of myocardial involvement. Within weeks or months the CNS may become involved (more acutely in the East African *T. b. rhodesiense* than the West African *T. b. gambiense*), with the gradual development of headache, psychological changes ('silent grief'), voracious appetite and weight loss, and finally coma ('sleeping sickness'; see Fig. 30.17) and death. Unlike malaria, cured trypanosomiasis can leave the patient with severe residual neurological and mental disability.

Immunity

The ability of the parasite to survive free in the blood is due to its remarkable degree of antigenic variation, based on switching between some 1000 different genes for the glycoprotein coat (see Chapter 14). High levels of IgM are found in the blood, and later in the CSF, manufactured by the plasma cells (Mott cells) that are a feature of the lymphocytic infiltrate seen as 'perivascular cuffing' around blood vessels in the brain (Fig. 30.18).

Diagnosis, treatment and prevention

Diagnosis is by the demonstration of parasites in lymph nodes (by puncture) or, in late cases, the CSF. A raised

serum IgM (up to 16-times normal levels) is highly suggestive of the disease (see above).

Arsenical drugs such as trypansamide and melarsen have been the mainstay of treatment, and several non-arsenicals are also effective, e.g. suramin, nitrofurazone, pentamidine. The latter is the drug of choice for prophylaxis. Control of the tsetse fly vector is difficult, though insecticides are widely used. Unfortunately, bed nets are ineffective as the flies feed during daylight hours.

Chagas' disease

Trypanosoma cruzi differs from the African trypanosomes in being transmitted by a non-flying vector, the reduviid ('kissing') bug, which restricts the disease to areas of poor-quality housing. Almost all species of mammal can act as reservoirs of infection. Moreover, the parasite can infect and inhabit the cells of the host, notably macrophages and cardiac muscle cells.

Clinical features and pathogenesis

As with African trypanosomiasis, one or more chancres ('chagomas') may develop at the site of infection, with a febrile illness, which is usually transient but may rarely lead to death by heart failure. Following invasion of the parasites into cells, the disease pursues an extremely slow and chronic course. The two major symptoms, which can

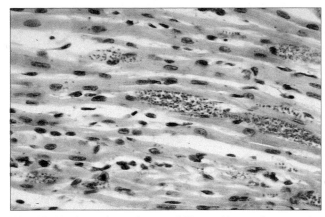

Fig. 30.19 Amastigote forms of *T. cruzi* in cardiac muscle in Chagas' disease. H & E stain. Courtesy of H Tubbs.

LEISHMANIA SPECIES AND CLINICAL SYNDROMES

species	distribution	disease
L. donovani L. infantum	Africa, India, Mediterranean	visceral leishmaniasis
L. chagasi	South America	
L. major L. tropica L. aethiopica	Africa, India, Mediterranean	cutaneous leishmaniasis
L. mexicana L. braziliensis L. peruviana	South and Central America	

Fig. 30.20 Leishmania species - their distribution and clinical syndromes.

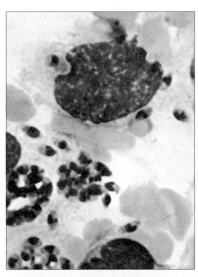

Fig. 30.21 Leishmania within macrophages in aspirate from a lesion of New World leishmaniasis. Courtesy of MJ Wood.

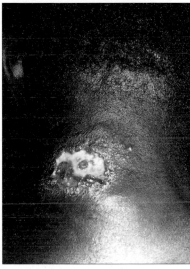

Fig. 30.22 Cutaneous lesion on the neck in *L. braziliensis* infection. Courtesy of PJ Cooper.

take years to appear, involve the heart and the intestinal tract. The major cause of death is myocarditis, with progressive weakening and dilatation of the ventricles, due to destruction of cardiac muscle by the parasite (Fig. 30.19) and probably also to autoimmune mechanisms induced by cross-reacting antigens. Dilatation of the hollow viscera is due to similar processes in nerve cells and leads to organs incapable of proper peristalsis; mega-oesophagus and megacolon are the two commonest manifestations.

Diagnosis

In the acute phase, parasites may be seen in a a blood film, but the chronic disease is usually diagnosed either serologically or by 'xenodiagnosis'. The latter involves allowing clean reduviid bugs to feed on the patient and examining the rectal contents 1–2 months later, or homogenizing them and injecting the contents into mice, in which even a single trypanosome will produce a patent infection. In the late stages, muscle biopsy may also be diagnostic.

Treatment and prevention

Chagas' disease is one of the most difficult protozoal infections to cure. Several drugs, including arsenicals, are effective against the blood stage (trypomastigote) but usually fail to eliminate the intracellular stage (amastigote). The role of the physician is chiefly to treat the heart failure and mega-syndromes that are such a miserable feature of this disease.

Prevention would ideally be achieved by improved housing and living standards. Vector control by insecticides is difficult and a vaccine, though under investigation, is in practical terms a long way off.

Leishmaniasis

Leishmania are related to, and somewhat resemble, trypanosomes. They are transmitted by sandflies and a variety of species of the parasite cause disease in South and Central America ('New World leishmaniasis'), India, the Middle East, Africa and the shores of the Mediterranean (Old World leismaniasis; Fig. 30.20). In the latter areas especially, dogs can act as an important reservoir of infection.

Clinical features and pathogenesis

Like *T. cruzi*, leishmania is an intracellular parasite, inhabiting macrophages (Fig. 30.21), in which it avoids elimination, except when they are strongly activated, e.g. by IFN-γ. The two principal sites of parasite growth are the liver and spleen (visceral leishmaniasis) and the skin (cutaneous leishmaniasis).

Visceral leishmaniasis usually develops slowly, with fever and weight loss, followed months or years later by hepatomegaly and, especially, splenomegaly; the spleen may reach to the right iliac fossa, and the untreated patient will die of liver failure. This form of the disease is known as 'kala azar'. Skin lesions may appear following treatment; these contain massive numbers of parasites and the syndrome is known as 'post-kala azar dermal leishmaniasis' (PKDL).

Classical cutaneous leishmaniasis also progresses insidiously, from a small papule at the site of infection to a large ulcer, which may eventually heal with considerable scarring (Fig. 30.22). Almost alone among protozoal infections, this type of primary lesion leaves the patient relatively immune to reinfection, which has encouraged the hope that an effective vaccine might be produced (see Chapter 36). The cutaneous lesions are known in the Old World as 'Oriental sores' (and also 'Baghdad boil,' 'Delhi sore') and in the New World as 'Espundia' (muco-cutaneous) and 'Chicero's ulcer' (of the ear). In immunodeficient patients, widespread chronic lesions can occur – diffuse cutaneous leishmaniasis – analagous to lepromatous leprosy.

Diagnosis
Demonstration of the organism in biopsy material, marrow or spleen and skin lesions depending on the clinical picture, is the definitive proof of leishmaniasis. A positive delayed hypersensitivity reaction to leishmania antigens (Montenegro test) can be useful where parasites are not found.

Treatment and prevention
Apart from the simple self-healing cutaneous lesion, leishmaniasis requires prolonged treatment with antimonial compounds (sodium stibogluconate, meglumine antimonate); if these fail, pentamidine or amphotericin B may be successful. If a very large spleen persists after treatment, it is usually removed.

Impregnated bed nets are effective against the sandfly vector, and the animal reservoir can be eliminated by proper dog control. As stated above, the prospects for vaccination against the cutaneous disease are quite promising.

HELMINTH INFECTIONS

Schistosomiasis
In contrast to the other infections covered in this chapter, where the vector is an arthropod, schistosomiasis is transmitted through a snail vector. All members of the group to which schistosomes belong (the digenetic trematodes or flukes, must pass through a mollusc intermediate host in order to complete their larval development. However, schistosomes are the only flukes in which larvae penetrate directly into the final host after release from the snail.

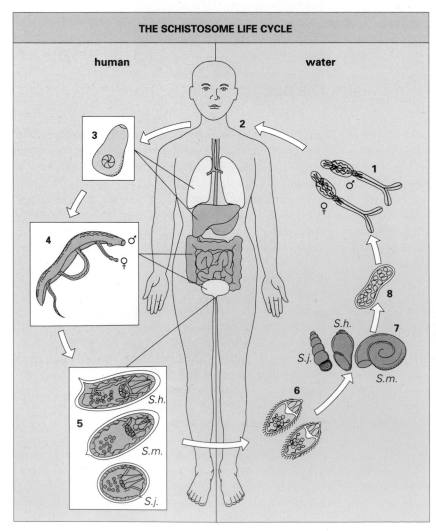

THE SCHISTOSOME LIFE CYCLE

human | water

Fig. 30. 23 Life cycle of schistosomes. Free-swimming cercariae in water (1) penetrate unprotected skin. (2) During penetration they lose their tails to become schistosomulae. (3) These migrate through the blood stream via the lungs and liver to the veins of the bladder (*S.haematobuim.*) or bowel (*S.mansoni, S. japonicum.*), where they mature (4) to produce characteristic eggs (5) within 6-12 weeks. The eggs then penetrate the bladder or colon, to be passed in the urine or the faeces (6). Eggs released into fresh water are taken up by snail intermediate hosts (7) where they mature into sporocysts (8). These release cercariae (1) into the water to complete the cycle.

The life cycle of schistosomes is illustrated in figure 30.23. Infected snails, which are always aquatic, release fork-tailed larvae into the surrounding water. These penetrate the host's skin, enter the dermis and pass via the blood, through the lungs to the liver, where they mature and form permanent male and female pairs before relocating to their final site. In the case of *S. haematobium* this is the veins surrounding the bladder, for *S. japonicum* and *S. mansoni* it is the mesenteric veins around the small intestine. The cycle is completed when eggs laid by the female worms move across the walls of the bladder or bowel and leave the body.

Clinical features and pathogenesis

The stages of skin penetration, migration and egg production are each associated with pathological changes, collectively affecting many body systems. Penetration can cause a dermatitis, which becomes more severe on repeated reinfection. The developmental stages are associated with the onset of allergic symptoms (fever, eosinophilia, lymphadenopathy, spleno- and hepatomegaly, diarrhoea) but the most severe pathology arises following the onset of egg laying. The body becomes hypersensitive to antigens released by the eggs as they pass through tissues to the outside world, or become trapped in other organs after being swept away in the bloodstream. In urinary schistosomiasis, caused by *S. haematobium*, movement of eggs through the bladder wall causes haemorrhage. With time the bladder wall becomes inflamed and infiltrated, polyps develop, and malignant changes may follow; nephrosis may also occur (see Chapter 23). Release of the eggs of *S. japonicum* and *S. mansoni* similarly causes intestinal haemorrhage and inflammation. A more serious consequence of these infections results from the inflammatory responses to eggs that become trapped in other organs of the body, primarily the liver, but also the lung and CNS. Not all patients suffer from these consequences, but in those that do severe disease may ensue (see Chapter 25). Formation of granulomata by delayed hypersensitivity reactions around eggs in the pre-sinusoidal capillaries interferes with blood flow, and this, together with extensive portal fibrosis (Symmer's pipestem fibrosis) leads to portal hypertension. As a consequence there is hepatosplenomegaly, collateral connections form between the hepatic vessels and fragile oesophageal varices develop. The collateral circulation can lead to eggs being washed into the capillary bed of the lungs. Intense inflammatory reactions are also provoked when worms killed by anthelmintic treatment are carried back from the mesenteric vessels into the liver.

Treatment and prevention

Treatment of individuals with praziquantel is effective in removing worms, but in advanced cases the pathology is irreversible. Control of infection at a population level is by breaking the transmission cycle, through avoidance of infected water and improvement in sanitation.

Filariasis

The filarial nematodes are characterized by their location in the deeper tissues of the body and their dependence upon blood-feeding arthropod vectors for transmission (see Chapter 3). The most important species in the group can be divided into those located in the lymphatics (*Brugia*, *Wuchereria*) and those in subcutaneous tissues (*Onchocerca*). A number of less harmful species also occur. In all, the female worms release live microfilaria larvae that are picked up by the vector from the blood (lymphatic species) or skin (*Onchocerca*). Both groups can cause severe inflammatory responses, reflected in a variety of pathological responses in the skin and lymph nodes, but each is associated with additional and characteristic pathology. Descriptions of the diseases caused by *Onchocerca* are given in Chapters 21 and 28.

Lymphatic filariasis

Infections with *Brugia* and *Wuchereria* are transmitted by mosquitoes, which introduce infective larvae into the skin as they feed. These larvae develop slowly into long, thin adult worms (females 80–100mm x 0.25mm) found in the lymph nodes and lymphatics of the limbs (usually lower) and groin. Infections become patent after about a year, when sheathed microfilaria appear in the blood. Infected individuals may show few clinical signs, or suffer acute manifestations such as fever, rashes, eosinophilia, lymphangitis, lymphadenitis (Fig. 30.24) and orchitis. Later chronic obstructive changes, caused by repeated episodes of lymphangitis, may block lymphatics, leading to hydrocoele and to the gross enlargement of breasts, scrotum and limbs, the latter condition being known as 'elephantiasis' (Fig. 30.25).

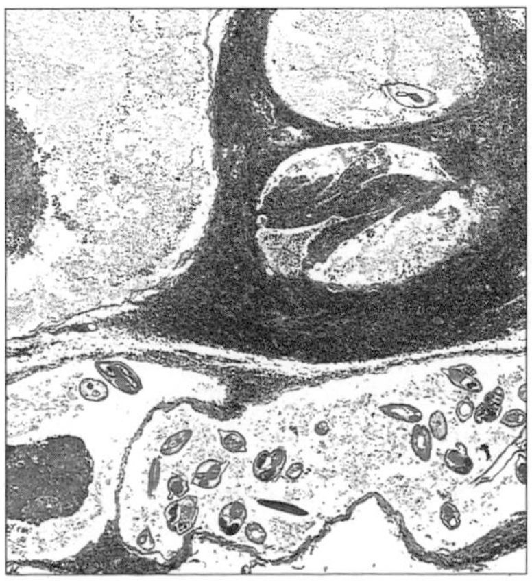

Fig. 30.24 Lymph node containing adult *Wucheria*, showing dilated lymphatics and tissue reaction in the vessel walls. Courtesy of R Muller and JR Baker.

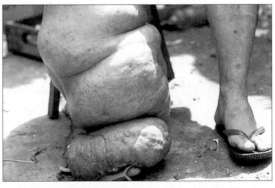

Fig. 30.25 Elephantiasis of the leg, caused by *Brugia malayi*. Courtesy of AE Bianco.

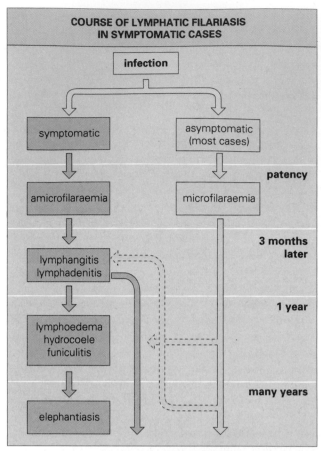

Fig. 30.26 Course of lymphocytic filariasis in symptomatic cases. Redrawn from Muller and Baker, 1990.

A feature of filarial infections in endemic regions is that not all persons exposed develop symptomatic infections. Many, although microfilaraemic, remain asymptomatic, and relatively few show gross pathology (Fig. 30.26). Some individuals develop pulmonary symptoms known as 'tropical pulmonary eosinophilia' (see Chapter 22).

It is difficult to prevent transmission of filariasis, although this can be minimized by vector control and prevention of biting. Few drugs are really satisfactory. Diethyl carbamazine has long been used, although this primarily kills microfilaria and can result in violent allergic responses (Mazzotti reaction). Suramin kills adult worms, but is toxic. Ivermectin is currently being used against onchocerciasis with some success.

SUMMARY

Many important infections are transmitted by insects, ticks or snails. These include some of the most chronic and potentially fatal infections. Often they are restricted to tropical countries because of the distribution of the vector, so that vector control can lead to disease eradication. In practice, however, this often proves to be very difficult. With very few exceptions, vaccines are not available for this group of diseases, despite the fact that strong immune responses are mounted, often leading to immunopathological complications. Treatment, therefore, is usually by chemotherapy.

Further Reading

Fisher-Hoch S. Viral hemorrhagic fever. *Med Int* 1988; **54**: 2240–2247.

Greenwood BM, Whittle HC. Immunology of medicine in the tropics. In: *Current topics in immunology*, Series. London: Edward Arnold, 1981.

Meyerhoff J. Lyme disease. *Am J Med* 1983; **75**: 663–670.

Muller R, Baker JR. *Medical parasitology*. London: Gower Medical Publishing, 1990.

Nimmanitya S. Dengue fever and dengue hemorrhagic fever. *Med Int* 1988; **54**: 2247–2251.

Warren KS, ed. *Immunology of parasitic infections*, 3rd edn. Oxford: Blackwell Scientific Publications, 1992.

Weiss E. The biology of rickettsiae. *Ann Rev Microbiol* 1982; **36**: 345–370.

Woodruff AW, ed. *Medicine in the tropics*. Edinburgh: Churchill Livingstone, 1974.

31 MULTISYSTEM ZOONOSES

Contents

INTRODUCTION

This chapter deals with those multisystem infections that exist as zoonoses, where a non-human vertebrate host acts as the reservoir of infection and humans are involved only incidentally. The human infection follows contact with the reservoir host but is not essential for the microbe's life cycle or for its maintenance in nature. One striking feature of zoonotic infections, and of the arthropod-borne infections described in Chapter 30, is that almost none are transmitted effectively from human to human.

Sometimes, however, the zoonotic definition of these infections is less clear. For example, tularaemia can be acquired either by direct contact with the reservoir host or from an arthropod vector, and is included in this chapter. Plague is included because it is transmitted from infected rats via the rat flea, although it is also transmissable directly from human to human.

Other zoonoses are dealt with in their relevant chapters, e.g. toxoplasmosis in Chapter 26, rabies in Chapter 27, salmonellosis in Chapter 25, psittacosis in Chapter 22.

ARENAVIRUS INFECTIONS

Many zoonoses are caused by enveloped ssRNA viruses called arenaviruses. On electron microscopy (Fig. 31.1)

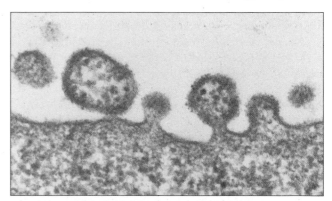

Fig. 31.1 Electronmicrograph of lymphocytic choriomeningitis virus budding from the surface of an infected cell. The sand-like granules in the virus particles are characteristic of arenaviruses. Courtesy of K Mannweiler and F Lehmann-Grübe.

VIRAL FEVERS AND HAEMORRHAGIC DISEASES ACQUIRED FROM VERTEBRATES OR FROM UNKNOWN SOURCES					
virus	**virus group**	**disease**	**animal of origin**	**lethality**	**geographical distribution**
Lymphocytic choriomeningitis (LCM)	arenavirus	LCM	mouse, hamster	–	world-wide
Lassa fever	arenavirus	Lassa fever	african bush rat (*Mastomys natalensis*)	+	West Africa
Machupo	arenavirus	Bolivian haemorrhagic fever	bush mouse (*Calomys callosus*)	+	NE Bolivia
Junin	arenavirus	Argentinian haemorrhagic fever	*Calomys* sp. mice	+	Argentina
Hantaan	bunyavirus	Haemorrhagic fever fever with renal syndrome (Korean haemorrhagic fever)	mice, rats	+	Far East, Scandinavia E. Europe
Marburg	filovirus	Marburg disease	unknown	+ +	Africa (lab. infections in Marburg etc.)
Ebola	filovirus	Ebola disease	unknown	+ +	Africa (Sudan, Zaire)

Fig. 31.2 Viral fevers and haemorrhagic diseases acquired from vertebrates or from unknown sources.

these pleomorphic virus particles can be seen to contain sand-like granules, giving rise to the name 'arena' (Latin *arena*, sand). Arenaviruses are parasites of various species of rodent, in which they cause a harmless life-long infection, with continuous excretion of virus in urine and faeces of apparently healthy infected animals. Humans infected from this source may develop severe and often lethal disease. The arenaviruses and the diseases they cause are included in figure 31.2.

As with most zoonoses, infection is not transmitted, or is transmitted with low efficiency, from human to human. However, doctors and nurses have been infected by direct contact with blood or secretions from patients infected with Lassa fever virus. The usual incubation period is from 5–10 days. Diagnosis by testing for specific antibodies (CF or IF tests) or by virus isolation can be carried out in special centres. Prevention of infection by reducing exposure to the virus was dramatically illustrated when rodent trapping terminated outbreaks of Bolivian haemorrhagic fever (see panel overleaf). Treatment with the antiviral ribavirin has been successful in Lassa fever, and human immune plasma in Lassa fever and Argentinian haemorrhagic fever.

Lymphocytic choriomeningitis (LCM) virus

This virus occurs throughout the world and has caused sporadic infection in people living in mouse-infested dwellings, and once or twice in children possessing apparently normal but infected hamsters. There is generally a non-specific febrile illness, but occasionally an aseptic (lymphocytic) meningitis occurs, with recovery.

Lassa fever

Lassa fever virus infects a bush rat (*Mastomys natalensis*) in parts of West Africa. Human exposure to infected rats or

their urine results in a febrile disease, which is generally not very severe. There are about 300 000 cases with 5000 deaths per year, and Lassa fever is the commonest febrile illness in hospitals in parts of Sierra Leone. Transfer of virus from hospital patient to nurse or doctor via blood or tissue fluids often gives rise to a more severe illness. This involves haemorrhage, capillary damage, haemoconcentration and collapse, and was seen when the disease was first recognized in Americans in the village of Lassa in 1969. So far there have been 10 deaths in 21 infected doctors and nurses. The incubation period of 7–18 days would allow an infected individual to carry the disease to anywhere in the world. However, person-to-person transfer via regular routes (droplets etc.), for instance in aircraft carrying infected patients, does not occur.

KOREAN HAEMORRHAGIC FEVER

This disease is due to Hantaan virus, a bunyavirus that causes a harmless persistent infection in various species of mice and rats. After exposure to the urine of infected animals there is a febrile illness, often with hypotension, haemorrhage and a renal syndrome. Many US soldiers suffered severe infections in Korea, and a milder disease is seen in Eastern Europe and Scandinavia. Related viruses are present in mice and rats in the USA, but cause little or no severe disease in humans. Laboratory diagnosis is by detecting specific IgM or IgG antibody.

MARBURG AND EBOLA HAEMORRHAGIC FEVERS

Both these diseases, present in Central and East Africa, are caused by filoviruses – long filamentous ssRNA viruses.

Bolivian haemorrhagic fever: A lesson in ecology

In 1962 there was an outbreak of a severe and often lethal infectious disease in the small town of San Joachim, Bolivia. Patients developed fever, myalgia, and an enanthem, followed by capillary leakage, haemorrhage, shock, and a neurological illness. This disease was termed 'Bolivian haemorrhagic fever', and had a mortality rate of 15%. Extensive investigations failed to incriminate an arthropod vector, but the evidence pointed to a role for mice in the epidemic. Acting on this possibility, hundreds of mouse traps were airlifted to the beleaguered town and it was soon shown that trapping mice had a dramatic effect on the incidence of the disease. The epidemic was completely halted. Quite separately, a virus was isolated from the tissues of a trapped local bush mouse (*Calomys callosus*). The virus was shown to cause a harmless life-long infection in this animal, with continued excretion of virus in urine and faeces. The virus (given the name 'Machupo') was an arenavirus, a group that includes LCM virus (infecting mice and hamsters) and Lassa fever virus (infecting an African bush rat). These viruses cause harmless persistent infection in the natural rodent host but an often severe disease in humans exposed to infected animals.

This outbreak of Bolivian haemorrhagic fever provides an important lesson in ecology. Because of the high incidence of malaria in the San Joachim area, extensive DDT spraying had been carried out to control mosquitoes. As a result geckos (small lizards that eat insects) accumulated DDT in their tissues, and the local cats, who preyed on geckos, began to die with lethal concentrations of DDT in their livers. The shortage of cats, in turn, allowed the bush mice to invade human dwellings. The close vicinity of infected mice to humans and human food led to the epidemic (Fig. 31.3).

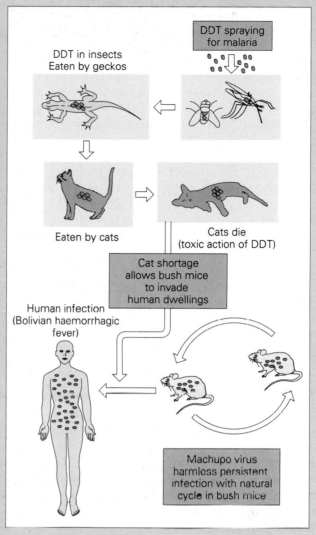

Fig. 31.3 Bolivian haemorragic fever - a lesson in ecology.

Patients develop fever, haemorrhage, rash, and probably disseminated intravascular coagulation (see Chapter 16). There is no specific treatment and no vaccine, and for both viruses the reservoir of origin and natural cycle of maintenance is unknown. Infection with Marburg virus was first recognized in 1967 in Marburg, Germany, after exposure of laboratory workers to infected African green monkeys from Uganda. But these monkeys are not the natural hosts, and the ultimate source of the infection is still unknown. Mortality was about 20% and, as with Ebola virus infection, it was noted that semen can remain infected for months after clinical recovery; one patient transmitted the infection to his wife in this way. One or two further cases have been reported, one of them in a European hitch-hiker in South Africa. Altogether 31 infections have been recorded, 8 of them fatal.

Outbreaks of a similar disease occurred in 1976 in Southern Sudan and in the region of the Ebola river in Zaire. There were more than 500 cases, and person-to-person transmission took place in local hospitals via contaminated syringes and needles. Overall mortality in this locally terrifying and mysterious outbreak of disease was 70%.

Q FEVER

The disease Q fever was first recognized in Australia in 1935, but the cause was unknown for several years – hence Q (query) fever. The name of the causative rickettsia is *Coxiella burneti*, reflecting the fact that it differs from other rickettsiae (see Chapter 30) in the following ways:

- It is not transmitted to humans by arthropods;
- It is relatively resistant to desiccation, heat and sunlight. Hence it is stable enough to be acquired from infected animals by the airborne route;
- Its main site of action is the lung rather than vascular endothelium elsewhere in the body, so that there is usually no rash.

In many countries (e.g. USA) infection of livestock with *C. burneti* is quite common, but there are nevertheless few human cases (less than 100 reported per year in the USA). People who come into in contact with infected animals, especially their placentas, unpasteurized milk and tissue fluids, are most at risk (veterinarians, farmers, abbatoir workers, etc.).

Clinical features and pathogenesis

After inhalation, the microbe multiplies in the terminal airways of the lung and about three weeks later the patient develops fever, severe headache, and often respiratory symptoms and an atypical pneumonia. The rickettsia can also spread to the liver, commonly causing hepatitis. Recovery is usually complete in two weeks, but the disease can become chronic. The heart (endocarditis) is sometimes involved, with thrombocytopenia and purpura in some patients; this condition is fatal if untreated.

Diagnosis, treatment and prevention

A four-fold or greater rise in CF antibody titre is significant. There are two antigenic forms, phase 1 and phase 2. Antibody to phase 2 is seen in ordinary Q fever, and to both phase 1 and phase 2 in chronic disease. The Weil-Felix test (see Chapter 30) is not used. The infection is treated with tetracycline or erythromycin, and a killed *C. burneti* vaccine is available for those at risk. The rickettsia are destroyed when milk is pasteurized.

ANTHRAX

Aetiology and transmission

Anthrax is caused by *Bacillus anthracis*, a large Gram-positive rod; it is aerobic and non-motile. Most members of the genus *Bacillus* are saprophytic (see Chapter 3), present in soil, water, air and vegetation. *Bacillus cereus* is a cause of food poisoning, but *B. anthracis* is the principal pathogen and is unique in having an antiphagocytic capsule made of D-glutamic acid. It forms spores which survive for years in soil.

Anthrax is primarily a disease of herbivores such as sheep, goats, cattle, horses, and bacilli are excreted in faeces, urine, and saliva. It is largely confined to developing countries (parts of Asia, Africa, Middle East), human infection occuring following direct contact with infected animals, or by contact with spores present in animal products. The spores enter the body via the skin or mucus membranes, and sometimes via the respiratory tract. In developed countries, where animal infection is rare, human infection is uncommon and has been due to exposure to contaminated imported hides, skin, wool, goat hair, bristles, bones, bonemeal in fertilizers, etc.

Clinical features and pathogenesis

The spores germinate in tissues at the site of entry. The bacteria then multiply and produce the anthrax toxin, which consists of an oedema factor (an adenylate cyclase), a lethal factor, and a protective antigen. All are plasmid-coded and have been purified and cloned. Host defences are inhibited by the antiphagocytic capsule surrounding the bacillus (see Chapter 12).

The skin is the usual site of entry. As the toxic material accumulates there is oedema, congestion, and a papule develops within 12–36 hours. This ulcerates, the centre becoming black and necrotic (Greek *anthrax*, coal) to form a 'malignant pustule' (although there is no pus), which is painless and is often surrounded by a ring of vesicles (Fig. 31.4). The bacilli spread to the lymphatics and in about 10% of cases reach the blood to cause septicaemia.

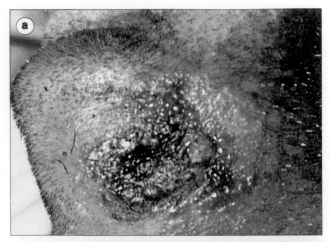
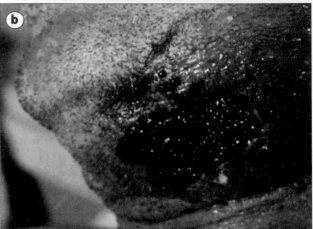

Fig. 31.4 Anthrax. (a) Characteristic black eschar surrounded by a ring of vesiculation. (b) Eight days later, the eschar has enlarged to cover the previously vesicular area, and the surrounding oedema has diminished. Courtesy of FJ Nye.

Continued multiplication and production of the toxin causes generalized toxic effects, oedema and death.

When the spores are inhaled and enter alveolar macrophages, bacterial growth in the lung leads to pulmonary oedema, mediastinal haemorrhage, with spread to blood, and death. Pulmonary anthrax is now very rare in most developed countries, where it was referred to as 'woolsorter's disease'.

Diagnosis

Films from skin lesions show Gram-positive bacilli, but the diagnosis is confirmed and non-pathogenic bacilli are distinguished after culture on blood agar. Serological tests are generally not helpful.

Treatment and prevention

Anthrax is successfully treated by penicillin, given early and in large doses. Cutaneous anthrax is fatal in 10–20% cases when untreated.

Animals can be protected by vaccination with live avirulent bacteria. Infected animals are isolated, killed, and buried or cremated without autopsy. A vaccine consisting of purified protective antigen is available for humans at high risk. Human infection is reduced by rigidly controlled disinfection of imported animal products such as hides, hair, and wool.

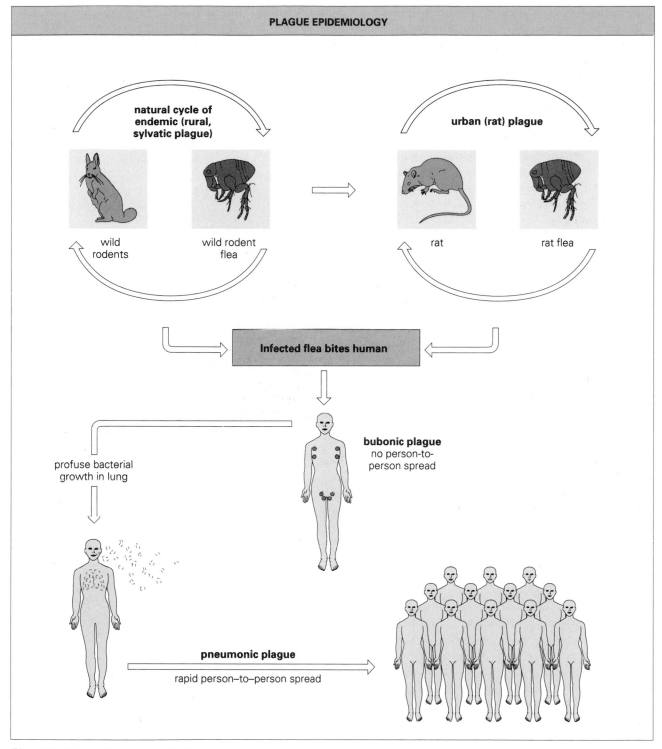

Fig. 31.5 The epidemiology of plague.

PLAGUE

Aetiology and transmission

The plague is caused by *Yersinia pestis*, a small Gram-negative rod with a surrounding capsule that is associated with virulence. The animal reservoirs are rodents such as rats, squirrels, gerbils, field mice etc., in which the infection is generally mild, the bacteria being spread between animals by fleas (Fig. 31.5). The bacillus has been endemic in wild rodents in Europe and Asia for thousands of years,

and the disease in humans has at times decimated populations and influenced the course of history. In the 14th century about one-quarter of the population of Europe died in plague epidemics (see panel overleaf). Early in the 20th century the disease arrived in North America and is at present endemic in wild rodents in western USA. Plague is now extremely rare in Europe and uncommon in the USA.

Major outbreaks in humans result from exposure to infected rats. The rat flea (*Xeopsylla cheopsis*) carries infection from rat to rat and from rat to human. The organism multiplies profusely in the gut of the flea, eventually blocking the lumen so that the flea regurgitates infected material as it attempts to feed. As infected rats sicken, their fleas seek other hosts and may bite nearby humans to cause 'bubonic' plague. This disease is not transmitted from person to person. However, when there is extensive replication of bacteria in the lung, with bronchopneumonia and large numbers of bacteria in the sputum, the infection can spread from person to person by droplets, causing 'pneumonic' plague, with extremely rapid onset.

Plague epidemics are preceded by increased infection in wild rodents and spread to rats. Rodent infection is endemic in India, S.E. Asia, S. Africa, S. America, Mexico and western states of USA. Sporadic plague continues to occur in these parts of the world, for instance in hunters exposed to infected prairie dogs in the USA and in rural populations elsewhere.

Clinical features and pathogenesis

The infecting bacteria multiply at the site of entry in the skin, and spread via the lymphatics to local and regional lymph nodes. They produce a number of virulence factors, including an antiphagocytic capsular antigen (F-1), endotoxin, and various other protein toxins. Two to six days after the flea bite occurs, lymph nodes in the armpit or groin become very tender, and enlarge to form 'buboes' (Greek *bubo*, groin), with haemorrhagic inflammation (Fig. 31.6). The patient develops fever. In mild forms the infection is arrested at this stage, but spread to the blood often occurs, with septicaemia, haemorrhagic illness and multisystem involvement (spleen, liver, lungs, CNS). Common complications are disseminated intravascular coagulation, pneumonia and meningitis. Death rate is about 50% in untreated bubonic plague, and nearly 100% in pneumonic plague. On recovery there is solid immunity and bacteria are eliminated from the body.

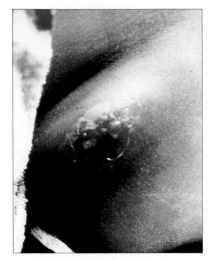

Fig. 31.6 Characteristic inguinal lymphadenitis (bubo) in which the lymph nodes have suppurated and drained spontaneously. Courtesy of JR Cantey.

The Black Death in Fourteenth Century England

For thousands of years *Yersinia pestis* has been endemic in rodents in the Far East, with occasional epidemic spread into Europe and elsewhere. In January 1348, three galleys, laden with spices from the East, brought the plague to the port of Genoa, Italy. The disease, which for reasons that are not clear became known as 'The Black Death', soon spread to the rest of Europe, arriving in London in December 1348. To the mediaeval mind, the speed and violence with which the illness passed from person to person (in the pneumonic form in the winter) was its most terrifying feature. The bubonic form (Fig. 31.7) was also important, especially in the warmer summer months, there being at least one family of black rats per household and three fleas to a rat.

The disease was attributed to earthquakes, to the movement of the planets, to a Jewish or Arab plot (350 massacres of Jews took place during the Black Death in Europe), and most commonly to God's punishment for human wickedness. You could become infected without touching a plague victim, and to many it seemed that there was something, a miasma, a poison, in the air. Physicians wore strange masks, infected houses were labelled and boarded up, together with the inhabitants. But it was impossible to isolate all those who were sick. Rich and poor perished. The population of England was about 4 million and, over a period of 2.5 years, approximately one-third (more than a million) died. The clergy, for unknown reasons, suffered an even greater mortality

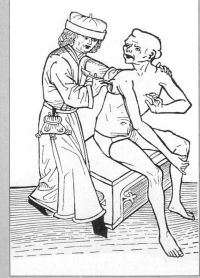

Fig. 31.7 Fifteenth century German woodcut showing incision of a bubo. Courtesy of The Wellcome Institute Library, London. With permission from Ciba-Zeitschift, Basel.

of nearly 50%. Altogether in Europe at least 25 million people died. The Black Death was a major human disaster, with lasting effects on economic and social structure. There were a further five, less severe outbreaks in England in the fourteenth century. The epidemic in 1665, the year before the Great Fire of London, was graphically described by Daniel Defoe (who was only five at the time) in his *Journal of a Plague Year in London*. The last pandemic arose in China and reached Hong Kong in 1894, where Yersin and (independently) Kitasato described the causative bacillus.

Diagnosis

Organisms are found in fluid aspirated from lymph nodes, or from sputum in pneumonic plague. They can be seen in smears after Giemsa, Gram or fluorescent-antibody staining (the staining is bipolar) and can also be cultivated.

Treatment and prevention

Streptomycin and/or tetracycline are used in treatment. Plague has been prevented by the following measures:

- Classically, by quarantine measures in ports and on ships. 'Quarantine', from the Italian *quarentina*, forty (days), refers to the original isolation period for ships suspected of carrying contagion;
- By rodent control, especially of rats, e.g. at the site of entry of ships and aircraft into plague-free countries;
- By strict isolation of patients with plague;
- By chemoprophylaxis (tetracycline) during an epidemic or visit to an affected area;
- By vaccination of military personnel or of certain workers in endemic areas. The vaccine consists of formalin-killed bacteria and gives partial protection.

YERSINIA ENTEROCOLITICA INFECTION

Aetiology and transmission

These Gram-negative bacteria have been isolated in Europe and USA from various rodents, from domestic animals and from freshwater sources. Human infection is by mouth from contaminated food or water.

Clinical features and pathogenesis

The infecting bacteria penetrate the intestinal mucosa, causing ulcerations in the terminal ileum (Fig. 31.8), with spread to local lymphoid tissue causing necrotic lesions in Peyer's patches and mesenteric adenitis. The commonest clinical appearance is an enterocolitis with fever, diarrhoea and abdominal pain. This lasts 1–3 weeks. A reactive arthritis is sometimes seen.

Diagnosis

Yersinia enterocolitica can be cultivated from stool, pharyngeal exudate etc., but this is not always easy. These organisms grow best at 25°C, so that biochemical tests are often positive at 25°C but not at 37°C.

Treatment and prevention

The condition usually resolves without treatment, but aminoglycosides, tetracycline or trimethoprim can be used.

TULARAEMIA

Aetiology and transmission

Tularaemia is caused by the small, Gram-negative rod *Franciscella tularensis* first isolated from rodents in Tular County, California in 1912. It is present in rodents and in a wide variety of other wild animals in many countries in the Northern Hemisphere, including the USA (especially Arkansas and Missouri), the CIS, Norway and Spain. In the infected animal it causes a plague-like disease and is spread via ticks, mites, lice and biting flies. In *Dermacentor*

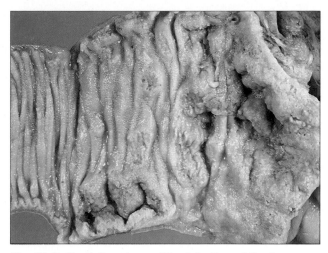

Fig. 31.8 *Yersinia enterocolitica* infection of the ileum, showing superficial necrosis of the mucosa and ulceration. Courtesy of J Newman.

ticks the bacteria are transmitted vertically to subsequent generations via the ovum. Human infection is sporadic and follows contact with an infected animal (e.g. skinning of hares, rabbits, muskrats) or with the arthropod vector. There is no spread from person to person.

Clinical features and pathogenesis

The organism grows at the site of entry, aided by its virulence-associated capsule, and after 3–5 days forms a skin ulcer. There is a febrile illness and lymphatic spread results in swollen, painful regional lymph nodes. Blood invasion and involvement of lungs, gastrointestinal tract etc. is not uncommon, with formation of granulomatous nodules around infected reticuloendothelial cells. There may be a rash. Mortality in untreated patients is 5–15%. The conjunctiva or oral mucosa can be infected via contaminated fingers to give ocular or oral manifestations. Infection by inhalation is less common and gives a febrile illness with respiratory symptoms.

Diagnosis

Infected tissues can be examined by fluorescent antibody staining, but isolation of bacteria is not often attempted due to the high risk of laboratory infection. Agglutination tests for antibody are more commonly used in diagnosis.

Treatment and prevention

Streptomycin is effective, and a live attenuated bacterial vaccine is available for people with occupational risk (e.g. fur trappers). Handling animals with gloves gives protection, and contact with ticks should be avoided.

PASTEURELLA MULTOCIDA INFECTION

Aetiology and transmission

This encapsulated Gram-negative rod is distributed worldwide, and is part of the normal oral flora in cats, dogs and other domestic and wild animals, in whom it can cause pneumonia, septicemia, etc. It is transmitted to humans by animal bites (especially cat bites), and other types of bacteria including anaerobes are often present in the lesion.

Clinical features and pathogenesis

Local multiplication of bacteria leads within a day or two to cellulitis. Virulence factors include endotoxin and the capsule.

Diagnosis

The organism can be cultivated and identified in material from the wound.

Treatment and prevention

Penicillin is effective and ampicillin has been used in prophylaxis after cat or dog bites. Bite wounds should be cleansed and debrided.

LEPTOSPIROSIS

Aetiology and transmission

Leptospira are tightly coiled spirochaetes 5–15 μm long. They show active rotational movement and have two flagella. Their delicate outline is best seen by darkfield microscopy because they are not very well stained by dyes. The ends of the species *Leptospira interrogans* are bent into a quesion-mark like hook – hence the name '*interrogans*' This species infects mammals such as rats in various parts of the world (Fig. 31.9), causing chronic kidney infection with excretion of large numbers of bacteria in urine. The spirochaetes are soon killed on drying, heating, exposure to detergents or disinfectants, but they remain viable for several weeks in stagnant alkaline water or wet soil. Humans are infected by ingestion of or exposure to contaminated water or food. The bacteria, aided by their motility, enter through breaks in skin or mucosae, so that infection can be acquired by swimming, working or playing in contaminated water (miners, farmers, sewage workers, watersport enthusiasts). There are about 60 cases a year in England and Wales and about 100 a year are reported in the USA. Bacteria are excreted in human urine but person to person transmission is rare. Immunity is serovar-specific.

Clinical features and pathogenesis

The bacteria reach the blood and after an incubation period of 1–2 weeks cause a febrile, influenza-like illness. In about 90% of cases this resolves uneventfully, but multiplication in the liver can lead to hepatitis, jaundice and haemorrhage, in kidneys to uraemia and bacteriuria, and in the CSF and the aqueous humor to aseptic meningitis and conjunctival or scleral haemorrhage (Fig. 31.10). The clinical picture depends to some extent on the particular type of leptospire. 'Weil's disease', the severe form with haemorrhagic complications and kidney and liver failure, occurs in only 5–10% of patients ill with leptospirosis.

Diagnosis

There is often a history of exposure. Bacteria can be isolated from blood, CSF and urine and a rise in agglutinating antibody can be demonstrated.

LEPTOSPIRA INTERROGANS DISEASES			
leptospiral serogroup	animal host	distribution	clinical features
canicola	dog	world-wide	influenza-like illness ('canicola fever', '7-day fever') is the commonest; can progress to aseptic meningitis, liver and kidney damage (Weil's disease)
ictero-haemorrhagiae	rat	world-wide	
hebdomadis	mice voles rats cattle	Japan, Europe	

Fig. 31.9 Diseases caused by the three main serogroups of *Leptospira interrogans*. There are 19 different serogroups of this organism, other serogroups including seroja (pigs) and pomona (swine and cattle in USA and Europe). Among the serogroups there are 172 different serotypes.

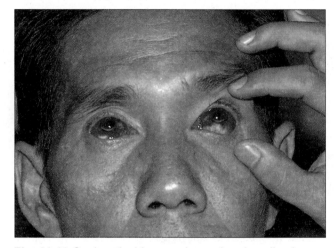

Fig. 31.10 Conjunctival haemorrhages in a jaundiced patient with leptospirosis. Courtesy of D Lewis.

Treatment and prevention

Penicillin and tetracyclines have been valuable in treatment when given within a day or two of onset of illness, and doxycycline will prevent disease in those exposed to infection. Measures for prevention include rodent control, and protective clothing and prophylactic penicillin after cuts and abrasions in those at risk (sewer and abbatoir workers).

RAT BITE FEVER

Aetiology and transmission

This uncommon but world-wide condition is caused by either *Spirillum minor*, a Gram-negative spiral-shaped organism, or by *Streptobacillus moniliformis*, a Gram-negative filamentous bacillus. These bacteria are found in the oropharyngeal flora of 50% of healthy wild and laboratory rats and also in other rodents. Transmission to humans is by biting.

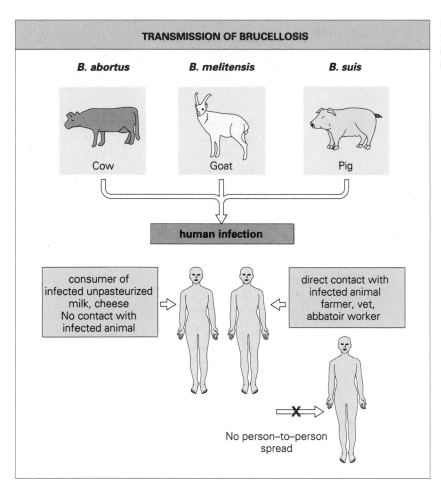

TRANSMISSION OF BRUCELLOSIS

B. abortus — Cow

B. melitensis — Goat

B. suis — Pig

human infection

consumer of infected unpasteurized milk, cheese
No contact with infected animal

direct contact with infected animal
farmer, vet, abbatoir worker

No person–to–person spread

Fig. 31.11 Transmission of brucellosis. Human infection follows contact with infected animals or consumption of infected animal products.

Clinical features and pathogenesis

After an incubation period of 7–10 days there is onset of fever, headache and myalgia. Bacteria multiply at the site of the bite and, in the case of *S. moniliformis,* cause an inflamed local lesion. Spread of infection to lymph nodes and the blood leads to lymphadenopathy, rash and arthralgia. Complications include endocarditis and pneumonia, with up to 10% mortality in untreated patients.

Diagnosis

Streptobacillus moniliformis can be cultured from the wound site, from lymph nodes and the blood, but *Sp. minor* cannot be cultivated and must be demonstrated in tissues by darkfield microscopy.

Treatment and prevention

Penicillin and streptomycin are effective. Measures for prevention include rodent control and prevention of rat bites in laboratory workers.

BRUCELLOSIS

Aetiology and transmission

Brucellosis, which has a world-wide distribution, is caused by bacteria of the genus *Brucella,* small Gram-negative, non-motile coccobacilli, adapted to intracellular replication. The principal antigens are A (*B. abortus*) and M (*B. melitensis*), and an endotoxin is involved in pathogenesis.

Brucellae are primarily animal pathogens, infecting humans after contact with infected animals or their products (Fig. 31.11). There are three important species, each with a predilection for a certain domestic animal, although capable of infection of a wider range of animals:

- *B. abortus* – infects cows; distribution is world-wide but has been eliminated from several developed countries;
- *B. melitensis* – infects goats; common in Malta (Latin *melita,* honey isle) and other Mediterranean countries, Mexico, South America. Tends to cause more severe disease in humans;
- *B. suis* – infects pigs; occurs in USA where it is the most important cause of brucellosis, and in South America and S.E. Asia.

In cows and goats brucella localize in the placenta, causing contagious abortion, and also in mammary glands from whence they are shed for long periods in milk. They are present in uterine discharges, faeces and urine.

Human brucellosis (undulant fever, Malta fever) occurs when the bacteria enter the body via abrasions in the skin, via the alimentary tract or, most commonly, via the respiratory tract. Infection is seen especially in those who are in close contact with infected animals (farmers, veterinary surgeons, abbatoir workers). Unpasteurized cows milk (UK, USA), goat's milk or cheese (Mediterranean countries) is a less frequent source of infection. There is no spread from person to person.

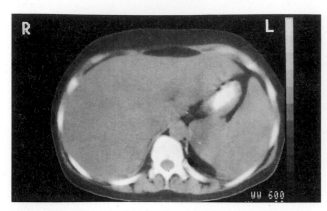

Fig. 31.12 CT scan showing hepatosplenomegaly in *Brucella melitensis* infection. Courtesy of H Tubbs.

Clinical features and pathogenesis

The infecting bacteria pass from the site of entry into local and regional lymph nodes, reaching the thoracic duct and thus the blood (septicaemic phase). Cells of the reticulo-endothelial system are then infected (liver, spleen, bone marrow, lymphoid tissues). It is in these cells and in monocytes and macrophages that the host's battle with the parasite is waged. The result is an inflammatory (granulomatous) reaction with epithelioid and giant cells, central necrosis and peripheral fibrosis. Quite commonly the infection is subclinical. The symptoms of acute brucellosis begin after an incubation period of 1–3 weeks, when there is gradual onset of malaise, fever, drenching sweats, aching and weakness. A rising and falling (undulant) fever is seen in a minority of patients. Enlarged lymph nodes and spleen may be detected and hepatitis can occur (Fig. 31.12). The bone marrow lesions may progress to osteomyelitis, and cholecystitis, endocarditis and meningitis are occasionally seen. Abortion occurs in infected cows, sows, goats, but not in humans. It is due to the presence in the placenta of erythritol, a sugar compound that stimulates bacterial growth. Erythritol is not present in the human placenta.

The patient generally recovers after a few weeks or months but a chronic stage (more than a year's illness) can develop with tiredness, aches and pains, anxiety, depression, and occasional fever. Relapses and remissions may occur. *Brucella* cannot be isolated at this stage, and chronic brucellosis is often a difficult diagnosis. Agglutinin titres are generally high but antibodies are less relevant than cell-mediated immunity for this intracellular parasite.

Diagnosis

The bacteria can be isolated in some cases from blood cultures (or from bone marrow, lymph nodes), and urine culture may be successful. This takes up to four weeks. In acute brucellosis agglutinating antibodies (IgM) are present but not generally in chronic brucellosis. CF tests and antiglobulin tests are also used, but radioimmunoassay tests are the most sensitive.

Treatment and prevention

Brucella are susceptible to tetracycline and streptomycin; cotrimoxazole is also used. But because of their intracellular location the bacteria are not easily eradicated and prolonged courses of treatment (3 months) are needed. Brucellae in milk are destroyed by pasteurization. In the USA and UK brucellosis has gradually declined (100–200 cases per year now reported in USA) following eradication programmes, involving the use in cattle of a live attenuated vaccine (S19) and slaughter of those already infected. For those in close contact with infected animals (farmers, vets, abattoir workers) protective clothing and goggles may be used on risky occasions. There is no satisfactory vaccine available for humans. Indeed vets may develop a mild illness when accidentally infected with the live S19 vaccine.

HELMINTH INFECTIONS

The allocation of a particular helminth infection to a chapter on multisystem infection is a somewhat arbitrary decision. Many of the worm parasites that can be acquired from animals, or through the bites of arthropod vectors, have stages that invade a number of the body systems. Others are primarily located in a particular organ, but cause pathological changes that can be widespread in their effects. Conversely, although stages of certain worms may be widely distributed in the body, their pathological effects are most commonly associated with a particular organ. For example, larvae of the pork tapeworm *Taenia solium*, which causes the disease 'cysticercosis', develop in a variety of tissues, including muscle. However, the most serious pathology is caused by larvae found in the CNS. Accordingly this infection is discussed in Chapter 27. After infection with eggs of the dog nematode *Toxocara canis*, larvae migrate throughout the body, causing the condition known as 'visceral larval migrans'. Again, the most serious effects are associated with larvae that localize in the CNS (see Chapter 27) and the eye (see Chapter 21). The filarial nematodes that localize in the lymphatics (*Wuchereria*, *Brugia*) or subcutaneous tissue (*Onchocerca*), give rise to lymphangitis, lymphadenopathy and pathological change in the skin, but their most dramatic pathology is seen as chronic obstructive lymphatic changes (see Chapter 30), and blindness (see Chapter 21), respectively.

However, three helminths can be considered as genuinely multisystem in their effects. These are the tapeworm *Echinococcus granulosus* and the nematodes *Trichinella spiralis* and *Strongyloides stercoralis*.

Echinococcus

The adults of this species live as tiny (3–5mm long) tapeworms in the intestine of the dog. Eggs laid by the worm leave the dog in faecal material and can survive in the outside world for long periods. If swallowed (under natural conditions by sheep, or accidentally by humans) the eggs hatch in the small intestine, releasing larvae which then penetrate the mucosa to enter a blood vessel. Chance determines where the larvae lodge in the capillary bed. This most often occurs in the liver, but it may occur in the body cavity, lung, brain, eye, spinal cord or long bones.

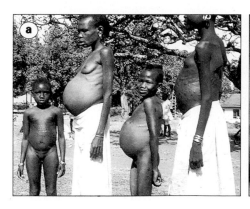

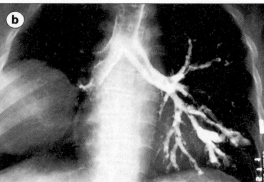

Fig. 31.13 Hydatid cysts. (a) Patients showing marked abdominal swelling caused by hydatid cysts in the liver. Courtesy of GS Nelson. (b) Bronchogram showing blockage of bronchus by a cyst of *E. granulosus* in lower left medial region. Courtesy of RB Holliman.

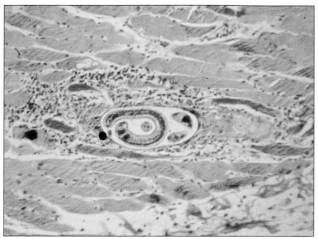

Fig. 31.14 Inflammatory reaction around a cyst containing a coiled larva of *Trichinella spiralis*. Trichrome stain. Courtesy of IG Kagan.

Once in the target organ the larvae slowly grow into large, thick-walled, fluid-filled (hydatid) cysts, the pathological signs being largely due to the mechanical pressures exerted by the cysts (Fig. 31.13). Laboratory diagnosis is by finding hooklets and scolices in the cyst fluid and demonstrating specific antibody (ELISA, indirect haemagglutination). Although drug treatment (praziquantel) is available, surgical removal, where possible, is the most satisfactory way of dealing with the infection. Great care must be taken during removal to prevent leakage of fluid from the cysts. Not only may this trigger anaphylactic responses in sensitized individuals, but the numerous larvae in the fluid (produced by asexual division) can cause metastatic infections in other sites.

Echinococcus multilocularis closely resembles *E. granulosus*, but causes a multilocular cyst consisting of hundreds of small vesicles, without a fibrous outer capsule. The parasite generally occurs as a fox-rodent cycle (N. Europe, Siberia, parts of N. America) and hunters or trappers are occasionally infected after ingesting food contaminated by fox faeces. Liver involvement leads to jaundice and weight loss, and the condition is usually inoperable.

Trichinella

Trichinella spiralis causes the disease 'trichinosis'. It is perhaps the most widely distributed of all nematode parasites, being capable of infecting almost any warm-blooded ani-

mal. In its natural cycle it is transmitted between predators (e.g. bears, seals) and their prey, and between scavengers and carrion, but a domestic cycle has become established in pigs and rats. Humans are infected by eating undercooked meat (pork or wild animal) containing the encysted, infected larval stages. These larvae mature rapidly into adults in the small intestine, their invasion of the mucosa causing an acute enteritis. Female worms release live larvae into the mucosa, and these invade the blood vessels 1–2 weeks after initial infection to become distributed around the body. Bacteraemia may occur at this stage. The larvae attempt to invade the cells of many organs (including the heart and CNS), although they can mature only in striated muscles, where they form the characteristic cysts (Fig. 31.14). This stage of infection is associated with a wide spectrum of pathological signs; fever, joint and muscle pains, eosinophilia and periorbital oedema; myositis, petechial haemorrhage, encephalitis and cardiac abnormalities may also occur. The majority of these are immunopathological in origin, caused by hypersensitivity and inflammatory responses. Diagnosis is by muscle biopsy and demonstration of specific antibody. Treatment is possible with anthelmintics (thiabendazole), but symptomatic treatment with anti-inflammatories may also be necessary.

Strongyloides

Like *Trichinella*, this nematode has an intestinal phase, but infection is acquired by the penetration of infective larvae through the skin. The larvae migrate to the lung, enter the alveoli, pass up the bronchi and trachea, and are then swallowed. Only females develop parthenogenetically in the host, and these lay strings of eggs into the intestinal mucosa (Fig. 31.15). The eggs hatch within the intestine to release larvae, which then pass out with the faeces. The larvae require warm, moist soil, and the geographic distribution of strongyloidiasis is similar to hookworm (especially in tropical areas and in rural southern states of USA).

Although not strictly a zoonosis in that infections are most often passed between humans, this species can develop in animal hosts including dogs. It possesses the unusual property that the faecal larval stages may, in a given patient, develop directly into the infective stage, and penetrate the perianal skin to reinfect the host; alternatively the larvae may complete a free-living, sexually reproducing generation in the soil, before once again producing infective larvae. This plasticity of behaviour means that the

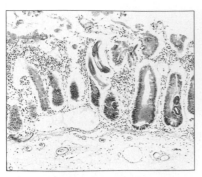

Fig. 31.15
Strongyloides stercoralis. Adults and larvae in the mucosa of small intestine, showing disruption of the villous surface.

species can undergo complete development within the host (autoinfection). Larvae released from eggs laid by females in the intestine can become infective in the bowel and reinvade the body, often in enormous numbers. This is unimportant in immunocompetent hosts and most infected individuals are asymptomatic, though vomiting or diarrhoea may occur. However, in those with T cell deficiencies or in malnutrition it can lead to the condition known as 'hyperinfection' or 'disseminated strongyloidiasis', the larvae invading almost all organs and causing severe, and sometimes fatal, pathology. Infected patients may show vomiting, abdominal pain, diarrhoea with malabsorption and dehydration, eosinophilia, pneumonitis and other 'allergic' signs. Disseminated strongyloidiasis can arise long after initial infection. It is firmly established that infections can persist for many years (more than 30), being maintained by low-level autoinfection until the patient's immune defences are reduced.

Laboratory diagnosis depends in finding the larvae in faeces. Treatment is by use of anthelmintics such as thiabendazole or levamisole.

SUMMARY

The multisystem infections described in this chapter are maintained naturally in a reservoir of non-human vertebrates. Humans are infected incidentally, and there is generally no transmission from person to person. Some of them are highly virulent, and when the reservoir host is common in crowded human communities (e.g. plague) disease epidemics have been major events in history. When humans have less extensive contact with the reservoir host, the infection, even when virulent, has less impact (e.g. Lassa fever, Ebola fever).

Most of these infections are now less common in developed countries (e.g. anthrax, brucellosis, hydatid disease) but remain as regular causes of disease in other parts of the world. In all cases the nature and the extent of human–animal contact is a determining factor.

There are satisfactory antimicrobial agents for most of the non-viral infections, but effective vaccines are generally not available.

Further Reading

Evans ME. *Francisella tularensis. Infec Control* 1985; **6**: 381-383.

Heath CW, Alexander AD, Galton MM. Leptospirosis in the United States: Analysis of 483 cases in man, 1949–1961. *New Engl J Med* 1965; **273**: 857-864, 915-922.

Heymann DL, Weisfeld JS, Webb PA *et al.* Ebola haemorrhagic fever: Tandala, Zaire, 1977–1978. *J Infect Dis* 1980; **142**: 372.

Howard CR, Simpson DIH. The biology of arenaviruses. *J Gen Virol* 1980; **51**: 1.

Kaufmann AF, Boyce JM, Martone WJ. Trends in human plague in the United States. *J Infect Dis* 1980; **141**: 522.

Mackenzie RB. Epidemiology of Machupo viruses infection I. Pattern of human infection, San Joaquin, Bolivia 1962-1964. *Am J Trop Med Hyg* 1965; **14**: 808.

Monath TP. Lassa fever: review of epidemiology and epizootiology. *Bull World Health Organ* 1975; **52**: 577.

Wise RI. Brucellosis in the United States: Past, present and future. *J Am Med Assoc 1980;* **244**: 2318.

Young EJ. Human brucellosis. *Rev Infect Dis* 1983; **5**: 821-842.

32 PYREXIA OF UNKNOWN ORIGIN

INTRODUCTION

The homeostatic mechanisms of the body maintain a constant body temperature with daily fluctuations (circadian temperature rhythm) of +/- 1 to 1.5°C. Although 37°C (98.6°F) is taken as 'normal', individuals vary in their body temperature; some may be as low as 36°C, others as high as 38°C. Fever is defined as an abnormal increase in body temperature – an oral temperature greater than 37.6°C (99.7°F), or a rectal temperature greater than 38°C (100.4°F), and may be continuous or intermittent. In continuous fever the body temperature is elevated over the whole 24-hour period and swings less than 1°C; this is characteristic of, for example, typhoid and typhus fever. In an intermittent fever the temperature is above normal throughout the 24-hour period but swings more than 1°C during that time. A swinging fever is typical of pyogenic infections and abscesses, and of tuberculosis.

Fever, or 'pyrexia', may be produced in response to an exogenous pyrogen, such as endotoxin in Gram-negative cell walls, or to endogenous pyrogen (e.g. interleukin-1) released from phagocytic cells. It is thought that fever may be a protective response of the host (Fig. 32.1)

PYREXIA (FEVER) OF UNKNOWN ORIGIN

Pyrexia is a very common complaint in patients presenting to a doctor. The cause is usually immediately apparent or is discovered within a few days, or the temperature settles spontaneously. If the patient's fever continues for 2–3 weeks or more, and the diagnosis is uncertain despite routine investigations performed during outpatient visits or in hospital, then a provisional diagnosis of 'pyrexia of unknown origin' (PUO), also known as 'fever of unknown origin' (FUO), is made. This is a classical definition of PUO, but as modern medicine successfully keeps alive an

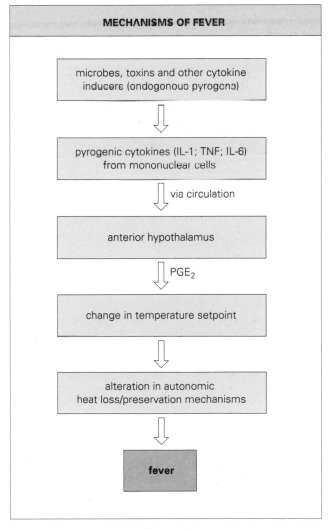

Fig. 32.1 Mechanisms of fever. Fever may be induced either by exogenous pyrogens such as microbes or their toxins, or by endogenous pyrogens released in the host, and may have a protective effect.

32.1

DEFINITIONS OF PYREXIA OF UNKNOWN ORIGIN		
definition	**symptoms**	**diagnosis**
Classical PUO	fever (> 38.3°C) on several occasions and more than **three weeks** duration	uncertain despite appropriate investigations after at least **three** outpatient visits or **three days** in hospital
Nosocomial (hospital-acquired) PUO	fever (> 38.3°C) on several occasions in a hospitalized patient receiving acute care; infection not present or incubating on admission	uncertain after **three days** despite appropriate investigations, including at least **two days** incubation of microbiological cultures
Neutropenic PUO	fever (> 38.3°C) on several occasions; neutrophil count < 500/mm³ in peripheral blood, or expected to fall below that number within 1-2 days	uncertain after **three days** despite appropriate investigations, including at least **two days** incubation of microbiological cultures
HIV-associated PUO	fever (> 38.3°C) on several occasions; fever of more than **three weeks** duration as an outpatient or more than **three days** duration in hospital; confirmed positive HIV serology	uncertain after **three days** despite appropriate investigations, including at least **two days** incubation of microbiological cultures

Fig. 32.2 Definitions of PUO. The classical definition of PUO requires the fever to be of three or more weeks duration, but in compromised patients infections frequently progress rapidly because of inadequate host defences. Consequently the pace of the investigations also needs to be rapid if appropriate therapy is to be initiated.

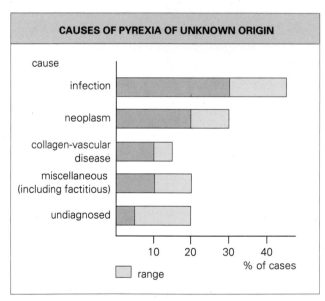

Fig. 32.3 Causes of PUO. The results of several retrospective studies show that infection is the single most common cause of PUO. In some studies a significant number of fevers remained undiagnosed.

increasing number of patients with serious underlying diseases, PUO in patients in particular risk groups has also been defined (Fig. 32.2).

CAUSES OF PUO

For centuries, fever has been recognized as a characteristic sign of infection, and infection is the single most common cause of PUO, accounting for 30-45% of PUO in adults and up to 50% in children. However, there are important non-infectious causes of fever, malignancies and collagen–

vascular diseases being the two main groups (Fig. 32.3). These need to be differentiated from infections during the investigation of a patient with a PUO. Despite intense and prolonged investigations, however, the cause of fever remains undiagnosed in as many as 10% of patients, and a further 10% may have a factitious fever (one produced artificially by the patient).

Infective causes of classical PUO

The most common infective causes of classical PUO are shown in figure 32.4. These can be divided into two main groups: 1) infections such as tuberculosis and typhoid fever, caused by specific pathogens; and 2) infections such urinary tract infections, biliary tract infections and abscesses, which can be caused by a variety of different pathogens. Most of these infections are described in detail elsewhere in this book. Bacterial endocarditis is discussed below.

Significant infection may be present in the absence of fever in some groups of patients, notably seriously ill neonates, the elderly, patients with uraemia, patients receiving corticosteroids and those taking antipyretic drugs continuously. In these people other signs and symptoms of infection have to be sought. This chapter deals only with patients whose presenting complaint is fever.

INVESTIGATION OF CLASSICAL PUO

Steps in the investigative procedure

Because of the many possible causes of PUO, both infectious and non-infectious, it will be apparent that it is not practicable to attempt specific investigations for each at the outset. The diagnostic pathway can be divided into a series of stages, each stage attempting to focus the investigation on the likely causes (Fig. 32.5):

INFECTIVE CAUSES OF PYREXIA OF UNKNOWN ORIGIN	
infection	**usual cause**
Bacterial	
Tuberculosis	*Mycobacterium tuberculosis*
Enteric fevers	*Salmonella typhi*
Osteomyelitis	*Staphylococcus aureus* (also *Haemophilus influenzae* in young children; *Salmonella* in patients with sickle-cell disease)
Endocarditis	oral streptococci, *Staph. aureus,* coagulase-negative staphylococci
Brucellosis	*Brucella abortus, melitensis and suis*
Abscesses (esp. intra-abdominal)	mixed anaerobes and facultative anaerobes from gut flora
Biliary system infections	Gram-negative facultative anaerobes e.g. *E. coli*
Urinary tract infections	Gram-negative facultative anaerobes e.g. *E. coli*
Lyme disease	*Borrelia burgdorferi*
Relapsing fever	*Borrelia recurrentis*
Leptospirosis	*Leptospira icterohaemorrhagiae*
Rat bite fever	*Spirillum minor, Streptobacillus moniliformis*
Typhus	*Rickettsia prowazekii*
Spotted fevers	*Rickettsia rickettsiae; Rickettsia conori*
Psittacosis	*Chlamydia psittaci*
Q fever	*Coxiella burnetii*
Parasitic	
Malaria	*Plasmodium* species
Trypanosomiasis	*Trypanosoma brucei*
Amoebic abscesses	*Entamoeba histolytica*
Toxoplasmosis	*Toxoplasma gondii*
Fungal	
Cryptococcosis	*Cryptococcus neoformans*
Histoplasmosis	*Histoplasma capsulatum*
Viral	
Infectious mononucleosis	Epstein-Barr virus
Hepatitis	Hepatitis viruses
CMV-infection	Cytomegalovirus

Fig. 32.4 Infective causes of PUO. A wide range of infections can present as PUO. Some, such as brucellosis are zoonoses, and many are vector-borne. Therefore the patient must have had appropriate exposure to contract these infections. For example, there are about 2000 cases of malaria annually in the UK but all are contracted outside the country. Thus a travel history is very important.

Stage 1

History. Careful history-taking is essential and should include questions about travel, occupation, hobbies, exposure to animals and to known infectious hazards, antibiotic therapy within the previous two months, drug-taking and other habits. Some of the infections listed in figure 32.4 are zoonoses (e.g. leptospirosis, spotted fevers), whereas others are vector-borne (e.g. malaria, trypanosomiasis) and/or of limited geographical distribution (e.g. histoplasmosis). Hence the importance of a travel history.

Physical examination. In the light of the history and the differential diagnosis, a complete physical examination of the patient with PUO is essential. In particular, skin, eyes, lymph nodes and abdomen should be examined and heart auscultation performed.

It is also important to confirm that the patient does have a fever. In some series, as many as a quarter of patients whose presenting complaint was a PUO did not have a fever but had a naturally exaggerated circadian temperature rhythm. Up to 10% may have a factitious fever.

Screening tests. Routine investigations such as chest x-ray and blood tests should be performed at this stage.

Stage 2

Review history and repeat physical examination. A review of the patient's history, particularly after discussion with colleagues and perhaps carried out by a second physician, is valuable to check for omissions such as exposure to particular risk factors in the recent or more distant past. The physical examination should also be repeated because rashes and other signs of infection may be transient.

Specific diagnostic tests . Because the most common cause of unexplained fever is infection, collection and careful examination of appropriate specimens is essential to the investigation. Skin tests may also be appropriate at this stage. Clues to the diagnosis elicited by careful history-taking should direct specific investigations.

The most important specimens include blood for culture and for examination for antibodies. A sample of serum collected when the patient presents should also be stored

INVESTIGATION OF CLASSICAL PUO	
Stage 1	history, physical examination, screening tests
Stage 2	review history, repeat physical examination, specific diagnostic tests, non-invasive investigations
Stage 3	invasive tests
Stage 4	therapeutic trials

Fig. 32.5 The diagnostic pathway for the investigation of a patient with PUO can be divided into several stages.

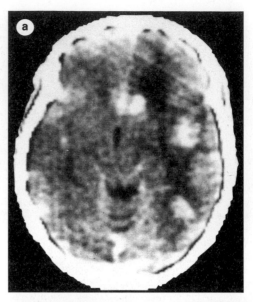

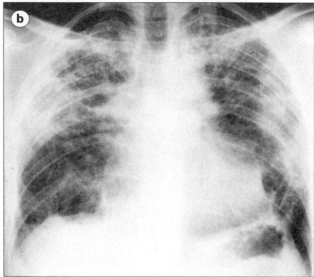

Fig. 32.6 Computerized tomography scans help in the demonstration of abscesses. The patient in (a) is suffering from a tuberculoma of the brain but the CT appearance is not sufficiently characteristic to distinguish this from a pyogenic abscess or a meningioma. Courtesy of J Ambrose. The chest x-ray in (b) shows a patient with sarcoidosis. The differential diagnosis between infective and non-infective causes of granulomata is important, and can be difficult in the early stages of the investigation. Courtesy of M. Turner-Warwick.

for comparison with later samples to detect rising antibody titres (even if the patient is some weeks into the infection). Serological tests are helpful, particularly in the diagnosis of cytomegalovirus and Epstein–Barr virus infection, toxoplasmosis, psittacosis and rickettsial infections. Positive results in syphilis serology should be regarded with caution, as other infections can cause biological false-positives (see Chapter 24). Direct examination of blood is required to diagnose malaria, trypanosomiasis and relapsing fever. Repeated sampling of blood, urine and other body fluids is often required and the laboratory should be alerted to search for unusual and fastidious organisms (e.g. nutritionally variant streptococci as a cause of endocarditis; see below). If possible, serial cultures should be collected before antimicrobial therapy is commenced.

Non-invasive investigations. Technical advances in diagnostic imaging techniques have provided the physician with a wide range of non-invasive investigative methods. Some radiological procedures, such as chest x-rays, are considered routine in the work-up of patients with PUO (Fig. 32.6); others such as gallium or technetium scans are applied in the light of the likely diagnosis (Fig. 32.7).

Stage 3
Invasive tests. Biopsy of liver and bone marrow should always be considered in the investigation of classical cases of PUO, but other tissues such as skin, lymph nodes, kidney, etc. may also be sampled. It is undesirable or impossible to repeat biopsies and therefore it is important to organize the laboratory examination of material carefully to maximize the information obtained.

Stage 4
Therapeutic trials. Trials of corticosteroids (e.g. prednisone, dexamethasone) or prostaglandin inhibitors (e.g. aspirin, indomethacin) may be indicated if a non-infectious cause is suspected. There are few indications for empiric antimicrobial or cytotoxic chemotherapy in the management of classical PUO. However, a trial of anti-tuberculous drugs may be advocated in patients with a history of tuberculosis,

even in the absence of supporting microbiological evidence. Infections may progress very rapidly in neutropenic and AIDS patients and 'blind' therapy is warranted (see below).

Treatment
The investigation and management of a patient with PUO requires persistence and an informed and open mind in order to reach the correct diagnosis. Because the range of infective causes of PUO is enormous the correct diagnosis is an essential prelude to the choice of appropriate treatment. As soon as the cause has been identified specific therapy, if available, should be given.

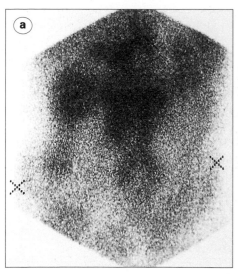
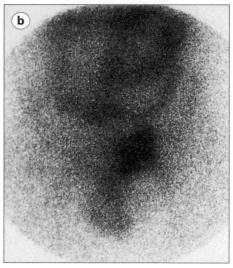
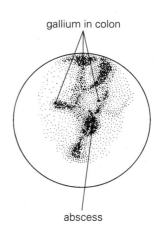

Fig. 32.7 Gallium concentrates in many inflammatory and neoplastic tissues and is a useful non-invasive technique in the investigation of a patient with PUO. (a) Retroperitoneal lymphadenopathy of Hodgkin's disease highlighted by gallium scan. Courtesy of H Tubbs. (b) Intra-abdominal abscess shown by a gallium scan. Courtesy of W E Farrar.

PUO IN SPECIFIC PATIENT GROUPS

As mentioned earlier, an increasing number of people are surviving with severe underlying disease which predisposes them to infection, or are receiving treatment (e.g. cytotoxic drugs) which compromises their defences against infection. These groups of patients are discussed in more detail in Chapter 33, but are included here because newer classifications of PUO define, in addition to the classical PUO described above, three other groups:
• nosocomial PUO
• neutropenic PUO
• HIV-associated PUO.

The main difference between PUO in these groups and classical PUO is the time course of the disease. Classically a PUO may exist for weeks or months before a diagnosis is made, whereas in hospital-acquired (nosocomial) PUO and in neutropenic patients the time course is much shorter, hours to days. The more common causes of PUO in these groups are shown in figure 32.8. The investigation should proceed in the stages listed above, but with particular emphases depending on the patient. In hospital patients these include the type of operative procedures performed, the presence of foreign bodies, especially intravascular devices, and drug therapy. Drug fevers are a common non-infective cause of PUO. In neutropenic patients the underlying disease and stage of chemotherapy should be noted. Fever is a common complaint in patients who have received transplants and may indicate graft-versus-host disease rather than infection. In HIV-positive patients particular attention should be paid to the known risk factors such as intravenous drug abuse, and to travel and contact with infected individuals. Although the major opportunist infections in AIDS patients are well-described (see Chapter 33) atypical presentations of common infections occur and new infections continue to emerge.

INFECTIVE ENDOCARDITIS

Infective endocarditis is an uncommon disease that often presents as a PUO and is fatal if untreated. The infection involves the endothelial lining of the heart, usually including the heart valves. It may occur as an acute, rapidly progressive disease or in a subacute form. In about two-thirds of patients there is a pre-existing heart defect, either congenital or acquired (e.g. as a result of rheumatic fever), or a prosthetic heart valve *in situ*. However, the patient may be unaware of any defect prior to the infection.

Aetiology and pathogenesis

Almost any organism can cause endocarditis, but infection of native valves is caused most commonly by species of oral streptococci (e.g. *Strep. sanguis, Strep. oralis, Strep. mitis*). About one-quarter to one-third of cases are caused by staphylococci, although this fraction is higher in intravenous drugs abusers. These patients also have a higher incidence of Gram-negative and fungal endocarditis arising from organisms that they inject into themselves. Coagulase-negative staphylococci are common causes of early prosthetic-valve endocarditis and are probably acquired at the time of surgery. The species causing late infections (>3 months) after cardiac surgery resemble more closely those seen in native valve endocarditis (Fig. 32.9).

Endocarditis is an endogenous infection acquired when organisms entering the bloodstream establish themselves on the heart valves. Thus, any bacteraemia may potentially result in endocarditis. Most commonly streptococci from the oral flora enter the bloodstream, for example during dental procedures or vigorous teeth cleaning or flossing, and adhere to damaged heart valves. It is thought that fibrin–platelet vegetations are present on damaged valves prior to the organisms implanting, and adherence is probably associated with the ability of the organisms to produce dextran as well as adhesins and fibronectin-binding

INFECTIVE CAUSES OF PUO IN SPECIFIC PATIENT GROUPS		
category of PUO	**infection**	**usual cause**
Nosocomial	vascular–line related	staphylococci
	other device related	staphylococci, *Candida*
	transfusion–related	hepatitis viruses cytomegalovirus (CMV)
	cholecystitis and pancreatitis	Gram-negative rods
	pneumonia (related to assisted ventilation)	Gram-negative rods, including *Pseudomonas*
	post-operative abscesses e.g. intra-abdominal	Gram-negative rods and anaerobes
	post gastric surgery	systemic candidiasis
Neutropenic	vascular-line related	staphylococci
	oral infection	*Candida*, herpes simplex virus
	pneumonia	Gram-negative rods, *Candida*, *Aspergillus*, CMV
	soft tissue, e.g. peri-anal abscess	mixed aerobes and anaerobes
HIV-associated	respiratory tract	CMV, *Pneumocystis*, *Mycobacterium tuberculosis*, *M. avium-intracellulare*
	central nervous system	*Toxoplasma*
	gastrointestinal tract	*Salmonella, Campylobacter, Shigella*
	genital tract or disseminated	*Treponema pallidum, Neisseria gonorrhoeae*

Fig. 32.8 Infective causes of PUO in specific patient groups. Patients who contract their PUO in hospital are most likely to be infected with 'hospital pathogens' either from their own normal flora or from the hospital environment. Neutropenic patients are similar in this regard if they are hospitalized, but some are treated as outpatients and thus may be exposed to a wider range of pathogens. AIDS patients commonly become infected with opportunist pathogens but an increasing range of organisms is associated with infections. It is important to take a detailed history as latent infections may become florid as the patient's immune status deteriorates.

proteins. Having attached themselves to the heart valve, the organisms multiply and attract further deposition of fibrin and platelets. In this position they are protected from the host defences and vegetations can grow to several centimetres in size. This is probably quite a slow process and correspondingly the time period between the initial bacteraemia and the onset of symptoms is around five weeks (Fig. 32.10).

Clinical features
The signs and symptoms are very varied but relate essentially to four ongoing processes:
- the infectious process on the valve and local intracardiac complications;
- septic embolization to virtually any organ;
- bacteraemia, often with metastatic foci of infection;
- circulating immune complexes and other factors.

The patient almost always has a fever and a heart murmur. He/she may also complain of non-specific symptoms such as anorexia, weight loss, malaise, chills, nausea, vomiting and night sweats, symptoms that are common to many of the causes of PUO listed in figure 32.4. Peripheral manifestations may also be evident in the form of splinter haemorrhages and Osler's nodes (Fig. 32.11). Microscopic haematuria resulting from immune complex deposition in the kidney is a characteristic (see Chapter 16).

Diagnosis
Microbiological and cardiological investigations are of critical importance. The blood culture is the single most important laboratory test. Ideally three separate samples of blood should be collected within a 24-hour period and before antimicrobial therapy is administered. Methods for processing blood cultures are described in the Appendix.

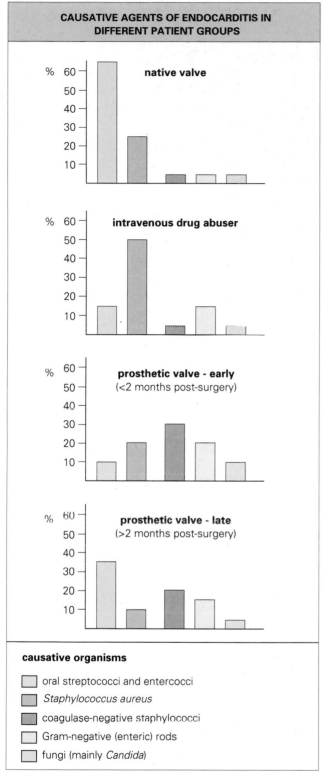

CAUSATIVE AGENTS OF ENDOCARDITIS IN DIFFERENT PATIENT GROUPS

native valve

intravenous drug abuser

prosthetic valve - early
(<2 months post-surgery)

prosthetic valve - late
(>2 months post-surgery)

causative organisms

- oral streptococci and entercocci
- *Staphylococcus aureus*
- coagulase-negative staphylococci
- Gram-negative (enteric) rods
- fungi (mainly *Candida*)

Fig. 32.9 Causative agents of endocarditis in different groups of patients. Although almost any organism can cause endocarditis the vast majority of cases are caused by a relatively small range of species. The relative importance of these species varies depending on whether the patient has his/her own heart valves or a prosthetic valve.

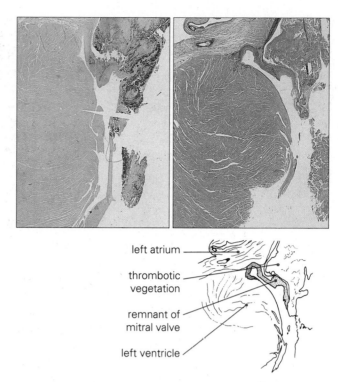

left atrium

thrombotic vegetation

remnant of mitral valve

left ventricle

Fig. 32.10 Bacteria circulating in the bloodstream adhere to and establish themselves on the heart valves. Multiplication of the microbes is associated with destruction of valve tissue and formation of vegetations which interfere with and may severely compromise the normal function of the valve. These histological sections show the virtual destruction of the leaflet at the mitral valve by staphylococci. (Left) Gram stain. (Right) E-VG stain. Courtesy of R H Anderson.

The isolation of the causative organism is essential to enable antibiotic susceptibility tests to be performed and optimal therapy to be prescribed. Nutritionally variant strains of oral streptococci are known to cause infective endocarditis. These may fail to grow in blood culture media unless pyridoxal is added to the broth. Alternatively they grow as satellite colonies around *Staphylococcus aureus* colonies on blood agar.

Treatment

Although the majority of species causing infective endocarditis are highly susceptible to a range of antibiotics, complete eradication takes several weeks to achieve and relapse is not uncommon. This is probably due to the relative inaccessibility (both to antibiotics and to host defences) of the organisms within the vegetations, their high population densities and relatively slow rate of multiplication. Prior to the advent of antibiotics infective endocarditis had a mortality of 100%, but even today mortality remains at 20–30% despite treatment with appropriate antibiotics.

For penicillin-susceptible streptococci, high doses of penicillin is the treatment of choice. Erythromycin should be used for patients with a history of penicillin allergy. However, MIC (minimum inhibitory concentration) and MBC (minimum bactericidal concentration) tests (see Chapter 35) should be performed to detect organisms that are tolerant to penicillin (inhibited but not killed; MBC > 4 x MIC). These and enterococci (which are always more resistant to penicillin) should be treated with a combination of penicillin (or ampicillin) and an aminoglycoside. Combinations such as these can be shown to act synergistically against streptococci and enterococci (see Chapter 35).

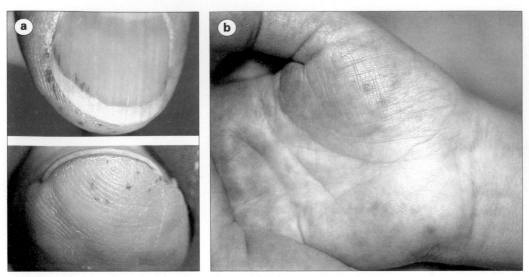

Fig. 32.11 Outward signs of endocarditis may be helpful in suggesting the diagnosis. These result from the host's response to infection in the form of immune-complex mediated vasculitis, focal platelet aggregation and vascular permeability. (a) Splinter haemorrhages in the nail-bed and petechial lesions in the skin. (b) Osler's nodes. These are tender, nodular lesions which tend to affect the palms and fingertips. Courtesy of H Tubbs.

Staphylococcal endocarditis often presents a more difficult therapeutic challenge, particularly in prosthetic valve endocarditis when the organisms may be hospital-acquired and consequently often resistant to many antibiotics. A beta-lactamase stable penicillin such as cloxacillin is often suitable and may be given in combination with an aminoglycoside, rifampicin or fusidic acid. Vancomycin or teicoplanin should be used for penicillin-allergic patients and for treating methicillin-resistant staphylococci. Detailed treatment regimens are published by the American Heart Foundation and the British Society for Antimicrobial Chemotherapy.

Prevention

People with known heart defects should be given prophylactic antibiotics to protect them during dental surgery and any other invasive procedure that is likely to cause a transient bacteraemia.

SUMMARY

The majority of patients presenting with a PUO have a treatable or curable disease presenting in an unusual manner. The clinical investigation needs to be individualized, but this chapter outlines the essential stages in the investigation of every patient and draws attention to the important infective causes of PUO.

Although classically a patient with PUO presents with a long history (weeks or months of fever), compromised patients also present with fevers that are not immediately diagnosed by routine laboratory investigations. For these groups (nosocomial, neutropenic and HIV-associated), new definitions of PUO have been proposed. The list of pathogens causing fever in these patients is growing.

The clinician's aim in the investigation of every patient with PUO should be to discover the cause, i.e. to change a PUO to a pyrexia of known origin, and to initiate appropriate treatment.

Further Reading

Deal WB. Fever of unknown origin: An analysis of 34 patients. *Postgrad Med J* 1971; **50**: 182.

Jacoby GA, Swartz MN. Fever of unexplained origin. *New Engl J Med* 1973; **289**: 1407.

Larson EB, Featherstone HJ, Petersdorf RG. Fever of undetermined origin: Diagnosis and follow up of 105 cases. 1970–1980. *Medicine (Baltimore)* 1982; **61**: 269.

Petersdorf RG, Beeson PB. Fever of unexplained origin. Report on 100 Cases. *Medicine (Baltimore)* 1961; **40**: 1.

Reese RE, Douglas RG,eds. *A practical approach to infectious diseases.* Boston/Toronto: Little, Brown & Co., 1986.

33 INFECTIONS IN THE COMPROMISED HOST

Contents

INTRODUCTION

The human body has a complex system of protective mechanisms to prevent infection, involving both adaptive (cellular and humoral) and innate (skin, mucous membranes, etc.) immune systems. These have been described in detail in earlier chapters (see Chapters 4 and 5). So far we have concentrated on the common and serious infections occurring in people whose protective mechanisms are largely intact. In these circumstances the interactions between host and parasite are such that the parasite has to use all its guile to survive and invade the host, and the healthy host is able to put up a fight against such an invasion. In this chapter we will consider the infections that arise when the host–parasite equation is weighted heavily in favour of the parasite. In other words when the host is compromised.

THE COMPROMISED HOST

A compromised host is an individual who has one or more defects in their body's natural defences against microbial invaders. Consequently they are much more liable to suffer from severe and life-threatening infections. Modern medicine has effective methods for treating at least half of all serious cancers, has perfected organ transplantation, and has developed technology which enables people with otherwise fatal diseases to lead prolonged and productive lives. A consequence of these achievements, however, is an increasing number of compromised people prone to infection. In addition there is a growing population of patients suffering from AIDS.

THE HOST CAN BE COMPROMISED IN MANY DIFFERENT WAYS

Compromise can take a variety of forms, falling into two main groups: 1) defects, accidental or intentional, in the body's innate immune defence mechanisms; and 2) deficiencies in the adaptive immune response. These disorders of the immune system can be further subclassified as 'primary' or 'secondary' (Fig. 33.1). Primary immunodeficiency is inherited or occurs by exposure *in utero* to environmental factors or by other unknown mechanisms. It is rare, and varies in severity depending on the type of

WHAT MAKES A HOST COMPROMISED	
factors affecting innate systems	
Primary	complement deficiencies phagocyte cell deficiencies
Secondary	burns, trauma, major surgery, catheterization, foreign bodies (e.g. shunts, prostheses), obstruction
factors affecting adaptive systems	
Primary	T cell defects, B cell deficiencies, severe combined immunodeficiency
Secondary	malnutrition, infectious diseases, neoplasia, irradiation, chemotherapy, splenectomy

Fig. 33.1 Factors that make a host compromised.

defect. Secondary, or acquired, immunodeficiency is due to an underlying disease state (Fig. 33.2), or occurs as a result of treatment of a disease.

Primary factors involving innate immunity

Congenital defects in phagocytic cells confer susceptibility to infection, and of these perhaps the best known is chronic granulomatous disease (Fig. 33.3), in which an inherited failure to synthesize cytochrome b_{245} leads to failure to produce reactive oxygen intermediates during phagocytosis (see Fig. 8.3). The central role of complement in the innate defence mechanisms is undisputed, and the inability to generate the classical C3 convertase (see Chapter 5) through congenital defects in synthesis of the early components, particularly C4 and C2, is associated with an undue frequency of extracellular infections.

Secondary factors involving innate immunity

A variety of factors can disrupt the mechanical, non-specific barriers to infection. For example, burns, traumatic injury and major surgery destroy the continuity of the skin and may leave poorly vascularized tissue near the body surface, providing a relatively defenceless site for microbes to colonize and invade. In health the mucosal barriers of the respiratory and alimentary tract are vital to prevent infection. Damage sustained, for example, through endoscopy, surgery, or irradiation therapy, provides easy access for infecting organisms. Devices such as intravascular and urinary catheters, or procedures such as lumbar puncture or bone marrow aspiration, allow organisms to bypass the normal defences and enter normally sterile parts of the body. Foreign bodies such as prostheses (e.g. hip joints or heart valves) and CSF shunts alter the local non-specific host responses and provide surfaces that microbes can colonize more readily than they can the natural equivalents.

The adage 'obstruction leads to infection' is a valuable reminder that the defences of many body systems work partly through the clearance of undesirable materials, e.g.

urine flow, ciliary action in the respiratory tract, peristalsis in the gut. Interference with these mechanisms as a result of pathological obstruction, central nervous system dysfunction or surgical intervention tends to result in infection.

Primary adaptive immunodeficiency

The major congenital abnormalities arising in the adaptive immune system are depicted in figure 33.4. A defect in the stromal microenvironment in which lymphocytes differentiate may lead to failure to produce B cells (Bruton-type agammaglobulinaemia) or T cells (DiGeorge syndrome).

Differentiation pathways themselves may be affected. For example, a non-functional recombinase enzyme will prevent the recombination of gene fragments which form the B cell antibody or the T cell receptor variable regions for antigen recognition, with a resulting severe combined immunodeficiency (SCID). The most frequent form of congenital antibody deficiency seen – common variable immunodeficiency – is characterized by recurrent pyogenic infections and is probably heterogenous. Although the number of immature B cells in the marrow tends to be normal, the peripheral B cells are either low in number or in some cases absent. Where present they are unable to differentiate into plasma cells in some cases or to secrete antibody in others. Transient hypogammaglobulinaemia of infancy, characterized by recurrent respiratory infections, is associated with low IgG levels, which often normalize abruptly by 3–4 years of age (Fig. 33.5). Immunoglobulin deficiency occurs naturally in human infants as the maternal IgG level decays and can become a serious problem in very premature babies.

INFECTIONS THAT CAUSE IMMUNOSUPPRESSION	
viral	**bacterial**
Measles	*Mycobacterium tuberculosis*
Mumps	*Mycobacterium leprae*
Congenital rubella	*Brucella* spp.
EBV	
CMV	
HIV1, HIV2	

Fig. 33.2 Infections that cause immunosuppression.

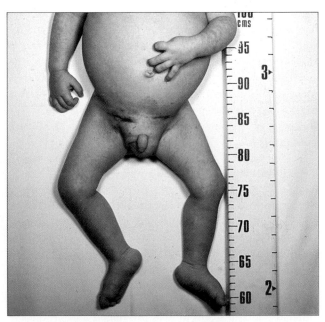

Fig. 33.3 Bilateral draining lymph nodes in an 18-month-old boy with chronic granulomatous disease. Abscesses caused by *Staph. aureus* had developed in both groins, which had to be surgically drained. Courtesy of AR Hayward.

Secondary adaptive immunodeficiency

World-wide, malnutrition is a common and most important cause of acquired immunodeficiency. The major form, protein–energy malnutrition (PEM) presents as a wide range of disorders, with kwashiorkor and marasmus at the two poles. There are drastic effects on the structure of the lymphoid organs (Fig. 33.6), gross reductions in synthesis of complement components, sluggish chemotactic responses of phagocytes, lowered secretory and mucosal IgA and reduced affinity of IgG. In particular there is a serious deficit in circulating T cell numbers (Fig. 33.7), leading to inadequate cell-mediated responses.

Infections themselves are often immunosuppressive (see Fig. 33.2), and none more so than human immunodeficiency virus (HIV1 and HIV2) infection which gives rise to the acquired immune deficiency syndrome (AIDS; see Chapter 24). Neoplasia of the lymphoid system frequently induces a state of reduced immunoreactivity and splenectomy, for whatever reason, results in impaired humoral responses.

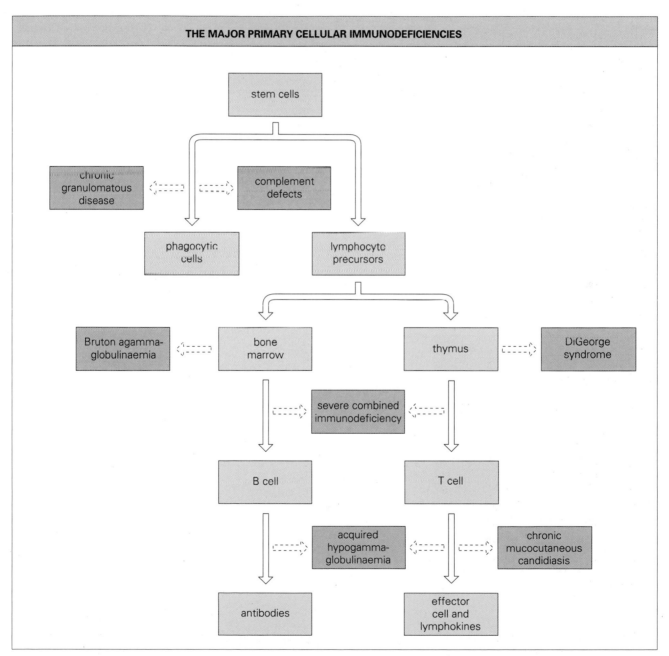

Fig. 33.4 The major primary cellular immunodeficiencies. The deficiency states (shown in purple boxes) derive either from defects in the primary differentiation environment (bone marrow or thymus) or during cell differentiation (shown as dashed arrows derived from the differentiation state indicated).

Treatment of disease can also cause immunosuppression. For example, cytotoxic agents (e.g. cyclophosphamide and azathioprine) cause leukopenia or derangement of T and B cell function. Corticosteroids reduce the number of circulating leucocytes, monocytes and eosinophils and suppress leucocyte accumulation at sites of inflammation. Irradiation therapy adversely affects the proliferation of lymphoid cells. Thus a patient receiving treatment for neoplastic disease will be immunocompromised both as a result of the disease and the treatment.

It is important to recognize immunodeficiencies and to understand which procedures are likely to compromise the natural defences of a patient. Through improvements in medical technology many immune defects (particularly immunosuppression resulting from irradiation or cytotoxic drugs) are transient, and if the patients survive the period of immunosuppression they have a good chance of a complete recovery.

WHICH MICROBES CAUSE INFECTION IN THE COMPROMISED HOST?

Compromised people can become infected with any pathogen able to infect the non-compromised individual, as well as with opportunist pathogens – microbes that are incapable of causing disease in a healthy person but able to infect when the host's defences are lowered, often with fatal consequences. Different types of defect predispose to infection by different pathogens, depending on the critical mechanisms operating in the defence against each particular microorganism (Fig. 33.8). Here we will concentrate mainly on the opportunist infections and refer to other chapters for information about other pathogens.

IgG IN TRANSIENT HYPOGAMMAGLOBULINAEMIA

serum IgG (mg/dl)

— mean — patient ▒ range

Fig. 33.5 Serum immunoglobulin levels in a boy with transient hypogammaglobulinaemia compared with the range of normal controls. The patient developed mild paralytic polio when immunized at 4 months of age with attenuated (Sabin) vaccine.

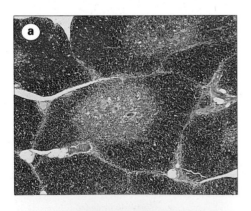
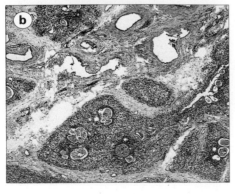
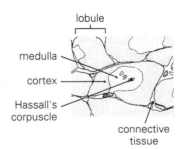
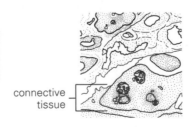

Fig. 33.6 Thymic histology in normal and protein–energy malnourished (PEM) children. (a) Normal thymus showing well demarcated cortex and medullary zones. (b) Acute involution in PEM characterized by lobular atrophy, loss of distinction between cortex and medulla, depletion of lymphocytes and enlarged Hassall's corpuscles. Courtesy of RK Chandra.

INFECTIONS IN PATIENTS WITH DEFICIENCY IN INNATE IMMUNITY DUE TO PHYSICAL FACTORS

Infections associated with burn wounds

Burn wounds are sterile immediately after the burn is inflicted but inevitably become colonized within hours with a mixed bacterial flora. Burn injuries cause direct damage to the mechanical barriers of the body and also cause abnormalities in neutrophil function and in immune responses. In addition there is major physiological derangement and loss of fluids and electrolytes. The burn provides a highly nutritious surface for organisms to colonize, and the incidence of serious infection varies with the size and depth of the burn and the age of the patient. Modern topical antimicrobial therapy should prevent infection of burns of less than 30% of the total body area but larger burns are always colonized. Non-invasive infection is confined to the eschar (the non-viable skin debris on the surface of deep burns). It is characterized by rapid separation of the eschar from the underlying tissue and a heavy exudate of purulent material from the burn wound. The systemic symptoms are usually relatively mild. However organisms can invade from heavily colonized burn eschars into viable tissue beneath and rapidly destroy the tissue, converting partial thickness burns into full-skin-thickness destruction. From here it is a small step to invasion of the lymphatics and thence to the bloodstream (or direct invasion of blood vessels), and to septicaemia. Septicaemia in burned patients is often polymicrobial.

The major pathogens in burn wounds are aerobic (and facultatively anaerobic) bacteria and fungi, the most important being *Pseudomonas aeruginosa* and other Gram-negative rods, *Staphylococcus aureus*, *Streptococcus pyogenes*, other streptococci and enterococci. *Candida* spp. and *Aspergillus* together account for about 5% of infections. Anaerobes are rare in burn wound infections. Viral infections, mostly herpes virus and CMV, have been reported but their clinical significance is uncertain.

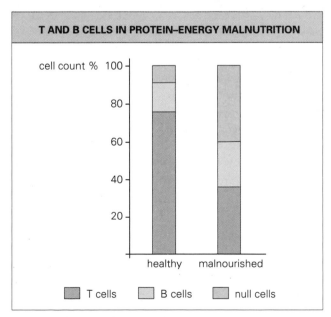

T AND B CELLS IN PROTEIN–ENERGY MALNUTRITION

Fig. 33.7 The proportion of T cells is decreased in malnourished patients compared with healthy controls. B cell counts are usually unaltered and null cells (non-T, non-B) are increased.

INFECTIONS ASSOCIATED WITH DEFECTS IN IMMUNE RESPONSES	
defect	**pathogen**
Induced by physical means (e.g. burns, trauma)	*Pseudomonas aeruginosa* *Staphylococcus aureus* *Staphylococcus epidermidis* *Streptococcus pyogenes* *Aspergillus* spp. *Candida* spp.
Granulocytes/monocytes defects in numbers, movement, phagocytosis, killing	*Staphyococcus aureus* *Streptococcus pyogenes* *Haemophilus influenzae* Gram-negative bacilli *Escherichia coli* *Klebsiella* spp. *Pseudomonas aeruginosa* *Nocardia* spp. *Aspergillus* spp. *Candida* spp.
Complement system individual components	*Staphylococcus aureus* *Streptococcus pneumoniae* *Pseudomonas* spp. *Proteus* spp. *Neisseria meningitidis* *Neisseria gonorrhoeae*
T cells	cytomegalovirus herpes simplex virus herpes zoster virus *Listeria monocytogenes* *Mycobacterium* spp. *Nocardia* spp. *Aspergillus* spp. *Candida* spp. *Cryptococcus neoformans* *Histoplasma capsulatum* *Pneumocystis carinii* *Strongyloides stercoralis*
B cells	enteroviruses *Staphylococcus aureus* *Streptococcus* spp. *Haemophilus influenzae* *Neisseria meningitidis* *Escherichia coli* *Giardia lamblia* *Pneumocystis carinii*
Combined immunodeficiency	as for T and B cells

Fig. 33.8 Infections associated with defects in immune responses.

Pseudomonas aeruginosa is an opportunist Gram-negative rod which has a long and infamous association with burn infections. It grows well in the moist environment of the burn wound, producing a foul, green-pigmented discharge and necrosis. Invasion is not uncommon and the characteristic skin lesions (ecthyma gangrenosum), which are pathognomic of *P. aeruginosa* septicaemia, may appear on non-burned areas (Fig. 33.9). Host factors predisposing to infection include both abnormalities in the antibacterial activities of neutrophils and deficiencies in serum opsonins. Added to these are the virulence factors of the organism which include the production of elastase, protease and exotoxin, a combination which makes *P. aeruginosa* the most devastating Gram-negative pathogen of burned patients. Treatment is difficult because of the organism's innate resistance to many antibacterial agents. A combination of aminoglycoside (usually gentamicin or tobramycin) with one of the newer beta-lactams (such as azlocillin or ceftazidime) is usually favoured, but several units have reported strains resistance to these agents. It is virtually impossible to prevent colonization. Prevention of infection depends largely on inhibiting the multiplication of organisms that are colonizing the burn by application of topical agents such as silver nitrate. Both active and passive immunization have been tried; the latter appears to hold more promise at present.

Staphylococcus aureus is now the foremost pathogen of burn wounds. The most important predisposing factor to this infection in the burn patient appears to be an abnormality of the antibacterial function of neutrophils. Infections follow a more insidious course than do streptococcal infections (see below) and it may be several days before the full-blown infection is apparent. The organism is capable of destroying granulation tissue, invading and causing septicaemia. *Staph. aureus* infections of skin have been discussed in detail in Chapter 28. Treatment with anti-staphylococcal agents such as cloxacillin or nafcillin should be administered if there is evidence of invasive infection. Every effort should be made to prevent the spread of staphylococci from patient to patient. Although transmissible by both airborne and contact routes, the latter is far by the more important.

Streptococcus pyogenes infections of skin and soft tissue have also be discussed in some detail in Chapter 28. This organism was the most common cause of burn wound infections in the pre-antibiotic era and is still to be feared in burns wards. *Strep. pyogenes* infection is usually seen within the first few days of injury. It is characterized by rapid deterioration in the state of the burn wound and invasion of neighbouring healthy tissue. The patient may become severely toxic and will die within hours unless treated appropriately. *Strep. pyogenes* rarely infects healthy granulation tissue, but freshly grafted wounds may become infected, resulting in destruction of the graft.

The high transmissibility of *Strep. pyogenes* makes it the scourge of burns wards and every effort should be made to prevent spread. Penicillin is the drug of choice for treatment, and erythromycin or vancomycin can be used for penicillin-allergic patients. Beta-haemolytic streptococci of other Lancefield groups (notably C and G; see Appendix)

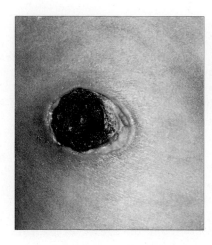

Fig. 33.9 Ecthyma gangrenosum in a child with *Pseudomonas* septicaemia associated with immunodeficiency. Courtesy of H Tubbs.

and enterococci are also important pathogens of burn wounds.

Infections associated with traumatic injury and surgery

Both accidental and intentional trauma destroy the integrity of the body surface and leave it liable to infection. Accidental injury may result in microbes being introduced deep into the wound. The species involved will depend on the nature of the wound, as discussed in Chapter 28.

Staphylococcus aureus is the most important cause of surgical wound infection (see Chapter 39). The organism may be acquired during surgery or post-operatively and may originate from the patient himself or from another patient or staff member. The wound is less well defended than normal tissue; it may have a damaged blood supply and foreign bodies (sutures) may be present. Classic studies of wound infections have shown that far fewer staphylococci are needed to initiate infection around a suture than in normal healthy skin. Wound infections can be severe and lead to invasion of organisms into the bloodstream with consequent seeding of other sites such as the heart valves (causing endocarditis; see Chapter 32) or bones (causing osteomyelitis; see Chapter 28), thereby further compromising the patient.

Patients with plastic *in situ*

The technical developments in plastics and other synthetic materials have enabled many advances in medicine and surgery, but in so doing have produced new groups of compromised patients.

Urinary catheters

Urinary catheters disrupt the normal host defences of the urinary tract and allow organisms easy access to the bladder. Catheter-associated infection of the urinary tract is very common, especially if catheters are left in place for more than 48 hours (see Chapter 23). The organisms involved are usually Gram-negative rods from the patient's own faecal or peri-urethral flora, but cross-infection also occurs (see Chapter 39).

Intravenous and peritoneal dialysis catheters

These catheters breach the integrity of the skin barrier and allow organisms from the skin flora of the patient or hands of the carer easy access to deeper sites. Staphylococci are the most common cause of infection but coryneforms, Gram-negative rods and *Candida* are also implicated. Coagulase-negative staphylococci, particularly *Staph. epidermidis,* account for more than half of the infections (Fig. 33.10). These opportunists are members of the normal skin flora and for many years were considered to be harmless. However, they have a particular propensity for colonizing plastic and thus can seed sites adjacent to plastic devices and thence cause invasive infections. Their virulence factors are not well understood, but the ability to produce an adhesive slime material and grow as biofilms on plastic surfaces is likely to be important. Infections are characteristically more insidious in onset than those caused by the more virulent *Staph. aureus,* and recognition is hampered by the difficulty in distinguishing the infecting strain from the normal flora. Treatment is also difficult because many *Staph. epidermidis* carry multiple antibiotic resistances and agents such as vancomycin and rifampicin may be required (see Chapter 35). Whenever possible the plastic device should be removed.

Prosthetic valves and joints

Patients with prosthetic heart valves or prosthetic joints are compromised both by the surgery to implant the prosthesis and by the continued presence of a foreign body. *Staph. epidermidis* is again the most common pathogen, either gaining access during surgery or from a subsequent bacteraemia originating from, for example, an intravascular-line infection. Endocarditis associated with prosthetic heart valves is discussed in Chapter 32. The most common complication of joint replacement is loosening of the prosthesis, but infection ranks second and is much more likely to lead to permanent failure of the procedure. The difficulties of treatment have been outlined above, but there is great reluctance to remove a prosthetic device, even though it is sometimes the only way to eradicate an infection.

Staphylococcus epidermidis is also an important cause of infection of cardiac pacemakers, vascular grafts and cerebrospinal fluid shunts.

Infection associated with compromises of the body's normal clearance mechanisms

Stasis predisposes to infection, and in health the body functions to prevent stasis from occurring. In the respiratory tract, damage to the ciliary escalator predisposes the lungs to invasion. This is a particular problem in patients with cystic fibrosis who are infected with *Staph. aureus* and *Haemophilus influenzae,* and later with *Pseudomonas aeruginosa* (see Chapter 22).

Obstruction and interruption of normal urine flow allows Gram-negative organisms from the peri-urethral flora to ascend the urethra and to establish themselves in the bladder. Septicaemia arising from a urinary tract infection superimposed on obstruction is an important complication.

INFECTIONS INVOLVING *STAPHYLOCOCCUS EPIDERMIDIS*	
infection of:	% of infections caused by *Staph. epidermidis*
prosthetic heart valve early (<2 months post-surgery) late (>2 months post-surgery)	30 – 70 20 – 30
Prosthetic hip	10 – 40
CSF shunt	30 – 65
Vascular grafts	5 – 20
Peritoneal dialysis related	30
Intravascular catheters	10 – 50

Fig. 33.10 Percentage of infections caused by *Staphylococcus epidermidis* in patients with plastic *in situ.* Data from Gemmell and McCartney, 1990.

INFECTIONS IN SECONDARY ADAPTIVE IMMUNODEFICIENCY

The underlying immunodeficiency state determines the nature and severity of infection, and in some cases infection is the presenting clinical feature in a patient with immunological deficit. However septicaemia and related infectious complications of immunodeficiency are encountered with greatest frequency in patients hospitalized for chemotherapy for malignant diseases or organ transplantation. In these groups, infection continues to be a major cause of morbidity and mortality (Fig. 33.11). Increasingly these infections are iatrogenic and caused by opportunist pathogens acquired in hospital.

Infections in patients with haematological malignancies and in bone marrow transplant recipients

Susceptibility to infection in patients with leukaemia is primarily due to the lack of circulating neutrophils that inevitably follows bone marrow failure. Septicaemia may be the presenting feature but is much more common when the patient has been exposed to chemotherapy to induce a remission of the disease (remission–induction chemotherapy). Neutropenia (defined as a count of $<0.5 \times 10^9$ neutrophils per litre) may persist for periods ranging from a few days to several weeks. Similarly, prolonged periods of neutropenia occur after bone marrow transplantation.

The length of time for which the patient is neutropenic influences the nature of the infections and the frequency with which they occur. For example, fungal infections are much more common in patients who are neutropenic for more than 21 days. Although Gram-negative rods such as *Escherichia coli* and *Pseudomonas aeruginosa* from the bowel flora have in the past been the most common cause of septicaemia in neutropenic patients, Gram-positive organisms – staphylococci, streptococci and enterococci – are gaining

OPPORTUNISTIC PATHOGENS IN NEUTROPENIC PATIENTS AND ORGAN TRANSPLANT RECIPIENTS
bacteria

Gram-positive
  Staphylococcus aureus
  coagulase-negative staphylococci
  streptococci
  Listeria spp.
  Nocardia asteroides
  Mycobacterium tuberculosis
  Mycobacterium avium-intracellulare

Gram-negative
  Enterobacteriaceae
  Pseudomonas aeruginosa
  Legionella spp.
  Bacteroides spp.

fungi
Candida spp. *Aspergillus* spp. *Cryptococcus neoformans* *Histoplasma capsulatum* *Pneumocystis carinii*
parasites
Toxoplasma gondii *Strongyloides stercoralis*
viruses
herpes viruses, e.g. HSV, CMV, V-ZV, EBV hepatitis B hepatitis C polyomaviruses, e.g. BKV, JCV HIV*
* HIV has been transmitted via organ   transplantation and unscreened blood

Fig. 33.11 Opportunistic pathogens in neutropenic patients and organ transplant recipients.

in importance. *Staphylococcus epidermidis* septicaemia associated with intravascular catheters (see above) is common. Infections caused by fungi are also on the increase, partly because, with the aid of modern antibacterial agents and granulocyte transfusions, more patients are surviving the early neutropenic period. Severe cytomegalovirus infections are an important feature of bone marrow transplantation, due to graft-versus-host reactions as well as immunosuppressive therapy.

Infections in recipients of solid organ transplants

Suppression of a patient's cell-mediated immunity is necessary to prevent rejection of the grafted organ and the cytotoxic regimens used usually suppress humoral immunity to some extent as well. In addition high doses of cortico-

steroids are required and the combination of these conditions results in a seriously compromised host. The factors which affect infection in recipients of solid organ transplants (e.g. kidney, heart, lung, liver) include:

* the underlying medical condition of the patient;
* their prior immune status;
* the type of organ transplant;
* the immunosuppressive regimen;
* the exposure of the patient to pathogens.

The organisms that cause the most common and most severe infections are shown in figure 33.11. Most infections occur within 3 or 4 months of transplantation (Fig. 33.12); after this period the risk of infection is reduced but remains present as long as the patient is immunosuppressed.

Infections in AIDS patients

The clinical definition of AIDS includes the presence of one or more opportunistic infections. AIDS patients are often infected concomitantly with multiple pathogens which they fail to eradicate despite prolonged, appropriate and aggressive antimicrobial chemotherapy (Fig. 33.13). Most of the pathogens involved are intracellular microbes that require an intact cell-mediated immune response for effective defence. As the patient progresses from HIV-seropositivity to full-blown AIDS the immunodeficiency deepens, and organisms that are usually controlled by cell-mediated immunity are able to reactivate to cause disseminated infections that are not seen in the immunologically normal individual.

Many of the pathogens that cause infections in the immunocompromised host (see Figs 33.11 and 33.13) have been described elsewhere in this book. Other opportunist pathogens are described in more detail below.

OTHER IMPORTANT OPPORTUNIST PATHOGENS

Fungi

Candida

This yeast is an opportunist pathogen in a variety of patients and in various body sites. It is the cause of vaginal and oral thrush (see Chapter 24), skin infections (see Chapter 28), and endocarditis, particularly in drug addicts (see Chapter 32), and is the most common fungal pathogen in compromised patients. It manifests itself in different ways depending on the nature of the underlying compromise.

Chronic mucocutaneous candidiasis. This rare disease is a persistent but non-invasive infection of mucous membranes and hair, skin and nails in patients (often children) who have a specific T cell defect rendering them anergic to *Candida* (Fig. 33.14). The condition may be controlled by intermittent courses of ketoconazole.

Oropharyngeal and oesophageal candidiasis. This condition is seen in a variety of compromised patients, including those with ill-fitting dentures, diabetics, those on antibiotics and

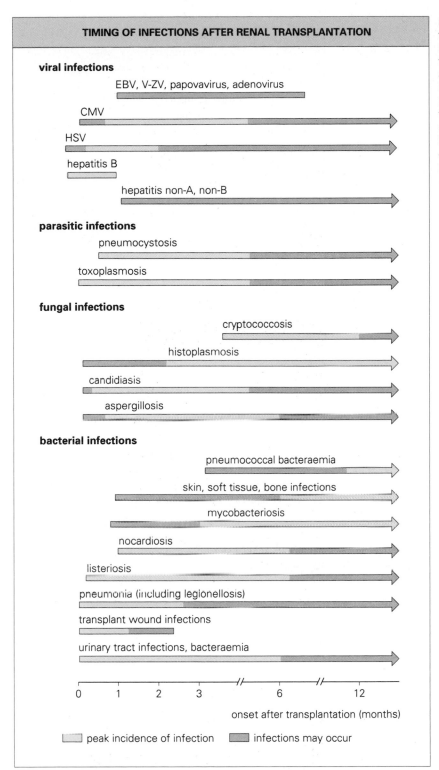

Fig. 33.12 This timetable shows the time of onset and peak incidence of infections in patients after renal transplantation. Note that the patient is at risk of some infections, particularly hepatitis B and wound infections, for a limited period only immediately post-transplant. Other infections may develop after several weeks of immunosuppression, but the majority constitute a risk throughout the period of immunosuppression. Adapted from Reese and Douglas, 1986.

steroids, and now characteristically in HIV-positive patients (Fig. 33.15.). Treatment with antifungal mouthwashes (nystatin or an azole compound) is recommended, particularly in the immunocompromised in whom the gastrointestinal tract probably serves as one of the routes to disseminated disease (see below).

Gastrointestinal candidiasis. This condition is seen in patients who have undergone major gastric or abdominal surgery, and in those with neoplastic disease. The organism can pass through the intestinal wall and spread from a gastrointestinal focus. Ante-mortem diagnosis is difficult and as many as a quarter of the patients do not have any symptoms in the early stages of disease. If dissemination from the gut occurs, blood cultures may become positive and candida antigens may be detectable in the serum. A high index of suspicion is required to initiate antifungal therapy early in these patients, but disseminated disease is often fatal.

PRINCIPAL OPPORTUNIST PATHOGENS IN AIDS PATIENTS
bacteria
Listeria monocytogenes *Nocardia asteroides* *Mycobacterium tuberculosis* *Mycobacterium avium-intracellulare* *Salmonella* spp. *Legionella pneumophila*
fungi
Candida spp. *Cryptococcus neoformans* *Histoplasma capsulatum* *Coccidioides immitis* *Pneumocystis carinii*
parasites
Toxoplasma gondii *Strongyloides stercoralis*
viruses
Herpes simplex Cytomegalovirus Varicella-zoster Measles JC virus Adenovirus

Fig. 33.13 Principal opportunistic pathogens in AIDS patients.

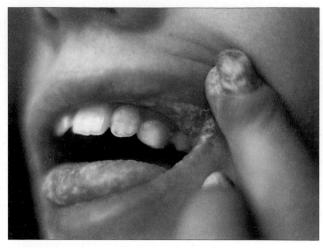

Fig. 33.14 Chronic mucocutaneous candidiasis in a child with impaired T cell response to antigens. Courtesy of MJ Wood.

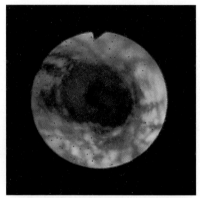

Fig. 33.15 *Candida* oesophagitis. Endoscopic view showing extensive areas of whitish exudate. Courtesy of I Chesner.

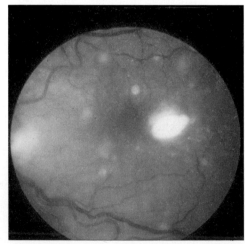

Fig. 33.16 *Candida* endophthalmitis. Fundus photograph showing areas of white exudate. Courtesy of AM Geddes.

Disseminated candidiasis. This condition is probably acquired via the gastrointestinal tract but also arises from intravascular catheter-related infections. Patients with lymphoma and leukaemia are most at risk. Blood-borne spread to almost any organ can occur. Infections of the eye (endophthalmitis; Fig. 33.16) and the skin (nodular skin lesions; see Chapter 28) are important because they provide diagnostic clues and without these the non-specific symptoms of fever and septic shock make early diagnosis difficult. Immunocompromised patients are often given antifungal therapy 'blindly' if they have a fever and fail to respond to broad-spectrum antibacterial agents (Fig. 33.17).

Cryptococcus neoformans

This is an opportunist yeast with a world-wide distribution. It can cause infection in the immunocompetent host but is seen more frequently in people with impaired cell-mediated immunity. The onset of disease may be slow and usually results in lung infection or meningoencephalitis; occasionally other sites such as skin, bone and joints are involved (see Chapter 28).

The organism can be demonstrated in the CSF and is characterized by its large polysaccharide capsule (see Fig. 27.12). Rapid identification can be made by antigen detection in a latex agglutination test using specific antibody-coated latex particles. Treatment requires a combination of amphotericin and flucytosine (see Chapter 35) and can be monitored by detecting a fall in CSF antigen levels. The prognosis depends largely on the patient's underlying disease and in the severely immunocompromised, mortality is around 50%.

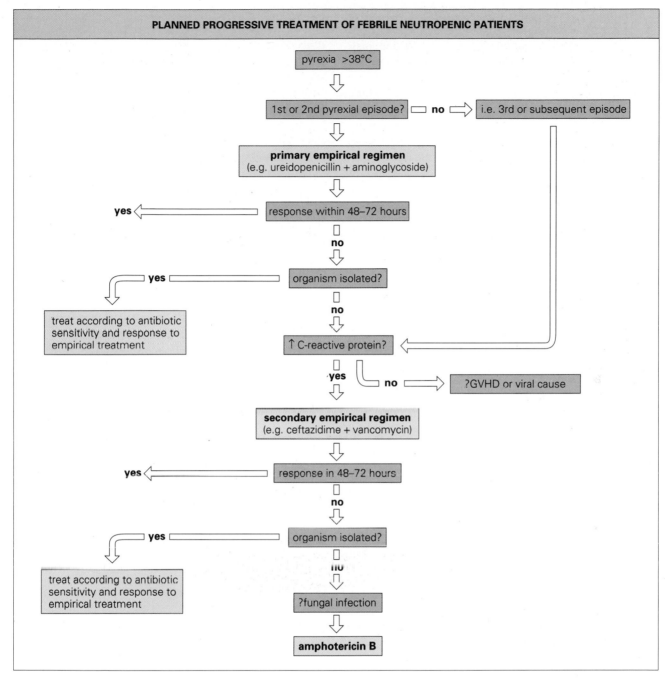

PLANNED PROGRESSIVE TREATMENT OF FEBRILE NEUTROPENIC PATIENTS

Fig. 33.17 Neutropenic patients succumb very rapidly to infections, and decisions to treat have to be made on an empiric basis. This figure shows one example of such a decision-making tree. GVHD, graft versus host disease. Adapted from Rogers, 1989.

Histoplasma capsulatum

This is a highly infectious fungus that causes an acute but benign pulmonary infection in healthy people, but which may produce a chronic progressive, disseminated disease in the compromised host. The organism is endemic only in tropical parts of the world and notably in the so-called 'histo belt' of the central United States particularly in the Ohio and Mississippi river valleys. The natural habitat of the organism is the soil. It is transmitted by the airborne route and the fungal spores are deposited in the alveoli, from whence the fungus spreads via the lymphatics to the regional lymph nodes. In immunocompromised patients disseminated disease may occur many years after the initial exposure. Thus it may present in patients who have long since left endemic areas. The infection is also seen in HIV-positive patients who have visited endemic areas.

Cultures of blood, bone marrow, sputum and CSF may yield *Histoplasma*, but biopsy and histological examination of bone marrow, liver or lymph nodes is often required to make the diagnosis (Fig. 33.18). Progressive disease in the immunocompromised should be treated with amphotericin and may be successful in about 50% of cases.

Aspergillus

The role of *Aspergillus* spp. in disease of the lung has been outlined in Chapter 22, but this fungus is reported increasingly as a cause of invasive disease in compromised patients, usually in profoundly neutropenic patients or those receiving high-dose steroids (Fig. 33.19) Like *Histoplasma*, aspergilli are found in soil, but have a worldwide distribution. Infection is spread by the airborne route and the lung is the site of invasion in almost every case. Dissemination to other sites, particularly the central nervous system (Fig. 33.20) and heart, occurs in about 25% of compromised individuals with lung infection. Because of the ubiquitous nature of the fungus, diagnosis depends on the demonstration of tissue invasion and this usually entails a lung biopsy.

Invasive aspergillosis is usually a fatal disease in the compromised patient but early diagnosis and institution of treatment (amphotericin is the drug of choice; see Chapter 35), together with a reduction in steroid and cytotoxic therapy wherever possible, appears to improve the prognosis. Outbreaks of hospital-acquired infection have been reported (see Chapter 39), related especially to recent building works.

Pneumocystis carinii

This is an organism of uncertain taxonomic status but currently considered to be a fungus. It appears to be widespread; a large proportion of the population have antibodies to the organism, but it only causes symptomatic disease in people whose cellular immune mechanisms are deficient. Thus there is a high incidence of *Pneumocystis carinii* pneumonia in patients receiving immunosuppressive therapy to prevent transplant rejection and in HIV-positive patients. It is very rare to find *Pneumocystis* infection in any other site in the body but the reason for this is unknown.

Diagnosis is not easy and requires a high index of suspicion. The symptoms are non-specific and can mimic a variety of other infectious and non-infectious respiratory disease. Added to this is the difficulty in finding the organism in expectorated sputum, and invasive techniques such as bronchoalveolar lavage or open lung biopsy are required. In samples obtained by these techniques the organism can be demonstrated by silver or immunofluorescent stains (Fig. 33.21). DNA amplification techniques (by the polymerase chain reaction) have been shown to improve the sensitivity of the diagnostic tests (and have raised doubts that disease results from reactivation of a childhood infection).

Treatment is with high dose cotrimoxazole or pentamidine (see Chapter 35), and cotrimoxazole has been used prophylactically with some success.

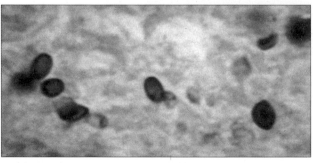

Fig. 33.18 Histologial section of the lung showing yeast forms of *Histoplasma capsulatum*. Methamine silver stain. Courtesy of TF Sellers, Jr.

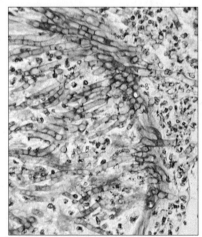

Fig. 33.20 Numerous septate hyphae invading a blood vessel wall in cerebral aspergillosis. Periodic acid-Schiff stain. Courtesy of WE Farrar.

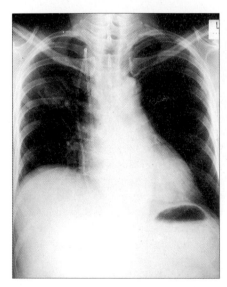

Fig. 33.19 Chest x-ray showing invasive aspergillosis in the right lung of a patient with acute myeloblastic leukaemia. Courtesy of C Kibbler.

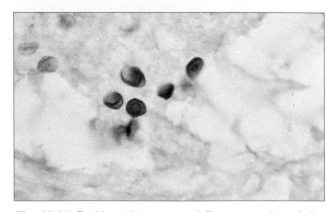

Fig. 33.21 Darkly staining cysts of *Pneumocystis carinii* in an open lung biopsy from an AIDS patient with pneumonia. Grocott silver stain. Courtesy of M Turner-Warwick.

Bacteria

Nocardia asteroides

The family Actinomycetes, relatives of the mycobacteria (but resembling fungi in that they form branching filaments), contain two pathogenic genera, *Actinomyces* and *Nocardia*. Actinomycosis has been discussed in Chapter 25. *Nocardia asteroides* is an uncommon opportunist pathogen with a world-wide distribution. Infections have been reported in the immunocompromised, especially in renal transplant patients. The lung is usually the primary site but infection can spread to the skin, kidney or central nervous system (Fig. 33.22). As with *Aspergillus*, hospital outbreaks of nocardiosis have been described.

Nocardia can be isolated on routine laboratory media but is often slow to grow and consequently easily overgrown by commensal flora. Thus the laboratory staff should be informed if nocardiosis is suspected clinically so that appropriate media are inoculated. The organism is a Gram-negative branching rod and weakly acid-fast (Fig. 33.23).

Sulphonamides or cotrimoxazole are the drugs of choice but treatment can be difficult and various other regimens involving tetracycline, aminoglycosides or imipenem have been described.

Mycobacteria

Although mycobacterial infections are well-documented in immunosuppressed patients, it is the association between AIDS and mycobacteria which is now the most prominent. This includes disseminated infection with *Mycobacterium tuberculosis* and *Mycobacterium avium-intracellulare,* and both of these can be isolated from blood cultures from AIDS patients. *Mycobacterium tuberculosis* has been described in detail in Chapter 22; *M. avium-intracellulare* belongs to the so-called 'atypical' mycobacteria or mycobacteria other than tuberculosis (MOTT). It resembles *M. tuberculosis* in that it is slow-growing, but it is resistant to the conventional antituberculous drugs. Multidrug therapy with combinations such as clofazamine or rifamycin derivatives together with isoniazid, ethambutol, cycloserine or pyrazinamide have been recommended.

Protozoa and helminths

Cryptosporidium (Fig. 33.24) is a protozoan parasite recognized only recently to be a cause of human disease, although it is well known to the veterinarians as an animal pathogen. It causes significant but self-limited diarrhoea in the normal person (see Chapter 25), but severe and chronic diarrhoea in AIDS patients. Effective treatment is difficult but the experimental drug spiramycin is currently the first choice (see Chapter 35). *Isospora belli* (Fig. 33.25)

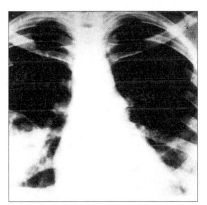

Fig. 33.22
Pulmonary nocardiasis. Chest x-ray showing a large rounded lesion in the right lower zone with multiple cavities. Courtesy of TF Sellers, Jr.

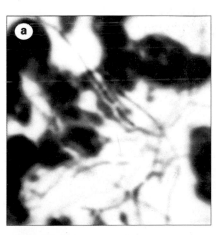

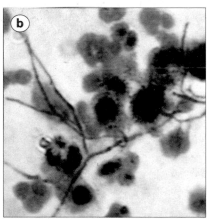

Fig. 33.23 *Nocardia asteroides* in sputum. (a) Acid-fast stain. Courtesy of TF Sellers, Jr. (b) Gram's stain. Courtesy of HP Holley.

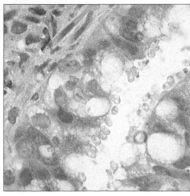

Fig. 33.24 Numerous organisms in the brush border of the intestine in cryptosporidiosis. Courtesy of J Newman.

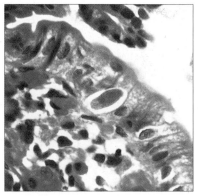

Fig. 33.25 Human coccidiosis, with a single *Isospora belli* organism within an epithelial cell and a chronic inflammatory reaction in the lamina propria. Courtesy of GN Griffin.

is a parasite very similar to *Cryptosporidium* and also produces severe diarrhoea in AIDS patients. Unlike *Cryptosporidium*, however, it is susceptible to cotrimoxazole.

Strongyloides sterocoralis is a parasitic roundworm which, following initial infection, remains dormant for years but may be reactivated to produce massive autoinfection in the immunosuppressed patient. Although rare in UK and most of the USA, it should be borne in mind in patients who have lived in endemic areas such as the tropics and southern USA, even if they were resident in the endemic areas many years before their immunosuppression.

Viruses

The virus infections which are more common or more severe in the compromised patient (see Figs 33.8, 33.11 and 33.13) have been described in detail elsewhere in this book. Many of these represent reactivation of latent infections, for example, polyomavirus infection (BK and JC virus) acquired via the respiratory tract and latent in the kidney (see Chapter 23), and JC virus, which can reactivate and disseminate to cause progressive multifocal leukoencephalopathy in AIDS patients. However, it is less common than other causes of lesions in the central nervous system, e.g. toxoplasmosis or herpes encephalitis.

SUMMARY

This chapter has attempted to draw together the many different ways in which humans can be compromised in their defence against infection and the enormous variety of microbes that take advantage of the compromised host. Despite therapeutic advances with potent antimicrobial agents, in the absence of assistance from the patient's own defence mechanisms, many otherwise trivial infections become life-threatening.

Early recognition of infections is important because they progress rapidly to a fatal outcome unless antimicrobial therapy is instituted promptly. However this requires an astute physician and an informed laboratory, as infections are often caused by unusual pathogens and by organisms which may be dismissed as 'harmless' commensals. Reactivation and dissemination of latent infections is also common.

The clinical presentation of infections is often unusual – absence of the usual signs and symptoms because of the inability of the patient to mount an appropriate immune response, unusual sites of infection, rapid progression to a fatal outcome – all are characteristics of infections in the immunocompromised host.

Further Reading

Brostoff J, Scadding GK, Male D, Roitt IM. *Clinical immunology*. London: Gower Medical Publishing, 1991.

Gemmell CG, McCartney AC. Coagulase-negative staphylococci within the hospital environment. *Rev Med Microbiol* 1990; **1:** 213–218.

Orr KE, Gould FK. Infection problems in patients receiving solid organ transplants. *Rev Med Microbiol* 1992; **3:** 96–103.

Reese RE, Douglas RG, eds. *A practical approach to infectious diseases*. Baltimore/Toronto: Little, Brown & Co., 1986.

Rogers TR. Management of septicaemia in the immunocompromised with particular reference to neutropenic patients. In: *Septicaemia and endocarditis*. Shanson DC, ed. Oxford: Oxford Medical Publications, 1989.

section 4

CONTROL

34 STRATEGIES FOR CONTROL: AN INTRODUCTION

Contents

INTRODUCTION

One of the great achievements of applied medical research has been its success in controlling so many infectious diseases, in one case even to the point of eradication. This has been accomplished in three main ways: by the use of drugs (chemotherapy), by vaccines (immunization), and by improving the environment (better sanitation, nutrition, etc.) (Fig. 34.1) These strategies for control will be described individually in the following chapters; here, we will briefly compare and contrast these methods, and evaluate their importance in the control of disease.

CHEMOTHERAPY VERSUS VACCINATION

Although they appear so different (Fig. 34.2), both chemotherapy and vaccination grew together out of the intensive study that followed the demonstration in the late 1800s that diseases could be caused by microbes. Pasteur (see panel) showed that killed or weakened microbes (e.g. anthrax, rabies) could be used to induce immunity that is specific to one disease, while Ehrlich's work with histological dyes led him to the idea that specific chemicals ('drugs') might bind to particular microbial structures and damage them (see Chapter 35). The concept of selectivity, or specificity, is therefore central to both approaches.

STRATEGIES FOR CONTROL OF INFECTIOUS DISEASES	
General features	water purification (waterborne diseases) sewage disposal (enteric infections) improved nutrition (host defence) improved housing (less crowding, dirt, etc.)
Food	cold storage pasteurization (milk, etc.) food inspection (meat, etc.) adequate cooking
Zoonoses and arthropod-transmitted infections	control of vectors (mosquitoes, ticks, lice etc.) control of reservoir animal (rabies, bovine TB)
Specific disease treatment or prevention	chemotherapy vaccines
Miscellaneous measures	changes in personal habits (reduced promiscuity, use of condoms, improved personal hygiene etc.) control of intravenous drug abuse screening of transfused blood and organs

Fig. 34.1 Strategies for the control of infectious diseases.

CHEMOTHERAPY AND VACCINES COMPARED		
	chemotherapy	**vaccination**
Specificity	usually high	very high
Toxicity	potentially high	usually low
Duration of effect	usually short	usually long
Duration of treatment	may be prolonged	usually short, but may need boosting
Effectiveness	bacteria: high viruses fungi ⎤ moderate parasites ⎦	viruses: high bacteria ⎤ low/ fungi ⎥ mode- parasites ⎦ rate

Fig. 34.2 Comparison of chemotherapy and vaccination.

SPECIFICITY

In the case of antimicrobial drugs, specificity resides in their ability to damage the microbe and not the host, so that the drug should ideally bind to a molecule present only in the microbe. The extent to which this can be achieved varies from microbe to microbe. Bacteria, with their procaryotic cell structure, are much more remote from humans than are fungi, protozoa, or worms (which are all eucaryotic). It is not surprising, therefore, that the most effective antibiotics are, generally speaking, those used against bacteria. There are four major sites in the bacterial cell that are sufficiently different from human cells that they can be targetted by antibacterial agents. These are the cell wall, the bacterial ribosome, the nucleic acid synthetic pathway and the cell membrane (Fig. 34.4).

What is more surprising, however, is that many antibacterial agents are products of microbes themselves, or derivatives of these products. It is presumed that they form part of the self-preservation mechanism by which the microbes prevent overcrowding with their own or other species.

Louis Pasteur (1822–1895)

The science of microbiology was established in the 19th century by the work of many distinguished scientists. However one such scientist, Louis Pasteur may legitimately be regarded as a founding father of this discipline (Fig. 34.3). He, along with Robert Koch, a German doctor (see Chapter 10), was able to show that living organisms or 'microbes' were the cause of disease, and provided a firm scientific basis for their study and control.

Pasteur began work at a time when spontaneous generation was still an accepted explanation for the appearance of microorganisms in decaying material. His elegant experiments showed that sterile organic infusions would not putrify or ferment if there was no subsequent contact with air-borne contaminants, proving that spontaneous generation does not occur, and that all microbes must come from pre-existing microbes. This discovery contributed to many fields of the science, both basic and applied. Perhaps most important was the contribution Pasteur made to the work of Lister on antiseptics, which revolutionized approaches to surgery.

Pasteur worked in an amazing variety of microbiological fields, from fermentation in the brewing of beers and production of wines, to identification of silk worm diseases, bringing to each a penetrating scientific insight and making discoveries which brought him national and international reknown. His understanding of the roles of organisms in causing diseases, and his acute scientific perception, enabled him to grasp, from a series of 'mishaps' with experiments on chicken cholera, that attenuated microbes could induce not disease but immunity from disease. His ideas generated powerful opposition, but his belief then was strong enough to encourage him in 1881 to take part in a public trial of his vaccine against anthrax in domestic animals. Later, he used his insights into rabies, caused by organisms he could not see or culture, to develop an attenuated vaccine made from the dried spinal cords of infected rabbits. This was proven effective in humans in 1885 when Pasteur inoculated a Joseph Meister, a 9-year-old boy who had been badly bitten by a rabid dog. Meister survived and Pasteur's views on vaccination became universally accepted.

Pasteur ended his life as a national hero in his native France, and with a world-wide reputation for his work. His name is immortalized not only in the process of sterilization -'pasteurization'- that he developed, but in the Institut Pasteur in Paris, which remains one of the most important international centres of microbiological work.

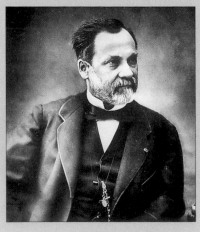

Fig. 34.3 Louis Pasteur (1822–1895).

35 ANTIMICROBIAL AGENTS AND CHEMOTHERAPY

Contents

INTRODUCTION

The interactions between host, microbial pathogen and antimicrobial agent can be considered as a triangle, and any alteration in one side will inevitably affect the other two sides (Fig. 35.1). In this chapter two sides of the triangle will be examined in greater detail – the interactions between antimicrobial agents and microorganisms, and between antimicrobial agents and the human host. Laboratory aspects of antibiotic susceptibility tests and assays will also be outlined. The third side of the triangle, the interactions between microorganisms and the human host, have been considered in detail in the preceding chapters. The concluding section of the present chapter will draw together the three sides of the triangle.

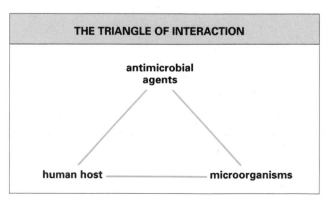

THE TRIANGLE OF INTERACTION

antimicrobial agents

human host —————— microorganisms

Fig. 35.1 The interactions between antimicrobial agents, microorganisms and the human host can be viewed as a triangle. Any effect on one side of the triangle will have effects on the other two sides.

Paul Ehrlich (1854–1915)

Just as Pasteur towers over immunomicrobiology, Ehrlich (Fig. 35.2) is the father figure of immunochemistry. His contributions to the science of medicine at all levels are quite extraordinary. He was the first to propose that foreign antigens were recognized by 'side-chains' on cells (1890), a brilliant insight that took seventy years to confirm. He also discovered the mast cell, invented the acid-fast stain for the tubercle bacillus and devised a method to manufacture and commercialize a strong diphtheria antitoxin. He pioneered the development of antibiotics with his work on '606' (or 'Salvarsan') a treatment for syphilis, for which he was denounced by the church for interfering with God's punishment for sin.

While working on the treatment of infections caused by trypanosomes he set forth the concept of 'selective toxicity':

> But, gentlemen, it should be made clear that in general this task is much more complicated than that using serum therapy. These chemical agents, in contrast to the antibodies, may be harmful to the body. When such an agent is given to a sick organism, a difference must exist between the toxicity of this agent to the parasite and its toxicity to the host. We must always be aware of the fact that these agents are able to act on other parts of the body as well as on the parasites.

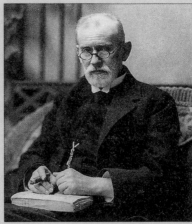

Fig. 35.2
Paul Ehrlich
(1854–1915).

Like Pasteur, he had a grasp of the continuum from the whole body to the cell, to the three-dimensional structure of molecules, and throughout his life he stressed the importance of molecular interaction as the basis of all biological function; this is summed up in his famous maxim "*corpora non agunt nisi fixata*" (things do not interact unless they make contact). A Nobel prize winner in 1908, his name was systematically eliminated from the records by the nazi regime on account of his Jewish birth, but he was restored to honour by a reconstruction of his laboratory at the Seventh International Congress of Immunology in Berlin, in 1989.

SELECTIVE TOXICITY

The term 'selective toxicity' was proposed by the immunochemist Paul Ehrlich (see panel). It is achieved by exploiting differences in the structure and metabolism of microorganisms and host cells; ideally the antimicrobial agent should act at a target site which is present in the infecting organism but absent from host cells. This is more likely to be achievable in microorganisms that are procaryotes than in those that are eucaryotes, as they are structurally more distinct from the host cells (a comparison of the cellular organization of procaryotic and eucaryotic cells is given in Chapter 1). At the other end of the spectrum, viruses are difficult to attack because of their obligate intracellular life-style; a successful antiviral agent must be able to enter the host cell but inhibit and damage only a virus-specific target. The desirable features of ideal antimicrobial agents are summarized in figure 35.3.

DISCOVERY AND DESIGN OF ANTIMICROBIAL AGENTS

Antibiotics are natural products of fungi, actinomycetes and bacteria which kill or inhibit the growth of microorganisms. Antibiotic production is associated particularly with soil microorganisms and in the natural environment is thought to provide a selective advantage for organisms

in their competition for space and nutrients. Although the majority of antibacterial and antifungal agents in clinical use today are derived from natural products of fermentation, most are then chemically modified to improve their antibacterial or pharmacological properties. However, some agents are totally synthetic, e.g. sulphonamides, quinolones. Thus the term 'antibacterial' (or 'antimicrobial') agent is often used in preference to 'antibiotic'.

The discovery of new antimicrobial agents used to be entirely a matter of chance. Pharmaceutical companies undertook massive screening programmes searching for new soil microorganisms which produced antibiotic activity. In the light of our greater understanding of the mechanisms of action of existing antimicrobials the processes have become rationalized, searching either for new natural products by target-site-directed screening or synthesizing molecules predicted to interact with a microbial target. The steps in a rational design programme are summarized in figure 35.4.

ANTIBACTERIAL AGENTS

Ways of classifying antibacterial agents
There are three ways of classifying antibacterial agents:
- whether they are bactericidal or bacteriostatic
- by target site
- by chemical structure.

DESIRED PROPERTIES OF A NEW ANTIMICROBIAL AGENT
antimicrobial properties
selectivity for microbial rather than mammalian targets broad spectrum of activity cidal activity (antibacterial and antifungal agents)
pharmacological properties
non-toxic to the host long plasma half-life (once-a-day dosing) good tissue distribution including CSF low plasma-protein binding oral and parenteral dosing forms no interference with other drugs

Fig. 35.3 In the design of new antimicrobial agents both antimicrobial activity and pharmacological properties of the antibiotic for the host have to be considered.

RATIONAL DESIGN OF AN ANTIMICROBIAL AGENT
select an appropriate target
identify a chemical lead (i.e. a new molecule with inhibitory activity on the target)
modify the lead compound to enhance potency
evaluate *in vitro* activity
evaluate *in vivo* activity and toxicity
test in clinical trials and develop

average 10 years

Fig. 35.4 The discovery process of new antimicrobial agents has moved away from the random screening of soil microorganisms towards a rational design programme. The figure identifies different steps in this programme. From discovery to development and marketing may take at least 10 years and cost about US$200 million.

Bactericidal versus bacteriostatic

Some antibacterial agents kill bacteria (bactericidal), while others only inhibit their growth (bacteriostatic). Bacteriostatic agents are successful in the treatment of infections because they prevent the bacterial population from increasing and host defence mechanisms can cope with the static population. In immunocompromised patients, bacteriostatic drugs may be less efficacious.

As a means of classification, the distinction between bactericidal and bacteriostatic agents has become blurred because some agents are capable of killing some species but are only bacteriostatic for others, e.g. chloramphenicol inhibits growth of *Escherichia coli* but kills *Haemophilus influenzae*.

Target site

A convenient way of classifying antibacterials is on the basis of their site of action. This classification does not allow an accurate prediction of which antibacterials will be active against which bacterial species, but it does help in the understanding of the molecular basis of antibacterial action (and conversely in the elucidation of many of the synthetic processes in bacterial cells).

There are four main target sites for antibacterial action:
• cell wall synthesis
• protein synthesis
• nucleic acid synthesis
• cell membrane function.

These targets differ to a greater or lesser degree from those in the host cells and so allow inhibition of the bacterial cell without concomitant inhibition of the equivalent mammalian cell targets (selective toxicity).

Each target site encompasses a series of synthetic reactions, each of which may be specifically inhibited by an antibacterial agent. A range of chemically diverse molecules may inhibit different reactions at the same target site (e.g. protein synthesis inhibitors).

Chemical structure

Antibacterial agents are very diverse chemical structures so classification on this basis alone is not of practical use. However a combination of target site and chemical structure provides a useful working classification and will be used in the later sections of this chapter. Each target site will be considered in turn and the antibacterial agents grouped in families according to their chemical structure.

RESISTANCE TO ANTIBACTERIAL AGENTS

Resistance to antibacterial agents is a matter of degree. In the medical setting we define a resistant organism as one which will not be inhibited or killed by an antibacterial agent at concentrations of the drug achievable in the body after normal dosage.

> Some men are born great, some achieve greatness,
> and some have greatness thrust upon them.
> Twelfth Night, William Shakespeare.

Likewise some bacteria are born resistant, others have resistance thrust upon them. In other words some species are innately resistant to some families of antibiotics, either because they lack a susceptible target or because they are impermeable to the antibacterial agent. The Gram-negative rods with their outer membrane layer exterior to the cell wall peptidoglycan are less permeable to large molecules than Gram-positive cells. However, within species that are innately susceptible, there are strains which have developed or acquired resistance.

The genetics of resistance

In parallel with the rapid development of a wide range of antibacterial agents since the 1940s, bacteria have proved extremely adept at developing resistance to each new agent that comes along. Resistance may arise by a single chromosomal mutation in one bacterial cell resulting in the synthesis of an altered protein (e.g. streptomycin resistance via the alteration in a ribosomal protein; a single amino acid change in the enzyme dihydropteroate synthetase resulting in a lowered affinity for sulphonamides). In the presence of antibiotic, these spontaneous mutants have a selective advantage and survive and outgrow the susceptible population (Fig. 35.5a). They can also spread to other sites in the same patient or by cross-infection to other patients and thus become disseminated.

Not content with surviving the antibacterial onslaught by relying on random chromosomal mutation, bacteria are also able to acquire resistance genes on transmissible plasmids (Fig. 35.5b; see also Chapter 3). Such plasmids often code for resistance determinants to several unrelated families of antibacterial agents. Thus a cell may acquire resistance to as many as six different drugs at once. This so-called 'infectious resistance' was first described by Japanese workers studying enteric bacteria but is now recognized to be widespread throughout the bacterial world. Some plasmids are promiscuous, crossing species barriers and thus the same resistance gene is found in widely different species. For example, TEM-l, the most common plasmid-mediated beta-lactamase in Gram-negative bacteria, is widespread in *E. coli* and other enterobacteria and also accounts for penicillin resistance in *Neisseria gonorrhoeae* and ampicillin resistance in *H. influenzae*.

Resistance genes may also occur on transposons; the so-called 'jumping genes', which are capable of integration into the chromosome or into plasmids. The chromosome provides a more secure position for the genes, but they will be disseminated only as rapidly as the bacteria divide. Transposons moving from the chromosome to plasmids allow chromosomal genes to be disseminated more rapidly. Transposons can also move between plasmids, for example from a non-transmissible to a transmissible plasmid again accelerating their dissemination (Fig. 35.5c).

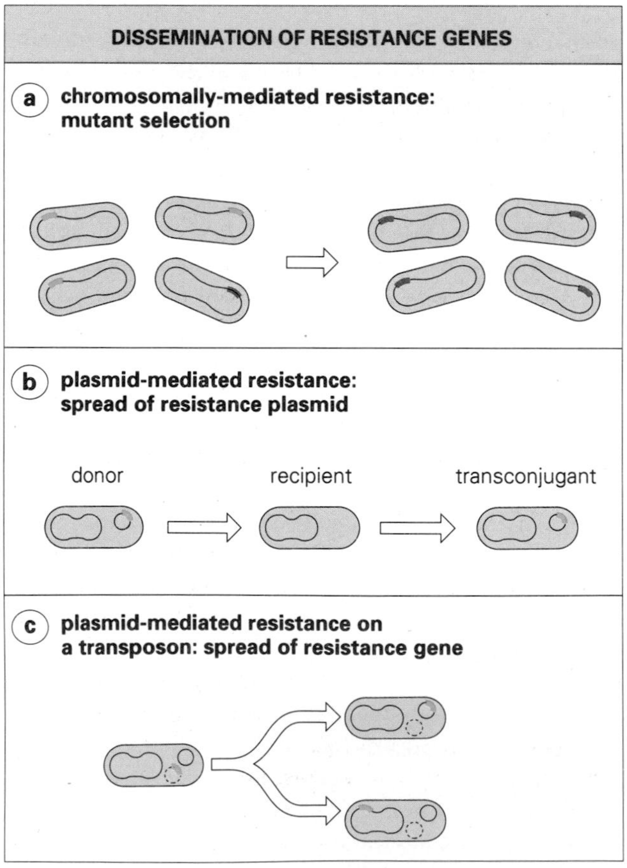

Mechanisms of resistance

Resistance mechanisms can be broadly classified into three main types. These are summarized below and in figure 35.6, and described in more detail where relevant for each antibiotic in later sections of this chapter.

DISSEMINATION OF RESISTANCE GENES

(a) chromosomally-mediated resistance: mutant selection

(b) plasmid-mediated resistance: spread of resistance plasmid

donor   recipient   transconjugant

(c) plasmid-mediated resistance on a transposon: spread of resistance gene

Fig. 35.5 A chromosomal mutation (a) can produce a drug-resistant target which confers resistance on the bacterial cell and allows it to multiply in the presence of antibiotic. Resistance genes carried on plasmids (b) can spread from one cell to another more rapidly then cells themselves divide and spread. Resistance genes on transposable elements (c) move between plasmids and the chromosome and from one plasmid to another, thereby allowing greater stability or greater dissemination of the resistance gene.

RESISTANCE TO ANTIBACTERIAL AGENTS

antibacterial	mechanism of resistance		
	altered target	altered uptake	drug inactivation
Beta-lactams	−	+	++
Glycopeptides	−		
Aminoglycosides	−	+	++
Tetracyclines	−	+	
Chloramphenicol		−	+
Macrolides	++		
Lincosamides	++		
Fusidic acid	++		
Sulphonamides	++	−	
Trimethoprim	++	−	
Quinolones	−	+	
Rifampicin	++		
Metronidazole		−	
Polymyxin	−	−	

− rare; occurs infrequently or only in few species
+ common
++ very common, in many species

Fig. 35.6 Mechanisms of resistance can be classified into three main types. Resistance to some antibiotics is more frequently found through alteration in the target site than other mechanisms. Drug inactivation mechanisms are most important for beta-lactams, aminoglycosides and chloramphenicol.

Alteration in target site

The target enzyme may be altered so that it has a lowered affinity for the antibacterial but still functions adequately for normal metabolism to proceed. Alternatively an additional target enzyme may be synthesized.

Alteration in access to the target site (altered uptake)

This mechanism involves decreasing the amount of drug that reaches the target, either by altering entry, for example by increasing the impermeability of the cell wall, or by pumping the drug out of the cell (known as an efflux mechanism).

Production of enzymes which modify or destroy the antibacterial agent (drug inactivation)

There are many examples of such enzymes, the most important being beta-lactamases, aminoglycoside-modifying enzymes, and chloramphenicol acetyl transferases. These will be described in the relevant sections on these antibiotics.

Where the mechanisms of resistance in bacteria have been elucidated they appear to involve the synthesis of new or altered proteins and, as mentioned above, the genes encoding these proteins may be either plasmid-mediated or on the chromosome.

CLASSES OF ANTIBACTERIAL AGENTS

The following sections of this chapter deal with groups of antibacterial agents arranged according to their target site, and subdivided on the basis of chemical structure. Each section attempts to summarize the answers (where known)

WHAT DO WE NEED TO KNOW ABOUT AN ANTIBACTERIAL AGENT?	
What is it ?	chemical structure natural or synthetic product
What does it do?	target site mechanism of action
Where does it go? (and therefore preferred route of administration)	absorption, distribution, metabolism and excretion of the drug in the body of the host
When is it used?	spectrum of activity and important clinical uses
What are the problems?	toxicity to the human host lack of toxicity, i.e. resistance of the bacteria
How much does it cost?	great variation between agents but cost is a serious limitation on availability of some agents in developing countries

Fig. 35.7 In order to understand the nature and optimum use of an antibacterial agent, several questions must be answered.

to the questions set out in figure 35.7, reviewing the interactions between antibacterial agent and bacteria and between the antibacterial and the host, in other words two sides of the triangle (see Fig. 35.1).

INHIBITORS OF CELL WALL SYNTHESIS

Peptidoglycan, a vital component of the bacterial cell wall (see Chapter 3), is a compound unique to bacteria and thus provides an optimum target for selective toxicity. Synthesis of peptidoglycan precursors starts in the cytoplasm, wall subunits are transported across the cytoplasmic membrane and finally inserted into the growing peptidoglycan molecule. Thus there are several different stages which are potential targets for inhibition (Fig. 35.8) The antibacterials which inhibit cell wall synthesis (Fig. 35.9) are very varied in chemical structure. The important groups are the beta-lactams and the glycopeptides; bacitracin and cycloserine have many fewer clinical applications.

Beta-lactams

Structure

This is a large family of different groups of compounds all containing the beta-lactam ring (Fig. 35.10). The different groups within the family are distinguished by the structure of the ring attached to the beta-lactam ring; in penicillins this is a five-membered ring, in cephalosporins a six-membered ring, and by the side chains attached to these rings.

Mechanism of action

Beta-lactams inhibit cell wall synthesis by binding to enzymes known as 'penicillin binding proteins' (PBPs). These proteins are carboxypeptidases and transpeptidases responsible for the final stages of cross-linking of the bacterial cell wall structure. Inhibition of one or more of these essential enzymes results in an accumulation of precursor cell wall units and this causes the cell's autolytic system to be activated and results finally in cell lysis (Fig. 35.11).

Absorption, distribution and excretion

The majority of beta-lactams have to be administered intramuscularly or intravenously but there are some orally active agents (see Fig. 35.13 below). Most achieve clinically useful concentrations in the CSF when the meninges are inflamed (as in meningitis) and the blood-brain barrier becomes more permeable. In general, they are not effective against intracellular organisms.

A few of the cephalosporins, notably cefotaxime, are metabolized to compounds with less microbiological activity. All beta-lactams are excreted in the urine; some, such as benzylpenicillin, very rapidly and hence the need for frequent doses. Probenicid can be administered concurrently to slow down excretion and maintain higher blood and tissue concentrations for a longer period.

Uses

There are more than 40 different beta-lactam antibiotics currently registered for clinical use. Some, such as penicillin, are active mainly against Gram-positive organisms,

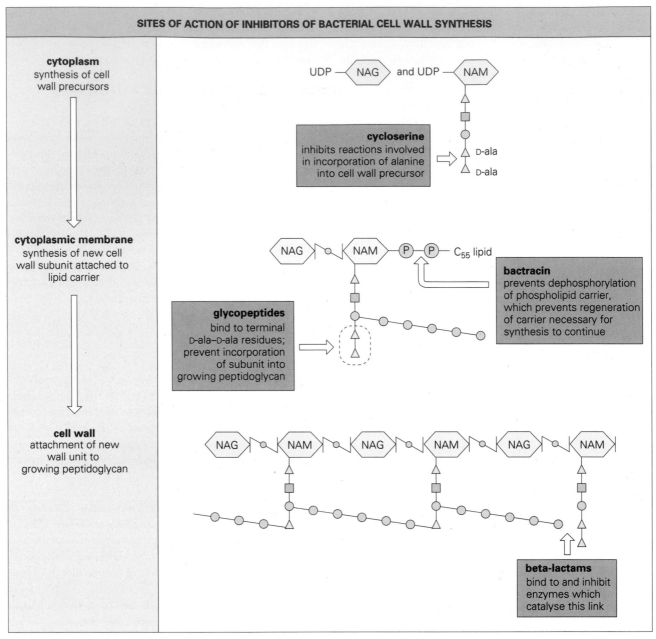

Fig. 35.8 The synthesis of peptidoglycan is a complex process which begins in the cytoplasm, proceeds across the cytoplasmic membrane and leads to the attachment of new wall units to the growing peptidoglycan chain. This synthetic pathway can be inhibited at a number of different points by antibacterial agents. The precise mechanism of inhibition caused by glycopeptides such as vancomycin is unknown but the mechanism of action of beta-lactams has now been fully elucidated (see below). UDP, uridine diphosphate; NAM, N-acetyl muramic acid; NAG, N-acetyl glucosamine.

INHIBITORS OF CELL WALL SYNTHESIS
beta-lactams   penicillins, cephalosporins, carbapenems, monobactams
glycopeptides   vancomycin, teicoplanin
cycloserine
bacitracin

Fig. 35.9 The beta-lactam group is by far the largest and most important of the cell wall synthesis inhibitors. Glycopeptides are active only against Gram-positive organisms. Cycloserine and bacitracin have very limited uses.

whereas others have been developed for their activity against Gram-negative rods such as the enterobacteria. Only the more recent beta-lactams are active against resistant organisms such as *Pseudomonas aeruginosa*. Some examples of the spectrum of activity of these agents is given in figure 35.12. The main clinical uses for important beta-lactams are shown in figure 35.13.

Toxicity

Serious allergy to beta-lactam drugs in the form of an immediate hypersensitivity reaction occurs in approximately 0.004–0.015% of treatment courses. Mild idiopathic reactions, usually in the form of a rash, occur more frequently (23% of treatment courses), and especially with

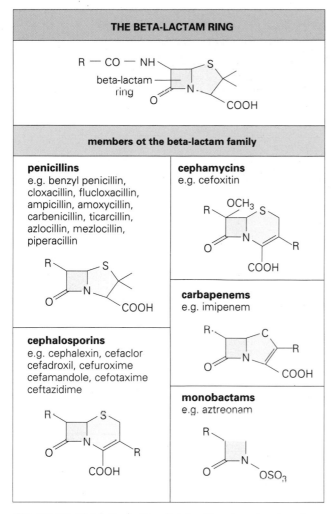

Fig. 35.10 The beta-lactam family. The ring structure is common to all beta-lactams and must be intact for antibacterial action. Enzymes (beta-lactamases) which catalyse the hydrolysis of the beta-lactam bond render the agents inactive. The penicillins and cephalosporins are the major classes of beta-lactam antibiotics, but other members of the family, particularly the carbapenems and monobactams, are the focus of new developments.

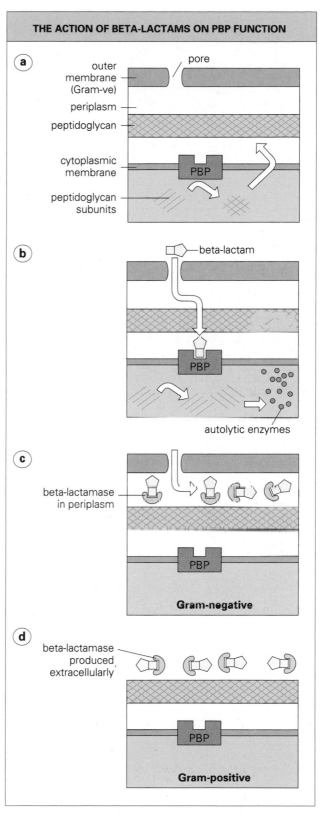

Fig. 35.11 Penicillin binding proteins (PBPs) play a key role in the final stages of peptidoglycan synthesis. They catalyse the cross-linkage of wall subunits, which are then incorporated into the cell wall (a). Beta-lactams are able to enter the cell through pores in the outer membrane (Gram-negatives) (b), and bind to the PBP. This prevents it from catalysing the cross-linkage of subunits, leading to their accumulation in the cell, and release of autolytic enzymes which cause cell lysis. Beta-lactamases, (c) and (d), can inactivate beta-lactams before they reach their target PBPs, thereby protecting the cell from the action of beta-lactams.

ampicillin. Patients who are allergic to penicillin are often also allergic to cephalosporins and vice versa, but aztreonam, a monobactam shows negligible cross-reactivity.

Benzylpenicillin can produce neurotoxicity if given in high doses particularly in patients with renal impairment. This toxicity is manifest as fits, unconsciousness, myoclonic spasms and hallucinations. Carbenicillin can cause platelet disfunction and sodium overload (because it is given as a sodium salt) especially in patients with liver failure, renal failure and congestive heart failure.

Resistance

Clinical isolates resistant to beta-lactams may exhibit any one (or more than one) of the three mechanisms of resistance.

PATTERNS OF SUSCEPTIBILITY TO BETA-LACTAMS

	penicillin§	cloxacillin‖	methicillin‡	ampicillin§	amoxycillin§	carbenicillin	azlocillin piperacillin	augmentin**§	cephalexin§	cefuroxime	cefotaxime	ceftazidime	imipenem	aztreonam
Staph. aureus βL+	R	S		R				S					S	R
Staph. aureus βL−	S	S		S				S					S	R
MRSA	R	R	R					R	R	R	R	R	R	R
Coagulase-negative staphs	R	S†		R				S†					S†	R
Strep. pneumoniae	S			S					S	S			S	R
Strep. pyogenes	S			S									S	R
Enterococcus faecalis	R			S				S					R	R
Enterococcus faecium	R			R				R					R	R
Oral streptococci	S			S										R
Listeria	S			S										R
Clostridium	S													R
Neisseria gonorrhoeae βL+	R			R				S						
Neisseria gonorrhoeae βL−	S			S				S						
Neisseria meningitidis	S													
Branhamella	R			R						S	S			
E. coli	R			R*	R*	S	S	S	S	S	S	S	S	S
Klebsiella	R			R	R	S	S	R	S	S	S	S	S	S
Proteus	R			R*	R*	S	S	S	S	S	S	S	S	S
Pseudomonas	R			R		S	S	R	R	R	R	S	S	S
H. influenzae βL+	R			R				S	R	S	S			S
H. influenzae βL−	R			S				S	R	S·	S			S
Brucella	R													
Campylobacter	R													
Legionella	R													
Bacteroides	R*			R*				S						
Mycoplasma	R													
Chlamydia	R													

R, resistant; S, susceptible

MRSA, methicillin-resistant Staph. aureus

* ≥ 50% strains resistant due to β-lactamase (βL) production

** augmentin is a combination of amoxycillin and a beta-lactamase inhibitor clavulanic acid

† but methicillin resistant coagulase-negative staphs will be resistant to all beta-lactams

‡ methicillin is tested in the laboratory because it gives more reliable results in in vitro tests, but it is not used for treatment, susceptibility to methicillin indicates susceptibility to cloxacillin, flucloxacillin and oxacillin

§ orally-active agents   ‖ flucloxacillin is usual choice for oral administration

Fig. 35.12 The most commonly used beta-lactams are shown, together with the usual susceptibility of bacteria of medical importance. The empty boxes indicate that the agents are not drugs of choice for the corresponding organism. It is important to note that the mycobacteria are uniformly resistant to beta-lactam agents, as are mycoplasma and chlamydia and other intracellular organisms.

USES FOR BETA-LACTAMS		
beta-lactam	**major clinical indications for use**	**route of administration**
Penicillins Benzyl penicillin	bacterial upper respiratory tract infection pneumonia meningitis endocarditis	IV/IM/oral
Cloxacillin Flucloxacillin	skin and soft tissue osteomyelitis and septic arthritis (Gram+ve)	IV/IM/oral
Ampicillin Amoxycillin	urinary tract infection meningitis enteric fever epiglottitis osteomyelitis (Gram-ve) bronchitis/pneumonia	IV/IM/oral
Carbenicillin	serious sepsis caused by *P. aeruginosa* (usually in combination with aminoglycoside); now largely replaced by newer agents	IV
Azlocillin Piperacillin	serious sepsis caused by *P. aeruginosa* or other antibiotic-resistant Gram-ve rods (usually in combination with aminoglycoside)	IV
Cephalosporins Cephalexin Cefaclor Cefadroxil	urinary tract infections	oral
Cefuroxime	respiratory tract and urinary tract infections	IV/IM
Cefotaxime	meningitis (in neonates) respiratory and urinary tract infections abdominal sepsis	IV/IM (oral cefixime)
Ceftazidime	serious sepsis caused by *P. aeruginosa* or other antibiotic-resistant Gram-ve rods (often in combination with aminoglycosides)	IV/IM
Cephamycins Cefoxitin	abdominal sepsis	IV/IM
Carbapenems Imipenem	serious sepsis caused by *P. aeruginosa* or other antibiotic-resistant Gram-ve rods	IV
Monobactams Aztreonam	urinary tract infections enteric fever Gram-ve sepsis not active against Gram+ve or anaerobes	IV

Fig. 35.13 The uses of beta-lactams. Although there are many beta-lactam agents available the most commonly used ones are listed, together with the main indications. Some of the agents are available for oral administration but most are given intravenously or intramuscularly. IV, intravenous; IM, intramuscular.

Alteration in target site. Methicillin resistant staphylococci synthesize an additional PBP which has a much lower affinity for beta-lactams than the normal PBPs, and is thus able to continue cell wall synthesis even when the other PBPs are inhibited. Although the gene coding for the additional PBP is present on the chromosome in all cells of a resistant population, it is only transcribed in a proportion of the cells resulting in the phenomenon of 'heterogeneous resistance'. In the laboratory, special cultural conditions are used to enhance expression and demonstrate resistance. Methicillin-resistant staphylococci are resistant to all other beta-lactams. The majority of strains also produce beta-lactamase (see below).

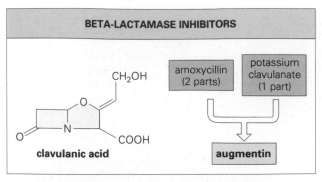

Fig. 35.14 Clavulanic acid, a product of *Streptomyces clavuligerus*, inhibits the most common beta-lactamases (e.g. TEM enzymes) and allows amoxycillin to inhibit cells producing these enzymes. Augmentin is the most widely used of these combination drugs.

Alteration in access to the target site. This mechanism is found in Gram-negative cells where beta-lactams gain access to their target PBPs by diffusion through protein channels (porins) in the outer membrane. Mutations in porin genes result in a decrease in permeability of the outer membrane and hence resistance. Strains resistant by this mechanism may exhibit cross-resistance to unrelated antibiotics which use the same porins.

Production of beta-lactamases. Beta-lactamases are enzymes which catalyse the hydrolysis of the beta-lactam ring to yield microbiologically inactive products. Genes encoding these enzymes are widespread in the bacterial kingdom and are found on the chromosome and on plasmids.

In Gram-positive bacteria beta-lactamases are released into the extracellular environment (see Fig. 35.11) and resistance will be manifest only when a large population of cells is present. In Gram-negative cells, the beta-lactamases remain within the periplasm (see Fig. 35.11).

There are many different beta-lactamase enzymes which have the same function but differ in their affinity for different beta-lactam substrates. Thus some beta-lactams, e.g. cloxacillin, ceftazidime, imipenem, are hydrolysed by very few enzymes (beta-lactamase stable), whereas others, e.g. ampicillin, are much more labile. Beta-lactamase inhibitors, such as clavulanic acid (Fig. 35.14), are molecules which contain a beta-lactam ring and which act as 'suicide inhibitors', binding to beta-lactamases and preventing them from destroying beta-lactams. They have little bactericidal activity of their own.

Glycopeptides

Structure
This group includes vancomycin and teicoplanin. Both are large molecules (see Fig. 35.9). Teicoplanin is a complex of five different but closely related molecules.

Mechanism of action
Glycopeptides interfere with cell wall synthesis by binding to terminal D-ala–D-ala at the end of pentapeptide chains that are part of the growing bacterial cell wall structure

(see Fig. 35.8). This binding inhibits the transglycosylation reaction and prevents incorporation of new subunits into the growing cell wall. Glycopeptides act at an earlier stage than beta-lactams, and thus it is not useful to administer them in combination in the treatment of infections.

Absorption, distribution and excretion
Vancomycin and teicoplanin are not absorbed from the gastrointestinal tract and must be given by injection for treatment of systemic infections. The drugs do not penetrate into the CSF in patients without meningitis but bactericidal concentrations are achieved in most patients with meningitis due to the increased permeability of the blood-brain barrier. Excretion is via the kidney.

Uses
Both vancomycin and teicoplanin are active only against Gram-positive organisms. They are used mainly for the treatment of infections caused by Gram-positive cocci and Gram-positive rods that are resistant to beta-lactam drugs, or in patients who are allergic to beta-lactams. Oral administration is used for the treatment of *Clostridium difficile* in antibiotic-associated colitis.

Toxicity
Vancomycin must be given by slow intravenous infusion to avoid 'red-man' syndrome (due to histamine release). The glycopeptides are potentially ototoxic and nephrotoxic. Blood concentrations should be monitored to achieve peak serum concentrations between 10 and 40 mg/l; particular care must be taken to prevent toxic concentrations accumulating in patients with renal impairment. Teicoplanin is less toxic than vancomycin.

Resistance
Acquired resistance to these agents is extremely rare among bacteria of medical importance but has now been reported among enterococci, where resistance is plasmid-mediated and transmissible. The mechanism of resistance is not clear.

INHIBITORS OF PROTEIN SYNTHESIS

Although protein synthesis proceeds in an essentially similar manner in procaryotic and eucaryotic cells, it is possible to exploit the differences to achieve selective toxicity. The process of translation of the mRNA chain into its corresponding peptide chain is complex and still incompletely understood. A range of antibacterial agents act as inhibitors of protein synthesis although the details of their mechanisms of action are not yet all known (Fig. 35.15).

Aminoglycosides

Structure
This is a family of related molecules containing either streptidine (streptomycin) or 2-deoxystreptamine (e.g. gentamicin (Fig. 35.16). The original structures have been modified chemically by changing the side chains to produce molecules (eg. amikacin, netilmicin) which are active

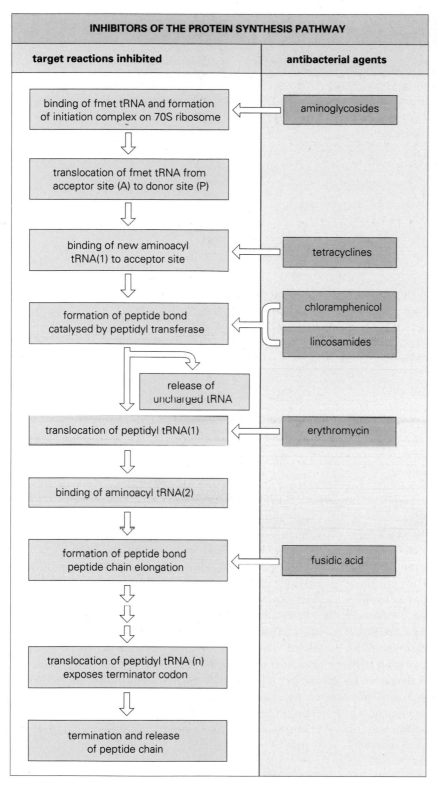

INHIBITORS OF THE PROTEIN SYNTHESIS PATHWAY

target reactions inhibited	antibacterial agents
binding of fmet tRNA and formation of initiation complex on 70S ribosome	aminoglycosides
translocation of fmet tRNA from acceptor site (A) to donor site (P)	
binding of new aminoacyl tRNA(1) to acceptor site	tetracyclines
formation of peptide bond catalysed by peptidyl transferase	chloramphenicol / lincosamides
release of uncharged tRNA	
translocation of peptidyl tRNA(1)	erythromycin
binding of aminoacyl tRNA(2)	
formation of peptide bond peptide chain elongation	fusidic acid
translocation of peptidyl tRNA (n) exposes terminator codon	
termination and release of peptide chain	

Fig. 35.15 The synthetic pathway leading to the production of new protein in bacterial cells is extremely complicated and still not fully elucidated. A number of different groups of antibacterial agents act by inhibiting proteins with specific reactions in this synthetic pathway. They can be grouped into those that act on the 30S subunit of the ribosome such as aminoglycosides and tetracyclines, and those that act on the 50S subunit, e.g. chloramphenicol, lincosamides, erythromycin and fusidic acid.

against organisms that have developed resistance to earlier aminoglycosides.

Mechanism of action

Aminoglycosides inhibit and kill organisms by interfering with the binding of formylmethionyl-tRNA (fmet-tRNA) to the ribosome (see Fig. 35.15) and thereby preventing the formation of initiation complexes from which protein synthesis proceeds. Streptomycin also causes misreading of mRNA codons.

Absorption, distribution and excretion

Aminoglycosides are not absorbed from the gut and must be given intravenously or intramuscularly for systemic treatment. They do not penetrate well into tissues and bone and do not cross the blood-brain barrier. Intrathecal administration of streptomycin is used in treatment of tuberculous meningitis, and gentamicin may be administered by this route for the treatment of Gram-negative meningitis in neonates. Aminoglycosides are excreted via the kidney.

CHEMICAL GROUPS OF AMINOGLYCOSIDES	
4, 6-disubstituted 2-deoxystreptamines	
Gentamicin*	complex of 3 closely related structures; first aminoglycoside with broad spectrum
Tobramycin**	activity very similar to gentamicin but slightly better against *P. aeruginosa*
Kanamycin **	no longer in clinical use
Amikacin	semi-synthetic derivative of kanamycin; active against many gentamicin-resistant Gram-negative rods;
Netilmicin*	activity spectrum similar to amikacin; probably least toxic of aminoglycosides
4, 5-disubstituted 2-deoxystreptamines	
Neomycin**	too toxic for parenteral use but has topical uses in decontaminating mucosal surfaces
streptidine-containing	
Streptomycin**	oldest aminoglycoside; now use restricted to treatment of tuberculosis
others	
Spectinomycin**	important for treatment of beta-lactam resistant *Neisseria gonorrhoeae*
* micins from *Micromonospora* species ** mycins from *Streptomyces* species	

Fig. 35.16 Aminoglycosides (or more properly aminoglycoside-aminocyclitols) can be classified according to their chemical structure. They are also differentiated by the genus of microorganisms that produces them and this is reflected in the spelling of the names.

Uses

Gentamicin and the newer aminoglycosides, tobramycin, amikacin and netilmicin are important for the treatment of serious Gram-negative infections including those caused by *P. aeruginosa* (Fig. 35.17). They are not active against streptococci, but do have activity against staphylococci. They are not active against anaerobes. Tobramycin is slightly more active than gentamicin against *P. aeruginosa*. Amikacin and netilmicin are both less active but may be active against strains resistant to gentamicin and tobramycin (see below). Streptomycin is now reserved almost entirely for the treatment of mycobacterial infections. Neomycin is not used for systemic treatment, but can be used orally in gut decontamination regimens in neutropenic patients. Spectinomycin is used to treat beta-lactam resistant *N. gonorrhoeae*.

Toxicity

The aminoglycosides are potentially nephrotoxic and ototoxic, and the therapeutic 'window' between serum concentrations required for successful treatment and those that are toxic, is small. Blood concentrations should be monitored regularly, particularly in patients with renal impairment. Netilmicin is reported to be of lower toxicity than the other aminoglycosides.

Resistance

Alteration in the ribosomal target site is not an uncommon mechanism for streptomycin resistance (where a single amino acid change in the P10 protein of the 30S subunit prevents streptomycin binding), but is very rare for other aminoglycosides.

Resistance may also arise in Gram-negative rods through alterations in cell wall permeability or in the energy-dependent transport across the cytoplasmic membrane.

Production of aminoglycoside-modifying enzymes is the most important mechanism of acquired resistance (Fig. 35.18). The genes for these enzymes are often plasmid-mediated and transferable from one bacterial species to another. The effect of the enzymes is to alter the structure of the aminoglycoside molecule which consequently changes the uptake of drug by the cell. The type of enzyme will determine the spectrum of resistance of the organism containing it.

Tetracyclines

Structure

Tetracyclines are a family of large cyclic structures which have several sites for possible chemical substitutions (Fig. 35.19). The members of the family differ mainly in their pharmacological properties rather than in their antibacterial spectra.

Mechanism of action

Tetracyclines inhibit protein synthesis by preventing aminoacyl transfer RNA from entering the acceptor sites on the ribosome (see Fig. 35.15). However this action is

INDICATIONS FOR AMINOGLYCOSIDE THERAPY
Basic rule: use only in severe, life-threatening infections
Gram-negative septicaemia (including *Pseudomonas*) usually in combination with beta-lactam
Septicaemia of unknown* aetiology arising from: hospital-acquired infection malignancy immunosuppressive therapy major trauma, major surgery or major burns intravenous catheter urinary catheter extremes of age
Bacterial endocarditis for synergy with penicillin
Staph. aureus septicaemia in combination with beta-lactam
Pyelonephritis for difficult cases
Post-surgical abdominal sepsis in combination with anti-anaerobe therapy
* every effort should be made to establish aetiology

Fig. 35.17 Aminoglycosides are valuable additions to the clinicians' armamentarium despite their potential toxicity. They are important agents active against Gram-negative facultative bacteria and are often used in combination with beta-lactams to broaden the spectrum to include streptococci and some anaerobes which are not susceptible to aminoglycosides alone. Resistance to aminoglycosides particularly among enterobacteria and staphylococci is mediated by the production of aminoglycoside-modifying enzymes which react with groups on the aminoglycoside molecule to yield an altered aminoglycoside product which competes with the unmodified aminoglycoside for uptake into the cell and binding to the ribosome.

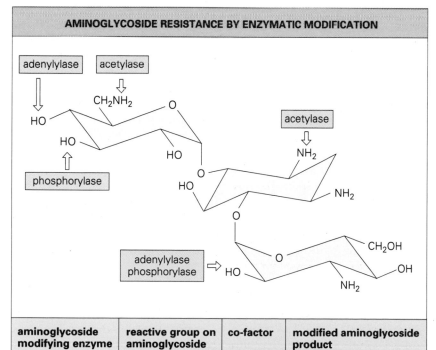

AMINOGLYCOSIDE RESISTANCE BY ENZYMATIC MODIFICATION

Fig. 35.18 Protoype structure of aminoglycoside, consisting of aminohexoses linked via glycosidic linkage to a central 2-deoxystreptamine nucleus. Hydroxyl and amino groups are sites at which these compounds can be inactivated by phosphorylation, adenylation or acetylation.

aminoglycoside modifying enzyme	reactive group on aminoglycoside	co-factor	modified aminoglycoside product
Acetylase	$-NH_2$	acetyl CoA	$-NHAc$
Adenylylase (nucleotidyl transferase)	$-OH$	ATP	$-O-AMP$
Phosphorylase	$-OH$	ATP	$-O-PO_2-OH$

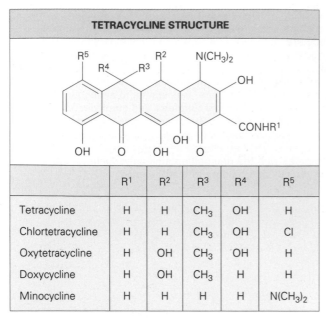

TETRACYCLINE STRUCTURE

	R¹	R²	R³	R⁴	R⁵
Tetracycline	H	H	CH₃	OH	H
Chlortetracycline	H	H	CH₃	OH	Cl
Oxytetracycline	H	OH	CH₃	OH	H
Doxycycline	H	OH	CH₃	H	H
Minocycline	H	H	H	H	N(CH₃)₂

Fig. 35.19 Tetracyclines are four-ring molecules with five different sites for substitution thereby giving rise to a family of molecules with different substituents at different sites. Members of the family differ particularly in their pharmacological properties more than their spectrum of activity.

not selectively toxic for procaryotes; tetracyclines will inhibit protein synthesis in cell free protein synthesis systems containing human ribosomes. The selective action of tetracyclines is based on their uptake by bacterial cells which is much greater than by human cells.

Absorption, distribution and excretion
These drugs are usually administered orally. Doxycycline and minocycline are more completely absorbed than tetracycline, oxytetracycline and chlortetracycline, resulting in higher serum concentrations and less gastrointestinal upset because there is less inhibition of normal gut flora. Tetracyclines are well distributed and penetrate host cells to inhibit intracellular bacteria. They are excreted via the kidneys.

Uses
They are used for treatment of infections caused by mycoplasmas, chlamydiae and rickettsiae. Tetracyclines are active against a wide variety of different bacterial species, but their use is now restricted by widespread resistance.

Toxicity
Suppression of normal gut flora causes gastrointestinal upset and diarrhoea and encourages overgrowth by resistant and undesirable bacteria (e.g. *Staph. aureus*) and fungi (e.g. *Candida*).

Interference with bone development and brown staining of teeth occurs in the foetus and in children and thus these drugs should be avoided in pregnancy and in children under 8 years of age.

Systemic administration may cause liver damage.

Resistance
Resistance is common, due partly to the widespread use of these drugs in humans and also to their use as growth promoters in animal feedstuffs. The resistance genes are carried on a transposon and, in the presence of tetracycline, the synthesis of new cytoplasmic membrane proteins is induced. The precise mechanism of resistance is unclear but tetracycline is accumulated less and may be positively pumped out of resistant cells (efflux mechanism).

Chloramphenicol

Structure
Chloramphenicol is a relatively simple molecule (Fig. 35.20) containing a nitrobenzene nucleus which is responsible for some of the toxic problems associated with the drug (see below). Other derivatives have been produced but none is in widespread clinical use.

Mechanism of action
Chloramphenicol blocks the action of peptidyl transferase thereby preventing peptide bond synthesis (see Fig. 35.15). It inhibits bacterial protein synthesis selectively because it has a much higher affinity for the transferase in the 50S subunit of the bacterial ribosome than it has for the transferase in the 60S subunit of the mammalian ribosomes. However it does have some inhibitory activity on human mitochondrial ribosomes and this may account for some of the dose-dependent toxicity to bone marrow (see below).

Absorption, distribution and excretion
The drug is well absorbed when given orally but can be given intravenously if the patient cannot take drugs by mouth. Topical preparations are also available. It is well distributed in the body and penetrates host cells. Chloramphenicol is metabolized in the liver by conjugation with glucuronic acid to yield a microbiologically inactive form that is excreted by the kidneys.

Uses
Chloramphenicol is active against a wide variety of bacterial species both Gram positive and Gram negative, aerobes and anaerobes, including intracellular organisms such as *Salmonella typhi*, chlamydiae and rickettsiae. It achieves satisfactory concentrations in the CSF and is valuable in the treatment of bacterial meningitis. Topical preparations are used for eye infections.

Toxicity
It is the rare but serious toxic effects of chloramphenicol that have tended to restrict use of this drug in countries where alternative agents are readily available. The most important toxic effects are in the bone marrow. Nitrobenzene itself is a bone marrow suppressant and the structurally similar chloramphenicol molecule has similar effects. This toxicity takes two forms:
- Dose-dependent bone marrow suppression, which occurs if the drug is given for long periods and is reversible when treatment is stopped;

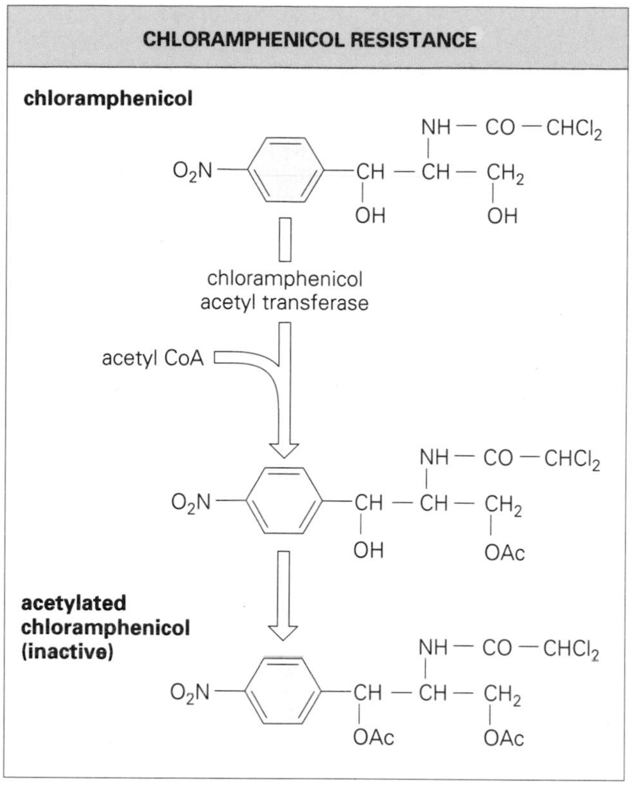

Fig. 35.20 Resistance to chloramphenicol is mediated in some organisms by the production of a chloramphenicol acetyl transferase enzyme which catalyses the addition of acetyl groups to the chloramphenicol molecule. This is a two-stage reaction producing acetylated chloramphenicol which is inactive.

- An idiosyncratic reaction causing aplastic anaemia; this is not dose dependent and is irreversible. It can occur after treatment has stopped but is fortunately very rare, occurring in about 1 in 30 000 patients treated.

Chloramphenicol is also toxic to neonates particularly premature babies whose liver enzyme systems are incompletely developed. This can result 'grey baby syndrome'. Chloramphenicol serum concentrations should be monitored in neonates.

Resistance

The most common mechanism involves inactivation of the drug catalysed by chloramphenicol acetyl transferases produced by resistant bacteria (see Fig. 35.20). These plasmid-mediated enzymes are intracellular but are capable of inactivating all the chloramphenicol in the immediate environment of the cell. Acetylated chloramphenicol fails to bind to the ribosomal target. Resistance is becoming increasingly common and this, together with the potential toxicity, has tended to reduce the use of the drug.

Macrolides, lincosamides and streptogramins

These three groups of antibacterial agents share overlapping binding sites on ribosomes, and resistance to macrolides confers resistance to the other two groups. The clinically-important drugs are the macrolide erythromycin, and the lincosamide clindamycin.

Macrolides

Structure

The macrolides are a family of large cyclic molecules all containing a macrocyclic lactone ring (Fig. 35.21). Erythromycin is the best known and most widely used but some of the newer agents such as azithromycin and roxithromycin, with improved activity and pharmacology, may take its place for specific indications. Spiramycin is another macrolide used almost exclusively for the treatment of cryptosporidiosis and in the prevention of congenital toxoplasmosis.

Mechanism of action

Erythromycin binds to the 23S rRNA in the 50S subunit of the ribosome and blocks the translocation step in protein synthesis, thereby preventing the release of tRNA after peptide bond formation (see Fig. 35.15).

Administration, distribution and excretion

Erythromycin is usually administered by the oral route but can also be given intravenously. The drug is well distributed in the body and penetrates mammalian cells to reach intracellular organisms. The drug is concentrated in the liver and excreted in the bile. A small proportion of the dose is recoverable in the urine.

Uses

Erythromycin is active against Gram-positive cocci and is an important alternative treatment of infections caused by streptococci in patients allergic to penicillin. It is active against *Legionella pneumophila* and *Campylobacter jejuni*. It is also active against mycoplasmas, chlamydiae and rickettsiae and is therefore an important drug for treatment of atypical pneumonia and chlamydial infections of the urogenital tract.

Toxicity

Erythromycin is a relatively non-toxic drug although it causes nausea and vomiting after oral administration in a significant number of patients. Jaundice is associated with some formulations of the drug.

Resistance

Resistance is due to alteration in the 23S rRNA target by methylation of two adenine nucleotides in the RNA. The methylase enzyme is plasmid-mediated and inducible. Erythromycin is a better inducer of resistance than the lincosamides but strains resistant to erythromycin will also be resistant to lincomycin and clindamycin, so-called 'MLS (macrolide lincosamide streptogramin) resistance'. Induction also varies between bacterial species.

Lincosamides

Structure

The two important molecules in this group are lincomycin and clindamycin. The latter (which is a chlorinated derivative of the former) is more active and has almost completely superseded lincomycin.

THE MACROLIDES

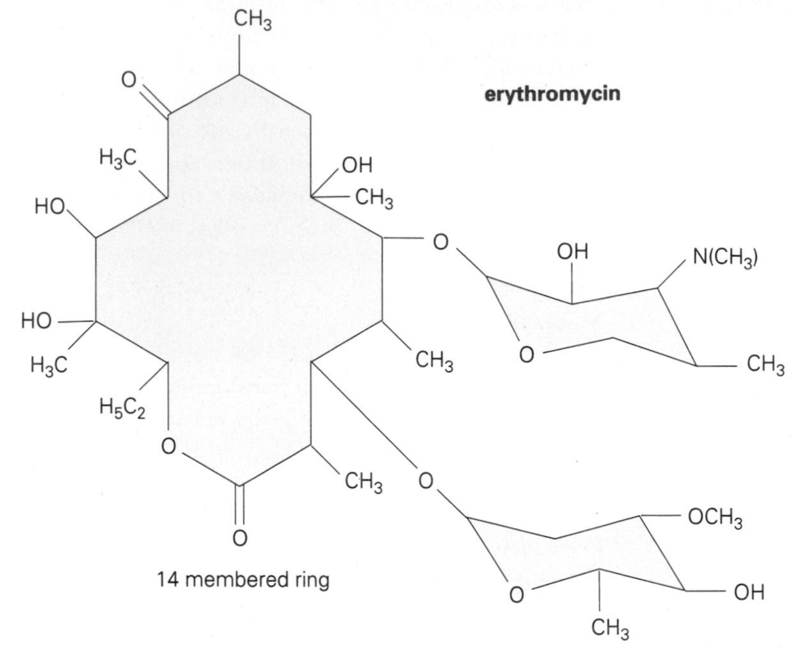

erythromycin

14 membered ring

New macrolide	*in vitro* activity compared with erthyromycin	human pharmacokinetics
Roxithromycin (14-membered ring)	comparable	high peak serum concentrations $T^{1/2} = 12h$
Azithromycin (15-membered ring)	improved against Gram-negative bacteria	high tissue concentrations, once-daily administration
Clarithromycin (14-membered ring)	improved against Gram-positive bacteria and *Legionella spp.*	improved peak serum concentration compared with erythromycin

Fig. 35.21 The macrolides are antibacterial agents composed of large structures which may be 14, 15 or 16 membered rings. Erythromycin is the oldest and most widely used of these but new agents are being developed which have improved activity and less toxicity than erythromycin.

Mechanism of action

Lincosamides bind to the 50S ribosomal subunit and inhibit protein synthesis by inhibiting peptide bond formation, but the mechanism is incompletely understood (see Fig. 35.15). The selectively toxic action results from failure to bind to the equivalent mammalian ribosomal subunit.

Administration, distribution and excretion

Clindamycin is usually given orally but can be administered intramuscularly or intravenously. The drug penetrates well into bone but not into CSF even when the meninges are inflamed. It is actively transported into polymorphonuclear leucocytes and macrophages. It is metabolized in the liver to several products with variable antibacterial activity and clindamycin activity persists in faeces for up to 5 days after a dose.

Uses

Clindamycin has a spectrum of activity similar to erythromycin but it is much more active against anaerobes, both Gram-positive e.g. *Clostridium* spp, and Gram-negative

e.g. *Bacteroides*. However, *Cl. difficile* is resistant and may be selected in the gut, causing pseudomembranous colitis (see below). The activity of clindamycin against *Staph. aureus* and its penetration into bone makes it a valuable drug in the treatment of osteomyelitis.

Toxicity

The association between antibiotic administration and pseudomembranous colitis (PMC) caused by *Cl. difficile* was first noted following clindamycin treatment but has subsequently been shown to follow treatment with many antibiotics. The pathogenesis of this complication is described in Chapter 25. Oral vancomycin or metronidazole should be used to treat PMC.

Resistance

See MLS resistance above. Because clindamycin is a less potent inducer of the 23S rRNA methylase, erythromycin-resistant strains may appear susceptible to clindamycin *in vitro*. However, resistance will be manifest *in vivo*.

INHIBITORS OF NUCLEIC ACID SYNTHESIS

inhibitors of synthesis of precursors
sulphonamides
trimethoprim

inhibitors of DNA replication
quinolones

inhibitors of RNA polymerase
rifampicin

Fig. 35.22 Inhibition of nucleic acid takes place at different stages in its synthesis and function and a number of different groups of antimicrobial agents are involved.

Fusidic acid

Structure and mechanism of action

This is a steroid-like compound which inhibits protein synthesis by forming a stable complex with elongation factor EF-G (the bacterial equivalent of the human EF-2), guanosine diphosphate and the ribosome.

Administration, distribution and excretion

Fusidic acid can be administered orally or intravenously. It is well-absorbed and penetrates well into tissues and bone but not into the CSF. Topical preparations are also available but their use should not be encouraged because of the rapid emergence of resistance (see below). Fusidic acid is metabolized in the liver and excreted in the bile.

Uses

Fusidic acid is active against Gram-positive cocci and its most important use is in the treatment of staphylococcal infections which are resistant to beta-lactams, or in patients who are allergic to alternative staphylococcal agents. Fusidic acid should be given in combination with another anti-staphylococcal agent (e.g. rifampicin or erythromycin) to prevent the emergence of resistant mutants.

Toxicity

Fusidic acid may occasionally cause jaundice and gastrointestinal upset.

Resistance

Resistant mutants with altered EF-G emerge rapidly in staphylococcal populations exposed to the drug.

INHIBITORS OF NUCLEIC ACID SYNTHESIS

Antibacterial agents which act as inhibitors of nucleic acid synthesis do so in one of three main ways as shown in figure 35.22. The inhibitory effects may be so fundamental to the cell that protein synthesis and other metabolic pathways may also appear to be targets.

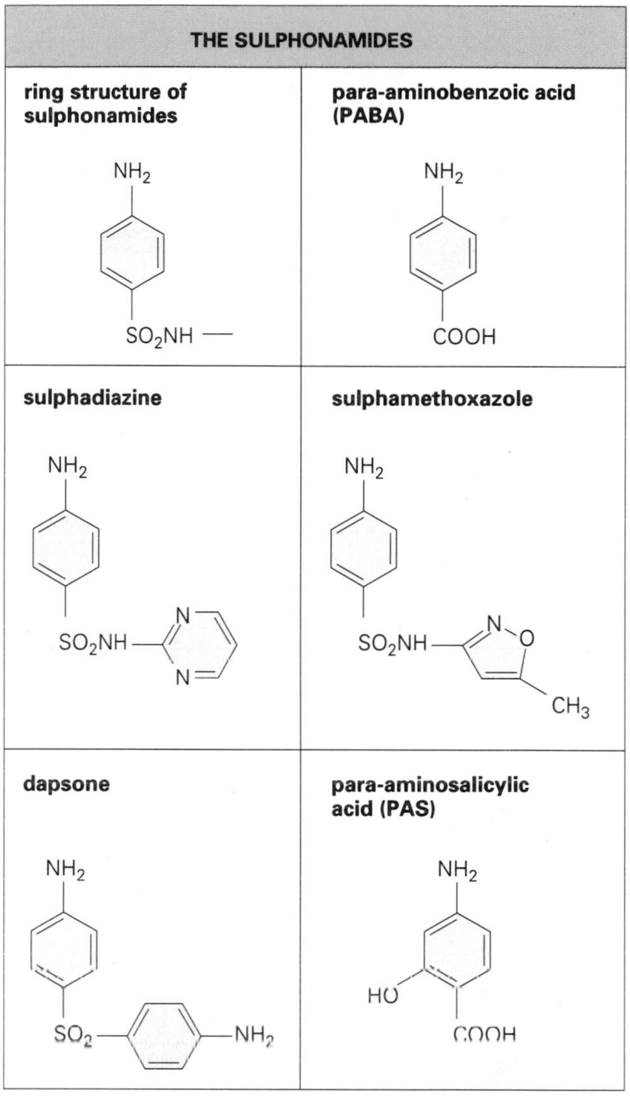

Fig. 35.23 The ring structure of the sulphonamides is very similar to the structure of the normal substrate (para-amino benzoic acid - PABA) of the dihydropteroate synthetase enzyme which the sulphonamides inhibit. There are many different sulphonamides available which differ in their pharmacological properties more than in their spectrum of activity. Relatively few are now in common clinical use. Dapsone is important in the treatment of *Mycobacterium leprae* and para-amino salicylic acid is a second line drug for the treatment of *Mycobacterium tuberculosis*.

Sulphonamides

Structure

This group of molecules are all structural analogues of para-amino benzoic acid (PABA), produced entirely by chemical synthesis (i.e. they are not natural products). In 1935, the parent compound sulphanilamide became the first clinically-effective antibacterial agent. The *p*-amino group is essential for activity but modifications to the sulphonic acid sidechain have produced a large number of related agents (Fig. 35.23).

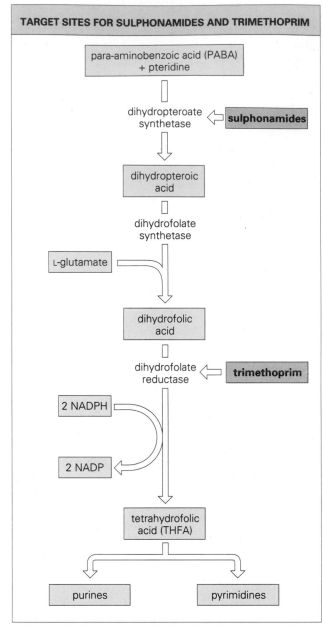

TARGET SITES FOR SULPHONAMIDES AND TRIMETHOPRIM

Fig. 35.24 Sulphonamides and trimethoprim inhibit in series the steps in the synthesis of tetrahydrofolic acid by interacting with key enzymes in the pathway.

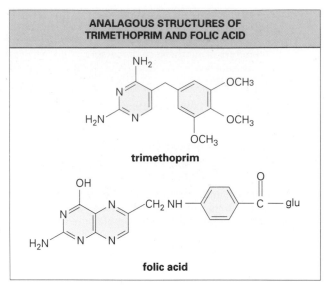

ANALAGOUS STRUCTURES OF TRIMETHOPRIM AND FOLIC ACID

Fig. 35.25 Trimethoprim resembles the aminohydroxy-pyrimidine moiety of folic acid and in this way antagonizes the enzyme dihydrofolate reductase.

Mechanism of action

Sulphonamides act in competition with PABA for the active site of dihydropteroate synthetase, an enzyme which catalyses an essential reaction in the synthetic pathway of tetrahydrofolic acid (THFA), required for the synthesis of purines and pyrimidines and thus for nucleic acid synthesis (Fig. 35.24). Selective toxicity depends on the fact that many bacteria synthesize THFA whereas human cells lack this capacity and depend on an exogenous supply of folic acid. Bacteria which can utilize preformed folic acid are similarly unaffected by sulphonamides.

Absorption, distribution and excretion

Sulphonamides are usually administered orally often in combination with trimethoprim as cotrimoxazole (see below). Different molecules within the family differ in their solubility and penetrability. Metabolism occurs in the liver and free and metabolized drug is excreted by the kidneys.

Uses

The sulphonamides have a spectrum of activity primarily against Gram-negative organisms (except *Pseudomonas*). Thus they are useful in the treatment of urinary tract infection (see Chapter 23). However resistance is widespread and susceptibility cannot be assumed.

Toxicity

Sulphonamides are relatively free of toxic side effects but rashes and bone marrow suppression can occur. Rarely they cause Stevens–Johnson syndrome (see Chapter 16).

Resistance

Plasmid-mediated genes code for an altered dihydropteroate synthetase which has a greatly decreased affinity for the sulphonamide but is essentially unchanged in its affinity for PABA. Thus a resistant cell possesses two distinct enzymes – the sensitive chromosome-encoded enzyme and the resistant plasmid-encoded enzyme.

Trimethoprim (and cotrimoxazole)

Structure

Trimethoprim is one of a group of pyrimidine-like structures analogous in structure to the aminohydroxypyrimidine moiety of the folic acid molecule (Fig. 35.25). Other agents with similar structure and mechanism of action include the antimalarial pyrimethamine and the anticancer drug, methotrexate.

Mechanism of action

Trimethoprim, like sulphonamides, also prevents the synthesis of THFA but at later stage by inhibiting dihydrofolate reductase (see Fig. 35.24). This enzyme is present in

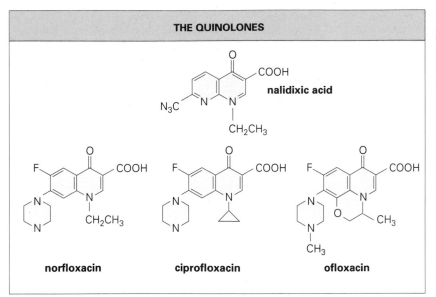

Fig. 35.26 The quinolones are a large group of synthetic antibacterial agents. This figure shows nalidixic acid and only a few of the many new agents that are being produced and evaluated at present.

mammalian cells as well as bacterial and protozoal cells and selective toxicity depends on the far greater affinity of trimethoprim for the bacterial enzyme.

Trimethoprim is often given in combination with sulphamethoxazole as cotrimoxazole. The advantages of this combination over either drug alone are:

- mutant bacteria which are resistant to one agent are unlikely to be resistant to the other (i.e. double mutation);
- the two agents act synergistically against some bacteria, i.e. the action of the combination is greater than the action of either agent alone.

Absorption, distribution and excretion
Trimethoprim can be given orally (either alone or as cotrimoxazole) or by intravenous infusion (alone or accompanied by sulphonamide in the same ratio as that given above). Trimethoprim is excreted in urine, and in patients with severe renal failure it is excreted more rapidly than sulphonamide so that the synergistic ratio of the combination may be lost.

Uses
Trimethoprim alone is active against Gram-negative rods with the exception of *Pseudomonas* species and its main use is in the treatment (and long-term prophylaxis) of urinary tract infection (see Chapter 23). However, it is now used for other Gram-negative infections where cotrimoxazole was used previously.

Cotrimoxazole is active against a wide range of urinary tract pathogens and against *S. typhi*. When given intravenously in high doses, this combination is valuable for the treatment of *Pneumocystis carinii* pneumonia. It is also useful for treatment of nocardiosis (see Chapter 33) and chancroid (see Chapter 24).

Toxicity
Trimethoprim alone and in combination with sulphameth-

oxazole can cause neutropenia. Nausea and vomiting may occur. AIDS patients seem to be more prone to toxic side effects.

Resistance
Plasmid-encoded dihydrofolate reductases with altered affinity for trimethoprim allow the synthesis of THFA to proceed unhindered by the presence of trimethoprim. The 'replacement enzymes' are approximately 20 000-fold less susceptible to trimethoprim whilst retaining their affinity for the normal substrate. Bacteria which are resistant to sulphonamide and to trimethoprim are also resistant to cotrimoxazole.

Quinolones

Structure
This is a large family of synthetic agents. Nalidixic acid is one of the earlier prototypes, but the synthesis of fluoroquinolones has led to an enormous number of chemical derivatives with improved antibacterial activity (Fig. 35.26).

Mechanism of action
Quinolones act by inhibiting the activity of DNA gyrase and thereby preventing supercoiling of the bacterial chromosome. As a result the bacterial cell can no longer 'pack' its DNA into the cell (Fig. 35.27). The inhibition is specific to bacterial gyrase and does not affect the equivalent topoisomerase enzymes in mammalian cells.

Absorption, distribution and excretion
Quinolones are administered orally, are well-absorbed from the gastro-intestinal tract and are excreted mostly in the urine but a small proportion in the faeces. Nalidixic acid does not achieve adequate serum concentrations for systemic therapy, but the newer fluoroquinolones achieve significant serum concentrations after oral dosage and are very well-distributed throughout the body compartments.

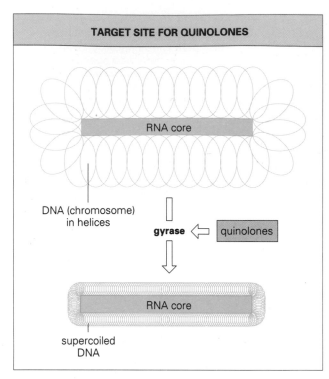

TARGET SITE FOR QUINOLONES

RNA core

DNA (chromosome) in helices

gyrase ⇐ quinolones

RNA core

supercoiled DNA

Fig. 35.27 Quinolones inhibit bacterial gyrase, the enzyme which is responsible for supercoiling bacterial DNA so that the chromosome can be packed into the bacterial cell.

Uses

Nalidixic acid is only active against enterobacteria and its use is confined to the treatment of urinary tract infection (see Chapter 23). The newer quinolones such as norfloxacin and ciprofloxacin have a greater degree of activity than nalidixic acid against Gram-negative rods. Ciprofloxacin is also active against *P. aeruginosa*. In addition to the treatment of urinary tract infection the newer quinolones are useful for systemic Gram-negative infections and may find a role in the treatment of chlamydial and rickettsial infections. They may also be useful in infections caused by other intracellular organisms such as *L. pneumophila*, *S. typhi*, and in combination with other agents for 'atypical' mycobacteria. They have activity against staphylococci but less against streptococci and enterococci are resistant.

Toxicity

Gastro-intestinal disturbances are the most common side effects. Neurotoxicity and photosensitivity reactions occur in 1–2% of patients. The fluoroquinolones are not licensed at present for use in children because of possible toxic effects on cartilage development.

Resistance

An important feature is that to date there have been no substantiated reports of plasmid-mediated resistance. However, chromosomally mediated resistance occurs and is exhibited in two forms:

- Changes in DNA gyrase subunit structure resulting in a lowered affinity for the drug.
- Changes in cell wall permeability, resulting in decreased uptake. This mechanism may also lead to cross resistance to other unrelated agents taken up by the same route.

Rifamycins

Structure

Rifampicin (Rifampin) is the most important member of this family in clinical use. It is a large molecule with a complex structure.

Mechanism of action

Rifampicin binds to RNA polymerase and blocks the synthesis of messenger RNA. Selective toxicity is based on the far greater affinity for bacterial polymerases than for the equivalent human enzymes.

Absorption, distribution and excretion

Rifampicin is administered orally, is well absorbed and very well distributed in the body. It crosses the blood brain barrier and reaches high concentrations in saliva, and also appears to have an affinity for plastics (which can be valuable in the treatment of infections involving prostheses). It is metabolized in the liver and excreted in bile. The compound is red and urine, sweat and saliva of treated patients turns orange. This is harmless although disturbing for the patient, but is good evidence of patient compliance.

Uses

The primary use for rifampicin is in the treatment of mycobacterial infections. Because of its distribution in the body (and because of bacterial resistance to other agents) rifampicin is now the drug of choice for the prophylaxis of close contacts of meningococcal and haemophilus meningitis. Short courses only (maximum 48 hours) should be given (see Chapter 27). Staphylococci are extremely susceptible to rifampicin but rapidly develop resistance (see below). However the drug can be efficacious if used in combination with another agent particularly in the treatment of prosthetic valve endocarditis (see Chapter 28).

Toxicity

Rashes and jaundice occur with rifampicin treatment. Intermittent dosage may lead to hypersensitivity reactions.

Resistance

Chromosomal mutations produce alterations in the RNA polymerase target which then has lowered affinity for rifampicin and escapes inhibition.

OTHER AGENTS THAT AFFECT DNA

Nitroimidazoles

Structure and mechanism of action
Metronidazole is a nitroimidazole with antiparasitic and antibacterial properties. It has also been used as a hypoxic cell sensitizer in radiotherapy. After entry into the microbial cell the molecule is activated by reduction and it is the reduced intermediate products are responsible for antimicrobial activity, probably through interaction with and breakage of the cell's DNA. The reactive intermediates are short-lived and decompose to nontoxic, inactive end-products. Metronidazole is active only against anaerobic organisms because only these can produce the low redox potential necessary for the reduction of the parent drug.

Absorption, distribution and excretion
Metronidazole is usually given orally or per rectum. It is well absorbed and well distributed into tissues and CSF. The drug is metabolized and most of the parent compound and the metabolites are excreted in the urine

Uses
Metronidazole was originally introduced for the treatment of the flagellate parasite *Trichomonas vaginalis* but it is also effective against other parasites such as *Giardia lamblia* and *Entamoeba coli*. It is an important agent for the treatment of infections caused by anaerobic bacteria.

Toxicity
The most serious side effects involve the central nervous system including peripheral neuropathy, but these are rare and usually seen only in patients on large doses or prolonged treatment.

Resistance
Metronidazole resistance is rare and in the few reports, the mechanism is unclear but appears to involve either an alteration in uptake or a decrease in cellular reductase activity which thereby slows the activation of intracellular drug.

INHIBITORS OF CYTOPLASMIC MEMBRANE FUNCTION

The cytoplasmic membranes which encompass all kinds of living cells perform a number of vital functions. The structure of these membranes in bacterial cells differs from that in mammalian cells and allows the application of some selectively toxic molecules but these are few in number compared with those acting at other target sites. The most important are the polymyxins which act on the membranes of Gram-negative bacteria. The polyene antifungal agents (amphotercin B, nystatin) also act by inhibiting membrane function(see below).

Polymyxins

Structure and mechanism of action
These are cyclic polypeptides. The free amino groups act as a cationic detergent which disrupts the phospholipid structure of the cell membrane. Colistin (polymyxin E) is the most common member of the family in clinical use.

Administration, distribution and excretion
Polymyxins are not absorbed orally; they have been used systemically but have now been superseded by less toxic agents.

Uses
Colistin is active against Gram-negative organisms except *Proteus* spp. As an oral agent it is used in some gut decontamination regimens for neutropenic patients. Other topical uses include wound irrigants and bladder washouts.

Toxicity
Colistin is nephrotoxic and its systemic use is no longer indicated for this reason.

Resistance
Chromosomally mediated alterations in membrane structure or antibiotic uptake have been reported.

URINARY TRACT ANTISEPTICS

Nitrofurantoin and methenamine are both synthetic compounds which when taken orally are absorbed and excreted in the urine in concentrations high enough to inhibit urinary pathogens. Nitrofurantoin has activity only in acid urine. Methenamine is hydrolysed at acid pH to produce ammonia and formaldehyde; it is the latter which has antibacterial activity. Nitrofurantoin is used to treat uncomplicated urinary tract infection and both agents are used to prevent recurrent UTIs. They have the advantage that resistance rarely develops.

ANTI-TUBERCULOUS AGENTS

The treatment of infections caused by *Mycobacterium tuberculosis* and other mycobacteria presents an enormous challenge to medicine and the pharmaceutical industry. Firstly, the waxy outer layer of these organisms means that they are naturally very impermeable and are difficult to penetrate with antibiotics. Added to this is their intracellular location, often in cells that are surrounded by a mass of caseous material. They grow and multiply extremely slowly and effective inhibition takes weeks or months to achieve. Secondly, there is the problem of drug delivery; long-term therapy means that orally administrable drugs are highly desirable and also means that the emergence of resistance among the mycobacteria and toxicity in the patient are more likely than with the 'short sharp shock' treatment more often administered for bacterial infections. Finally, there is the problem of cost of the drugs for treatment of patients in the developing world where the incidence of mycobacterial infection is high.

A number of anti-tuberculous agents are now available. Most are restricted to this use to prevent resistance emerging in other species and potentially being transferred to mycobacteria, or because the toxicity of the drugs makes them unattractive for general use.

First-line therapy

Treatment regimens may vary between countries but in general first-line (i.e. first-choice) therapy is a combination of isoniazid, ethambutol and rifampicin for 6 to 9 months. Streptomycin may be added in treatment of tuberculous meningitis. The structure and mechanism of action of rifampicin and streptomycin have been described in preceding sections.

Isoniazid

This is isonicotinic acid hydrazide, a compound which inhibits mycobacteria but does not affect other species of bacteria, or humans to any great extent. Despite use for over 30 years its mechanism of action is unclear but may involve inhibition of mycolic acid synthesis which would account for its specificity. The drug is well-absorbed after oral administration and a single daily dose is sufficient, except in the treatment of meningitis or miliary tuberculosis when the frequency of dosage should be increased to three times daily. The main toxic effects in humans are neurological complications (which can be prevented by the concurrent administration of pyridoxine), and hepatitis.

Ethambutol

Ethambutol is a synthetic molecule which inhibits but does not kill mycobacteria. Its mechanism of action is unknown but it may interfere with RNA synthesis. It is well absorbed after oral administration and well distributed in the body including the CSF. Resistance appears fairly rapidly if the drug is used alone and it should be combined with other drugs in anti-tuberculous therapy. An important toxic side-effect is optic neuritis and visual acuity should be monitored during therapy.

Second-line therapy

Despite the use of antibiotics in combination, the incidence of resistance among mycobacteria is increasing and a cure may not be achieved by the first-line drugs. Infections with mycobacteria other than *M. tuberculosis* are on the increase as opportunist infections in AIDS patients and these organisms tend to be innately more resistant than *M. tuberculosis*.

Second-line therapy for drug resistant *M. tuberculosis* includes drugs such as paraminosalicylate, pyrazinamide and thiacetazone. Their selection and administration requires specialist knowledge.

Treatment of leprosy

Infection caused by *M. leprae*, characterized by persistence of the organism in the tissues for years, necessitates very prolonged treatment to prevent relapse. For many years dapsone, a sulphone derivative (see Fig. 35.23) has been used. This drug has the advantages that it is given orally and it is cheap and effective. However, widespread use as monotherapy has resulted in the emergence of resistance and multidrug regimes are therefore preferable. Rifampicin can be combined with dapsone. Alternatively, clofazime, a phenazine compound, is active against dapsone-resistant *M. leprae* but it is expensive.

ANTIFUNGAL AGENTS

In contrast to the antibacterial drugs, the number of antifungal drugs suitable for treatment of infections is very limited. Selective toxicity is much more difficult to achieve in the eucaryotic fungal cells than in the procaryotic bacteria and although the available antifungals have greater activity against fungal cells than they do against human cells the difference is not as marked as it is for most antibacterial agents. Treatment of fungal infections is further hampered by problems of solubility, stability and absorption of the existing drugs.

Classification of antifungal drugs

Antifungals can be classified by the same scheme used for the antibacterials, i.e. on the basis of target site and chemical structure. This immediately reveals a major difference in emphasis between antibacterial and antifungal activity, with the majority of the latter acting on the synthesis or function of the cell membrane. The exceptions are flucytosine (5-fluorocytosine) and griseofulvin (Fig. 35.28). There are no inhibitors of fungal protein synthesis which do not also inhibit the equivalent mammalian pathway.

Spectrum of activity

Griseofulvin binds specifically to newly formed keratin and is active *in vivo* only against dermatophyte fungi (see Chapters 3 and 28). Other antifungals have a wider spectrum of activity, in particular amphotericin B, which remains the drug of choice for the treatment of serious systemic fungal infections, despite its serious toxic side effects. The azole antifungals act by inhibiting lanosterol C14-demethylase, an important enzyme in sterol biosynthesis. Inhibition of the fungal enzyme in preference to the human one is the key to selective toxicity. Clotrimazole and miconazole are useful as topical preparations. Ketoconazole has become the agent of choice for many serious fungal infections (Fig. 35.29), and fluconazole is increasingly used in the treatment of *Candida* infections. Further azole compounds are currently under development.

The main uses and adverse effects of the antifungals are summarized in figure 35.29. No single antifungal is ideal; the relative merits of the systemic agents are summarized in figure 35.30.

Development of new antifungal agents

Superficial fungal infections are extremely common but usually mild. Although there are several effective preparations available, some conditions e.g. ringworm infection of the nails or recurrent vaginal candidiasis are frequently intractable to treatment. Systemic fungal infections are uncommon and often present as opportunistic infections in immunocompromised people. However, the incidence of these infections is increasing in parallel with the increasing numbers of such patients and their improved survival due to effective antibacterial therapy. The number of agents available is severely limited and their adverse effects are considerable. Thus there is an urgent need for safer, more efficacious antifungal agents, and considerable resources are being channeled into the search for new agents.

CLASSIFICATION OF THE IMPORTANT ANTIFUNGAL AGENTS

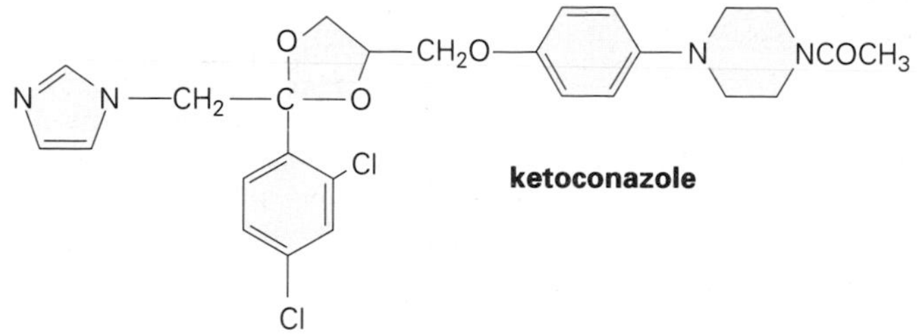

ketoconazole

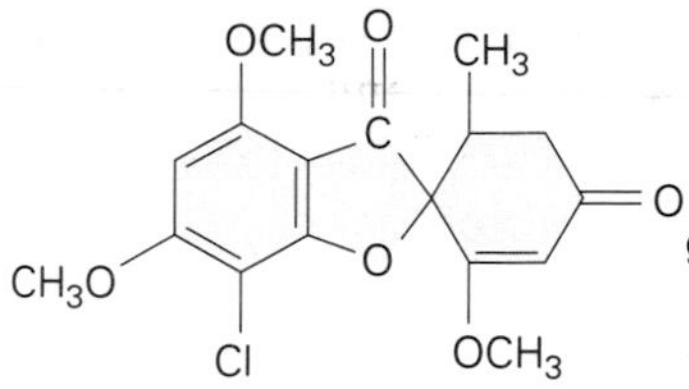

griseofulvin

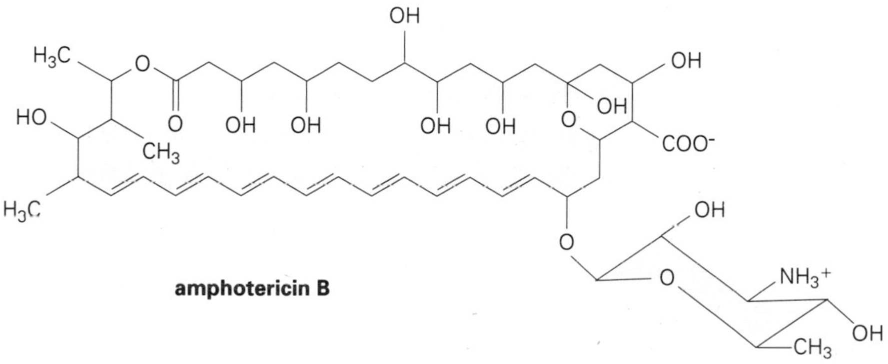

amphotericin B

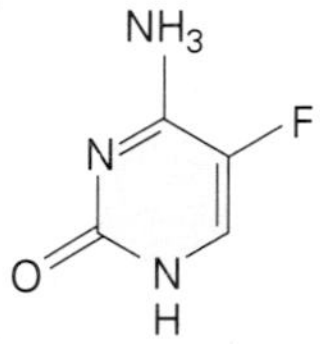

5-fluorocytosine

target	chemical group	examples	mechanism of action
Cell membrane Synthesis	azoles	miconazole ketoconazole fluconazole	inhibit lanosterol C14-demethylase by binding to cytochrome P450, resulting in inhibition of ergosterol synthesis
Function	polyenes	amphotericin B nystatin	bind to sterols (ergosterol >> cholesterol) in cell membrane, causing leakage of cellular components and cell death
Nucleic acid Synthesis	pyrimidines	flucytosine (5-fluorocytosine)	deaminated in cell to 5-fluorouracil which ultimately inhibits DNA synthesis and causes disturbance of protein synthesis
	benzofurans	griseofulvin	appears to inhibit nucleic acid synthesis and to have anti-mitotic activity possibly by inhibiting microtubule assembly, may also have effects on cell wall by inhibiting chitin synthesis

Fig. 35.28 In contrast to the target sites for antibacterial agents, target sites for antifungal agents are more limited. This reflects the difficulty in inhibiting reactions in the eucaryotic fungal cell and not in the human cell. A variety of other agents such as Whitfield's ointment (a mixture of benzoic and salicylic acids), tolnaftate, ciclopirox, haloprigin and naftifine, are available as creams for the topical treatment of superficial mycoses. These are generally available without prescription and there is little to choose between them.

ANTIVIRAL THERAPY

For most viral infections there is no specific treatment. Effective antiviral drugs are few in number (Fig. 35.31), in contrast to the great range of successful antibiotics available for bacterial infections. The shortage of antivirals is partly due to the difficulty of interfering with viral activity in the cell without adversely affecting the host. However, the advent of AIDS has stimulated intensive research, and new antiviral drugs will undoubtedly appear. Also, virus-specific replication steps can be identified (Fig. 35.32) and more of these will doubtless be exploited.

There are two other problems with the therapy of virus infections:

THERAPEUTIC APPLICATIONS OF ANTIFUNGAL AGENTS			
infection	antifungal of choice	route of administration	adverse effects
superficial mycoses			
Ringworm (dermatophytes)	griseofulvin	oral	nil
	ketoconazole	oral	anorexia, nausea vomiting; dose-dependent depression of serum testosterone leading to gynecomastia
Candidiasis	fluconazole	oral	inhibits metabolism of cyclosporin when given at high doses
	nystatin	topical	nil
systemic mycoses			
Histoplasmosis	ketoconazole	oral	see above
Blastomycosis	ketoconazole	oral	see above
Coccidioidomycosis	ketaconazole (amphotericin B for CNS involvement)	oral	do not use ketaconazole and amphotericin B together (some evidence of antagonism)
Paracoccidioido-mycosis	ketoconazole	oral	see above
Aspergillosis	amphotericin B	IV (now available in liposomes)	nephrotoxicity and potassium loss; acute reactions within 1/2 - 1 1/2 hrs of injection include rigors and hypotension
Candidiasis	fluconazole amphotericin B + flucytosine	oral IV oral	flucytosine may cause neutropenia and jaundice; emergence of resistant mutants is common if drug is used alone; combination with amphotericin B can be synergistic
Cryptococcosis	amphotericin B + flucytosine	IV oral	
Zygomycosis	amphotericin B	IV	

Fig. 35.29 The major therapeutic applications of antifungal drugs. Orally active agents are important for the treatment of superficial mycoses which are often minor but troublesome infections and may require prolonged treatment. Amphotericin is the most important agent for the treatment of severe systemic mycoses, but this agent is toxic and the advent of azole antifungals particularly ketoconazole and some of the newer agents may provide suitable alternative therapy in some instances.

RELATIVE MERITS OF SYSTEMIC ANTIFUNGALS			
	amphotericin	flucytosine	ketoconazole
Broad spectrum of antifungal activity	+	−	+
Emergence of resistance	−	+	?*
Ease of maintaining high concentrations at site of infection	−	+	−
High concentrations in urine	−	+	−
Oral formulation	−	+	+
Serious toxic side effects	+	−	±
* data on emergence of resistance not yet clear			

Fig. 35.30 Antifungal agents suitable for use in systemic infections fall into three groups. The most serious drawbacks with amphotericin are the problems of toxicity whereas flucytosine has relatively narrow range antifungal activity and the emergence of resistance is common. Ketoconazole represents the newer azole antifungal drugs and there will be further developments in this field.

THE STRUCTURE OF ANTIVIRAL AGENTS

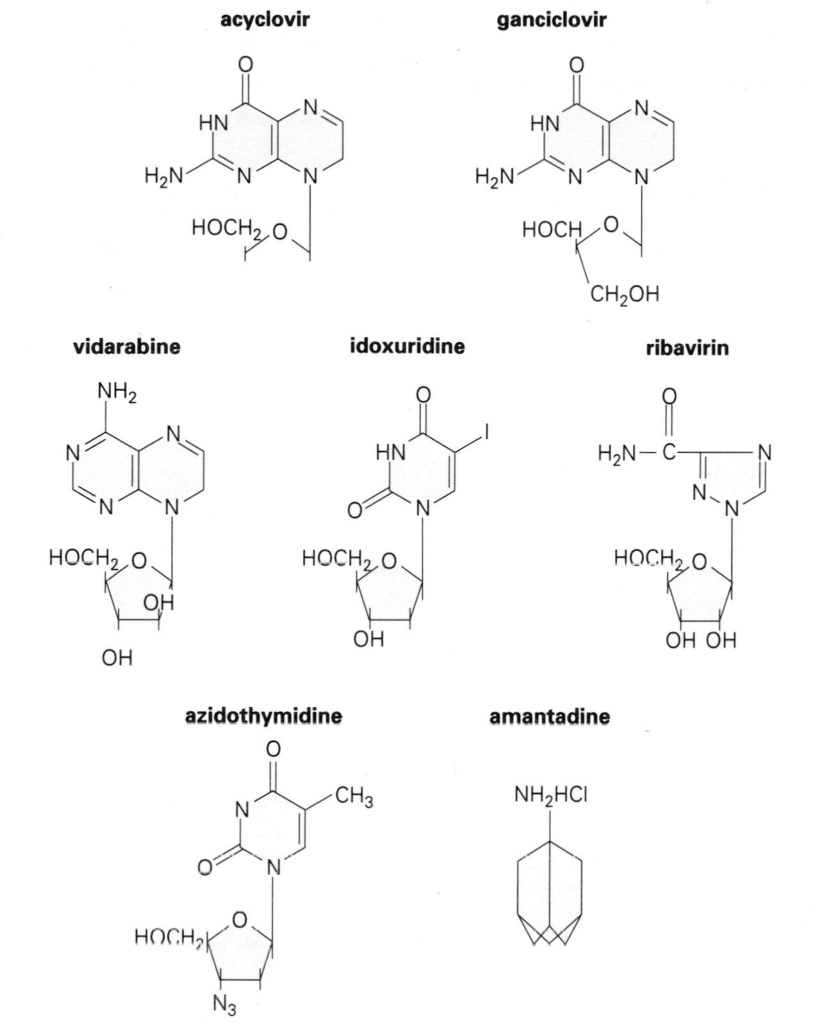

acyclovir

ganciclovir

vidarabine

idoxuridine

ribavirin

azidothymidine

amantadine

Fig. 35.31 Antiviral agents are few in number and narrow in their spectrum of activity, e.g. amantadine is effective against influenza A but not other myxoviruses, acyclovir is effective against HSV and V-ZV but not CMV or EBV.

SITE OF ACTION OF ANTIVIRAL AGENTS

replication stage	drugs available	
1 Adsorption	none available	
2 Penetration and uncoating	amantadine	
3 Viral DNA/RNA synthesis	idoxuridine vidarabine acyclovir zidovudine ribavirin	
4 Viral protein synthesis	interferons	
5 Assembly	none available	
6 Release	none available	

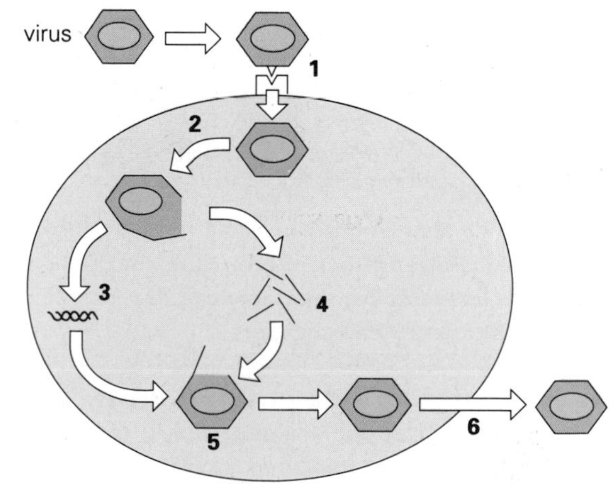

Fig. 35.32 The site of action of antiviral agents. Resistance to agents is uncommon, but does occur, e.g. CMV strains resistant to ganciclovir, HSV strains resistant to acyclovir.

- The incubation period is often a week or more, and by the time the patient becomes ill most of the spread and replication of virus has already taken place (e.g. mumps, polio). Infection cannot be diagnosed during the incubation period and even after the patient becomes ill laboratory diagnosis often takes several days. Some of the rapid (24 hour) diagnostic methods currently being developed will help overcome this problem;
- Viruses that are latent in cells and not actively replicating (e.g. latent herpes viruses) are generally insusceptible to antivirals.

Viruses are resistant to antibacterial antibiotics, although the latter may be needed to control secondary bacterial infection, for instance in influenzal pneumonia.

Acyclovir (acycloguanosine)

This drug has virtually replaced the other nucleosides in the treatment of herpes virus infections.

Mode of action

Acyclovir (Fig. 35.33) is phosphorylated by the herpes virus thymidine kinase and the monophosphate is then converted by cellular kinases to the triphosphate, which acts by inhibiting the herpes virus DNA polymerase. The drug is also incorporated into viral DNA, resulting in chain termination. Because acyclovir is inactive until phosphorylated and is efficiently phosphorylated only in infected cells, toxic side effects (neutropenia, thrombocytopenia) are usually not severe. The drug acts on herpes simplex and varicella-zoster viruses but is almost inactive against CMV and EB virus.

Use

Acyclovir is used topically to treat primary genital herpes, herpes simplex virus dendritic ulcers and, less effectively, for cold sores and zoster. Systemic acyclovir has revolutionized the treatment of herpes simplex encephalitis, and herpes simplex and V-ZV infections in immunocompromised patients.

Ganciclovir (dihydroxypropoxymethylguanine, DHPG)

This drug is active against cytomegalovirus, and is valuable in disseminated CMV infections and in CMV retinitis in AIDS patients.

Vidarabine

This nucleoside analogue is converted to the triphosphate by cellular kinases and then inhibits the viral DNA polymerase. It is less effective than acyclovir, but can be used topically for herpetic dendritic ulcers.

Iododeoxyuridine (idoxuridine, IDU).

This is another nucleoside analogue that is triphosphorylated by cellular kinases and then incorporated into viral DNA. The virus produced is therefore defective. But it is also incorporated into cellular DNA which makes it too toxic to be used systemically. It can be used for dendritic ulcers.

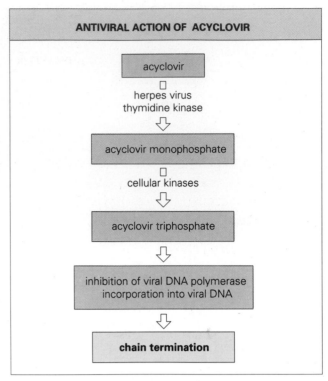

Fig. 35.33 The activity of an antiviral agent against different herpes viruses is correlated with their ability to induce a thymidine kinase, hence acyclovir is most active against HSV, least active against CMV.

Zidovudine (azidothymidine, AZT, 'Retrovir')

Zidovudine is another nucleoside analogue in which the hydroxyl group on the ribose is replaced by an azido group. After conversion to the triphosphate by cellular enzymes (Fig. 35.34) it acts as an inhibitor of and substrate for, the viral reverse transcriptase. Proviral DNA formation is blocked because the drug is incorporated into the DNA with resulting chain termination. Zidovudine is currently the most useful drug for patients with AIDS-related complex (ARC) and AIDS, and when used in the earlier asymptomatic stages of HIV infection will decrease progression to ARC and AIDS.

Zidovudine is given orally. Toxicity is a problem, with bone marrow suppression (anaemia, neutropenia, leucopenia) and less commonly nausea, vomiting, myalgia, malaise, etc.). Regular tests are given for anaemia and myelosuppression. It is also very expensive. Drug resistance has not so far been a clinical problem, but resistant mutants have been isolated in the laboratory.

Deoxycytidine (ddc) and deoxyinosine (ddi)

Trials on these related drugs are in progress, with the hope that side effects may be less marked. Synergism with acyclovir has been shown, and combined drug schedules may be developed.

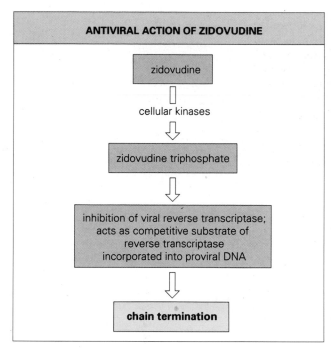

Fig. 35.34 HIV reverse transcriptase is 100 times more sensitive to zidovudine triphosphate than is host cell DNA polymerase, but toxic effects are not uncommon.

Ribavirin

This guanosine analogue has various actions including inhibition of production of guanosine triphosphate pools needed for viral nucleic acid synthesis. It is used clinically as an aerosol for severe RSV infection in infants, for severe influenza B and for arenavirus infections such as lassa fever (see Chapter 31).

Amantidine

It has been known since the 1960s that this drug specifically inhibits the replication of influenza A viruses, but influenza B and other respiratory viruses are unaffected. It acts by inhibiting the penetration of virus into the cell or its uncoating. With the standard dose (200 mg/day orally) there are minor neurologic side effects (insomnia, dizziness, headache etc.), especially in elderly patients, and this has discouraged its widespread use. When given prophylactically during community outbreaks amantidine is about as effective as influenza vaccine in preventing illness. It can also be used for treatment, and if taken within 48 hours of symptoms there is a reduction in disease that far outways the drug's toxic effects.

Uses of interferons in human infection

Interferons (IFNs; see Chapter 12) show a dramatic effect on virus replication *in vitro* (at picograms of IFN per ml) and are active against certain experimental virus infections. However, their clinical use has been disappointing. One problem has been that their very short half-life in the circulation makes it difficult to deliver adequate amounts of IFN to sites of infection. Very large intravenous doses have an established role in the treatment of chronic hepatitis B and C infection. IFNs can be shown to have an effect on papillomavirus infections (intralesional injection) and on certain herpes virus infections, but are not routinely used.

Side effects

Many patients experience flu-like symptoms (fever, myalgia, headache), even with genetically engineered IFNs. Indeed such symptoms in virus infections have been attributed to the action of endogenously produced IFNs. Leucopenia, thrombocytopenia, and CNS effects have also been noted, especially with high dose treatment.

ANTIPARASITIC AGENTS

Any consideration of antiparasitic agents must take into account the vast number of different parasites capable of infecting man, the complexities of their life cycles and differences in their metabolism. Parasites can be divided into two groups – the protozoa and the helminths (see Chapter 3). The protozoa are unicellular organisms, often with complicated life cycles, whereas the helminths have highly developed internal structures and integuments. Thus it is no surprise that the drugs acting against protozoa are usually inactive against helminths, and vice versa.

A wide array of different drugs have been developed, and these are summarized in figures 35.35 and 35.36. The problems of finding agents that are toxic to the parasite and not to man are considerable, and many of the agents have unpleasant side effects. Some antibacterial agents also have antiprotozoal activity, indicating that their toxicity is not limited to procaryotic cells.

LABORATORY ASPECTS OF ANTIBACTERIAL AGENTS

It will be clear from the preceding sections of this chapter that although there are certain 'rules of thumb' about resistance of bacteria to an antibiotic, it is often impossible to do more than guess in the absence of laboratory tests. Susceptibility tests performed in the laboratory examine the interaction between antibiotics and bacteria in an isolated and rather artificial fashion. At best the results are a helpful guide to the likely outcome of therapy; at worst they are misleading. Patient factors such as age, underlying disease, renal and liver impairment, must be taken into account in the the antibiotic management of an infection.

Susceptibility tests

Laboratory tests for antibiotic susceptibility fall into two main categories:
- Diffusion tests
- Dilution tests

THERAPEUTIC APPLICATIONS OF MAJOR ANTI-PROTOZOAL DRUGS			
disease/site	**agent**	**route of administration**	**safety**
Amoebiasis			
Lumen	diloxanide furoate	oral	safe
Tissue	metronidazole	oral	treatment of chronic mild infection and of extra-intestinal infections, all safe
	tinidazole	oral	
	dehydroemetine	IM	treatment of acute and hepatic infections
	chloroquine	oral	dehydroemetine has some toxicity
Amoebic meningoencephalitis	amphotericin B	IV	nephrotoxic, fever
Cryptosporidiosis	spiramycin	oral	experimental, effective agent awaited
Giardiasis	metronidazole	oral	safe
	tinidazole	oral	safe
	furazolidone	oral	toxic; hypersensitivity reactions
Leishmaniasis	antimonials	IV/IM	toxic
	pentamidine	IM	
	amphotericin B	IV	
Malaria			
Pre-erthyrocytic stages	primaquine	oral	radical cure, some toxicity (risk of favism in G6PDH deficient patients)
Blood stages	chloroquine	oral	generally safe
	quinine	oral, IM	some toxicity, used against drug resistant *P. falciparum*
	proguanil	oral	used with chloroquine
	pyrimethamine		used in combination with sulphadoxine
	tetracycline	oral	used against drug resistant *P. falciparum*
	mefloquine	oral	mild side effects
Pneumocystis	trimethoprim + sulphamethoxazole	oral	side effects, e.g. rash, neutropenia
Toxoplasmosis	pentamidine	IM and aerosolized	toxic IM, shock
Trichomoniasis	pyrimethamine sulphadiazine	oral	safe, but long-term treatment may produce anaemia
	metronidazole	oral	safe
	tinidazole	oral	safe
Trypanosomiasis			
African	suramin	IV	toxic
	pentamidine	IM	toxic
	melarsoprol	IV	toxic, passes blood–brain barrier
	tryparsamide	IV	toxic, passes blood–brain barrier
American	nifurtimox	oral	side effects common
	benznidazole	oral	side effects common

Fig. 35.35 Therapeutic applications of the major antiprotozoal drugs. Several are potentially toxic and must be given under supervision. Some also have antibacterial activity and have been described in detail earlier in the chapter. Drug resistance is a problem, particularly in the treatment of malaria.

THERAPEUTIC APPLICATIONS OF MAJOR ANTHELMINTIC DRUGS		
disease	**agent**	**safety**
cestodes (tapeworms)		
Adult stage infection	niclosamide	safe
	praziquantel	safe, can prevent cysticercosis following infection with *T. solium*
Larval stage (e.g. hydatid disease, cysticercosis)	benzimidazole carbonates	safe, but limited use
trematodes (flukes)		
Schistosomiasis and intestinal flukes	praziquantel oxamniquine	safe, mild side effects
Liver and lung fluke infection	praziquantel	
nematodes (roundworms)		
Ascariasis and pinworm infection	mebendazole albendazole flubendazole	all are safe drugs[†], mebendazole drug of choice
	pyrantel pamoate	safe[†], mild side effects, not used in children <1 year
	piperazine	safe[†], except in epilepsy
Hookworm infection	mebendazole albendazole flubendazole	all are safe drugs[†] mebendazole drug of choice
	pyrantel pamoate	safe[†], mild side effects, not used or children <1 year
Strongyloidiasis	thiabendazole	mild side effects[†]
Trichinosis	mebendazole albendazole flubendazole	all are safe drugs[†] mebendazole drug of choice
	thiabendazole	mild side effects[†]
Trichuriasis	mebendazole	safe[†]
Cutaneous larva migrans (infection with animal hookworm)	albendazole thiabendazole*	safe[†] mild side effects[†]
Toxocariasis (visceral larva migrans)	thiabendazole mebendazole	mild side effects[†] safe[†]
Lymphatic filariasis	diethyl carbamizine ivermectin	allergic side effects mild side effects
Aberrant or unusual species	mebendazole thiabendazole	drugs of choice for majority of infections

* topical administration
[†] not used in pregnancy

Fig. 35.36 Therapeutic applications of the major anthelmintic drugs. All are administered orally except thiabendazole for larva migrans, which is administered topically. Note that many of these drugs are not safe in pregnancy.

Diffusion tests

The isolate to be tested is seeded over the entire surface of an agar plate and filter paper discs containing the antibiotics are applied. After overnight incubation the plate is observed for zones of inhibition around each antibiotic

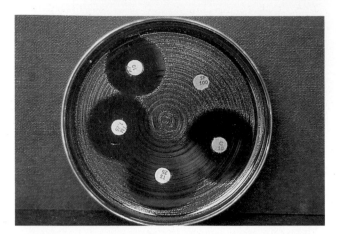

Fig. 35.37 The antibiotic susceptibility of an organism can be tested by the application of filter paper discs impregnated with antibiotic onto a lawn of the organisms seeded on an agar plate. After overnight incubation during which time the organism grows and the antibiotics diffuse from the discs, a zone of inhibition of develops indicating the degree of susceptibility of the organism. This plate shows the antibiotic susceptibility of *Shigella*, indicating sulphonamide resistance. (SF100 is the sulphonamide disc.) Courtesy of DK Banerjee.

disc (Fig. 35.37). The amount of antibiotic in the disc is related to, among other things, the achievable serum concentration and therefore differs for different antibiotics. In addition, antibiotics differ in their ability to diffuse in agar, so that the size of the inhibition zone, and not simply its presence, is an indicator of susceptibility of the isolate. The zone sizes are compared with those for reference organisms and the result recorded as S (susceptible), I (intermediate) or R (resistant). An 'I' result indicates that the isolate is less susceptible than the norm but may respond to higher doses of antibiotic or in sites where the antibiotic is concentrated (e.g. in the bladder urine for antibiotics excreted by the kidneys).

Dilution tests

A more quantitative estimate of susceptibility can be achieved by performing an MIC ('minimum inhibitory concentration') test, i.e. a test to find the lowest concentration that will inhibit visible growth *in vitro*. A series of dilutions of the test antibiotic is prepared in broth or agar medium and inoculated with a suspension of the test organism. After overnight incubation, the MIC is recorded as the highest dilution in which there is no macroscopic growth (Fig. 35.38). MIC tests are clearly more costly in terms of time and materials and are not required for every isolate from every patient, but they yield information which is useful in the management of difficult infections such as bacterial endocarditis or in patients who are failing to respond to apparently appropriate therapy.

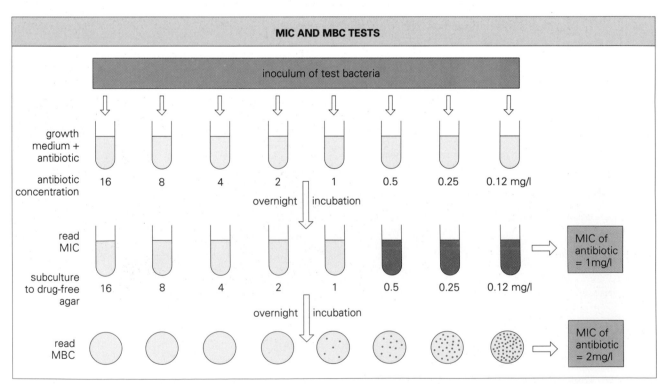

Fig. 35.38 More precise measures of the amount of antibiotic required to inhibit and kill a bacterial population can be estimated by establishing the minimum inhibitory concentration (MIC) and minimum bactericidal concentration (MBC) of the antibiotic. Using the standard method as outlined in the figure, the MIC result is available after 24 hours and the MBC result after 48 hours. A number of variables such as the inoculum size, the growth medium and the interpretation of the results will affect the results of MIC tests.

An advantage of an MIC test is that it can be extended to determine the MBC ('minimum bactericidal concentration', the lowest concentration of an antibiotic required to kill the organism) of an antibiotic. In order to discover whether the agent has actually killed the bacteria rather than simply inhibited their growth, the test dilutions are subcultured onto fresh, drug-free medium and incubated for a further 18-24 hours (see Fig. 35.38). The antibacterial agent is considered to be bactericidal if the MBC is equal to or not greater than four-fold higher than the MIC.

Killing curves

One of the disadvantages of MIC and MBC tests is that the result is read at only one point in time. A more dynamic estimate of bacterial susceptibility can be gained by measuring the decrease in viability of the population with time. (Fig. 35.39). As with MIC tests, it is not feasible to perform killing curves manually for every test isolate but they can provide useful information for difficult treatment problems. A number of the automated susceptibility test systems utilize a measure of bacterial viability (e.g. turbidity, electrical impedance) in the presence of antibacterial as their indicator system. These machines can produce results more rapidly (about 5 hours) than conventional susceptibility tests.

COMBINATIONS OF ANTIBACTERIAL AGENTS

Hospital patients frequently receive more than one antibacterial agent and these agents may interact with each other (and also with other drugs such as diuretics).

Antibacterial combinations are described as:
- 'synergistic', if their activity is greater than the sum of the individual activities; or
- 'antagonistic', if the activity of one drug is compromised in the presence of the other.

Both diffusion and dilution tests allow the action of combinations of antibiotics to be studied (Fig. 35.40). Although synergy can often be demonstrated *in vitro*, it is difficult to

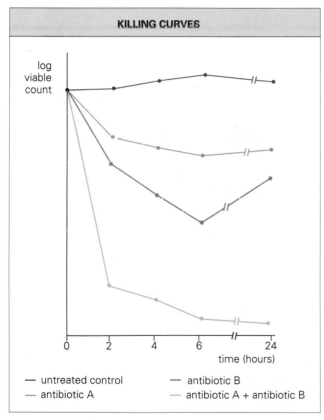

Fig. 35.39 A more dynamic picture of the interaction between an antibiotic and a bacterial population can be gained from performing killing curves. In these experiments a culture of 2 x 10⁶ c.f.u./ml was treated with antibiotics A and B alone and in combination. Compared with the untreated control both A and B inhibited the growth of the bacterial culture but B is more active than A. However in combination the activity of A plus B is synergistic, i.e. it is more active than the sum of the activities of the two antibiotics alone. The combination also prevents the regrowth which is seen between 6 and 24 hours when the antibiotics are used singly.

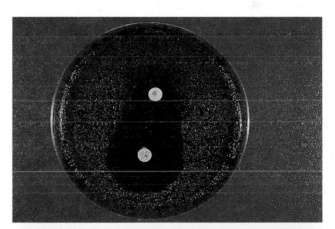
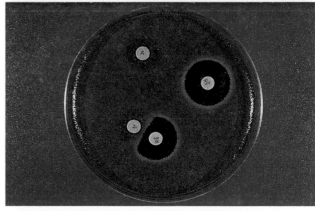

Fig. 35.40 Discs containing sulphonamide and trimethoprim (top) have been placed to demonstrate the synergistic activity of these two agents against *Escherichia coli*. Synergy can be recognized by the fact that the zones of inhibition become continuous between the two discs. Nitrofurantoin is capable of antagonising the activity of nalidixic acid, as shown (bottom). When the discs are placed far apart nalidixic acid inhibits the test organism but when placed close together this inhibition is antagonized by the presence of nitrofurantoin, evidenced by the foreshortening of the zone of inhibition.

35.31

USE OF ANTIBIOTIC COMBINATIONS
to obtain a synergistic effect e.g. cotrimoxazole
to prevent or delay emergence of persistent organisms e.g. isoniazid, rifampicin and ethambutol for tuberculosis
to treat polymicrobial infections e.g. intra abdominal abcesses where the different microbes have different susceptibilities
to treat serious infections in the stage before the infectious agent is identified

Fig. 35.41 Reasons for use of antibiotic combinations. Ideally, single drugs are used, but antibiotic combinations are justifiable under certain circumstances.

ANTIBIOTIC ASSAYS ARE IMPORTANT
When an antibiotic has a narrow therapeutic index e.g. aminoglycosides
When the normal route of excretion of antibiotic is impaired e.g. in patients with renal failure for agents excreted via the kidney
When the absorption of the antibiotic is uncertain e.g. after oral administration
To ascertain concentrations in sites of infection into which penetration of antibiotic is irregular or unknown e.g. in CSF
In patients receiving prolonged therapy for serious infections e.g. endocarditis
In neonates with serious infections
In patients who fail to respond to apparently appropriate therapy
To check on patient compliance

Fig. 35.42 Assays of antibiotics in clinical practice are particularly important when the antibiotic is potentially toxic, but there are a number of other situations in which assays are important.

confirm *in vivo*. Cotrimoxazole is an example if a combination frequently used (see above). Another example is in the treatment of endocarditis caused by *Enterococcus* spp. where the combination of penicillin (or ampicillin) with gentamicin has been shown to be clearly superior to the beta-lactam alone (Fig. 35.41).

Antagonism can be demonstrated between some pairs of antibiotics in vitro but is rarely evident in vivo.

ANTIBIOTIC ASSAYS

In the preceding sections of this chapter the pharmacokinetic properties (absorption, distribution, excretion) of antibacterial agents have been summarized. Some antibacterials have a narrow 'therapeutic index' i.e. the concentration required for successful treatment and the concentration toxic to the patient are not very different. The concentrations of such antibiotics should be monitored both to prevent toxicity and to ensure that therapeutic concentrations are achieved. Other less toxic agents should be monitored in some circumstances in some patients (Fig. 35.42). Concentrations are usually measured in serum but urine, CSF and other body fluids can be assayed where applicable.

Antibiotic assays can be performed in a manner similar to that described above for diffusion susceptibility tests. The method lends itself to the assay of almost any antibiotic but it requires technical skill and time before the result is available (about 18 hours). Nowadays most laboratories use automated techniques based on immunological methods employing labelled antibodies to each antibiotic. Such methods are rapid, require only small volumes of serum, and are highly specific. However they are available only for a limited range of antibiotics.

USE AND ABUSE OF ANTIMICROBIAL AGENTS

Much has been said in this chapter about the interactions between antimicrobial agents and microbes: the mechanisms of selective toxicity and the defences put up by resistant organisms. The distribution, metabolism and excretion of agents by the host has been considered briefly, together with the important toxic side effects of the agents. The choice of antimicrobial for treating specific infections is dealt with in the appropriate systems chapters (see Chapters 19 to 33). Dosage regimes have not been included because they vary with the agent, the infection, the age and underlying condition of the patient, and sometimes from one country to another. Practitioners should consult appropriate local pharmacy guidelines.

In conclusion we should stand back and ask "Is antimicrobial therapy necessary for this patient, and if so which agent is appropriate?" Antimicrobial agents can be used to help prevent infection (prophylaxis) or to treat infection. Prophylactic use of antibiotics is appropriate only in a few clearly-defined circumstances and is usually of limited duration (1–2 days) (Fig. 35.43). For example peri-operative antibiotic 'cover' for patients with known cardiac defects to prevent endocarditis or in abdominal surgery, when the risk of faecal soiling of the peritoneal cavity and the wound is high. In the community, the main uses are for close contacts of bacterial meningitis or tuberculosis.

If treatment is necessary then several factors must be considered and these are summarized in figure 35.44. It is important to recognize that during treatment not only the infecting microbe but the patient and all his normal microbial flora are being exposed to the effects of the antimicrobial agent. Use of antimicrobials has been clearly shown to select for resistant strains both in the individual and in the community and overuse or inappropriate use only increases this risk. History suggests that microbes will never run out of ways of developing resistance.

INDICATIONS FOR PROPHYLACTIC USE OF ANTIBIOTICS
patients of normal susceptibility exposed to specific pathogens
Rifampicin to eradicate carriage of *Neisseria meningitidis* and *H. influenzae* type b in people who have had close contact with a case of meningitis
Isoniazid to asymptomatic contacts of a case of active tuberculosis
patients with increased susceptibility to infection
Penicillin (or erythromycin if penicillin-allergic) for patients with damaged or prosthetic heart valves undergoing dental or other operations, to prevent endocarditis
Penicillin (long-term) for patients who have had rheumatic fever, to prevent recurrent streptococcal infections
Oral, non-absorbable antibiotics (e.g. framycetin and colistin) for neutropenic patients – to reduce aerobic gut flora and help to prevent endogenous Gram-negative bacteraemia
patients undergoing surgery
Penicillin or metronidazole for patients having implantation or amputation operations on the lower limbs, to prevent clostridial infection
Ampicillin and metronidazole (or other appropriate combination) or cefoxitin (or other broad-spectrum cephalosporin) for patients having abdominal operations when faecal soiling of the peritoneum is likely – to prevent endogenous infection with gut organisms
Cloxacillin and gentamicin for patients having major cardiovascular, *orthopaedic or neurosurgical operations – to prevent infection particularly with skin organisms
* local antibiotic policies may differ on choice of agents

Fig. 35.43 Antibiotics should not be used indiscriminately with a view to eradicating organisms, but in well-defined situations prophylaxis is valuable and may be life-saving.

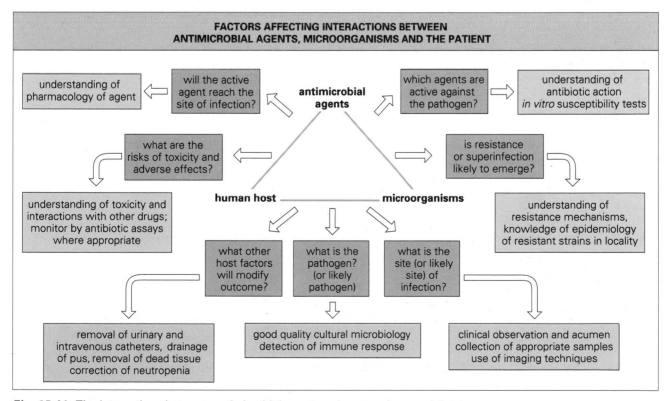

Fig. 35.44 The interactions between antimicrobial agents, microorganisms and the human host can be summarized by posing several questions affecting each side of the triangle of interaction, and examining the answers to these questions.

SUMMARY

There are now many different antibacterial agents, which can be classified into groups on the basis of their site of action in the bacterial cell and their chemical structure. There are fewer antifungal and antiviral agents and development of further agents in these classes is hindered by the difficulty of discovering and designing agents with appropriate selective toxicity.

Antimicrobial agents are undoubtedly valuable in the treatment of, and in well-defined circumstances in the prevention of, infection. However, their inappropriate use carries with it potential risks to the patient of toxicity and superinfection, and to the community of selection of resistant organisms. Finally, of course, there is also the consideration of cost.

Further Reading

Brock TD. *Milestones in microbiology.* London: Prentice-Hall International Inc., 1961.

Dolin R. Antiviral chemotherapy and chemoprophylaxis. *Science* 1985; **227;** 1296–1303.

Franklin TJ, Snow GA. *Biochemistry of antimicrobial action.* London: Chapman and Hall,1989.

Garrod GLP, Lambert HP, O'Grady F. *Antibiotic and chemotherapy.* London: Churchill Livingstone, 1992.

Lorian V, ed. *Antibiotics in laboratory medicine.* Maryland: Williams & Wilkins, 1980.

Marriott MS. Rational design of a magic bullet: antifungal drugs. *Rev Med Microbiol* 1990: **1:** 151–159.

36 VACCINATION

Contents

INTRODUCTION

"Never in the history of human progress," wrote the pathologist Geoffrey Edsall, "has a better and cheaper method of preventing illness been developed than immunization at its best." It is a sobering thought that the greatest success story in medicine, the elimination of smallpox, began before either immunology or microbiology were recognized as disciplines – indeed before the existence of microbes or the immune system was even suspected. It is in honour of the pioneering work of Jenner with vaccinia (see panel) that all forms of specific, actively induced immunity are nowadays referred to as 'vaccination'.

The principle of vaccination is simple: to induce in the patient a 'primed' state such that on first contact with the relevant infection, a more rapid and effective secondary immune response will be mounted, leading to prevention of disease. Vaccination depends on the ability of lymphocytes, both B and T, to respond to specific antigens and develop into memory cells, and thus represents a form of actively enhanced adaptive immunity. The passive administration of pre-formed elements such as antibody is considered in Chapter 37.

THE AIMS OF VACCINATION

The most ambitious aim, so far only realized for smallpox, is obviously the eradication of the disease in question. Which other diseases will follow smallpox into oblivion depends on many subtle features of host-parasite balance (discussed in Chapter 37), but there has clearly been a dramatic downward trend in the incidence of most of the diseases against which vaccines are currently in use (Fig. 36.2). But as long as any focus of infection remains in the community, the main effect of vaccination will be the protection of the individual against infection. In certain cases an even more limited aim may suffice, namely to protect the individual against symptoms or pathology, where the simple presence of the microbe is not itself harmful: diphtheria and tetanus are examples of 'anti-disease' rather than anti-microbial vaccines. And finally, in the case of vector-borne diseases with a well-defined infective stage, e.g. malaria, one can visualize a vaccine that will block transmission without benefiting the vaccinated individual at all - the 'altruistic' vaccine.

REQUIREMENTS OF A GOOD VACCINE

Whichever of the above aims it is designed to achieve, a vaccine should as far as possible be effective, safe, stable and of low cost.

- To be *effective* a vaccine must not only induce an adequate response, but the response must also be of the right type. Thus, a purely antibody response is unlikely to be of benefit against tuberculosis, or a purely cell-mediated one against streptococcal pneumonia, while high levels of serum antibody may be irrelevant to mucosal protection against polio, and activation of cytotoxic T cells may be positively harmful in hepatitis.

The duration of the response is also of prime importance. For short-term protection, e.g. a tourist about to visit a disease area, the presence of antibody arising from the vaccine itself may be perfectly adequate and memory cells may not be strictly necessary. On the other

Edward Jenner (1749–1823)

The English physician Edward Jenner is regarded as the founder of modern vaccination, but he was by no means the first to try the technique. The ancient practice of 'variolation' goes back to tenth century China, and arrived in Europe in the early 18th century by way of Turkey. The technique involved the inoculation of children with dried material from healed scabs of mild smallpox cases, and was a striking foretaste of the principles of modern attenuated viral vaccines. This practice was, however, both inconsistent and dangerous, and Jenner's innovation was to show that a much safer and more reliable protection could be obtained by deliberate inoculation with cowpox (vaccinia) virus. Milkmaids exposed to this infection were traditionally known to be resistant to smallpox and so retain their smooth complexions. In 1796, Jenner tested his theory by inoculating eight-year-old James Phipps with liquid from a cowpox pustule on the hand of Sarah Nelmes. Subsequent inoculation of the boy with smallpox produced no disease. (Note that such an experiment would today be considered extremely unethical!). Jenner's book *"An inquiry into the causes and effects of the Variolae Vaccinae, a disease discovered in some of the Western counties of England, particularly Gloucestershire, and known by the name of The Cow Pox."*, published in 1798, is a classic of its kind –

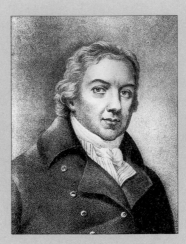

Fig. 36.1 Edward Jenner (1749-1823).

lively, stylish and well-argued. Although greeted with scepticism at first, Jenner's ideas soon became accepted and he went on to inoculate thousands of patients, in a shed in the garden of his house at Berkeley, Gloucestershire. He ultimately achieved world fame, though his fellowship of the Royal Society was conferred for a quite different piece of work on the nesting habits of the cuckoo! His house at Berkeley is now preserved as a museum, and is used for small symposia by the British Society of Immunology.

hand, for protection against exposure at some time in the future, the induction of memory is essential; here the benefit will be correspondingly greater the longer the incubation period of the infection, because the immune system has more time to mount a secondary response. Fortunately, memory is often naturally boosted by periodic outbreaks of disease in the community (e.g. the annual measles and mumps epidemics), but as diseases gradually die out this can no longer be relied on. Paradoxically, therefore, the less disease there is in the population, the more important it is to keep up vaccination – a point that parents often do not appreciate.

In general, living vaccines induce stronger and more lasting immunity than non-living ones (see below).

- The *safety* of vaccines has become a major consideration in recent years; indeed, the very high cost of the awards that can follow successful litigation for vaccine-induced damage has been an element in the retreat of several commercial organisations from vaccine production and development (coupled with the fact that vaccination is inherently less profitable than chemotherapy, see below). Moreover, vaccines are the only compounds routinely given to perfectly healthy people.

In fact, considering the enormous number of vaccine administrations (at least 20 000 000 a year in the USA alone), the safety record is extremely good. Nevertheless there have been a few serious vaccine accidents, such as the Lubeck disaster of 1926 (see Chapter

13), and safety testing is now very rigorous, requiring extensive quality control and animal trials. The problems encountered in assuring the safety of vaccines are summarized in figure 36.3

- *Stability* is, of course, a requirement of all compounds destined to remain on the shelf for long periods, but is particularly critical with living attenuated vaccines. Maintenance of the 'cold chain' between the factory and the clinic – which may be a small field hospital thousands of miles away – is not easy, and in one study with measles vaccine in Cameroon, only one dose in six actually reached the patient in an active form. The attenuated polio vaccine has been shown to be stable for a year at 4°C but only a few days at 37°C.

- The *cost* of a vaccine is of course relative, and one might even think that $80 spent on a vaccine that prevented hepatitis B, a potentially fatal infection and one of the major causes of liver carcinoma, was money well spent. However in terms of the health budget of a typical developing country, such vaccines – and indeed many much cheaper ones – are clearly out of reach of the ordinary population. Fortunately the World Health Organization has set up several programmes which specifically direct international funding towards vaccines against diseases of particular importance in the developing world (Fig. 36.4).

The question of whether vaccines made by new technology will be less, or more, expensive, is discussed below.

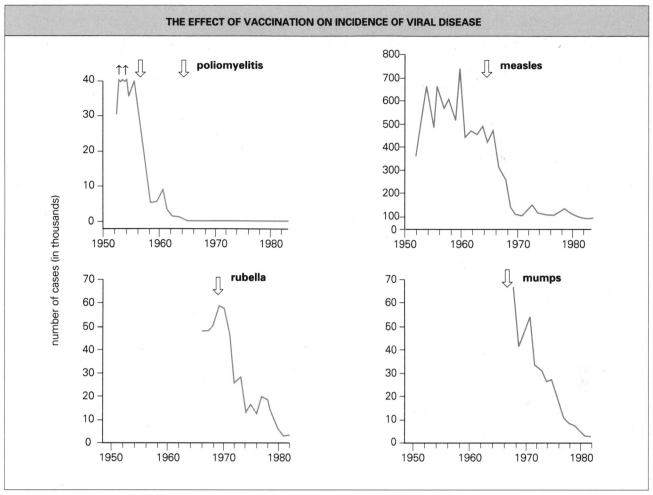

Fig. 36.2 The effect of vaccination on the incidence of various viral diseases in the USA. Most infections have shown a dramatic downward trend after the introduction of a vaccine (arrows). Redrawn from Mims and White, 1984.

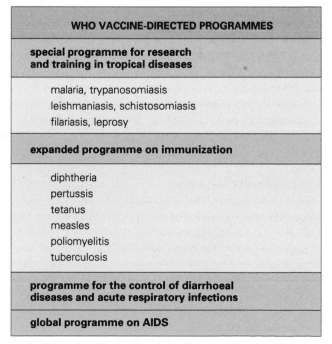

PROBLEMS WITH VACCINE SAFETY

live attenuated vaccines

insufficient attenuation
reversion to wild type
administration to immunodeficient patient
persistent infection
contamination by other viruses
foetal damage

non-living vaccines

contamination by live organisms
contamination by toxins
allergic reactions
autoimmunity

genetically engineered vaccines

?inclusion of oncogenes

Fig. 36.3 Both living and non-living vaccines require rigorous quality and safety control. Some of the commoner problems are listed.

WHO VACCINE-DIRECTED PROGRAMMES

special programme for research and training in tropical diseases

malaria, trypanosomiasis
leishmaniasis, schistosomiasis
filariasis, leprosy

expanded programme on immunization

diphtheria
pertussis
tetanus
measles
poliomyelitis
tuberculosis

programme for the control of diarrhoeal diseases and acute respiratory infections

global programme on AIDS

Fig. 36.4 The World Health Organisation has been responsible for identifying diseases where vaccine research is required, and channels internationally raised funding.

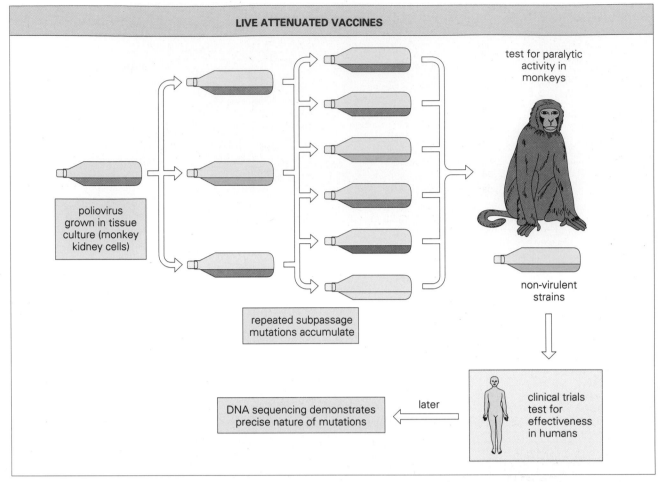

LIVE ATTENUATED VACCINES

poliovirus grown in tissue culture (monkey kidney cells)

repeated subpassage mutations accumulate

test for paralytic activity in monkeys

non-virulent strains

clinical trials test for effectiveness in humans

later

DNA sequencing demonstrates precise nature of mutations

Fig. 36.5 Live attenuated vaccines (e.g. polio) were originally produced by allowing viruses to grow in unusual conditions, and selecting the randomly occuring mutants which had lost virulence.

TYPES OF VACCINE

The minimal requirement of a vaccine is that it should contain some (or at least one) of the protective antigens of the microbe in question. With the single exception of vaccinia – a natural animal ('heterologous') virus sharing antigens with smallpox but of low virulence in man – the vaccines in use today consist of either microbes whose virulence has been artificially reduced ('attenuated'), killed organisms, or subcellular fragments. Each type has its merits and drawbacks.

Heterologous vaccines

Vaccinia was in many ways the ideal vaccine, but it is not impossible that another equally good heterologous vaccine may be found. In animal experiments, for instance, non-virulent strains of some parasites will induce protection against virulent ones, and several veterinary vaccines are based on the same idea. For example, herpes virus from turkeys has been used to protect chickens, and monkey and calf-derived rotavirus has been tried with some success in human infants. The ancient Middle Eastern practice of 'leishmanization', in which children are deliberately infected with *Leishmania tropica* from a mild case in an inconspicuous skin site, resulting in a self-healing lesion ('oriental sore') and subsequent immunity to more widespread disease, could work in the same way, though an experiment in which volunteers were infected with a squirrel-derived strain of *L. donovani* did not give significant protection against the natural infection.

Live attenuated vaccines

These make up the bulk of successful viral vaccines and there is one well-established attenuated bacterial vaccine – BCG (bacille Calmette-Guerin; see below).

The attenuated virus vaccines in current use have been produced by the selection of mutants induced painstakingly but ultimately at random – 'genetic roulette' as it has been termed (Fig. 36.5). Two principal methods are used: serial passage in cells cultured *in vitro* and adaptation to low temperatures. With the development of recombinant DNA technology it is now possible to deliberately induce the required genetic change where this is known. The use of a virus as a carrier of complete genes from another source is considered in the following section.

The unpredictable character of random mutants is illustrated by the three serotypes of attenuated poliovirus (the 'Sabin' oral vaccine). Type 1 has subsequently been shown to contain 57 separate base substitutions and types 2 and 3 only a few, of which all but two are probably unrelated to the loss of virulence. This explains why

LIVE ATTENUATED VACCINES	
organism	**method of attenuation**
Viruses	
Standard	
Poliovirus	passage in monkey kidney, human embryo
Measles	passage in human kidney, amnion, chick embryo
Rubella	passage in rabbit kidney, human diploid cells
Mumps	passage in chick fibroblasts
Yellow fever	passage in monkey, mouse, egg
Hepatitis A	passage in human embryo fibroblasts
Experimental	
Influenza	
Respiratory syncitial virus	cold adaptation
Rotavirus	
Cytomegalovirus	
Herpesvirus	passage in human embryo fibroblast
Varicella	
Bacteria	
Standard	
Mycoplasma tuberculosis (BCG)	passage for 10 yrs in glycerol-bile-potato medium
Salmonella typhi	chemical mutagenesis
Experimental	
Shigella	chemical mutagenesis
V. cholerae	toxin deleted

Fig. 36.6 Several different approaches are used to produce today's live attenuated vaccines.

reversion to the wild-type virulent virus is commoner with types 2 and 3 (though still rare at less than once per million vaccinations). In this case, attenuation was by passage through monkey kidney cells or human embryo fibroblasts, virulence being checked by signs of neurotoxicity in monkeys. Analogous methods have been used for measles, rubella, mumps and yellow fever (Fig. 36.6).

Interestingly, the polio and measles vaccines produced in this way have also turned out to be temperature sensitive mutant strains. In other cases, temperature sensitivity has been deliberately selected for by the process of cold adaptation, during which the virus is encouraged to grow at low temperatures, for example 25°C, which usually means that it grows less well, if at all, at body temperature. Such a virus might then colonize the upper respiratory tract but not warmer tissues such as the lungs. An influenza vaccine made in this way has given promising results. Another temperature sensitive influenza mutant induced by a chemical mutagen was unfortunately found to revert rather easily to the wild type, and the same occurred with a respiratory syncytial virus vaccine.

Randomly induced attenuation of bacteria has not been achieved to the same extent, but the development by Calmette and Guérin of an attenuated strain of bovine tuberculosis after more than 10 years (1908–1918) of culture on glycerol-bile-potato medium shows that it is possible. The 'bacille Calmette-Guérin' (BCG) has not reverted to virulence in over 70 years and in effect it constitutes a new species of mycobacterium. Its effectiveness is, however, still in dispute (see below). A more recent development is the production of an attenuated strain of Salmonella typhi, produced by exposure to chemical mutagens, which has proved to be at least as good as the older killed typhoid vaccine.

Genetically engineered or 'site-directed' mutation, on the other hand, shows great promise in both viruses and bacteria. The majority are deletion mutants in which a gene related to virulence has been put out of action. Examples range from an experimental poliovirus type 2 strain with a single base change, through salmonella strains with mutations in the aroA or galE enzyme genes, to pseudorabies virus lacking the entire thymidine kinase gene and cholera organisms lacking the gene for the A toxin subunit.

Killed vaccines

Killed or 'inactivated' organisms are used where living ones are not available, e.g. where attenuation has not been achieved or reversion to the wild type occurs too easily (Fig. 36.7). They have the advantage of non-infectivity and therefore relative safety, but the disadvantage of generally lower immunogenicity and the consequent need for several doses.

A variety of methods are available for inactivation. With the older viral vaccines, e.g. influenza and polio (Salk), formaldehyde was used, but more recently, b-propiolactone and various ethylenimines and psoralens are replacing it, e.g. for the current rabies vaccine. Ultraviolet light is not regarded as fully reliable because the damage it causes in the viral nucleic acid is selective and can be repaired. For bacteria formaldehyde, phenol, acetone, or simple heating are all used and are equally successful.

Subcellular fractions

When protective immunity is known to be directed against a particular part of an organism, it is sometimes possible to use this as the vaccine. Established examples include the polysaccharide capsules of pneumococci, haemophilus, and meningococci, and the surface coat of the hepatitis B virus, which is produced in excess by the virus and can be purified from the plasma of carriers or, preferably, by recombinant DNA technology. Still experimental are vaccines based on the protein filaments (pili) used by *E. coli* and *N. gonorrhoeae* to attach to urinary tract epithelium. Removal of all live infectious material is obviously a vital element in safety control of such vaccines.

Toxoids

Bacterial toxins, inactivated (usually by formaldehyde) so that they are no longer toxic but still induce protective antibody are called toxoids. Two of these, diphtheria and tetanus, are among the most successful and widely used of all vaccines. In combination with killed *B. pertussis*, they constitute the well-known triple vaccine ('DPT'). There is some evidence that omission of the pertussis component reduces the antibody response to the two toxoids; thus pertussis is acting as an 'adjuvant' as well as a specific vaccine.

With the use of small peptides as potential vaccine antigens (see below) tetanus toxoid has come to the fore as a useful 'carrier' protein; the idea is that most patients, having previously been immunized to the toxoid, will possess tetanus-specific T memory cells which will help the peptide-specific B cells to make antibody. This approach is useful for inducing a good primary response but less so for memory responses, in which T cells will need to be recalled by the proteins of the infection in question rather than by those of tetanus.

The other common toxin-inducing bacterium is *Vibrio cholerae*, and vaccines containing the B subunit of cholera toxin plus killed organisms have had some success. Vaccines have also been made against the neurotoxin of *Clostridium botulinum*.

Microorganisms as vectors for cloned genes

The idea of using expression vectors (*E. coli*, yeast etc.) to clone genes coding for potentially immunogenic proteins is as old as recombinant DNA technology itself. More

INACTIVATED VACCINES	
organism	**method of inactivation**
Viruses	
rabies	β-propiolactone
influenza	β-propiolactone
polio (Salk)	formaldehyde
Bacteria	
Salmonella typhi	heat plus phenol or acetone
Vibrio cholerae	heat
Bordetella pertussis	heat or formaldehyde
E. coli (experimental)	colicin
Yersinia pestis	formaldehyde

Fig. 36.7 Several methods are in use to produce inactivated vaccines. One of the most famous, the rabies vaccine, dates back to the time of Pasteur.

recently, however, an ingenious modification has been introduced in which the expression vector, complete with inserted gene(s), is itself the vaccine. Following injection into the patient, it would proliferate sufficiently to release an immunizing amount of the foreign protein, but without, of course, inducing disease itself.

The first vector to be proposed, in 1982, was the vaccinia virus. This had the advantage of being already established as a highly effective vaccine and of possessing a large enough (DNA) genome for the insertion of several foreign genes without disrupting virus structure or function. However, it also had the disadvantage that a large proportion of the world's population was already immune to vaccinia and would probably eliminate the virus before it had produced the desired amount of the foreign gene product. There was also the problem that vaccinia itself was known to induce complications (principally encephalitis) in about 1 case in 100 000. Nevertheless in a pioneer experiment in chimpanzees, vaccinia containing the gene for hepatitis B surface antigen (HBsAg) gave excellent protection against a challenge infection (Fig. 36.8), and similarly with influenza and herpes simplex.

Several other viruses have subsequently been considered as vectors, including attenuated yellow fever, adenovirus, herpes and varicella-zoster; successful insertion has been achieved of genes from respiratory syncitial , Epstein-Barr, rabies, dengue and Lassa fever viruses, among others.

Bacteria are also good candidates as vectors, the two leading ones being the attenuated salmonellae mentioned earlier and BCG. *Salmonella typhi* has the advantage of being an intestinal infection, so that when given orally (with a dose of bicarbonate to prevent inactivation by gastric acid) it will induce mucosal immunity in the gut. Avirulent mutants of *S. typhi* might therefore act as general vectors for vaccines against all enteric diseases – a field in which current vaccines are far from adequate.

BCG is the latest vector to be proposed; here the advantages are firstly the very large genome and secondly the fact that BCG is now the most widely used of all vaccines, being given, usually just after birth, to about 75% of all

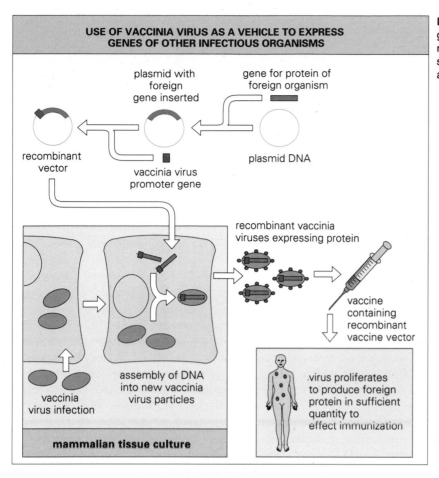

USE OF VACCINIA VIRUS AS A VEHICLE TO EXPRESS GENES OF OTHER INFECTIOUS ORGANISMS

plasmid with foreign gene inserted

gene for protein of foreign organism

recombinant vector

plasmid DNA

vaccinia virus promoter gene

recombinant vaccinia viruses expressing protein

vaccine containing recombinant vaccine vector

assembly of DNA into new vaccinia virus particles

vaccinia virus infection

virus proliferates to produce foreign protein in sufficient quantity to effect immunization

mammalian tissue culture

Fig. 36.8 It is now possible to insert genes coding for antigens of one or more microorganisms into a large virus such as vaccinia so that they replicate and are released into the host.

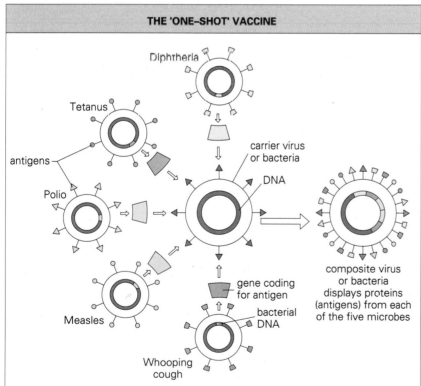

THE 'ONE-SHOT' VACCINE

Diphtheria

Tetanus

antigens

Polio

Measles

Whooping cough

carrier virus or bacteria

DNA

gene coding for antigen

bacterial DNA

composite virus or bacteria displays proteins (antigens) from each of the five microbes

Fig. 36.9 The vaccines of the future may consist of a single viral or bacterial vector containing genes for all required vaccines – the 'one-shot' vaccine. This illustration first appeared in New Scientist, London, the weekly review of science and technology.

children in the world. Another special merit is that it induces predominantly cell-mediated immunity, both to itself and to other antigens given with it, so that it could be the ideal vector for antigens from all persistent intracellular organisms – a large and important category that includes, in addition to tuberculosis and leprosy, brucella, leishmania, toxoplasma, histoplasma, listeria, rickettsia and chlamydia, many viruses, and possibly (in its liver stage) malaria. Perhaps in the future a single vector containing all the required antigens may be available (Fig. 36.9)

Antigens produced by gene cloning and peptide synthesis

These new approaches may be considered together since they both aim to produce immunogenic peptides for use as vaccines. The technologies involved are now reasonably standard, though there is considerable debate as to which expression vector to use for cloning genes. The first successful vaccine made in this way was against foot and mouth disease. First by gene cloning in *E. coli* and soon afterwards by chemical synthesis, it was shown that a 20-aminoacid peptide from one of the capsid proteins could protect guineapigs against infection.

Cloned or synthetic peptides are now available from a wide range of microbes, and there is extensive research into the question of how to select the right peptide and how to make it as immunogenic as possible. One approach is to attach peptides to larger carrier molecules such as tetanus toxin (see above), but whenever possible the attempt is made to include sequences in the peptide which can themselves trigger T cells. These 'T cell epitopes' can to some extent be predicted from the known sequence of the molecule. Where they are not available, the strategy is to construct new sequences including one or more T cell epitope as well as the epitope against which antibody is required (the 'B cell epitope'). A further refinement has been to couple together several copies of separate T and B epitopes into 'multiple antigen peptides', using a branching core of lysines and up to eight attached peptides – the so-called 'octopus' molecule. In one study four each of the T cell and B cell epitopes gave the best results. Even then, it has usually been found that an adjuvant is needed to enhance immunogenicity.

One problem with these small peptides is the variation in response from patient to patient and the existence of genetic non-responders. The role of MHC antigens in this is discussed below.

Another problem arises with those glycosylated proteins in which the carbohydrate portion constitutes part or all of the antigen. Glycosylation is very different in different expression vectors, *E. coli* being generally unsuitable. Yeast, insect, and mammalian cells are all used to produce more correctly glycosylated proteins.

Anti-idiotype vaccines

The most novel proposal for preparing antigens is to use antibody molecules which are themselves copies of the antigen. This is possible because antibodies can recognize structures related to each other's combining sites (idiotypes; see Chapter 7), just as they can recognize antigens; thus a first antibody against an antigen can be used to raise second antibodies, some of which will have idiotypes resembling the original antigen (Fig. 36.10). Considerable selection is required and monoclonal antibody technology is essential. One advantage of such 'surrogate antigens' is that, being large proteins, they behave as T-dependent antigens, even when the original antigen was T-independent – a polysaccharide for example. This strategy has been successfully applied to the vaccination of mice against streptococcal and trypanosomal antigens, and to raise secondary antibody responses to endotoxin. At present it looks as though it could be of value with carbohydrate or glycolipid antigens, which cannot be cloned or synthesized in bulk as proteins can.

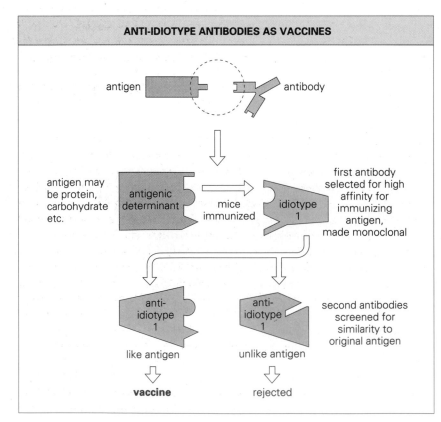

ANTI-IDIOTYPE ANTIBODIES AS VACCINES

antigen   antibody

antigen may be protein, carbohydrate etc.

antigenic determinant   mice immunized   idiotype 1   first antibody selected for high affinity for immunizing antigen, made monoclonal

anti-idiotype 1   anti-idiotype 1   second antibodies screened for similarity to original antigen

like antigen   unlike antigen

vaccine   rejected

Fig. 36.10 Monoclonal antibody technology and the discovery of the 'idiotype network' has meant that immunoglobulins can now be used as 'surrogate' antigens. In the case of a carbohydrate or lipid antigen, this allows a protein 'copy' to be made, which may have certain advantages as a vaccine.

SPECIAL CONSIDERATIONS

Living versus non-living vaccines

On this topic, one of the most keenly debated in vaccinology, some general points may be made, as well as some which apply specifically to particular vaccines. These are summarized in figure 36.11

The issue can be appreciated most clearly with those diseases that normally induce good long-term immunity following recovery from infection (e.g. the common childhood viruses). Here live attenuated vaccines are much more likely to be effective, since they reproduce many of the features of the infection itself, including replication of the virus, localization to the appropriate part of the body (gut, lung etc.), and the efficient induction of cytotoxic T cells. The latter may be related to the fact that for microbial peptides to become associated with MHC class I molecules it is usually necessary for the peptides to have been synthesized in the cell rather than taken in by endocytosis, as a non-living vaccine antigen would be. A further theoretical advantage is the possibility that attenuated strains will spread through the population by normal transmission routes protecting even those who have not been vaccinated ('herd immunity').

The principal disadvantages of living attenuated vaccines are the possibility of reversion to virulence and the danger that in immunocompromised patients they may cause severe disease.

Many natural infections do not leave the patient with solid immunity (e.g. influenza). This can be for a variety of reasons, as discussed in Chapter 14, prominent among them being antigenic diversity, antigenic variation, immunosuppression, and the induction of responses that

protect the microbe. In such cases the rationale for a living attenuated vaccine is weaker, and a subcellular component that induces strong immunity which attacks the microbe at a weak spot (e.g. a polysaccharide capsule or a vital attachment molecule), possibly in the form of a mixture of antigenic types, is more likely to work. The problem of correct localization will then need to be addressed by other means, such as aerosols for the lung, enteric capsules for the gut, etc.

There is only one disease at present for which live and killed vaccines are competing on more or less equal terms, and this is discussed below (see Poliomyelitis).

T-independent antigens

Most complex antigens contain both T and B cell epitopes, so that T cells are induced which co-operate with B cells, leading to T and B cell memory, immunoglobulin switching (e.g. IgM→IgG), and affinity maturation – all features of the secondary response and essential for a vaccine to be effective. However many polysaccharide antigens fail to stimulate T cells, so that they induce only primary responses no matter how often they are administered. Such antigens are also particularly ineffective in children below the age of two. The current strategy is to conjugate the polysaccharide to a suitable protein, preferably from the same microorganism. The results of this are discussed below in relation to pneumococcal and meningococcal vaccines.

Another approach to this problem, although still largely experimental, is the use of anti-idiotypic antibody as a 'surrogate' antigen (see above).

MHC restriction

Antigens that do stimulate T cells may still be less effective in some individuals than in others. This is especially a feature of small peptides and is due to the very precise binding required between the peptide, the MHC class II (HLA-D) molecule on the antigen presenting cell, and the T cell receptor. HLA antigens are extremely polymorphic and it is quite common to find that a particular HLA molecule fails to bind a particular peptide. If, among an individual's available MHC class II molecules (two each of DP, DQ, and DR) there is none that binds a particular peptide, that person will be a 'non-responder' and will not mount T cell responses.

It is not known how much MHC restriction contributes to the failure of a certain percentage of individuals to respond well to almost all standard vaccines, and it may be that the problem has been over-emphasized even where small peptides are concerned. For example, a 21 amino acid malaria peptide has been found from which peptides of 11–14 amino acids stimulate only T cells from a few DR types, whereas a 15 amino acid sequence stimulates all the DR types tested. This suggests that it may often be possible to confer a broader range of MHC responsiveness by adding a few amino acids to a peptide.

Pathological consequences of vaccination

These may be due to extrinsic elements in the vaccine or to features intrinsic to the immune response. Examples of

LIVING VERSUS NON-LIVING VACCINES		
	living	non-living
Preparation	attenuation (not always feasible)	inactivation
Administration	may be natural route (e.g. oral) may be single dose	injection usually multiple doses
Adjuvant	not required	usually required
Safety	may revert to virulence	pain from injection
Heat lability (for tropical use)	requires cold chain	satisfactory
Cost	low	high
Duration of immunity	usually years	may be long or short
Immune response	IgG, IgA cell-mediated	mainly IgG, little or no cell-mediated

Fig. 36.11 Live and killed vaccines each have their advantages and disadvantages.

PATHOLOGICAL COMPLICATIONS OF VACCINATION	
complication	vaccine
hypersensitivity to egg antigens to viral antigens	live measles, mumps killed measles, RSV
convulsions, encephalitis	pertussis, measles (1 per million)
meningitis	mumps (1 per million)
arthritis	rubella

Fig. 36.12 With modern vaccines, complications are rare, but the physician must always be aware of the possibility.

the former are contamination of attenuated viruses with other viruses growing in the same cell lines, particularly since monkey cells are often used and several monkey viruses are lethal for humans. Another problem arises with living viral vaccines grown in chick embryo cells, namely hypersensitivity to egg proteins. Children with a history of egg sensitivity should be skin-tested with diluted vaccine and may have to be immunized in stages with lower than usual doses, or, where anaphylaxis is expected, not at all.

A more complicated situation arises where the vaccine antigen itself induces a pathological response, such as hypersensitivity or autoimmunity. Hypersensitivity reactions to the older killed measles vaccines were a stimulus to the development of a living attenuated replacement. What appears to have happened is that the killed vaccine induced good non-neutralizing antibodies to the haemagglutinin, but failed to induce antibody to the fusion (F) protein, which was destroyed by the inactivation process. The F protein is responsible for viral cell-to-cell spread, and as a consequence during infection large amounts of virus are produced together with high titres of non-neutralizing antibody. The resulting immune complexes caused severe type III hypersensitivity during the attack of measles, so that the patient was actually made worse. A similar response occurred to the killed RSV vaccine. The fever and malaise that follow vaccination with killed typhoid organisms is due to the endotoxin, and mediated by cytokines such as IL-1 and TNF.

Autoimmunity during infections can sometimes be traced to antigenic similarity ('mimicry') between host and microbe, and the same is theoretically possible with vaccine antigens. However this does not seem to have been observed with the present vaccines, but could clearly occur if strong T cell epitopes are conjugated to weak antigens, such as polysaccharides, which might cross-react with host molecules. Where the cross-reacting component can be identified, it should clearly be removed before a vaccine is considered for use; Chagas' disease is a case in point.

Perhaps the most widely publicized complication of vaccination is the occurrence of fits and brain damage, notably after vaccination for pertussis (see Chapter 22). Whether or not this is truly due to the vaccine is discussed below. Figure 36.12 lists the major reported complications of other vaccines.

The immunocompromised host

The need to avoid living vaccines in the immunocompromised has been mentioned, but is subject to some qualifications. The most absolute contraindications are the use of vaccinia or BCG in patients with severe T cell deficiency. Indeed it was the spreading and eventually fatal vaccinia infections which alerted the New York paediatrician Di George to the occurrence of the athymic syndrome that bears his name. However, in less severe T cell deficiency states, including HIV infection, the use of the live measles vaccine is now recommended, the risk of complications being, on balance, less than the risk of death from the natural infection. In other T-cell deficiencies of childhood, including treatment with steroids or immunosuppressive drugs, MMR vaccine is generally not advised.

Non-living vaccines are less of a problem since while they may be ineffective they are unlikely to be dangerous. Vaccines aimed specifically at the induction of antibody (e.g. capsular polysaccharides, hepatitis B) are recommended in all but the most severe B-cell deficiencies, but the alternative of passive immunization (see Chapter 37) should also be considered.

Adjuvants

It has been known since the 1920s that certain substances, when administered simultaneously with antigen, will enhance the consequent immune response. The first such substances shown to be safe, convenient and effective were aluminium salts. These constitute the principal vaccine adjuvants in use today, though numerous other materials are being considered or tried experimentally for clinical use. It should be noted that the word 'adjuvant' is also sometimes used in a slightly different sense to denote a substance which, given alone, enhances some immune function such as the inhibition of tumour growth or recovery from infection. This type of non-specific immunostimulant is discussed in the following chapter.

Many years of work in animals have established that a wide range of materials are effective as vaccine adjuvants and these will be briefly described since the clinical adjuvants of the future are likely to be drawn from among them (Fig. 36.13).

The powerful adjuvanticity of aluminium salts has not been fully explained. Some of it is no doubt due to the formation of small inflammatory lesions, which may progress to granulomata, with consequent trapping of antigen and slow release with exposure to large numbers of macrophages and other antigen-presenting cells. Antigens (e.g. toxoids) were originally entrapped in 'floccules' of the salt by adding them during its chemical preparation. Such antigens are described as 'alum precipitated'. Now, however, it is more usual to add the antigen to

VACCINE ADJUVANTS		
inorganic salts		
aluminium hydroxide (alhydrogel)*		
aluminium phosphate*		
calcium phosphate*		
beryllium hydroxide		
delivery systems		
liposomes**		
ISCOMS**		
block polymers		
slow release formulations**		
bacterial products		
BCG		
Mycobacterium bovis and oil (complete Freund's adjuvant)†		
MDP†		
*Bordetella pertussis** (with diphtheria, tetanus toxoids)		
natural mediators*		
IL-1		
IL-2		
IFN-γ		
* routinely used in man ** experimental † too toxic for human use		

Fig. 36.13 A variety of foreign and endogenous substances can act as adjuvants, but only aluminium and calcium salts and pertussis are routinely used in clinical practice.

a preformed gel of aluminium hydroxide or phosphate. Alum precipitated antigens are especially effective at inducing antibody responses but much less active in inducing cell-mediated immunity.

A similar 'depot' effect is thought to account for the adjuvanticity of a variety of novel formulations in which the antigen is presented on the surface of small spherical structures. These include liposomes, which are single- or multiple-walled phospholipid vesicles, ISCOMS (immune-stimulating complexes), which are micelles composed of a saponin derivative, QUIL A, which traps amphipathic proteins, and block polymers of polyoxyethylene and polyoxypropylene. Depending on the precise formulation and the nature of the antigen used, these have all been shown to be highly effective and many are in veterinary use. It is too early to say which, if any, will become standard clinical adjuvants, and this may depend on safety testing as much as immunological efficacy.

The adjuvanticity of mycobacteria is remarkable, and was made use of by Freund in his famous preparation 'complete Freund's adjuvant' (CFA), in which mycobacteria are emulsified with water in an oil vehicle. CFA is particularly effective in boosting cell-mediated responses such as delayed hypersensitivity to antigens that are normally

weak inducers. Unfortunately, as several accidental injections have shown, CFA is too toxic for use in man, causing chronic non-healing granulomas. The oil-in-water emulsion without mycobacteria is known as 'incomplete Freund's adjuvant' (IFA), and this has been used in man with no apparent undesired side-effects, but without the great potency of CFA for cell-mediated responses. An extensive study of the role played by the mycobacteria in CFA has yielded the small water-soluble molecule muramyl dipeptide (MDP), which is claimed to retain most of the benefit of mycobacteria without the toxicity.

Numerous other bacterial derivatives are being investigated as adjuvants and, as already mentioned, the killed pertussis organisms in the 'triple' DPT vaccine appear to act as adjuvants for the diphtheria and tetanus toxoids.

The most recent development in the adjuvant field has been the use of cytokines. It had always been suspected that adjuvants such as CFA and MDP acted partly by inducing cytokines important for lymphocyte triggering differentiation and function such as IL-1, and when purified recombinant cytokines became available it was found that at least three, IL-1, IL-2 and IFN-γ were indeed effective adjuvants when added to vaccines. IL-1 and IFN-γ have been shown to be particularly useful in cases where the response to a vaccine is impaired, for example in haemodialysis patients immunized against hepatitis B.

When to vaccinate

Since most of the diseases that vaccines are designed to prevent affect young children, vaccination is carried out as early as possible, bearing in mind certain considerations. The presence of maternally-derived antibody reduces the effectiveness of some vaccines, which are therefore usually delayed until the third month of life or later (see Chapter 38). Live attenuated vaccines (including vaccinia when it was used) can cause severe disease in immunodeficiency states, which may not be diagnosed immediately after birth. Where the disease is mainly a risk to the elderly (e.g. pneumococcal pneumonia) vaccination is usually given at a late age. Figure 36.14 gives the immunization schedule for vaccines in current use. Further details will be found in sections on individual vaccines (see below).

Other means of control

In the search for new vaccines, we must not lose sight of the fact that some diseases can be controlled equally well by other means. In the developed world it was public health measures rather than vaccines (or antibiotics) which eliminated malaria and cholera and weakened the hold of tuberculosis, and it could be argued that tropical maladies such as schistosomiasis or Chagas' disease, might also be better controlled by reducing contact with the snail or insect vector. It has to be admitted however, that vector control is much easier said than done and, like chemotherapy but unlike vaccination, it needs to be maintained more or less indefinitely.

With certain diseases the chance of infection is so slight that a vaccine, however successful, would never justify the cost and effort of producing it, and passive immunization after exposure may be a better approach (as it is for snakebite).

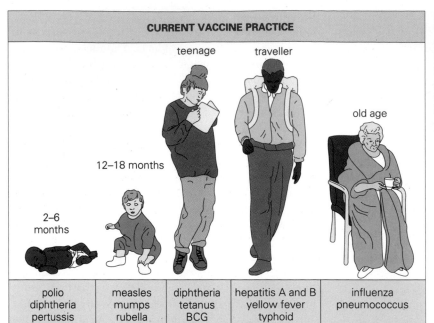

CURRENT VACCINE PRACTICE

teenage

traveller

old age

12–18 months

2–6 months

| polio diphtheria pertussis tetanus | measles mumps rubella | diphtheria tetanus BCG | hepatitis A and B yellow fever typhoid cholera | influenza pneumococcus |

Fig. 36.14 Current vaccine practice. While the administration of most vaccines is fairly standard world-wide, there are important local differences due to variations in risk of infection or in government health policy. *BCG vaccine also gives some protection against leprosy.

ADMINISTRATION SCHEDULE		
vaccine	**UK and USA**	**elsewhere**
'Triple' (DTP) vaccine: diphtheria, tetanus, pertussis	primary: given to all at 2–6 months (3 doses at 4 week intervals); booster: 15 months (USA) and 4 years (UK and USA); DT every 10 years (USA)	Japan: primary at 2 years
Polio vaccine: Sabin (live, oral) Salk (killed)	primary: given to all concomitantly with DTP vaccine; boost: 4 and 16 years (UK), 15 months, 4 years and high-risk adults (USA) immunocompromised	
'MMR' vaccine: measles, mumps rubella	given to all at 12–18 months; rubella given to seronegative girls at 10–14 years	Africa (WHO programme), children at 6 months
BCG: tuberculosis, leprosy*	given to all at 10-14 years (UK); high-risk groups only (USA)	Tropics, given at birth
Hepatitis B	travellers, high-risk groups (e.g. neonates of carriers, homosexuals, health workers)	Africa and Far East, given to infants
Hepatitis A	travellers to endemic areas (e.g. Africa, India, Far East)	
Rabies	pre-exposure in high-risk groups (e.g. laboratory, kennel workers); post-exposure in those bitten or licked by animals in endemic areas	
Yellow fever Typhoid Cholera	travellers to endemic areas	Tropics, given to infants; yellow fever: boost every 10 years for residents and frequent visitors
Meningitis (A+C)	travellers to endemic areas (e.g. parts of Africa, India)	
Pneumococcal disease	aged, high-risk groups	
Haemophilus	given to infants at 18 months	
Varicella	given to the immunocompromised and neonates at risk	
Influenza	aged, high-risk individuals	

CURRENT VACCINE PRACTICE

Vaccines in general use

Diphtheria

Despite the fact that diphtheria toxin loses some antigenicity when converted (by formaldehyde) to the toxoid, it remains a highly effective vaccine. Surprisingly, for a vaccine aimed at the disease rather than the bacterium, it has also reduced the number of carriers of diphtheria, which may imply that the toxin plays a role in the survival or spread of the organism. Diphtheria toxoid is almost universally given with tetanus toxoid and alum, usually with pertussis, in three injections starting at 2–3 months of age plus a later boost. If required, the success of vaccination can be measured by the serum antibody level, or by skin testing. In the Schick test, both toxin and toxoid are injected; an absence of reaction implies a satisfactory level of antibody, an erythematous response to the toxin at 5–7 days indicates inadequate antibody, while an early response (1–2 days) denotes hypersensitivity. Protection is usually 90% or better.

Tetanus

Tetanus toxoid is also highly effective, and is in universal use, though there are some differences in policy as regards booster injections and the treatment of patients after exposure. In most countries, following the three injections of young children, a booster is given at entry to school, and another is recommended every 5–10 years. Where exposure is suspected and a booster has not been given within 5 years, one is given combined with antitoxin if the wound is a dirty one (see passive immunization, Chapter 37). Reactions to the vaccine are limited to mild hypersensitivity in repeatedly boosted patients, so that tetanus toxoid can be considered one of the safest and most effective vaccines.

Pertussis

Mass vaccination against whooping cough was introduced in Britain in 1957, using the whole heat- or formalin-killed vaccine developed during the 1940s. This is given with diphtheria and tetanus toxoid as part of the DTP or 'triple' vaccine, though the later boosts are not given since whooping cough is only a serious disease in young children.

Controversy has surrounded the use of this vaccine. There is no doubt that the incidence of whooping cough has diminished dramatically where the vaccine has been used, but several trials were required to establish statistical evidence for a protective effect. This was partly due to the omission of one of the three serotypes from some batches. Moreover, there is no standard vaccine in general use.

A more serious controversy concerns undesirable reactions to the vaccine. Mild reactions such as pain, inflammation, and fever are quite common, probably due to the endotoxin and other toxins. But in the 1970s studies were published in the UK which claimed that severe screaming attacks, fits, and permanent brain damage could follow pertussis vaccination in approximately 1 case per 100 000 injections. The debate still continues on whether this is genuinely cause and effect, but meanwhile the understandable alarm of parents led to a fall of vaccine acceptance to as low as 30%. Predictably, a severe epidemic of whooping cough soon followed, in the winter of 1978/9, with over 100 000 cases and many deaths (Fig. 36.15). This perhaps constitutes the best evidence that the vaccine was in fact effective, but the controversy undoubtedly damaged the reputation of this vaccine, and of vaccines generally, in the mind of the public.

Not surprisingly, vigorous attempts are now being made to produce a safer vaccine. Among the components of the organism that are considered to be candidates are pertussis toxin (which is responsible for both bacterial adhesion and toxicity), and various other adhesion or toxic molecules, and these are being tried out separately as well as in combination. Some have already come into limited use, for example a two-component vaccine in Japan, which is claimed to be 80–90% effective. Another trial in Sweden also showed encouraging results. Most recently, a genetically engineered mutant version of the pertussis toxin molecule lacking all toxicity has been proposed as the ideal vaccine, and it seems likely that one or other of these new vaccines will soon be accepted for general use.

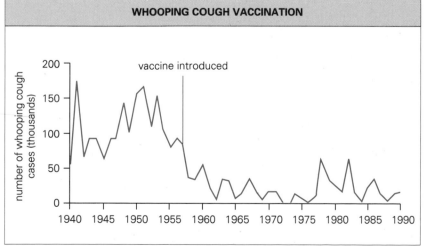

WHOOPING COUGH VACCINATION

vaccine introduced

number of whooping cough cases (thousands)

200 — 150 — 100 — 50 — 0

1940 1945 1950 1955 1960 1965 1970 1975 1980 1985 1990

Fig. 36.15 The number of cases of whooping cough notified fell steadily after the introduction of mass immunization in 1958, although epidemics continued to occur at approximately four year intervals. Following the scare about the possible adverse effects of pertussis vaccine, the number of cases rose, and the epidemic in the winter 1978–79 was the largest since the introduction of immunization.

Measles

Live attenuated measles vaccine was introduced in the USA in 1962 and since that time the incidence of the disease, which used to kill over 500 children a year, has shrunk to almost nil, so that measles is now being considered as a candidate for eventual worldwide eradication. However this will require a considerably better uptake in most other countries than at present.

The principal debate concerns the best age at which to give the vaccine. Maternal antibody can prevent proper immunization with measles, so it is necessary to wait until at least 6 months of age. However, even by the age of 9 months the vaccine gives only about 80% protection, so in countries where measles is uncommon it is usual to wait until about 1 year. But in developing countries, where measles is still widespread, children are likely to be exposed before this age, so the vaccine is generally given at around 6 months, followed by another dose at 1 year to protect those who responded poorly to the first. The duration of protection against measles appears to be at least 21 years, though this may be partly due to boosting during natural epidemics, so that as measles disappears from the population, adults may become susceptible again. If so, a logical strategy would be to give a boost as a routine, perhaps at primary or secondary school entry.

Mumps

What has been said about measles also applies to the live attenuated mumps vaccine. Some countries have questioned the need for a mumps vaccine, but in its absence about 1000 cases per year of mumps meningitis can be expected in the UK, while another calculation predicted 40 deaths and 95 cases of deafness per year in the USA. Mumps vaccine is most conveniently given with measles and rubella vaccines (MMR vaccine).

Rubella

This relatively mild disease illustrates vividly the issues that can arise when setting the benefit to the individual against that of the population. In the UK it has until recently been felt that boys do not need vaccinating against rubella and so should not be exposed to the slight risk of vaccine complications; moreover, circulation of wild rubella in the population as a whole is useful in boosting immunity in girls. Therefore the live attenuated vaccine was given only to girls at adolescence, to protect them against developing the disease while pregnant and transmitting it to the foetus, resulting in the congenital rubella syndrome.

However, because of its high reproduction rate (see Chapter 37), rubella would maintain its presence in the population indefinitely unless well over half of the population are protected. In the USA, therefore, rubella vaccine has been given to boys as well, and this approach (i.e. immunizaton with MMR vaccine at about 1 year) has recently been adopted in the UK. Unfortunately there is the danger that as the level of infection, in the community fell, cases would occur at a later age, thus actually increasing the chance of foetal damage. Until the disease is eradicated, therefore, vaccine strategy needs to be carefully tailored to the prevailing situation in each country.

Poliomyelitis

The remarkable decline in poliomyelitis is due to the use of one or other of two vaccines: the killed virus (Salk 1954) or the live attenuated virus (Sabin 1957). Both are effective and each has its advantages and disadvantages (Fig. 36.16).

The live attenuated oral polio vaccine (OPV) has become the first choice in most countries. Its main advantages are its lower cost, the fact that (as with all live vaccines) immunity is induced in the right place, namely the mucosal surfaces, and the prediction that by spreading within the population, it will induce 'herd' immunity. This is borne out by the fact that vaccine strains are now commoner (e.g. in sewage) in the USA than wild strains.

Against this is the risk of reversion to virulence, particularly by types 2 and 3 which, as described earlier, are not as different from the wild strains as might be desired. Wild virus has been isolated from the stools within days of vaccination, and there have been several cases of paralytic poliomyelitis, especially in contacts of the vaccine; one estimate put these at 1–2 cases per million. OPV is, of course, not used in immunocompromised patients.

ORAL AND INACTIVATED POLIO VACCINES COMPARED		
	inactivated (IPV)	attenuated (OPV)
Introduced	Salk 1954	Sabin 1957
In use	Sweden, Finland Holland, Iceland	most other countries
Dosage schedule	injection plus alum	oral at 2,4,6, months
Risks	inadequately killed (very rare) otherwise safe	in immunodeficiency reversion to virulence ?interference by other viruses cold chain failure
Advantages	?herd immunity can be added to other childhood vaccines	IgA boosted herd immunity cheaper than Salk vaccine

Fig. 36.16 Poliomyelitis is unusual in that both live attenuated and killed vaccines are available and widely used. Three doses of the attenuated virus vaccine are given as the three types of virus present in the vaccine interfere with each others replication in the intestine. The repeated doses ensure an adequate response to each type.

The above considerations have led to the rejection of OPV in favour of the inactivated polio vaccine (IPV) in certain countries, notably Sweden, Finland, Holland and Iceland. Here it is argued that in practice, IPV induces equally good immunity, and that it might even be more effective in developing countries, where OPV has been somewhat disappointing, presumably because, as was shown for measles, the 'cold chain' between factory and clinic was not adequately maintained. Surprisingly, the duration of immunity following OPV is not demonstrably longer than with IPV, perhaps reflecting the relatively shorter duration of mucosal than systemic immunity. But in the absence of substantial herd immunity, a high rate of IPV uptake would be essential if eradication was being contemplated.

Clearly, then, although polio vaccination has been highly successful, there is room for further improvements. Two current lines of development are the production of better and cheaper vaccines - both attenuated and inactivated - and the use of combined regimes, e.g. IPV followed by OPV in various sequential combinations.

Tuberculosis

Calmette and Guerin's attenuated tubercle bacillus (BCG) has been in use for 70 years, but still inspires fierce debate as to its usefulness. The matter is of some importance, considering that tuberculosis still kills some 3 million people a year world-wide, and is on the increase in countries where AIDS is pandemic.

In its favour is the fact that BCG has given clear protection in controlled trials, such as that carried out in the UK (1950), and in the USA on American Indians and Puerto Ricans in the 1970s. Efficacies of 70% or better have also been reported from several South American and African countries. Moreover, the same vaccine appeared to be equally effective against leprosy in Uganda and, to a lesser extent, in other countries.

Immunization strategy varies according to the likelihood of infection: at birth in high-risk countries, at entry to secondary school in the UK and USA (and then only in patients with a negative Mantoux test; see Chapter 9). One disadvantage of using BCG in countries where tuberculosis is rare is that, by causing Mantoux (tuberculin) conversion, it destroys the diagnostic value of this test.

One problem with such trials is the shifting background level of infection, which is dependent on factors other than vaccination, notably general public health and anti-tuberculous chemotherapy. In countries with a low incidence of disease it would now be impossible to carry out a satisfactory trial based on clinical protection, and unfortunately there is no rapid test which accurately predicts protection. The tuberculin skin test, widely used as such, has been shown to vary independently of actual protection, and is probably better regarded as a measure of prior exposure rather than immunity.

Another problem is that in other equally well controlled trials BCG had little or no protective effect. Indeed in two trials, in southern India (1980) and southern parts of the USA, BCG actually seemed to increase the incidence of tuberculosis. Numerous explanations have been put forward for these extraordinary discrepancies, which are unmatched by any other vaccine. These include differences between vaccine strains (there is no agreed world standard), genetic differences between the human populations, differences in the prevalent clinical pattern of disease, and differences in the type and number of 'environmental' mycobacteria which might modulate the level of immunity in the population.

Quite apart from these debatable effects on tuberculosis, BCG has three other potential uses: as an adjuvant for other vaccines, as a vector for cloned genes from other organisms (referred to in an earlier section) and as a general non-specific immunostimulant (see Chapter 37).

Vaccines in limited use

Hepatitis B

This vaccine, the most recent to come into large-scale use, is unusual in several ways. Despite the fact that hepatitis B virus (HBV) has not been grown in culture, a non-living antigenic preparation can be derived from the blood of carriers. This is because the surface coat antigen (HBsAg) is over-produced by the virus, and circulates as free non-infectious 22nm spherical particles (up to 10^{13} per ml of blood; see Fig. 36.17). These, purified and inactivated so as to be scrupulously free of DNA, were shown in a controlled trial in American male homosexuals (1980) to be at least 95% protective. The vaccine was licensed for use in the following year, and was given in three doses of $20\,\mu g$ at intervals of one and six months. It has three disadvantages. Being derived from human blood, it has to be purified with exceptional care because of the risk of transmitting live HBV or other viruses. Even after three doses antibody levels start to fall 1–2 years later, so that boosting may be necessary. A level of 100 units per litre is considered to be protective. Finally, it is extremely expensive to make and supplies are limited.

Meanwhile, a second vaccine has been produced via recombinant DNA technology – the first such vaccine to go into human use. The same antigen (HBsAg) is involved, the gene being cloned into a yeast vector which produces large amounts of the antigenic protein. Safer and cheaper (about half the cost when introduced, though the plasma-derived vaccine has now come down to the same price), this recombinant vaccine appears to be equally effective. Recent refinements include the insertion

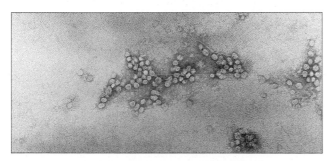

Fig. 36.17 Electronmicrograph of purified 22nm hepatitis B surface antigens expressed in yeast cells. Courtesy of J R Pattison.

of other ('pre-S') genes into the vector, to code for proteins involved in the infectious process. The idea of incorporating HBV genes into a living attenuated vector is also under consideration.

While HBV is now clearly a candidate for eventual eradication, current strategies have to take account of the prevailing level of infection. In the developed world, the vaccines are currently recommended for high-risk groups (Fig. 36.18). Since these include a number of likely low- or non-responders (e.g. immunocompromised patients), attention is being directed at the need for further boosts and the use of special adjuvants such as cytokines: both IL-2 and IFN-γ have been shown to improve responses to the vaccine in haemodialysis patients.

In Africa, HBV is typically acquired during early childhood, so the vaccine is given at the same time as the usual childhood ones, the major problem being to keep the cost within affordable limits. At present, $1 per dose is about the minimum.

In the Far East, on the other hand, HBV is commonly transmitted to newborns by mothers who are chronic carriers. Here a course of vaccine injections (at 1 week, 5 weeks, 9 weeks and 1 year), is combined with passive immunization with immune globulin. Early results show good protection and it is hoped that the number of carriers will fall progressively, and with it the incidence of liver carcinoma.

Other hepatitis viruses

A vaccine against hepatitis A, derived from human diploid cells and formaldehyde inactivated, is now available for travellers to countries where the disease is endemic. Until now, passive immunization with pooled normal human immunoglobulin, which gives good but transient protection, has been the standard method, it is hoped that a vaccine will ultimately be available for the newly discovered hepatitis C virus

Rabies

The rabies vaccine is famous for Pasteur's courageous demonstration in 1885 that a dessicated (air-killed) preparation of spinal cord from rabid rabbits would protect humans against rabies, even after infection with the virus (see Chapter 34). He was indeed fortunate, since rabies remains the only disease where post-exposure vaccination is successful, due to the unusually long incubation period.

Over a century later, neuro-tissue vaccine (NTV) is still the standard preparation, but is being replaced by virus grown in human diploid cells, and then inactivated with propiolactone. No safe attenuated virus is yet available, though an attenuated, or a genetic engineered, vaccine is still a possibility.

For post-exposure cases, a course of 5–6 intramuscular infections, starting as soon as possible, the first combined with an injection of human hyperimmune globulin (20 IU per kg), gives virtually complete protection. Pre-exposure (i.e. for travellers to high-risk areas), 2–3 doses are usually sufficient, with a boost every few years where the risk is maintained (e.g. vets and other animal handlers). Eradication might seem an unattainable goal, but schemes

HIGH RISK GROUPS IN WHICH HBsAg VACCINE IS RECOMMENDED

family contacts of known carriers
babies born to HBeAg-positive mothers
medical and nursing staff in high-risk institutes
   e.g. haemodialysis units
      blood banks
      serology laboratories
      dental surgeries
      mental homes
male homosexuals
drug addicts
immunocompromised patients
patients requiring repeated blood transfusion

Fig. 36.18 Hepatitis B vaccines are expensive, and are currently recommended only for people at high risk of infection.

to introduce an attenuated virus to wild-life via infected food bait, have been tried out in Switzerland and neighbouring countries, as well as Canada, and have had some remarkable successes.

Yellow fever and other arbovirus infections

This group of vector-borne fevers, which includes yellow fever, dengue, SE Asian haemorrhagic fever, and Japanese encephalitis, are among the most virulent virus infections (see Chapter 31), and good vaccines would be most desirable.

By good fortune an attenuated yellow fever virus was developed in 1937, and this '17D' strain remains the standard, and highly effective, vaccine. A single subcutaneous dose, with a boost every 10 years for residents in the tropics or frequent visitors, gives excellent protection, and is a requirement for all travellers to endemic countries .

Vaccines are also available against Japanese encephalitis (killed virus), and Rift Valley fever. However, no vaccine is currently available for dengue fever, and this is now recognized as a high priority. One problem is the existence of four serotypes, but a more serious complication is the possibility that one manifestation of the disease may be immunopathological. This is the 'haemorrhagic shock syndrome' seen in patients infected with a second serotype following earlier exposure to a first. Whatever the mechanism of this condition, there is an obvious possibility that a vaccine which did not protect fully against all serotypes might precipitate the condition.

Influenza

Unlike most of the diseases considered so far, influenza does not induce good long-lasting immunity even after recovery from infection in healthy people. This is mainly due to its ability to undergo antigenic 'shift' and 'drift' (see Chapter 22), but also to the curious tendency for responses to different strains to be dominated by antibody against the strain first encountered by the individual ('original antigenic sin'). However, influenza is such an important cause of morbidity and mortality (estimated at 150 per million in the USA), that a range of only partially effective vaccines is in use, pending the development of something better.

The most widely used are formalin- or β-propiolactone-killed viral vaccines, usually including two subtypes of influenza A and one of B, and containing the haemagglutinin (H) and neuraminidase (N) prevalent or anticipated in the population. This vaccine is offered to high-risk groups such as nursing and ancillary staff, the elderly, and patients with chronic respiratory, cardiac, or renal disease, anaemia, diabetes, or immunodeficiency. In such patients, efficacy is estimated at about 70% in terms of reducing severity, but only about 30% if total prevention is the criterion. Revaccination in subsequent years is required to maintain antibody levels but, whether with the same or a different strain, does not give a further boost of titre.

Trials with live cold-adapted strains have shown some protection, but up to 30% of normal patients may fail to produce antibody and would presumably not be protected. Temperature-sensitive mutants designed to grow in the upper but not the lower respiratory tract have been disappointing, due to reversion to wild-type.

An alternative is a recombinant virus containing portions of RNA coding for appropriate H and N antigens. A theoretical advantage of all these live vaccines would be the induction of cytotoxic T cell memory, which is generally poor or absent with killed viruses. However, viral antigens entrapped in ISCOM's have recently been shown to induce good cytotoxic T cell responses.

Varicella-zoster infection

Chicken-pox, caused by varicella-zoster virus (V-ZV), can occasionally lead to severe complications and is a life-threatening disease in children with leukaemia. A live attenuated V-ZV vaccine has been shown to be highly protective – up to 95% protection lasting 7 years in healthy patients but considerably less in leukaemic children on chemotherapy. However, some early cases where severe chicken-pox followed vaccination, the uncertainty as to whether the risk of zoster (shingles) would be decreased, or even increased, and the availability of alternative methods of treating chicken-pox in leukaemics (zoster immunoglobulin plus acyclovir) has discouraged the widespread use of V-ZV vaccine. Nevertheless many authorities consider that it should be added to the triple MMR vaccine for routine use.

Pneumococcal infection

Here again, antigenic diversity is a problem, but since the 84 serotypes of *Strep. pneumoniae* are stable in the population and do not show the rapid changes of influenza, it is theoretically possible to produce a complete vaccine containing them all. In practice it has been found that less than half this number is sufficient to protect against the majority of infections, and current vaccines contain 23–35 serotypes.

The antigen used is the capsular polysaccharide, prepared from large-scale bacterial culture. The indications for vaccination are similar to those for influenza, and in the USA the vaccine is strongly recommended for the elderly, being appreciably cheaper than the treatment for pneumonia. In children under two, the other main high risk group, the response to the vaccine is generally poor, since the IgG2 class of antibody, which predominates in responses to carbohydrate antigens, develops late, and the polysaccharides behave as T-independent antigens.

Conjugation to a protein carrier has been shown to improve the response, presumably by allowing T cells to participate, and trials of protein-polysaccharide conjugates are under way. To conjugate all the available serotypes is, however, a mammoth task, and it is likely that a smaller number, perhaps about eight, will be used initially.

There is clearly room for improvement, and other approaches are being seriously considered, including protein-based vaccines and the anti-idiotype strategy.

Meningococcal infection

Here the principle is the same as with the pneumococcus, though only three serotypes are needed – types A, B and C. Again the response is less than optimal, particularly in younger children and particularly to the type B polysaccharide, which is a very poor antigen being largely composed of sialic acid. Current trials of type B conjugated to either tetanus toxoid or to a meningococcal protein (which should theoretically be better) should show how much improvement can be expected. Meanwhile, only types A and C are used routinely.

A problem that has been noted with both pneumococcal and meningococcal vaccines is that other infections, notably even quite mild malaria, interfere with the normal response to the vaccine. Thus it was found in a Nigerian trial that treatment of the patients with chloroquine one week earlier improved the anti-polysaccharide responses. This emphasizes the desirability of a malaria vaccine (see below).

Haemophilus influenzae infection

This is the third type of bacterium for which a capsular polysaccharide vaccine is available. The b serotype (Hib) is responsible for the most serious disease and its capsule, a phosphodiester-linked polymer of ribose and ribitol, suffers from the same problems as the other polysaccharides-especially low immunogenicity in children under two. A variety of polysaccharide-protein conjugates are now available, using either tetanus or diphtheria toxoid, given either alone (2–3 doses subcutaneously at 2–6 months) or with the triple DPT vaccine. These appear to induce good antibody and memory responses and, encouragingly, poor initial responders may still respond well to later boosting.

A large-scale trial in Finland showed 94% efficacy, though this level has not always been achieved elsewhere.

Typhoid

For nearly a century travellers to the tropics, and particularly military personnel, have been subjected to the 'TAB' vaccine, consisting of heat-, phenol-, alcohol- or acetone-killed whole *Salmonella typhi* and *S. paratyphi* organisms, injected intramuscularly once or twice.

Not only is the vaccine fairly unpleasant, with local pain and general malaise due to the endotoxin content, but its efficacy has repeatedly been questioned. In various controlled trials protection has been estimated at between 10% and 70%, depending partly on the size of the infecting dose. There is therefore a considerable demand for new and better typhoid vaccines.

Two candidates have emerged: a live attenuated organism and a capsular polysaccharide. The first attenuated typhoid bacillus (Ty21a) was produced by random chemical mutagenesis, but current attention focuses on enzyme-deficient strains with mutations in either the galactose epimerase (Gal E) or the aromatic aminoacid synthesis pathway (AroA). These mutations allow the bacilli to survive and proliferate for a few days only, so that when given orally they induce local immunity in the intestine but not systemic disease. All these mutant strains appear to be safe and effective, and the latter two have the added advantage of being suitable vectors for inserted genes derived from other organisms. The TY21a strain has given 60–90% protection lasting at least 5 years, being given either with a tablet of sodium bicarbonate or in enteric-coated capsules.

The polysaccharide vaccine is composed of purified 'Vi' (virulence) antigen. A single dose of 25mg has given protection in the 70% range but, as with the other polysaccharides, conjugation to protein is required for the induction of T-dependent responses and memory.

Cholera

Heat-killed whole *Vibrio cholerae* vaccines suffer from the same disadvantages as the older typhoid vaccines – unpleasant reactions and poor protection (roughly 50% for 6 months), but several replacements are under active study.

Since cholera is essentially a toxin-induced disease, one might expect a toxoid-based vaccine to be sufficient. Some success has been obtained with the B (binding) subunit of the toxin given in combination with whole killed organisms. Another strategy is to construct an attenuated cholera organism with a deletion in the 'A' (toxic) subunit gene. A third idea is to express cholera genes in an attenuated *S. typhi* vaccine which, if it also contained genes from *Shigella* and *E. coli*, (see below) would constitute a formidable vaccine against enteric bacterial infection. Trials of these different vaccines are under way and should ultimately lead to significantly improved control of cholera.

Experimental vaccines

Rotavirus infection

As mentioned earlier, rotavirus infection might be amenable to a live heterologous vaccine, as was the case with smallpox. Bovine and monkey strains of the virus have been tried as oral vaccines in infants, with 70–80% reported protection. The possibility of using the 'naturally' attenuated human strains that can appear in nurseries is also being explored. Prospects are therefore quite favourable for the eventual availability of a rotavirus vaccine.

Shigellosis

Live, randomly attenuated *Shigella* organisms, though fairly effective as oral vaccines, never came into general use because of the short duration of protection and occasional side-effects. Current research is concentrated on deliberately mutated strains and on the insertion of shigella antigens into *S. typhi* or other vectors.

Escherichia coli infection

Because of the serotypic diversity of both surface antigens and toxins, no fully successful vaccine against *E. coli* infection has yet emerged. However trials have been conducted with toxoids based on the enterotoxins, purified fimbriae, whole killed organisms, and live attenuated strains, all of which give some protection. The combined killed cholera/B toxin-subunit vaccine mentioned above also gave significant protection against *E. coli*, due to cross-reaction between the two toxins.

Leprosy

The effect of BCG in protecting against leprosy (notably in a Ugandan trial) has already been mentioned. Meanwhile trials of combined BCG and killed *M. leprae* are under way, and *M. leprae* protein antigens are being cloned for insertion into vectors.

Malaria

At the time of writing, three clinical trials of a malaria vaccine have been published, and more will certainly follow. Two were with peptides derived from the major surface protein of the sporozoite (pre-hepatic stage) and one with a hybrid of peptides, mainly from the asexual blood stage. Despite individual cases of protection against a subsequent challenge, the overall results were unimpressive. Other potential targets for attack within the unusually complex malaria life-cycle (see Chapter 30) include the liver stage itself, the merozoite (infective for the red cell) the sexual stages (gametocytes and gametes) and the soluble molecules thought to be responsible for inducing pathology (Fig. 36.19). This wide range of choices clearly increases the chance of success, but each approach has its problems: for example, extensive antigenic variation in the blood stage, and the need for 100% efficacy with the hepatic and prehepatic stages; also the sexual stage vaccines would only block transmission, protecting the community but not the vaccinee.

While each approach has its vigorous proponents, it seems likely that a really successful vaccine will contain antigens from several or all stages.

Leishmaniasis

Three quite separate approaches have given some degree of protection against cutaneous leishmaniasis. One, 'leishmanization' with material from active lesions, has already been mentioned; it had some popularity in the former Soviet Union and Israel, but protection was variable and non-virulent disease could never be guaranteed. A second idea was killed promastigotes (the invasive stage), 2–3 times intramuscularly. Up to 80% protection was claimed in a Brazilian trial, but this was of uncertain duration. The

MALARIA VACCINE STRATEGIES

stage	vaccine strategy
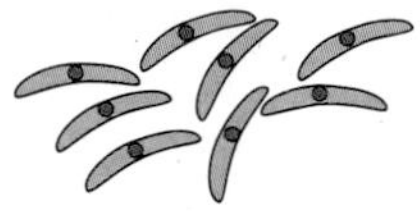 sporozoites	sporozoite vaccine to induce blocking antibody, already field-tested in humans
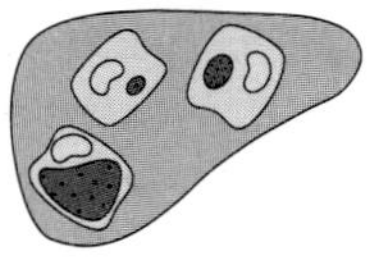 liver stage	sporozoite vaccine to induce cell-mediated immunity to liver stage
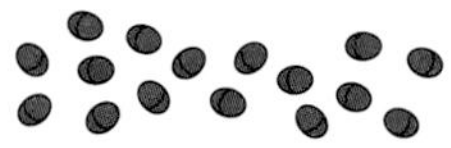 merozoites	merozoite (-antigen) vaccine to induce blocking antibody
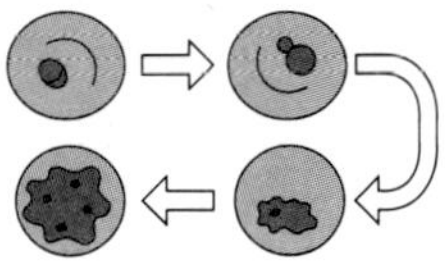 asexual erythrocyte stage	asexual stage (-antigen) vaccine to induce other responses to red cell stage, and against toxic products ('anti-disease' vaccine)
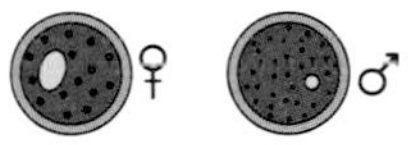 gametocytes	vaccines to interrupt sexual stages – 'transmission blocking' vaccine
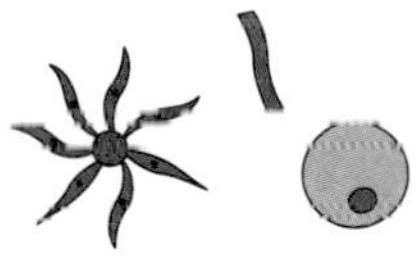 gametes	

Fig. 36.19 Malaria vaccine strategies. A number of different approaches are being investigated, reflecting the complexity of the life cycle and of immunity to this parasite (see also Chapter 30).

IMPORTANT INFECTIOUS DISEASES FOR WHICH THERE IS NO SATISFACTORY VACCINE

organism	disease
HIV	AIDS
Herpes simplex virus	genital infection
Cytomegalovirus	effect on foetus
EB virus	glandular fever
Rhinoviruses	common cold
Neisseria gonorrhoeae	gonorrhoea
Mycobacterium leprae	leprosy
Treponema pallidum	syphilis
Chlamydia trachomatis	trachoma, urethritis
Plasmodium sp.	malaria
Trypanosoma sp.	trypanosomiasis
Schistosoma sp.	schistosomiasis

Fig. 36.20 Important infectious diseases for which a satisfactory vaccine is not yet available.

most dramatic results came from a Venezuelan trial with injection of killed promastigotes plus BCG; over 90% protection was induced, but again it is too soon to say how long this lasts.

Vaccines still awaited

There remains a long list of important infectious diseases for which vaccines, although desirable, are not yet available (Fig. 36.20). In some cases it is probably only a matter of time, but in others there are fundamental problems. With the adenoviruses and rhinoviruses, for example, the serotypic diversity (about 40 and 110 respectively) make it hard to imagine a fully effective vaccine. With the live herpes virus vaccines there is the danger of latency with reactivation, and with the killed vaccines the difficulty of obtaining large amounts of virus (except with herpes simplex). With respiratory syncytial virus the problem has been reversion of attenuated strains and enhancement of disease by killed vaccines. With the bacterial diseases in figure 36.20, it is the lack of convincing immunity following natural infection that is discouraging, syphilis perhaps being the outstanding example. The same applies to the protozoa and helminths, though research is proceeding in a variety of directions, and some quite effective vaccines have been produced for veterinary use (e.g. hookworm in dogs, lungworm in cattle).

Perhaps the most concentrated effort is being directed agoinst HIV, where the production of a vaccine to limit the spread or progression of AIDS is literally a race against time. Most workers have focussed on the gp160 molecule by which the virus attaches and fuses itself to cells, and some promising results have been obtained in monkeys with the analogous molecule from simian immunodeficiency virus (SIV), a near relative of HIV2. Several human trials are in progress, but it will be some time before the results are clear, and at present the extraordinarily extensive antigenic variation of this molecule makes success quite problematic.

SUMMARY

Vaccination aims to prime the adaptive immune system to the antigens of a particular microbe, so that a first infection induces a secondary response. Vaccines are either live attenuated organisms, killed whole organisms, subcellular fractions, or antigens produced artificially by gene cloning or chemical synthesis. In general, live vaccines are more effective, but are subject to the danger of reversion to virulence or the induction of disease in immunocompromised patients. The details of vaccine choice, route, dose and risks have to be considered disease by disease, and there is room for considerable improvement in producing safe, effective, affordable vaccines.

Further Reading

Battle JL, Murphy FL, eds. *Vaccine biotechnology*. London: Academic Press, 1989.

Gregoriadis G, Allison AC, Poste G. *Vaccines. Recent trends and progress*. NATO ASI Series A, volume 215. London: Plenum Press, 1991.

Joint committee on vaccination and immunisation. *Immunisation against infectious disease*. London: HMSO, 1988.

Mims CA, White DO. *Viral pathogenesis and immunity*. Oxford: Blackwell Scientific Publishing, 1984.

Synthetic peptides as antigens. CIBA symposium, 1986; 119.

37 PASSIVE AND NON-SPECIFIC IMMUNOTHERAPY

INTRODUCTION

The most dramatic and successful form of immunotherapy is vaccination, as described in the previous chapter. However, there are some situations where a different approach may be necessary. For instance, the patient may already have been infected so that a more rapid build-up of immune effector mechanisms than occurs naturally may be called for. Alternatively, the patient's immune system may be inadequate, unable to respond either to the infection or to a vaccine, through immunodeficiency or some specially resistant property of the parasite. This brief chapter deals with such situations.

PASSIVE IMMUNIZATION WITH ANTIBODY

Before the introduction of antibiotics, acute infectious diseases were often treated by the injection of preformed antibody, on the principle that with the patient already ill it was too late for 'active' vaccination. Indeed, the demonstration that immunity to tetanus and diphtheria could be transferred to mice with serum from vaccinated rabbits was a key experiment in the discovery of antibody in the 1890s. Subsequently, the production of antiserum for passive treatment of diphtheria, tetanus and pneumococcal pneumonia, and against the toxic effects of streptococci and staphylococci, became an important industry, and generations of horses that had retired from active duty were kept on as the source of 'immune serum'. The introduction of anti-tetanus serum in the early months of World War I reduced the incidence of tetanus dramatically by up to 30-fold (Fig. 37.1).

The advent of penicillin and other antibiotics has, of course, changed the picture considerably, and passive immunotherapy is now used only in a select group of diseases (Fig. 37.2). The serum may be specific or non-specific and of human or animal origin.

Specific antibody

The use of antiserum raised in horses or rabbits has largely been abandoned because of the complications resulting from the immune response to the antibody, which is of course a foreign protein. These include progressively more rapid elimination (and therefore reduced clinical effectiveness) and, more seriously, serum sickness due to immune complex deposition in the kidney, skin, etc. (see

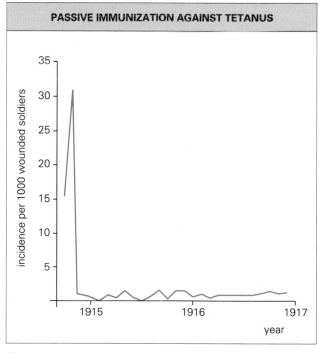

Fig. 37.1 Passive immunization significantly reduced the incidence of tetanus in the early months of the First World War. The figure shows the incidence of tetanus per 1000 wounded soldiers in British hospitals during 1914-16. There was a dramatic fall after the introduction of anti-tetanus serum in October 1914.

SPECIFIC PASSIVE IMMUNOTHERAPY WITH ANTIBODY		
infection	source of antibody	indication
Diphtheria	human, horse	prophylaxis, treatment
Tetanus	human, horse	
Varicella-zoster	human	treatment in immunodeficiencies
Gas gangrene	horse	post exposure
Botulism		
Snake bite Scorpion bite		
Rabies	human	post-exposure (plus vaccine)
Hepatitis B	human	post-exposure
Hepatitis A	pooled human immunoglobulin	prophylaxis (travel)
Measles		post-exposure

Fig. 37.2 Specific passive immunotherapy with antibody. Though not so commonly used as 50 years ago, passive injections of specific antibody can still be a life-saving treatment.

INDICATIONS FOR NORMAL IMMUNOGLOBULIN THERAPY
X-linked agammaglobulaemia/hypogammaglobulinaemia
common variable deficiency
Wiskott–Aldrich syndrome
ataxia telengiectasia
IgG subclass deficiency with impaired antibody response
chronic lymphocytic leukaemia
post-bone marrow transplantation (for CMV)
?AIDS
liver transplant in HBsAg-positive recipients

Fig. 37.3 Indications for normal immunoglobulin therapy. Sufficient antibody to protect immunocompromised patients against common infections can be obtained from pooled normal human plasma.

Chapter 16), and even anaphylaxis. However, horse antisera against diphtheria and gas gangrene are still sometimes used.

Such complications can be avoided by the use of human serum, taken during convalescence or following vaccination, to prevent infection after exposure (e.g. rabies) or to minimize its severity (e.g. varicella in immunodeficient children).

Theoretically the best form of specific antibody would be a monoclonal antibody, the specificity of which is precisely known. However, a mixture of several monoclonals might be required in situations where individual antigens are expressed in low amounts on the microbe, or where binding to more than one epitope is required for full effectiveness. Despite some success in animal experiments (e.g. pneumococcal infection in mice and dental caries in monkeys), therapeutic monoclonal antibodies have not yet made a great impact on the treatment of infection. However, a monoclonal antibody against the non-variant lipid portion of Gram-negative bacterial endotoxin is currently undergoing extensive trials for the treatment of septic shock, with some promising results.

Non-specific antibody

With reasonably common infections, it can be assumed that most normal people have antibody to the pathogen in their serum. The clearest proof of this is that patients with hypogammaglobulinaemia can be kept free of recurrent infection by regular injections of IgG from pooled normal serum, and that immunodeficient children can be protected against measles in the same way (Fig. 37.3).

Immunoglobulin is prepared from batches of plasma from 1000–6000 healthy donors after screening for hepatitis B and C, and HIV. With improvements in methods of preparation, intravenous injection is now preferred to intramuscular injection in most cases. Dosages for this type of therapy range from 100 mg to 400 mg IgG per kg monthly. In normal individuals the probability of contracting hepatitis A in an endemic area is enormously reduced by a single injection of as little as 5 ml of IgG. The immunity conferred by mothers on their newborn infants by placental transfer of IgG and subsequently by colostral IgA (though the latter is not absorbed but remains in the intestine) is further evidence for the protective effect of relatively small amounts of antibody.

NON-SPECIFIC CELLULAR IMMUNOSTIMULATION

The demonstration by William Coley almost a century ago that crude extracts of bacteria could induce remission and sometimes cure of cancers, indicates the extent to which the immune system can be nonspecifically 'overstimulated' with potentially beneficial results. Until recently, many of the compounds used in this way have been of microbial origin, but current interest is directed mainly at cytokines and other molecular mediators, on the principle that their induction was probably the basis of action of the older crude materials (Fig. 37.4).

Most of the applications of this type of immunostimulation have been in the tumour field, but some infectious diseases respond to treatment with cytokines (Fig. 37.5).

NON-SPECIFIC IMMUNOSTIMULATORS	
microbial	Coley's toxin (filtered cultures of *Streptococci* and *Serratia marcescens* used against tumours)
	BCG (Bacillus Calmette-Guérin)
	Corynebacterium parvum
	endotoxin (lipopolysaccharide)
	streptococcal-derived OK432
endogenous	thymus factors and hormones
	cytokines
	?transfer factor

Fig. 37.4 A variety of foreign and endogenous materials have been used in an attempt to raise the general level of immunological competence.

POTENTIALLY THERAPEUTIC CYTOKINES	
IFN-α, IFN-β	hepatitis B (chronic) hepatitis C herpes zoster papillomavirus rhinovirus (prophylactic only) ?HIV warts
IFN-γ	lepromatous leprosy leishmaniasis toxoplasmosis (brain) chronic granulomatous disease (CGD)
IL-2	leprosy (local treatment to skin lesions)
TNF	anti-TNF in septic shock
IL-1	receptor antagonist in septic shock
IL-10, TGF-β	septic shock
CSFs	bacterial infection due to neutropenia in irradiated patients

Fig. 37.5 Cytokines are increasingly used to improve immunity to infection, as well as in some cancers and haematological disorders.

SOME COMMON SIDE-EFFECTS OF CYTOKINE THERAPY	
Interferons	fever malaise fatigue muscle pains toxicity to: kidney liver bone marrow heart
IL-2	vascular leak syndrome hypotension oedema ascites pulmonary oedema renal failure hepatic failure mental changes; coma
TNF	shock (as IL-2, with hypotension particularly marked)

Fig. 37.6 Treatment with cytokines, especially if prolonged, can lead to serious side-effects.

Foremost among these are the interferons, notably IFN-α, which is effective in a number of virus infections, though less so than might have been predicted from the importance of their normal role in inhibiting viral replication. IFN-γ has recently been found to benefit many cases of chronic granulomatous disease (CGD), though the mechanism is unclear. The unpleasant side-effects of high dose therapy with interleukins, interferons or tumour necrosis factor (TNF), restricts their casual use (Fig. 37.6).

Mention should also be made of 'transfer factor' (TF), a dialysed extract of peripheral leucocytes. It has been claimed for many years that TF from normal patients will restore T cell responses in unresponsive recipients, and some dramatic cures, for example of chronic mucocutaneous candidiasis, have been reported. Whether this restoration is antigen-specific or non-specific has been the subject of great controversy, and in the absence of proper molecular characterization, TF is no longer regarded as an orthodox treatment.

Equally unorthodox but attracting increasing attention are a variety of plant products (saponins, Ginseng, chinese herbal remedies, etc.). These substances appear to improve resistance to infection and in some cases, also act as adjuvants when combined with vaccines – highlighting the very interesting 'grey area' where immunostimulation and nutrition overlap.

CORRECTION OF HOST IMMUNODEFICIENCY

This subject is discussed in more detail in Chapter 33, and will only be briefly summarized here. As mentioned above, antibody defects are the easiest to treat, since immunoglobulin can be transferred and has a reasonably long half-life (about three weeks for IgG). Treatment of T cell defects is much less successful, though thymus or bone-marrow grafting has been tried in certain cases (Fig. 37.7). Phagocytic defects are the most difficult of all to correct and in practice antibiotics remain the mainstay of therapy, though the future may lie in gene replacement.

TREATMENT OF IMMUNODEFICIENCY: AN OVERVIEW				
	B cell defects	**T cell defects**	**phagocyte defects**	**complement defects**
Correction of defect	bone marrow graft (SCID)	thymus graft (Di George) ?thymus hormones	?bone marrow graft (CGD)	—
Replacement therapy	pooled normal IgG specific IgG	blood transfusion (ADA, PNP deficiency) ?cytokines ??transfer factor	?cytokines	not successful
Symptomatic therapy	antibiotics	antivirals	antibiotics	antibiotics steroids (for immune complex disease)

SCID, severe combined immunodeficiency   ADA, adenosine deaminase
CGD, chronic granulomatous disease   PNP, purine nucleoside phosphorylase

Fig. 37.7 The treatment of immunodeficiency depends on a knowledge of the element at fault, some being more easily restored than others.

SUMMARY

Transfer of normal pooled IgG is the most widely practised type of passive immunotherapy, used to treat most forms of antibody deficiency, while specific antibodies can be used for certain defined conditions. Non-specific stimulation of T cell mediated immunity is still experimental but cytokines show some promise, particularly interferon for virus infections.

Further Reading

Allison AC. Immunopotentiation. In: *Clinical immunology.* Brostoff J, Scadding GK, Male D, Roitt IM, eds. London: Gower Medical Publishing, 1991.

Coley WB. The therapeutic value of the mixed toxins of erysipelas and *Bacillus prodigiosus* in the treatment of inoperable malignant tumours. *Am J Med Sci* 1896; **112:** 251.

Parker MT, Collier LH, eds. *Topley and Wilson's principles of bacteriology, virology and immunity.* Vol. 1. 8th edn. London: Edward Arnold, 1990.

38 EPIDEMIOLOGICAL ASPECTS OF THE CONTROL OF INFECTION AND DISEASE

Contents

INTRODUCTION

Medical practitioners are primarily concerned with the factors that make each infection unique. However, when considering infection and disease within populations, and their control by vaccination or chemotherapy, a number of general epidemiological principles emerge. This chapter discusses these principles and explores their relevance to the design of control policies based on vaccination or chemotherapy. It focusses on infection and disease in the community as opposed to the individual. In most cases what is best for the individual is also best for the community, but this is not always the case. If vaccination carries some risk of inducing serious disease, the optimum policy for the individual is to avoid vaccination whilst encouraging everyone else to be vaccinated! Conflicts between the interests of the individual and those of the community arise in a number of areas in infectious disease epidemiology. Their resolution is aided by a clear understanding of the precise circumstances in which they arise.

BASIC CONCEPTS

Microparasites and macroparasites

'Microparasites' are infectious agents such as viruses, bacteria and some protozoans which reproduce directly – often at very high rates – within the host. They are usually small and have a short generation time. Recovery from infection usually gives immunity against reinfection and this, in the case of viral infections, may be life long. With some important exceptions, the duration of infection is short relative to the lifespan of the host. Microparasite infections are, therefore, typically transient.

In defining the epidemiology of these infections it is useful to divide the host population into four classes of individuals: 1) susceptible; 2) infected but latent (i.e. non-infectious); note that this is a different type of latency to that described for persistent infections in Chapter 15; 3) infected and infectious; 4) recovered and immune (Fig. 38.1), and to quantify the incubation period (time between infection and disease) and the latent period (time

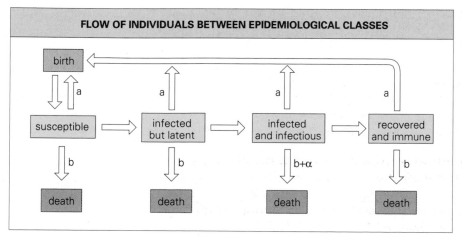

Fig. 38.1 The flow of individuals between susceptible, infected and immune classes in a population exposed to a directly transmitted microparasite. Reproduction at a per capita rate 'a' provides new susceptibles, whilst death at a per capita rate 'b' removes individuals from the flow. Disease related death rate 'α' is additional to 'b' in the infectious group. New infections arise as infectious and susceptible individuals mix.

THE SCIENCE OF EPIDEMIOLOGY

Epidemiology is the study of the occurrence, spread and control of diseases. It is based upon the collection of detailed statistical information and can be undertaken at several levels, from the purely descriptive to the analytical and experimental, in which mathematical modelling plays an increasingly important part. Epidemiological data can be used to record the diseases affecting a population and, where infectious, to identify their causes and modes of transmission. It can also be used to predict the future likelihood of infection, to identify risk factors, and to plan control programmes involving chemotherapy and vaccination. It is a science with professional practitioners – *epidemiologists* – who collaborate closely with clinicians and health workers. Like all sciences, epidemiology has its own jargon and specialized use of terms, and explanation of these is a necessary introduction to the topic.

Infection is the term used to indicate the presence of an infectious organism in an individual or population. The term *disease* is used only when infection has detectable clinical consequences, whether mild or severe. The time interval between exposure to infection and appearance of disease is the *incubation period*. Individuals who are infected and can transmit infection to others are *infectious*. Infectiousness may persist after disease has disappeared, the individuals concerned being known as *carriers*. The carrier state may also occur without disease ever having been apparent. Spread of infection – *transmission* – occurs in many ways, but depends upon direct or indirect contact between infectious individuals and individuals who are susceptible (see Chapter 11). Transmission may be vertical (e.g. from mother to foetus or new-born infant), or horizontal (spread by contact between individuals). Experience of infection may lead to an acquired immunity, and immune individuals are then often *resistant* to further infection.

In populations, infection or disease is described as *endemic* if it occurs regularly at low or moderate frequency, or *hyperendemic* if frequency is high. *Epidemics* occur when there are sudden increases in frequency above endemic levels; *pandemics* are global epidemics. *Prevalence* describes the number of cases of infection or disease in members of a population, either at a given point in time (*point* prevalence) or over a given period (*period* prevalence). *Seroprevalence* refers to the number of individuals who are antibody positive for a particular infection. The appearance of such antibodies in individuals is called *seroconversion*. *Incidence* refers to the number of new cases arising in a population over a defined period of time. *Age-specific* prevalence or incidence refers to infection or disease within particular age groups. Prevalence and incidence may show periodic fluctuations or trends over time (often referred to as longitudunal trends). *Secular* trends are long-term changes over periods of years, whereas *periodic* trends are shorter term (months to a few years). *Seasonal* trends are annual or monthly changes, reflecting climatic or behavioural factors, and *acute* trends are those that result in epidemic outbreaks.

Descriptive epidemiological data can be collected during outbreaks or collected subsequently. The more complete the data, the more fruitful analysis is likely to be. Accordingly, it is necessary to record not only data relating to the infection itself, but also demographic, geographic, climatic, socio-economic, behavioural and personal data. Division or *stratification* of a population by such parameters is a useful way of seeing whether infection is associated with particular characteristics.

Analytical epidemiology uses two basic approaches, case control and cohort studies. Case control studies are *retrospective*, taking a group in which infection or disease is present and comparing with a matching control group in which it is absent in order to identify cause and effect. Cohort studies are normally *prospective*. They monitor the appearance of infection or disease in carefully defined groups over a prolonged period. Again, comparison with a control group is used to identify cause and effect. A third form of analysis is *epidemiological investigation*, the study of epidemics as they occur. This involves collection of all relevant data in an attempt to identify the infectious agent and its transmission and to define control measures.

Experimental epidemiology applies epidemiological methods to experimental systems, such as drug or vaccine trials, in which individuals with or without disease, or exposed or non-exposed to infectious agents, are given specific therapy, and the results compared with individuals given placebos or alternative therapy. Experimental epidemiology requires detailed statistical planning and analysis. Mathematical modelling of infection and disease in populations is applied in descriptive, analytical and experimental epidemiology and is a powerful interpretive as well as a predictive tool with very wide applicability to disease control.

Surveillance

In many countries, public health authorities carry out continuing epidemiological surveys of particular diseases in the national population, e.g. the Centres for Disease Control (CDC) of the US Public Health Service and the Communicable Diseases Surveillance Centres (CDSC) of the Public Health Laboratory Service in the UK. The World Health Organization performs a similar role internationally. At a national level, surveillance is often based on notifiable diseases, practitioners being obliged to report these diseases when they occur in their patients (*morbidity* data). Surveillance records can also be taken from notified causes of death (*mortality* data), from reports sent in by diagnostic laboratories, from population surveys and from detailed case investigations. Such data are then published regularly, for example in the American Morbidity and Mortality Weekly Report (MMWR), and the weekly UK Communicable Diseases Report (CDR), so that the medical community is alerted to trends in patterns of disease, and recommendations for control made quickly and efficiently.

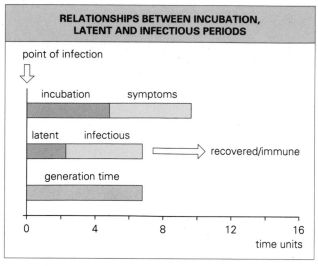

Fig. 38.2 The relationships between the incubation, latent and infectious periods for a hypothetical microparasitic infection. Note that the infectious period and the duration of symptoms of disease are not necessarily synchronous. The generation time is the sum of the latent and infectious periods (see text).

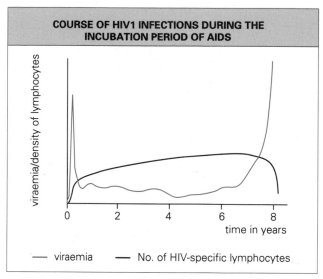

Fig. 38.3 Fluctuations in HIV1-induced viraemia in an infected patient who developed AIDS 8 years from the point of infection. Two major peaks in viraemia are recorded, one soon after infection and the second as symptoms of immunodeficiency develop and AIDS is diagnosed. The graph also shows changes in the abundance of lymphocytes specific for HIV1 antigens.

between infection and infectiousness) (Fig. 38.2). For some infections, e.g. the herpes viruses, intermittent bouts of infectiousness may occur; for others, e.g. the AIDS viruses, the degree of infectiousness may vary widely throughout the incubation period. With HIV1, viraemia (which is closely correlated with infectiousness) has an early peak a few weeks after infection, followed by a long period of a few to many years of relatively low infectiousness and a final period of very high infectiousness as symptoms of immunodeficiency appear (Fig. 38.3). The sum of the latent and infectious periods is referred to as the 'generation time' of the infection (see Fig. 38.2), a value which helps to determine the frequency with which epidemics may occur (see below). Average latent and infectious periods of some common microparasitic infections are listed in figure 38.4, and distributions of observed incubation periods for hepatitis B viral infection and AIDS in figure 38.5.

'Macroparasites', such as helminths and arthropods, have no direct reproduction within the definitive host, producing transmission stages that pass to the exterior to complete their life cycle. They are typically large and their generation times can often be a significant fraction of the host's life span. Immunity tends to be of a relatively short duration once the parasites are removed, and infections are often persistent, with hosts continually being reinfected. Infections are rarely uniformly or even randomly distributed (Fig. 38.6), most people harbouring few parasites and a few harbouring many. Models based on dividing populations into susceptible and infected persons are therefore inappropriate. The most useful epidemiological framework records the prevalence, average intensity and distribution of infection within the population.

TIME COURSE OF COMMON INFECTIONS			
infectious disease	incubation period (days)	latent period (days)	infectious period (days)
Measles	8–13	6–9	0–7
Mumps	12–26	12–18	4–8
Whooping cough (pertussis)	6–10	21–23	7–10
Rubella	14–21	7–14	11–12
Diphtheria	2–5	14–21	2–5
Varicella	13–17	8–12	10–11
Hepatitis B	50–110	13–17	19–22
Poliomyelitis	7–12	1–3	14–20
Influenza	1–3	1–3	2–3

Fig. 38.4 Incubation, latent and infectious periods for a variety of viral and bacterial infections.

Calculating the spread of infection – the basic reproductive rate

For a microparasite the basic reproductive rate, R_0, is defined as the average number of secondary cases of infection produced by one primary case in a susceptible population. R_0 is also referred to as the 'case reproductive rate' or the 'transmission potential'. When an infection becomes established in a population and 'herd' immunity develops, the proportion of susceptible individuals will

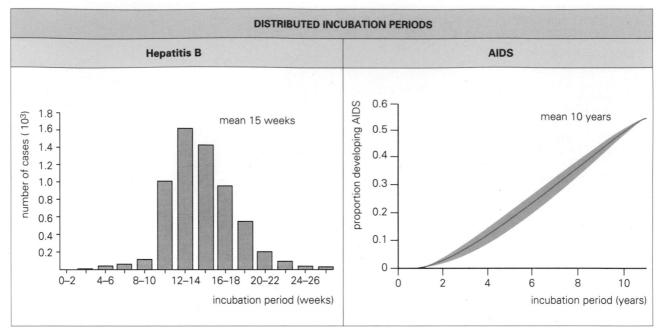

Fig. 38.5 Incubation periods (time since seroconversion) of (a) hepatitis B and (b) AIDS, in sexually active adults. (b) Shows the range of data from different studies in various urban centres in Europe and North America.

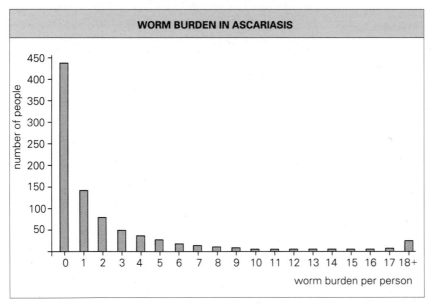

Fig. 38.6 The frequency distribution of the human roundworm *Ascaris lumbricoides*, in a rural community in Korea.

decrease. Eventually some sort of equilibrium is reached (endemic infection), although there may be fluctuations of a seasonal or longer term nature. One example is the seasonal cycle in the incidence of measles, imposed on a regular 2-year cycle, clearly observable prior to the introduction of mass vaccination (see Fig. 38.13, below).

At equilibrium the rate at which susceptible individuals are infected is exactly balanced by the rate at which new susceptibles are born into the community, each infection on average producing one secondary case, i.e. the effective reproductive rate is R=1. In a homogeneously mixed community the effective reproductive rate R is equal to the basic reproductive rate R_0 discounted by x, the fraction of the community that is susceptible, i.e. R=R_0x. Given that at equilibrium R=1, then

$$R_0=1/x^*$$

where x^* is the fraction susceptible at equilibrium. This simple relationship provides a method of estimating the value of R_0 from serological or other data on age-specific susceptibility.

For a macroparasite, R_0 is the average number of female offspring produced throughout the lifetime of a mature female parasite, which themselves achieve reproductive maturity in the absence of density-dependent regulation

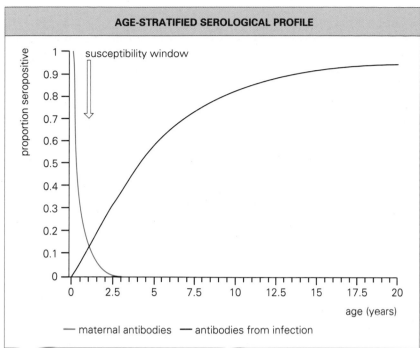

AGE-STRATIFIED SEROLOGICAL PROFILE

— maternal antibodies   — antibodies from infection

Fig. 38.7 An age-stratified serological profile recording the presence or absence of antibodies specific to the antigens of a directly transmitted childhood viral infection (average age at infection, 5 years). There is a susceptibility window between the decay in maternally derived antibody and the rise in seroprevalence due to infection.

(e.g. competition for space or other resources, and acquired immunity). Theoretically, in the absence of these regulatory mechanisms parasite numbers within the population would grow without constraint, provided $R_0 > 1$. In practice, because of such constraints, macroparasite populations tend to be rather stable.

We can sometimes observe an infection in its initial phase of invasion, such as with the AIDS virus HIV1 or when macroparasites begin to re-establish themselves after chemotherapy. In both cases the initial exponential rise in the proportion of people infected depends on the magnitude of R_0. The rate of this rise, Λ, is simply given by:

$$\Lambda = (R_0 - 1)/D$$

where D is the average duration of infectiousness of an individual with a microparasitic infection, or the average life expectancy of an adult macroparasite. This provides a further method of estimating the transmission potential of an infectious agent (R_0).

For most common viral and bacterial infections, serological tools are available to establish whether or not a person has acquired and recovered from infection at some time in their life. Age-stratified cross-sectional serological surveys or longitudinal cohort studies provide the best data for estimating the magnitude of R_0 in a given community. Figure 38.7 shows the decay in maternally derived antibodies and the subsequent rise in antibody-positive individuals due to infection in an unvaccinated population. The magnitude of R_0 can be estimated from this profile by calculating the fraction of the total population susceptible to infection, or equally simply from the following expression:

$$R_0 = (L - M)/(A - M)$$

where L is life expectancy, M is the average duration of maternal-antibody-derived protection (typically 6 months for many common viral infections such as measles) and A is the average age at infection. The key quantity is A, which

AVERAGE AGE AT INFECTION FOR DIFFERENT INFECTIONS IN DIFFERENT LOCALITIES		
infectious disease	**average age at infection A (years)**	**source of data**
Measles	5–6	USA, 1955–58
	4–5	England and Wales, 1948–68
	1–2	Thailand, 1967
	2–3	India, 1978
Rubella	9–10	Sweden, 1965
	9–10	Manchester, UK, 1970–82
	2–3	Gambia, 1976
	6–7	Poland, 1970–88
Varicella	6–8	USA, 1921–28
Poliomyelitis	12–17	USA, 1955
Pertussis	4–5	England and Wales, 1948–68
	4–5	USA, 1920–60
Mumps	6–7	England and Wales, 1975–77
	6–7	Netherlands, 1977–79

Fig. 38.8 Average age at infection (A) for different infections at different localities prior to widescale immunization.

can be estimated directly from the serological profile. If A is small, R_0 is large and the infection has high transmission efficiency; if A is large, R_0 is small and transmission efficiency is low. Figure 38.8 lists some estimates of A for a variety of common infections in unvaccinated communities. Transmission success can vary widely; in developing countries values of A are typically much lower than those in the UK or the USA.

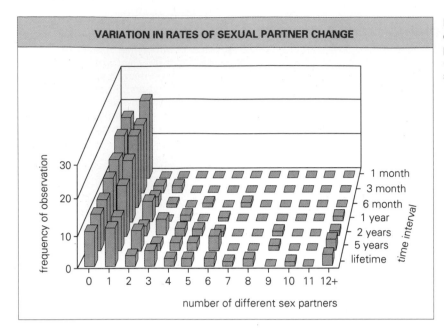

Fig. 38.9 Frequency distribution of claimed number of different sexual partners over various time periods (1 month to lifetime) recorded in a survey of male and female students in 1987 in the UK.

Serological surveys provide valuable information about the transmission dynamics of infectious agents. They not only provide information on the duration of maternally derived protection and average age at infection, but they can also indicate the optimum age at which to vaccinate and the fraction that should be immunized to block transmission. However, problems can arise if the duration of measurable antibody production following infection is not life long, as is the case for many bacterial and protozoan infections, and more sophisticated techniques to detect immunological markers of past infection are needed.

Spread of infection and behaviour

In the case of a directly transmitted respiratory viral infection, R_0 is simply:

$$R_0 = \beta XD$$

where X is the density of susceptible people, β is the transmission coefficient, a composite term defining the rate of mixing *and* the probability of transmission per contact between susceptible and infectious persons, and D is the average duration of infectiousness. For the infection to take hold R_0 must be equal or greater than 1, which implies that the density of susceptible people must exceed a critical value X_T given by:

$$X_T = 1/(\beta D)$$

This concept clarifies the target for mass vaccination programmes. To eradicate the infection the density of susceptibles must be reduced below X_T.

Infections that are transmitted by intimate contacts within a defined group of people, such as sexually transmitted diseases (STDs), are important exceptions. Here R_0 depends on the average rate at which new sexual partners are acquired, which is usually independent of population size. STDs, which often produce long-lasting infections (e.g. herpes virus, HIV and untreated gonorrhoea) are therefore ideally suited to persisting in low density human communities.

Many behavioural or spatial factors can influence the transmission of infectious agents. These are of particular importance for sexually transmitted infections such as gonorrhoea or HIV since there is great variability in the rate at which individuals acquire different sexual partners (Fig. 38.9). If sexually active individuals acquire partners in different sexual activity classes in proportion to their representation in the population, then the value of R_0 depends on the rate at which new sexual partners are acquired multiplied by the probability of transmission at each partner contact multiplied by the average duration of infectiousness. The value of R_0 can be greatly influenced by the variance in sexual activity. Those who have many sexual partners are both more likely to acquire and to transmit infection and therefore play a key role in the persistence of such infections in the community of sexually active individuals, the majority of whom have very few sexual partners (see Fig. 38.9).

Transmission between groups

Populations can be stratified using many factors, such as age, sex, sexual activity, residence location, etc. Intensity of transmission will differ within different groupings but, equally importantly, contact between groups can also play a key role in determining patterns of infection and disease. In these circumstances R_0 will be influenced by both within- and between-group transmission rates, i.e. by the likelihood of an individual in one group making contact with someone in the same group or in another group. In the case of STDs, the sexual partner contact pattern may be described as a 'mixing matrix'. The importance of these mixing matrices as determinants of epidemiological trends is illustrated in figure 38.10. This records a simulated epidemic of HIV1 in a male homosexual community in the UK, assuming either random choice of sexual partners or highly assortative choice (like-with-like) in which those who change partners frequently choose the majority of

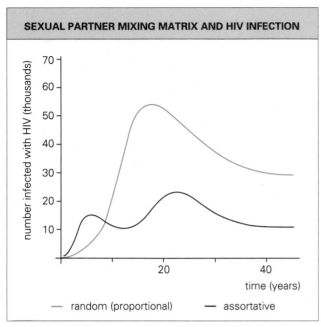

SEXUAL PARTNER MIXING MATRIX AND HIV INFECTION

— random (proportional)　　— assortative

Fig. 38.10 Influence of the sexual partner mixing matrix (preferences) on the predicted changes with time in the number of HIV1 infected individuals in a population of homosexual men. One trajectory assumes random (proportional) mixing between the different sexual activity classes (defined according to rates of sexual partner change) while the other assumes assortative (like-with like) mixing; all other parameters were kept the same.

INTER-EPIDEMIC PERIOD OF SOME COMMON INFECTIONS		
infectious disease	**inter-epidemic period T (years)**	**source of data**
Measles	2 1 1	England and Wales, 1948–68 Yaounde, Cameroun, 1968–75 Ilesha, Nigeria, 1958–61
Rubella	3–5	Manchester, UK, 1961–83
Mumps	3	England and Wales, 1960–80
Poliomyelitis	3–5	England and Wales, 1948–82
Pertussis	3–4	England and Wales, 1948–85

Fig. 38.11 Inter-epidemic period (T) of some common infections, at different localities.

their sexual partners within their own sexual activity class. All other parameters remain the same. Random choice generates a slowly developing epidemic, with wide dissemination of infection within the community. In contrast, assortative mixing, generates a rapidly growing epidemic which is of smaller magnitude (largely restricted to the high activity groups) and may show multiple peaks in the incidence of infection, as waves of infection gradually pass from high to lower sexual activity classes.

Different patterns of mixing, whether due to spatial, behavioural or demographic factors, are of great importance in the design of policies for the control of infection. For common, directly transmitted viral and bacterial infections (measles, rubella, mumps and pertussis) high rates of transmission occur among young children attending primary or secondary schools (5–15 year olds), and this age group serves to seed infection via family contacts in younger and older persons. Patterns of mixing are greatly influenced by the timing of school terms and vacations. Spatial factors are also important. In many developed countries, with generally high-level vaccination coverage, pockets of infection persist in poor communities or ethnic minorities in major urban centres with low rates of vaccine uptake. Targetting vaccination at children before they enter primary school and at young children in poor urban centres is an effective way of minimizing between-group transmission. For STDs, those who change sexual partners frequently serve as a core group of transmitters who main-

tain infection in the larger population of sexually active people. This group is an obvious target for treatment (in the case of gonorrhoea and syphilis) and education about safer sex practices (most importantly in the case of HIV1).

Changes in incidence of infection

Many countries have public health surveillance systems that record the incidence of certain notifiable diseases. These often extend back to the early part of this century, providing excellent long-term data with which to assess changes in incidence of particular infections.

What can be learned from these notification records? First, they enable one to ask whether observed changes in incidence are more regular than would be expected from chance alone. Long runs of data make it possible to measure the mean inter-epidemic period (the time interval between major peaks in incidence). A striking feature of many common directly transmitted viral and bacterial infections is the regularity of such peaks in incidence. They are usually of two kinds: seasonal (e.g. the effects of school terms and vacations on childhood infections), and longer term. Prior to mass vaccination the longer term inter-epidemic period for measles in the UK was 2 years, while for pertussis it was 3–4 years (see Fig. 38.11 and Chapter 36). These intervals are determined not by chance but by interactions between the infectious agent and its host. They are generated by fluctuations in the value of the effective reproductive rate, R, below and above unity. At the start of an epidemic cycle the infectious agent spreads rapidly. As the epidemic progresses, and the susceptible pool is depleted, more and more contacts are with individuals who are immune, so that eventually the effective reproductive rate falls below unity and incidence begins to decline. This decline continues until the pool of susceptibles is replenished by new births, the density of susceptibles eventually rising to a level sufficient to trigger the next epidemic. Simple theory predicts that the average inter-epidemic period for those infections that induce lasting

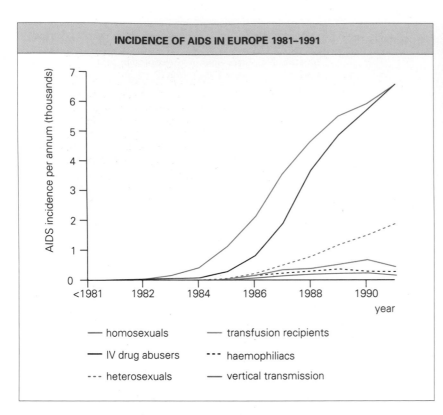

Fig. 38.12 The recorded incidence of AIDS (per annum) in Europe, stratified by risk group. The figures in the most recent years have been adjusted for delays in reporting. In transfusion recipients and haemophiliacs, the incidence is beginning to decline as a consequence of the screening of blood and blood products for HIV infection.

immunity to reinfection is related to the average age at infection and the duration of the average latent and infectious periods, i.e. the average generation time (see Fig. 38.2). This theoretical prediction agrees with observed trends for a wide variety of infections and emphasizes two important general points. First, the average age at infection is inversely related to the transmission potential of the organism concerned (the value R_0); hence infections with high transmission potential have short inter-epidemic periods and vice versa. Second, those infections with short generation times will have short inter-epidemic periods if they also have high transmission success, and vice versa (see Fig. 38.11). These factors, combined with the ability to induce lasting immunity in those who recover from infection, determine whether or not an infectious disease will exhibit longer-term fluctuations in incidence. Infectious diseases like gonorrhoea will not do so (apart from seasonal fluctuations) because of their inability to induce lasting immunity. The same is true for AIDS, but this disease has an additional factor that mitigates against recurrent epidemics, namely a very long incubation period (an average period of at least 10 years; see Fig. 38.5). As recorded in figure 38.12 the AIDS epidemic in Europe has not yet reached its peak, although at least 15 years have passed since the arrival of HIV1.

The transmission success of an infection (inversely measured by the average age at infection) will vary between communities because of differences in demographic parameters (net birth rate) and behavioural factors (patterns of mixing). For example, the inter-epidemic period for measles in large urban centres in Africa or India prior to the introduction of mass vaccination was often one year.

In contrast, in the UK and the USA the period was typically two years. The difference is a direct reflection of difference in the average age at infection (see Fig. 38.8).

Mass vaccination reduces transmission success and therefore acts to increase the average age at infection. The implications of this are discussed in a later section, but one consequence is an increase in the inter-epidemic period (Fig. 38.13). Mass vaccination, therefore, not only alters the incidence of infection, but it will affect the age distribution of cases and the temporal pattern of fluctuations.

COMMUNITY BASED CONTROL BY VACCINATION: HOW MANY PEOPLE SHOULD BE VACCINATED?

Mass vaccination

Other things being equal, the larger the value of R_0, the harder it will be to eradicate an infection by mass vaccination from the community in question. In a 'homogeneously mixing' population, eradication will be achieved if the proportion successfully immunized, p, exceeds a critical value, p_C, where:

$$p_C = (1 - 1/R_0)$$

so that too few susceptibles remain to perpetiate transmission (i.e. $X < X_T$ or $x < x^*$). Thus, the larger the value R_0 the higher the coverage (p_C) needed to eliminate infection. p_C values for various vaccine-preventable childhood viral and bacterial infections are listed in figure 38.14.

Global eradication of measles, with its R_0 of 15–17 and p_C of 92–95%, will almost certainly be more difficult than was eradication of smallpox (R_0 2–4). In the USA, where measles/mumps/rubella (MMR) vaccination is essentially

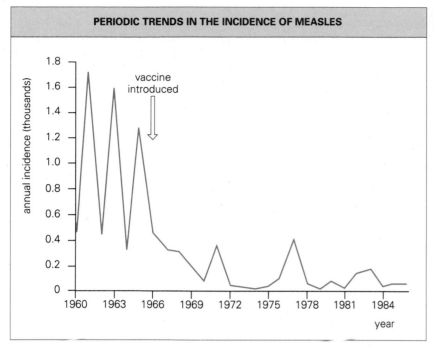

PERIODIC TRENDS IN THE INCIDENCE OF MEASLES

Fig. 38.13 Annual measles notification in an urban population over the period 1960 to 1985. Prior to mass vaccination, two-year cycles are clearly apparent in the fluctuations in incidence. The introduction of measles vaccination in 1966 combined with high levels of vaccine uptake in young children resulted in a significant increase in the period between epidemics. Data from the Office of Population Censuses and Surveys, UK.

CRITICAL VACCINATION COVERAGE TO BLOCK TRANSMISSION OF CERTAIN CHILDHOOD INFECTIONS

infectious disease	average age at infection before immunization* (years)	case reproductive rate R_0	critical vaccination coverage, p_c
Measles	4–5	15–17	92–95%
Pertussis	4–5	15–17	92–95%
Mumps	6–7	10–12	90–92%
Rubella	9–10	7–8	85–87%
Diphtheria	11–14	5–6	80–85%
Poliomyelitis	12–15	5–6	80–85%
* in developed countries			

Fig. 38.14 Estimates of vaccination coverage necessary to block transmission of certain vaccine-preventable childhood viral and bacterial infections.

compulsory prior to entry to primary school (see Chapter 36), the average age at infection for rubella before immunization was about 9 years, compared with around 5 years for measles. The R_0 value for rubella is roughly half that for measles, and rubella has been effectively eradicated by the vaccination programme. The incidence of measles on the other hand has declined more slowly and continues to show local flare-ups in poor urban centres with low vaccine uptake.

What is the optimum age at which to immunize?

Much depends on the influence of maternally derived antibodies against the infectious agent, and on the likelihood that vaccination will give good protection. For most live vaccines (e.g. MMR) efficacy is reduced if high titres of maternal antibodies are present. These typically decay to undetectable levels at around 6 months to 1 year (see Fig. 38.7). The subsequent rise in seropositivity in an unvaccinated community reflects immunity acquired via natural infection. The trough in seropositivity at about 1 year is obviously the optimum age to vaccinate, but high efficacy or high potency vaccines, such as those recently developed against measles and mumps, allow effective vaccination at younger ages when maternal antibodies are still present. This is particularly important in high transmission areas in developing countries, where the susceptibility age window for vaccination may be very narrow (see Fig. 38.7) and, more importantly, where the fraction susceptible at this age to infection may be less than the critical proportion of infants that must be immunized to block transmission.

When vaccination does not take place soon after birth, or when a broad age range of children is immunized, the estimation of the critical fraction to be immunized to

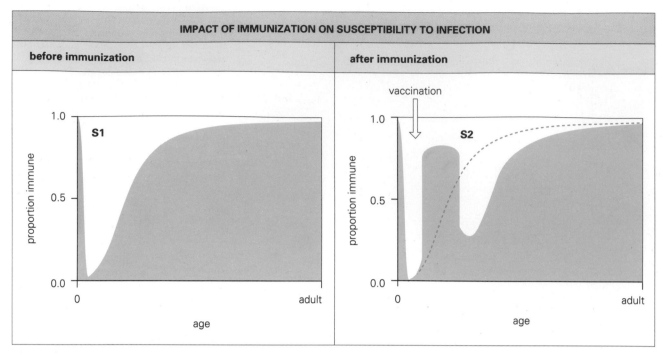

Fig. 38.15 Predicted impact of mass immunization against a typical childhood viral or bacterial infection on the age distribution of susceptibility in a population. Before immunization there is a 'valley' of susceptibility (S1) in the young age classes. Vaccination reduces the rate of transmission, creating an upward shift in the age at which susceptibles acquire natural infection. Paradoxically, mass childhood vaccination does not alter the fraction of the population which is susceptible (i.e. area S2=S1).

eliminate infection must take account of the average age at vaccination. For eradication to be possible the average age at vaccination must be less than the average age at infection, and cohort vaccination should therefore focus on young infants, taking account of vaccine performance in those with maternal antibodies. This highlights the difficulties of eradicating infections such as measles in major urban centres in some developing countries, where the average age at infection is often between 1–2 years (see Fig. 38.8). To block transmission, more than 97% of infants would have to be effectively immunized before their first birthday. In practice this is impossible. An alternative approach is a two-stage vaccination programme, for example, targetted at infants around 1 year of age and then young children at around 2–3 years of age. The first stage acts to reduce transmission efficacy (but not to block transmission) and hence widens the age window of susceptibility in which vaccine can be administered. The second stage attempts to block transmission via the creation of very high levels of herd immunity.

Why do we not require 100% coverage to eradicate an infection? Immunization has both a direct and an indirect effect. The direct effect protects those successfully immunized, and results in fewer infected individuals to transmit infection to those still susceptible. The latter therefore benefit indirectly from those who have been immunized. The effective proportion of susceptibles will eventually fall below the level required to maintain $R_0>1$ ($X<X_T$), even though immunization coverage is less than 100%.

Mass immunization at levels below those needed to block transmission obviously reduces the incidence of infection. Surprisingly, it has little impact on the total number of individuals remaining susceptible (Fig. 38.15). As long as the infection remains endemic the fraction remaining susceptible depends only on R_0, and not on whether those losing susceptibility did so as a result of immunization or of natural infection.

Indirect effects of mass vaccination

Mass vaccination at below eradication levels reduces the probability of an unimmunized individual acquiring infection. In consequence, infection tends to be acquired at an older average age than was the case prior to vaccination (see Fig. 38.15). If the risk of disease associated with infection increases with age, a programme of immunization at levels below that required to block transmission (i.e. below p_c) can have perverse complications. The outcome depends on precisely how the risk of serious disease per case of infection changes with age (Fig. 38.16). For example measles can lead to encephalitis in a small fraction of those infected. The risk does increase with age at infection but all levels of vaccination coverage reduce both the incidence of infection and the incidence of disease. Rubella and mumps are different since mass vaccination at certain levels of coverage will reduce the incidence of infection but increase the incidence of serious disease.

Rubella can damage babies whose mothers are infected in the first trimester of pregnancy. The risk of this damage

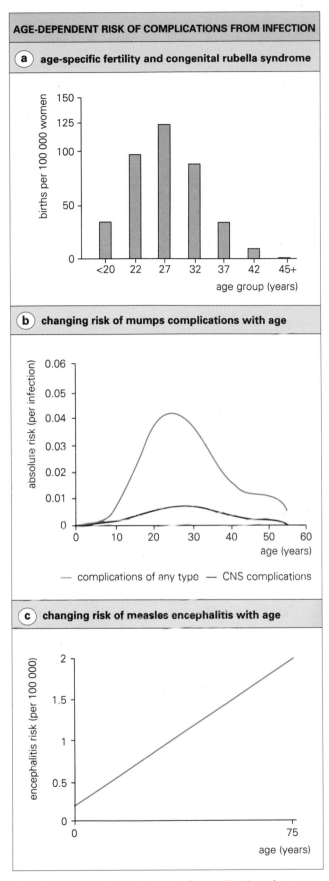

Fig. 38.16 Age-dependent risk of complications from infection. (a) Age specific fertility of women, as shown, directly influences the risk of congenital rubella syndrome in infants. Data for the UK, 1985. (b) Changes in the absolute risk of complications from mumps infection, in the UK, relative to age. (c) Changes with age in the risk of measles encephalitis in the US.

is therefore proportional to the age-specific fertility profile for a given country (Fig. 38.16a). Vaccinating, say, 50% of all 2 year olds would reduce the total number of cases of rubella but push the average age of the small number who become infected towards the child-bearing years. If very high levels of coverage can be attained (under a compulsory programme, as in the USA, or a highly coordinated system of recall, incentives and surveillance, as in the UK), eradication can be achieved by vaccinating successive cohorts of 1–2 year olds. If levels of vaccine uptake under a voluntary scheme only reach 60–70% (as in the UK earlier in the rubella vaccination campaign) vaccination should be confined to early teenage girls before they join the 'pregnancy' age classes, so that infection can spread and confer immunity at younger ages. How can we tell at what level of coverage to switch from one strategy to the other? Epidemiological calculations suggest that a switch to the mass cohort strategy (where MMR is offered to 1–2 year olds) is advisable provided that more than 70% of boys and girls can be immunized by 2 years of age. A two-stage programme of adding vaccination of 1–2 year-old boys and girls to an existing strategy focused on teenage girls would have little effect on disease, provided uptake in 12–13 year-old girls was high (80–90%) before MMR was added to the programme. Some benefit will accrue over 10 years or more once the uptake of MMR in 1–2 year olds reaches very high levels (90%).

Mumps can lead to complications (Fig. 38.16b) such as meningitis and/or encephalitis, which occur in approximately 10% of all diagnosed cases, and orchitis, which occurs in about 27% of clinical cases in post-pubertal males. Case complication rates are age- and sex-related. Inclusion of the mumps vaccine in the child immunization programme in the UK began in October 1988 with the introduction of MMR. Analysis shows that the incidence of serious disease will increase if vaccine uptake levels are less than approximately 60–70% of 1 to 2 year olds. Higher levels of uptake, as have now been achieved, should reduce both the incidence of infection and infection-related complications.

Abrupt introductions or changes in immunization programmes perturb the nature of herd immunity in the population because of sudden reductions in the transmission potential of the infectious agent. As stated above, the fraction susceptible remains the same, it is simply the distribution of susceptible individuals across age classes that changes.

FACTORS INFLUENCING THE SUCCESS OF VACCINATION

Spatial factors

The design of immunization programmes, particularly in developing countries, is influenced by variations in population density. In small villages in rural areas, population density and the associated net birth rates may be too low for the endemic maintenance of infections such as measles or pertussis (see Chapter 11). However, people living in those regions are at risk from contact with large urban centres. One solution is to target vaccination coverage in

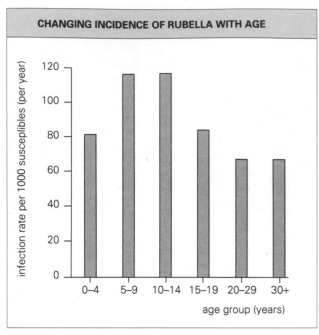

CHANGING INCIDENCE OF RUBELLA WITH AGE

Fig. 38.17 Age-related changes in the rate of infection with the rubella virus.

relation to group size, with dense groups receiving the highest levels of coverage. In some circumstances transmission can be blocked by high levels of mass immunization in the urban centres alone, since they provide the reservoir of infection for the low density rural regions.

Programmes in developed countries may be influenced by regional variation in vaccine uptake. In the USA, poor and ethnic minorities in large urban centres create pockets of susceptibility (due to low vaccine uptake) that prevent the virtual elimination of infections such as measles and pertussis. High vaccine coverage in infants and children, particularly in poor communities, must be a central aim in national immunization programmes. Serological surveillance, in both urban and rural areas, is a key component in the identification of weaknesses in current programmes.

Age-dependent transmission

For many common vaccine-preventable childhood infections, such as measles, mumps and rubella, the per capita rate at which susceptibles acquire infection varies with age. For rubella (Fig. 38.17) the rate changes from a low level in the 0–4 year-old class, via a high level in the 5–15 year-old classes, back to a lower level in the adult classes. This reflects social patterns of behaviour, the high rates in the 5–15 year-olds reflecting frequent and intimate contact within school environments. These age-dependent variations can reduce the predicted level of cohort vaccination required to block or eliminate transmission. This is because immunization increases the average age at infection (see above). Susceptibles who avoid vaccination and infection may move from an age class with a high rate of infection to an older one with a lower rate.

Vaccine potency

Most vaccines have some small risk of inducing serious complications. Any assessment of the benefit from an immunization programme must therefore include a comparison of the number of cases of serious disease prevented by mass vaccination with the number of cases due to vaccination itself. Such calculations are not straightforward because they depend on the interrelation between various factors, e.g. vaccine efficacy and safety, proportion of each cohort of children immunized, average age of immunization and the indirect effects of mass vaccination on the rate of transmission of the infectious agent. Typically, the risks from infection and from vaccination change as vaccination coverage increases. When infection is common and vaccination rare, the risks due to the former are invariably greater, often by many orders of magnitude. When infection is very rare as a result of vaccination, the reverse may be true. Ultimately, the risk of vaccination will always be greater once vaccination has eliminated infection. A factor relevant to concerns about vaccine-associated complications is the development of high potency live virus vaccines which provide protection for the vast majority of those immunized and allow vaccination at an age (around 6 months) when maternally derived antibodies are still present. These new, more immunogenic vaccines provide better protection, but their use may be associated with increased reactogenicity or lower safety, exacerbating the conflict between individual and community interests. Are there circumstances in which a higher efficacy vaccine should be used, even though it may lead to more cases of vaccine-associated disease? In the case of mumps, for example, the high potency 'Urabe Am 9' vaccine is estimated to have an efficacy of approximately 98% while the lower potency 'Jeryl Lynn' vaccine has an efficacy of around 94%, and evidence suggests higher complication rates with the former. At levels of vaccine cover high enough to block transmission, the sensible option is to use the lower potency vaccine. However, if high uptake cannot be achieved then the total incidence of serious disease (both vaccine- and infection-produced) is reduced to a greater extent by the high potency vaccine.

CONTROL OF SEXUALLY TRANSMITTED DISEASES

In this section we examine the community-wide control of sexually transmitted diseases (STDs) by reference to vaccination to protect against hepatitis B virus (HBV), chemotherapy for the control of gonorrhoea, and education and chemotherapy for the control of HIV1 (see Chapter 24).

Hepatitis B

There are some 300 million carriers of HBV world-wide, of whom approximately 25–30% will die of HBV-induced cirrhosis or hepatocellular carcinoma (see Chapter 25). The virus can be transmitted vertically, by transmission from mother to infant, or horizontally via sexual contact, injection of contaminated blood and blood products, or by accidental exposure to infected body fluids. In developed

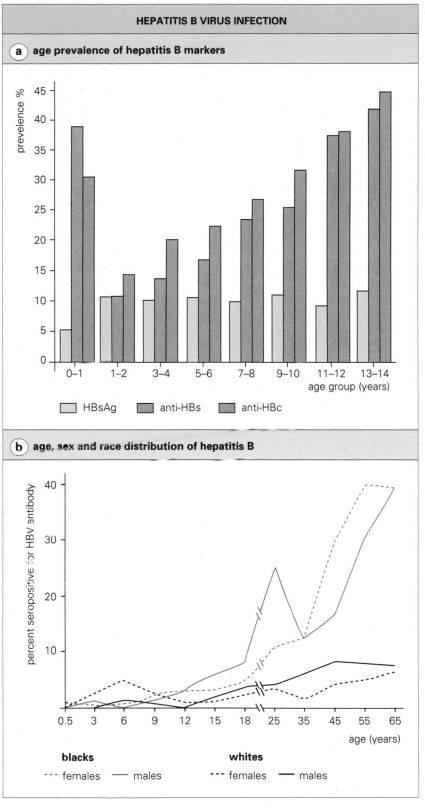

Fig. 38.18 Hepatitis B virus (HBV) infection. (a) Age prevalence of hepatitis B virus markers: surface antigen (HBsAg), antibodies to HBs (anti-HBs) and core antigen (anti-HBc), in Taiwan in 1984. Initially, maternal antibodies are present, which then disappear; later, antibodies levels rise as the immune response develops. Levels of HBsAg remain more or less constant throughout, reflecting persistent infection (see also Chapter 25). (b) Age, race and sex distribution of hepatitis B in the USA during 1976–1980, showing seroprevalence of HBV antibodies in different groups.

countries sexual contact and transmission between injecting drug users who share syringes appear to be the commonest routes. In developing countries, vertical transmission, sexual contact and horizontal transmission not involving sexual contact all appear to be important. Accordingly, there are great differences in the prevalence of serological markers of HBV infection in different age, ethnic and social groups (Fig. 38.18). Epidemiological study is further complicated by the presence of carriers of infection, who

harbour the virus for long periods of time and are infectious to others. In Taiwan, for example, the frequency of the carrier state in females may reach 15% at sexual maturity, and among infected male infants development of the carrier state is associated with a 50% lifetime cumulative probability of hepatic carcinoma. Serological and virological methods in surveillance are needed to estimate the proportion of individuals with antibodies to HBs (anti-HBs) and hepatitis core (anti-HBc), and HBs antigen

(HBsAg); the prevalence of the latter approximating to the proportion of carriers (see Fig. 38.18).

In areas of 'high' or 'intermediate' endemicity of HBV, control of transmission is dependent on the mass immunization of infants with plasma derived HBsAg or the genetically engineered vaccine based on HBsAg. Hepatitis B immune globulin administered within 24 hours of birth, followed by vaccination, appears to prevent the children of infected mothers from becoming carriers. Selective treatment of children born to infected mothers, and mass immunization of other infants, effectively limits transmission in areas of high endemicity. In developed countries with low levels of HBV infection, and where infection of infants is uncommon, control strategies involve the identification and selective immunization of high-risk individuals (intravenous drug users, male homosexuals, female and male heterosexuals who have many sexual partners, and health care workers). However, effective control may not be achieved by targetting high-risk individuals alone. There are difficulties in identifying such individuals, in diagnosing inapparent or mild HBV infections, and in delivery to socio-economically disadvantaged people (given that three doses of vaccine administered over a period of two months are required for 90% seroconversion in those who receive the full course of vaccination). The most effective strategy may therefore be mass immunization of infants or of young adolescents before they become sexually active. This would take some years to have an impact, but over a timescale of a decade would reduce the incidence of infection to very low levels. However, no detailed cost-benefit analyses have been performed for very low incidence areas, and costs may be prohibitive. Selective vaccination of attendees at STD clinics is predicted to be effective provided the compliance of core groups is high and that a very high proportion of individuals complete the full course of vaccination.

Gonorrhoea

Neisseria gonorrhoea is prevalent in many regions of the world with poor health care infrastructure. Where the prevalence of untreated infection in young sexually active men and women is high, gonococcal infection is a major determinant of fertility. In most developed countries, the situation is much less serious because of the impact of early diagnosis and drug treatment, and contact tracing to halt chains of transmission.

Some insight into the effectiveness of different control interventions can be obtained by identifying the factors that determine the magnitude of the case reproductive rate of infection R_0. For heterosexual transmission, where the typical course of infection differs between the sexes, R_0 is influenced by the probability of transmission from men to women, and from women to men, by the average durations of infection in men and women respectively, and by the effective rates of sexual partner change. Chemotherapy after early diagnosis reduces the average duration of infection (and hence the average period during which transmission can occur). For untreated gonorrhoea the typical duration of infection in women is thought to be around 6 months – treatment can reduce

this period to around 1 month. Effective treatment of a significant fraction of those infected can therefore reduce the value of R_0 by as much as five-sixths. This observation alone goes a long way towards explaining the relatively low prevalence of gonorrhoea in many developed countries such as Sweden and the Netherlands, compared with its high prevalence in some poor African countries. Condom use reduces the probability of transmission, while education can reduce the effective rate of sexual partner change.

AIDS and HIV infection

There are as yet no vaccines or drugs that are effective in the long-term suppression of HIV infections. In this section we consider the community-wide use of chemotherapeutic agents such as zidovudine (see Chapter 35) and control through changes in sexual behaviour.

Estimation of R_0 for HIV is fraught with problems. Typical epidemiological surveys record prevalence through time in specified risk groups such as male homosexuals, female prostitutes or pregnant women (Fig. 38.19). By ignoring differences in the transmission probability from men to women and women to men (twice as likely from men to women) a rough guide to the magnitude of R_0 can be obtained in the early stages of the epidemic from a simple relationship that relates the magnitude of R_0 to the doubling time of the epidemic, t_d:

$$R_0 = \{D(\ln 2)/t_d\} - 1$$

A doubling time in the prevalence of infection within a cohort of pregnant women of roughly 2 years (see Fig. 38.19) and an average infectious period of 10 years, gives an R_0 value of approximately 2.5 in the urban heterosexual population in some of the worst afflicted regions in Africa. The average infectious period may be somewhat less than the average incubation period; virological data (see Fig. 38.3) suggests that viraemia (and thus infectiousness) fluctuates widely over the period. The average incubation period may also be less than 10 years in developing countries, where continuous exposure to a wide range of infectious diseases may speed the development of severe immunodeficiency. If this is the case, the estimate of R_0 is reduced. However, taking the pessimistic view that R_0 is around 2–3 (one primary case generating 2 to 3 secondary cases) then the target of education programmes is to reduce the combined influence of epidemiological and behavioural parameters by at least a half to two-thirds.

Control options include the use of condoms to reduce the probability of transmission, and behavioural changes to reduce both the rate of, and the variation in, sexual partner change in the population. The latter factor is of particular importance, since variance in sexual partner change rates is usually much greater than the mean value (see Fig. 38.9), because of the small fraction of individuals who change sexual partners frequently. These individuals are also likely to experience higher than average levels of infection with other STDs, such as genital ulcers and gonorrhoea. These may act as cofactors to enhance the likelihood of HIV transmission, and contribute disproportionately to transmission within a community, underlining further the importance

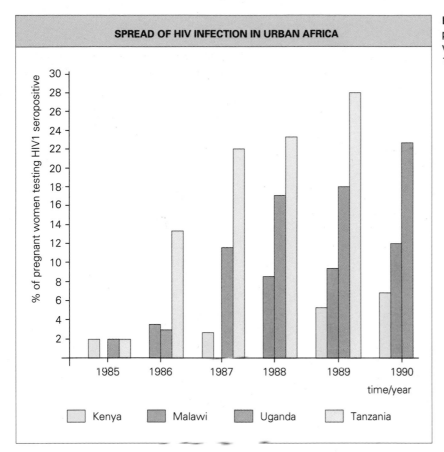

Fig. 38.19 The spread of HIV1 in pregnant women from urban centres in various African countries over the period 1985 to 1990.

of control measures. Enhanced STD control in general, particularly if targetted at this group, is therefore likely to slow the spread of HIV.

In developed countries drugs such as zidovudine are used to delay the onset of symptoms of AIDS in infected individuals. However, this may, under certain circumstances, have negative effects. Firstly, widespread use by asymptomatic individuals at low dosage levels may promote the spread of drug resistant strains of HIV. Secondly, and more importantly, it may prolong the period of infectiousness and could enhance the net rate of transmission. Treatment might therefore be good for the individual, but detrimental to the community at risk. There is a clear need for research to measure the impact of drug treatment on infectiousness and for reduced infectiousness to be part of the protocol of drug development. At present protocols are primarily concerned with safety and efficacy, but population level considerations concerning transmissibility are also of great importance.

SUMMARY

The development of a safe, effective and cheap vaccine or drug is only the first step – albeit a vital one – towards control of an infectious disease within a community. The interaction between a population of hosts and an infectious agent is inherently non-linear. For example, when population density doubles the prevalence of many directly transmitted viral and bacterial infections may increase more than twofold. Complex patterns of change in the incidence of infection can arise when immunization programmes with partial coverage are initiated. The many variables that influence rates of transmission often hinder the assessment of the likely impact of a given control programme. Epidemiological analysis at the level of the population biology of the interaction between host and infectious agent is critical for the development of community-based programmes. Appreciation of the components that determine the transmission potential of an infectious agent, as measured by the basic or case reproductive rate R_0, is vital.

In the design of control policies, most attention is presently directed towards what is best for the individual to be treated or vaccinated. However, what is best for the individual is not always best for the community and there can be genuine tensions between the interests of these two that are not easily resolved. However, the resolution of these tensions is eased greatly by a clear understanding of the precise circumstances that generate such conflicts.

Further Reading

Anderson RM, May RM. *Infectious diseases of humans: dynamics and control.* Oxford: Blackwell Scientific Publications, 1991.

Anderson RM, Nokes DJ. Mathematical models of transmission and control. In: *Oxford textbook of public health.* 2nd edn. Holland WW, Detels R, Knox G, eds. Oxford: Oxford Medical Publications, 1991.

Nokes DJ, Anderson RM. The use of mathematical models in the epidemiological study of infectious diseases and in the design of mass immunization programmes. *Epidemiol Infect* 1988; **101**:1–20.

Contents

INTRODUCTION: WHAT IS HOSPITAL INFECTION?

Amassing a large number of sick people together under one roof has many advantages but some disadvantages, notably the easier transmission of infection from one person to another. Hospital infection (also known as 'nosocomial' infection) is defined as any infection acquired whilst in hospital. Most of these infections become obvious while the patient is in hospital but some (as many as 25% of post-operative wound infections) are not recognized until after the patient has been discharged. This latter category may increase as earlier discharges are encouraged in this cost-conscious age, although a shorter pre-operative stay reduces the chance of acquisition of hospital pathogens (see below).

Hospital infection may be acquired from an exogenous source, for example from another patient (cross-infection) or from the environment, or from an endogenous source i.e. another site within the patient (self or auto-infection) (Fig. 39.1). An infection that is incubating in a patient when he/she is admitted into hospital is not a hospital infection.

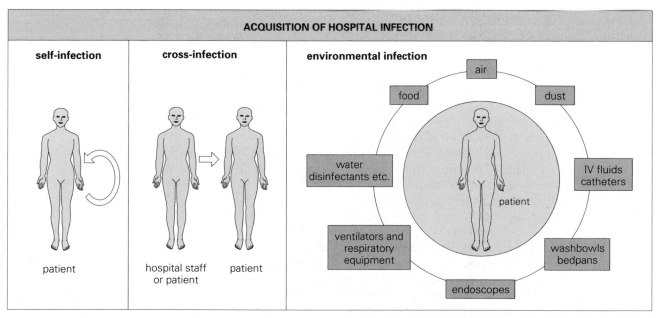

Fig. 39.1 Hospital-acquired infection can be endogenous, i.e. self-infection from another site in the body, or exogenous, from another person or from an environmental source. The sorts of organisms acquired from environmental sources depend on the nature of the source; e.g. moist areas tend to be colonized with Gram-negative rods whereas air and dust-borne organisms are those that can withstand drying (e.g. streptococci, staphylococci and mycobacteria).

However, community-acquired infections brought into hospital by the patient may subsequently become hospital infections for other patients and hospital staff.

Many hospital infections are preventable, as demonstrated by Semmelweiss in 1850 when he made the unpopular suggestion that puerperal fever, an infection in women who have just given birth (see Chapter 26), was carried on the hands of physicians who came directly from attending an autopsy to the delivery ward, without washing. A death rate of 8.3% was reduced to 2.3% by introducing the simple measure of hand washing before and after any clinical examination in the clinic. Extensive studies in the USA in the 1970s showed that the direct costs arising from hospital infection were around one billion dollars per year and that about one-third of all infections acquired in hospital could have been prevented.

WHICH INFECTIONS ARE MOST COMMON?

The infections most commonly acquired in hospitals are surgical wound infections, infections of the urinary and respiratory tracts, and bacteraemia. The relative frequency of these infections is illustrated in figure 39.2. Each may be acquired from an exogenous or endogenous source, and even the 'self-source' may be derived from outside by the patient becoming colonized with pathogens during his/her stay in hospital. Bacteraemia may arise from a variety of sources and may be primary, i.e. by direct introduction of organisms into the blood (e.g. from contaminated intravenous fluids), or secondary to a focus of infection already present in the body (e.g. urinary tract infection). Other infections which may cause outbreaks in the hospital setting include gastroenteritis and hepatitis.

WHICH ORGANISMS ARE IMPORTANT CAUSES OF HOSPITAL INFECTION?

Almost any microbe can cause a hospital-acquired infection (although protozoal infections are rare). The pattern of hospital infection has changed over the years, reflecting advances in medicine and the development of antimicrobial agents. In the pre-antibiotic era the majority of infections were caused by Gram-positive organisms, particularly *Streptococcus pyogenes* and *Staphylococcus aureus*. With the advent of penicillin and other antibiotics active against staphylococci, Gram-negative organisms such as *Escherichia coli* and *Pseudomonas aeruginosa* emerged as important pathogens. More recently, the development of more potent and broad-spectrum antimicrobials and the increase in invasive medical techniques has been accompanied by an increase in the incidence of antibiotic-resistant Gram-positive organisms such as *Staph. epidermidis*, enterococci and methicillin-resistant *Staph. aureus* (MRSA), and *Candida*. Many of these organisms are considered as 'opportunists', microbes that are unable to cause disease in healthy people with intact defence mechanisms but which infect compromised patients or when introduced during the course of invasive procedures. Currently, *E. coli* accounts overall for more hospital infec-

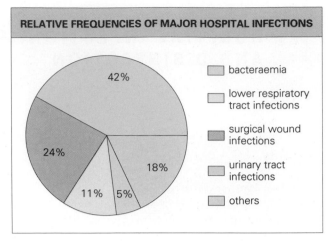

RELATIVE FREQUENCIES OF MAJOR HOSPITAL INFECTIONS

42%
24%
11%
5%
18%

- bacteraemia
- lower respiratory tract infections
- surgical wound infections
- urinary tract infections
- others

Fig. 39.2 The relative frequencies of different kinds of hospital infection vary for different patient groups, but overall urinary tract infections (UTI) are the most common hospital-acquired infections.

tion than any other single species but *Staph. aureus* is a close second (Fig. 39.3).

Viral infections probably account for more hospital-acquired infections than previously realized. The most important are respiratory viruses, especially influenza and respiratory syncytial virus (RSV), viruses acquired by the respiratory route such as measles and rubella, herpes viruses, especially varicella-zoster virus, rotavirus, hepatitis viruses, and HIV in countries where blood and blood products are not screened. The risks of viral infections in hospital are summarized in figure 39.4.

SOURCES OF HOSPITAL INFECTION

As stated above, the source of infection may be human, i.e. other patients or hospital staff (and occasionally visitors), or environmental, from contaminated objects ('fomites'), food, water or air (see Fig. 39.1). The source may become contaminated from an environmental reservoir of organisms, e.g. contaminated antiseptic solution distributed for use into sterile containers (Fig. 39.5). Eradication of the source will also require eradication of the reservoir.

Human sources may be people who are themselves infected or who are incubating an infection, or they may be healthy carriers. The time period for which a human source is infectious varies with the disease (see Chapter 38). For example, some infections can be spread during their incubation period, others in the early stages of clinical disease and others are characterized by a prolonged carrier state even after clinical cure (e.g. hepatitis B, typhoid fever) (Fig. 39.6). Carriers of virulent strains of, for example, *Staph. aureus* or *Strep. pyogenes* may act as

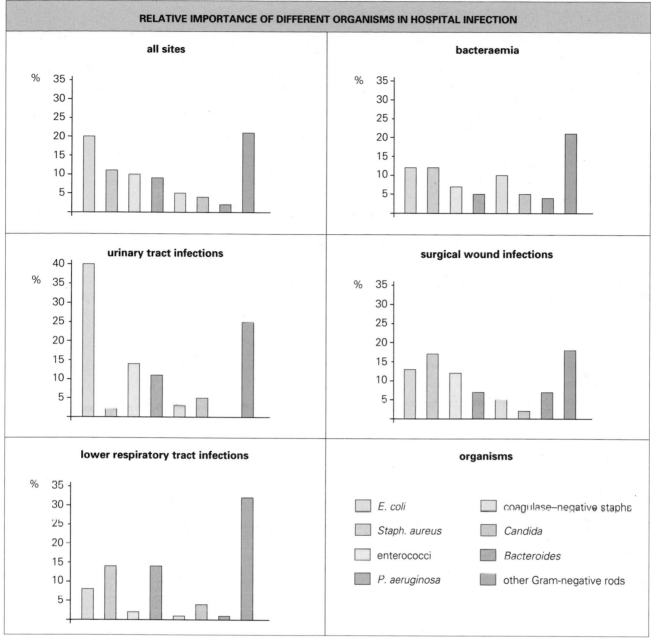

Fig. 39.3 Although a few species are the most important in all kinds of hospital infection, the rank order of their importance varies in different infections. Thus *Staph. aureus* is very important in surgical wound infections and bacteraemias but much less so in urinary tract infections.

The importance of Gram-negative rods other than *E. coli* has increased since the advent of broad-spectrum antibiotics. These organisms often carry multiple antibiotic resistances.

sources of hospital infection, although they themselves do not develop clinical disease. The carrier state may persist for a long time and go unnoticed unless there is an outbreak of infection which is traced to a carrier.

ROUTES OF SPREAD OF INFECTION

The important routes of spread of infection in hospitals are those common to all infections: airborne, contact and common vehicle. Examples of organisms spread by these routes in hospitals are illustrated in figure 39.5. Vector-borne spread, whilst theoretically possible, is very unusual in the hospital setting as is sexually-transmitted infection. It is important to remember that the same organism may be spread by more than one route. For example, *Strep. pyogenes* can be spread from patient to patient by the airborne route in droplets or dust, but it is also transmitted by contact with infected lesions, for example on a nurse's hand.

VIRUSES AS CAUSES OF HOSPITAL-ACQUIRED INFECTION			
virus	transmissibility	susceptibility of other patients and staff	resultant risk of hospital infection
Influenza	+ +	+/−*	+ +
Respiratory syncytial virus	+ +	+ +*	+ +
Parainfluenza ⎤ Adenovirus ⎬ Rhinovirus ⎦	+	+*	+
Varicella-zoster (V-ZV)	+ +	−*	−
V-ZV (localized)	+	− −	− −
Cytomegalovirus	−	+	− −†
Rubella	+ +	+**	+ +
Measles	+ +	− −	− −
Exotic viruses (Lassa, Marburg, Ebola, rabies)	− −	+ +	− −
Rotavirus	+ +	+	+
Enteroviruses	+	+	+
Hepatitis A	+	+	+
Hepatitis B	+ +§	+ +	+ +
HIV (in countries where not screened)	+ +‡	+ +	+ +

* high in paediatric age groups	** decreased since immunization programme initiated
† except for blood transfusion and organ transplantation	§ from needle-stick injuries ‡ from blood or blood product

Fig. 39.4 Viruses are probably more important causes of hospital infection than generally recognized. The risk of hospital infection is a sum of the transmissibility of the virus and the susceptibility of the patient group. Some viruses, such as varicella-zoster, are of low risk in general but are very important in paediatric units and particularly in immunocompromised children.

HOST FACTORS AND HOSPITAL INFECTION

Host factors play a fundamental role in the infection equation, all the more so in hospitals because of the high proportion of hospital patients whose natural defences against infection are compromised. The spread of an infectious agent to a new host can result in a spectrum of responses from colonization, through subclinical infection, to clinically apparent disease which may be fatal. The degree of host response differs in different people depending on their degree of compromise. The very young are particularly susceptible because of the immaturity of their immune system. Likewise, the elderly suffer a greater risk of infection because of predisposing underlying disease, impaired blood supply, and immobility which contributes to stasis and thus to infection in, for example, the lungs. In all age-groups, underlying disease and the treatment of that disease (e.g. cytotoxic drugs, steroids, etc.) may predispose to infection (Fig. 39.7), and invasive procedures allow organisms easier access to previously protected tissues (Fig. 39.8). The important host factors to be considered in hospital infection are summarized in figure 39.9; infections in the compromised host are discussed in more detail in Chapter 33.

Extensive studies of post-operative wound infection have identified a number of factors that predispose to this type of infection. (Wound infection or wound sepsis is characterized by the presence of inflammation, pus and discharge in addition to the isolation of organisms such as *Staph. aureus.*) Prolonged pre-operative stay increases the opportunity for the patient to become colonized with antibiotic-resistant hospital pathogens. Studies have shown that the nature and length of the operation also have an effect (Figs 39.10 and 39.11; see also Chapter 28). Wet or

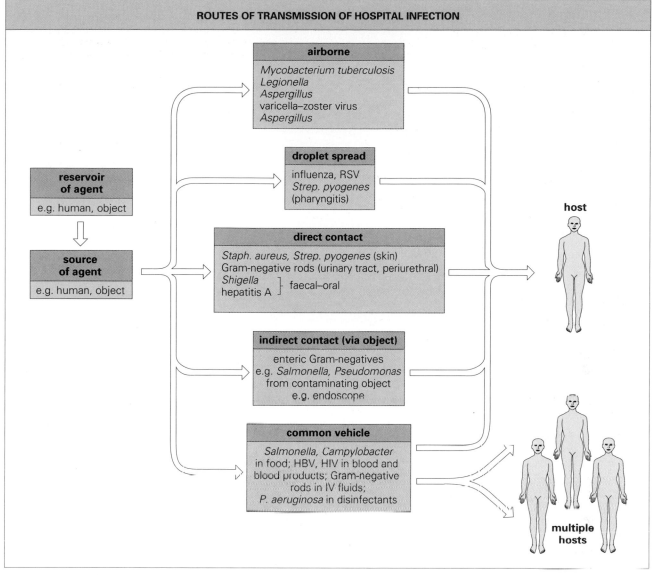

ROUTES OF TRANSMISSION OF HOSPITAL INFECTION

airborne
Mycobacterium tuberculosis
Legionella
Aspergillus
varicella–zoster virus
Aspergillus

droplet spread
influenza, RSV
Strep. pyogenes
(pharyngitis)

reservoir of agent
e.g. human, object

source of agent
e.g. human, object

direct contact
Staph. aureus, Strep. pyogenes (skin)
Gram-negative rods (urinary tract, periurethral)
Shigella
hepatitis A } faecal–oral

indirect contact (via object)
enteric Gram-negatives
e.g. *Salmonella, Pseudomonas*
from contaminating object
e.g. endoscope

common vehicle
Salmonella, Campylobacter
in food; HBV, HIV in blood and
blood products; Gram-negative
rods in IV fluids;
P. aeruginosa in disinfectants

host

multiple hosts

Fig. 39.5 Hospital infections are spread by the same routes as infections spread in the community. The reservoir and the source of infection may be human or inanimate and may be one and the same (e.g. a nurse with infected skin lesion). If the reservoir and source are distinct (e.g. contaminated distilled water supply used to prepare a variety of pharmaceuticals), both must be eliminated if the spread of infection is to be halted, otherwise the reservoir may continue to contaminate new sources.

open wounds are more liable to secondary infection. From these studies it has been possible to identify the patients and operations with greatest risk and apply preventive measures such as prophylactic antibiotic regimens and ultra-clean air in orthopaedic operating theatres (see below).

THE CONSEQUENCES OF HOSPITAL INFECTION

The consequences of hospital infection are several, both for the patient and for the community. Hospital infection may:
- result in serious illness or death;
- prolong hospital stay, which costs money, and results in loss of earnings and hardship for patient and his/her family;
- require additional antimicrobial therapy, which is costly, exposes the patient to additional risks of toxicity, and

increases selective pressure for resistance to emerge among hospital pathogens;
- result in the infected patient becoming a source from which others may become infected, both in hospital and in the community.

PREVENTION OF HOSPITAL INFECTION

For the reasons outlined above, the prevention of hospital infection deserves a very high priority. There are three main strategies for preventing hospital infection:
- excluding sources of infection from the hospital environment;
- interrupting the transmission of infection from source to susceptible host (breaking the chain of infection);
- enhancing the host's ability to resist infection.

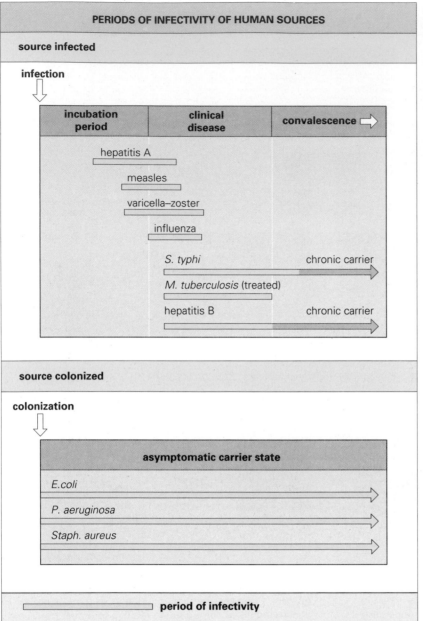

PERIODS OF INFECTIVITY OF HUMAN SOURCES

source infected

infection

incubation period	clinical disease	convalescence

hepatitis A

measles

varicella–zoster

influenza

S. typhi   chronic carrier

M. tuberculosis (treated)

hepatitis B   chronic carrier

source colonized

colonization

asymptomatic carrier state

E.coli

P. aeruginosa

Staph. aureus

period of infectivity

Fig. 39.6 Pathogens differ in the periods for which they can be disseminated from an infected person. For some it is during the incubation period when the person may not realize they are ill and infectious. Some people continue to carry organisms such as *Salmonella typhi* and hepatitis B virus long after they have recovered from the clinical disease. Opportunist pathogens are often members of the normal flora and thus may be carried for long periods without the host experiencing any adverse effects.

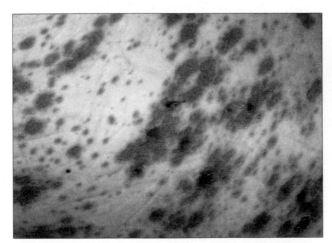

Fig. 39.7 Varicella in a patient with chronic myeloid leukaemia, showing purpuric confluent lesions on the trunk. Courtesy of GDW McKendrick.

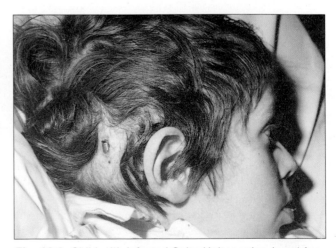

Fig. 39.8 Child with infected Spitz-Holter valve (used for the relief of hydrocephalus). Courtesy of JA Innes.

FACTORS WHICH PREDISPOSE PATIENTS TO HOSPITAL INFECTION	
Age	patients at extremes of age are particularly susceptible
Specific immunity	patient may lack protective antibodies to e.g. measles, chicken-pox, whooping cough
Underlying disease	other (non-infectious) diseases tend to lead to enhanced susceptibility to infection, e.g. hepatic disease, diabetes, cancer, skin disorders, renal failure, neutropenia (either as a result of disease or of treatment)
Other infections	HIV and other immunosuppressing virus infections, patients with influenza prone to secondary bacterial pneumonia, herpes virus lesions may become secondarily infected with staphylococci
Specific medicaments	cytotoxic drugs (including post-transplant immunosuppression) and steroids both lower host defences, antibiotics disturb normal flora and predispose to invasion by resistant hospital pathogens
Trauma accidental	burns, stab or gunshot wounds, road traffic accidents
intentional	surgery, intravenous and urinary catheters, peritoneal dialysis

(Trauma: disturb natural host defence mechanisms)

Fig. 39.9 Hospital patients are not all at equal risk of infection. Some factors that predispose to infection can be influenced by, for example, treating underlying disease, improving specific immunity and avoiding inappropriate use of antibiotics. Other factors such as age, are unalterable.

Exclusion of sources of infection

Exclusion of inanimate sources of infection is both desirable and to a large extent achievable. For example the provision of sterile instruments and dressings, sterile medicaments and intravenous fluids, use of blood and blood-products screened for infectious agents, clean linen and uncontaminated food. However, many of the sources of infection are human or are objects which become contaminated by humans, so that exclusion is more difficult. Hospitals must attempt to prevent patient contact with staff who are carriers of pathogens. The problem of course is the identification of these individuals and their relocation to less hazardous positions. Staff must undergo health screening before employment and should have regular health checks; they should also be encouraged to report any incidences of infection (e.g. an infected cut or a bout of diarrhoea). Appropriate immunizations should be offered and in some instances made mandatory. Work restrictions for personnel with selected infectious diseases are summarized in figure 39.12. However, healthy carriers of, for example, virulent staphylococci are difficult to identify unless bacteriological screening is undertaken, which is not feasible on a routine basis. In addition, staff are sources

RISK FACTORS FOR POST-OPERATIVE INFECTIONS	
Length of pre-operative stay	longer stay – more likely to become colonized with virulent and antibiotic-resistant hospital bacteria and fungi
Presence of intercurrent infection	operating on an already infected site more likely to cause disseminated infection
Length of operation	longer – greater risk of tissues becoming seeded with organisms from air, staff, other sites in patient
Nature of operation	any operation which results in faecal soiling of tissues has higher risk of infection (e.g. post-operative gangrene), 'adventurous' surgery tends to carry greater risks
Presence of foreign bodies	e.g. shunts, prostheses, impairs host defences
State of tissues	poor blood supply encourages growth of anaerobes, inadequate drainage or presence of necrotic tissue predisposes to infection

Fig. 39.10 The risks of infection after surgery have been studied in considerable detail and as a result surgeons are much more aware of the problems. 'High-tech' surgery, however, is often long and difficult and predisposes the patient to post-operative infection.

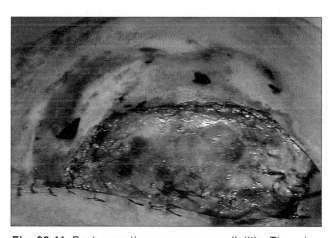

Fig. 39.11 Post-operative gangrenous cellulitis. There is a huge area of ulceration filled with gangrenous skin, with sloughing adjacent to the wound and surrounding cellulitis. Courtesy of MJ Wood.

of opportunist organisms such as coagulase-negative staphylococci or enterobacteria which are part of their normal flora and cannot be excluded.

Breaking the chain of infection

There are two elements to be considered here: the structural and the human. The structure of the hospital and its equipment can play a role in preventing airborne spread of infection and in facilitating aseptic practices by the staff but this is to no avail if staff do not use the facilities correctly and do not themselves act positively to prevent the spread of infection.

INFECTIOUS DISEASES WHERE STAFF CONTACT WITH PATIENT SHOULD BE AVOIDED
Diarrhoea
Hepatitis A
Herpes simplex on hands (herpetic whitlow)
Strep. pyogenes infections
Staph. aureus skin lesions
Measles
Mumps
Whooping cough
Rubella
Varicella-zoster infections
Upper respiratory tract infections (high-risk patients)

Fig. 39.12 Recommended work restrictions for staff with infectious diseases. In the event of a member of staff becoming infected either in the hospital or outside, he/she should be relieved from direct contact with patients. Kitchen staff should also be relieved from duty if they are suffering from diarrhoea or hepatitis A, or have infected lesions on their hands.

Control of airborne transmission of infection

Ventilation systems and air flow can play an important role in the dissemination of organisms by the airborne route. Wards comprising separate rooms have been shown to afford some protection against airborne spread and rooms with controlled ventilation are even better. However, neither prevent the carriage into the room of organisms on staff and their clothing, and some studies suggest that this is a more important route of infection than airborne spread. There is no doubt, however, that *Legionella* infection is acquired by the airborne route, and air conditioning systems throughout the hospital should be maintained so as to prevent the multiplication of these organisms (see Chapter 22).

Ventilation systems in operating theatres must be properly installed and maintained to prevent the ingress of contaminated air and to minimize air currents carrying organisms from the staff in the operating room to the operation site. 'Ultra-clean' air (air passed through high-efficiency filters to remove bacteria and other particles) has been shown to contribute positively to the reduction in the number of post-operative wound infections developing after long orthopaedic operations.

Airborne transmission of infection can be reduced significantly by isolation of patients. This may be done to protect a particularly susceptible patient from exposure to pathogens i.e. protective isolation, or to prevent the spread of pathogens from an infected patient to others on the ward, i.e. source isolation. Isolation also helps to prevent

transmission of infection by other routes by limiting access to the patient and reminding staff of the importance of contact in the spread of infection.

Protective isolation. This can be provided by a single room on a ward or by enclosing the patient in a plastic isolator. With appropriate positive-pressure ventilation, air should flow from the 'clean' patient area out of the room or isolator. Staff entering the room or in contact with the patient should wear sterile gowns, gloves and masks to prevent organisms which they are carrying, or have picked up from other patients, from coming in contact with the patient.

Source isolation. This, ideally, is arranged by accommodation in an isolation unit in a separate building (viz the tuberculosis sanatoria of the past). In a general hospital isolation is more often arranged in a separate ward or in side rooms off the main ward. To prevent airborne transmission of organisms from the patient's room to the ward, air should flow from the ward to the isolation room. In practice it is difficult to maintain the correct air flows without sophisticated designs, including double doors and air locks.

Facilitation of aseptic behaviour

A general state of cleanliness throughout the hospital is essential, and the design of hospital facilities affects the ease with which the environment can be kept clean and the staff can practise good techniques.

The human factor – hands spread diseases!

The hands of staff convey to patients organisms from septic lesions and healthy carrier-sites of other patients, from equipment contaminated from these sources and from carrier sites of the staff themselves (Fig. 39.13). Bacteriologically effective handwashing is one of the most important ways of controlling infection in the hospital. Staff should wash their hands before any procedure for which gloves or forceps are necessary, and after contact with an infected patient or one who is colonized with multiply-resistant bacteria and after touching infective material. Soap and water are adequate in most circumstances, but when dealing with infected patients disinfectant soaps are recommended. Drying hands after washing is also important. A more prolonged and thorough scrub is required before commencing surgery.

The design of taps, soap-dispensers and other washing facilities, including bedpan washers has reached a high degree of sophistication. However, human behaviour can be influenced by architectural design only to a limited degree and there is often a disappointingly low compliance with the simple technique of handwashing. Therefore training, and regular reinforcement, in proper behaviour is essential.

Enhancing the host's ability to resist infection

Although attempts can and should be made to control and prevent hospital infection by removing sources of infection and preventing transmission from sources to susceptible

<a>**CONTACT SPREAD OF OPPORTUNIST PATHOGENS**</a>		
patient	nursing activity	number of klebsiellae recovered per hand*
A	physiotherapy	10–100
	taking blood pressure and pulse	100–1000
	washing patient	10–100
	taking oral temperature	100–1000
B	taking radial pulse	100–1000
	touching shoulder	1000
	touching groin	100–1000
C	touching hand	10–100
D	extubation	100–1000
	touching tracheostomy	1000

* Control hand washings taken prior to procedure yielded no klebsiellae

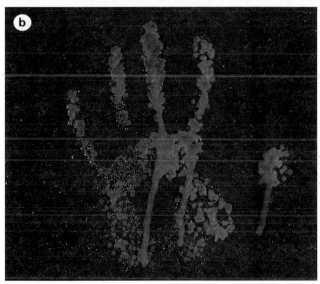

Fig. 39.13 (a) Nursing procedures involving skin contact resulting in contamination of staff hands. These data are derived from experiments performed during an outbreak of *Klebsiella* infection among urology patients. Data from Casewell and Phillips, 1977. (b) Gram-negative rods are not usually part of the resident skin flora (except in moist environments) but they are readily carried on hands and can be transferred from a source to a susceptible patient. This picture shows an impression of a hand that was inoculated with about 1000 *Klebsiella aerogenes*.

BOOSTING SPECIFIC IMMUNITY OF PATIENTS		
patient group	immunization	
	active	passive
Elderly (especially those with multisystem disease)	influenza vaccine	–
Pre-splenectomy Pre-renal or bone marrow transplant	pneumococcal vaccine	–
Haemodialysis patients	pneumococcal vaccine	–
Infants born to HBs Ag positive mothers	hepatitis B vaccine	–
Immunocompromised: exposed to varicella–zoster	live attenuated V-ZV vaccine in trials	zoster immune globulin (ZIG) within 3 days prevents severe disease
Exposed to measles	–	normal human immune globulin within 5 days

Fig. 39.14 Many patients will have been protected against some infections by routine immunization during childhood, but sometimes it is helpful to boost specific immunity by immunization of patients at particular risk of infection.

- Care of invasive devices which breach the natural defences, e.g. urinary catheters, intravenous lines;
- Attention to the risks predisposing to post-operative infection.

Boosting specific immunity by immunization has been discussed in Chapter 37. The problem for the immunocompromised patient is that he/she may not be able to mount an antibody response. Passive immunization can afford short-term protection, for example in patients who are neutropenic as a result of cytotoxic therapy and whose white cell count should recover after successful treatment. With the advent of efficacious hepatitis B vaccines it is recommended that all seronegative patients in dialysis units (and all staff in such units) should be immunized. Other immunizations for protecting hospital patients are summarized in figure 39.14.

The use of prophylactic antibiotics has been discussed in Chapter 33. There are several well-documented uses for prophylactic antibiotics in 'dirty' surgery and when the consequences of infection would be disastrous, e.g. in cardiac, neuro- and transplant surgery. However, there is a tendency to abuse antibiotics, first, by using them too often or for too long, thereby increasing the selection pressure for emergence of resistant organisms, and second, by choosing inappropriate agents.

Treatment (as opposed to prophylaxis) of patients and staff who are carriers of pathogens such as *Staph. aureus* or

hosts, neither of these strategies is failsafe. In addition, they do not protect the host from endogenous infection. A way of tipping the balance in favour of the host is to enhance his/her ability to resist infection, both by boosting specific immunity and by reducing personal risk factors. The following aspects should be considered:

- Boosting specific immunity by active or passive immunization;
- The proper use of prophylactic antibiotics;

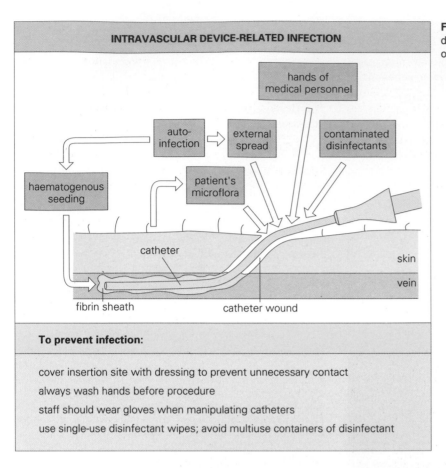

Fig. 39.15 Sources of intravascular device-related infection and opportunities for prevention of infection.

Strep. pyogenes has been used successfully to prevent endogenous infection and to control outbreaks of infection with these organisms. Topical preparations of antibiotics such as neomycin and fucidin have been used but there is no doubt that the emergence of resistance is a problem. More recently pseudomonic acid (Mupirocin), a fermentation product of *Pseudomonas fluorescens*, has been shown to be efficacious. It is unrelated to any other class of antibiotic in clinical use (thus diminishing the concern over emergence of resistant strains with cross resistance to other agents) and it is very active against Gram-positive cocci. In recent years it has played an important role in eradicating carriage of methicillin-resistant staphylococci (MRSA).

Gut decontamination regimes to reduce the aerobic Gram-negative flora of neutropenic patients has been practised for some time. More recently the use of selective bowel decontamination (SBD) in intensive care patients has become fashionable in some centres. The aim is to reduce the reservoir of potential pathogens in the gut by oral administration (or via a naso-gastric tube) of a high concentration of a mixture of antibiotics (polymyxin plus tobramycin plus amphotericin, or similar combination) to intensive care unit (ICU) patients throughout their stay in the unit. At the present time there is still controversy about the efficacy and safety of SBD.

Care of invasive devices is essential to reduce the risk of endogenous infection from skin organisms in the case of intravascular devices, and from the periurethral flora causing infection of the bladder in catheterized patients. Guidelines for the care of urinary catheters have been discussed previously (see Chapter 23). Up to one-third of hospital-acquired bacteraemias and the majority of candidaemias are infusion-related and derive mainly from vascular catheters. Most bacteraemias associated with invasive devices are caused by the patient's own skin flora (although this may be a more resistant flora acquired during the patient's stay in hospital and replacing his/her 'community-acquired' flora). *Staphylococcus epidermidis* accounts for more than 50% of infections but other aerobic bacteria including *Staph. aureus*, enterococci, coryneforms, various Gram-negative rods, and *Candida* are also implicated. These infections are largely preventable if appropriate steps are taken. The sources of infection and measures for prevention are shown in figure 39.15.

Reducing the risks of post-operative infection involves an understanding of the risks and the ways in which they can be circumvented. For example the pre-operative length of stay in hospital should be kept to a minimum, and intercurrent infections should be treated appropriately prior to surgery whenever possible, e.g. treatment of urinary tract infection prior to resection of the prostate.

Operations should be kept to the minimum duration consistent with good operating technique. Adequate debridement of dead and necrotic tissue is essential, together with adequate drainage and maintenance, or re-establishment, of a good blood supply to allow the body's natural defences optimum working conditions.

Good nursing techniques should ensure that all patients are prevented from developing pressure sores and that the risks of infection of the respiratory and urinary tracts are minimized by preventing stasis. Active physiotherapy is important in post-operative patients.

INVESTIGATING HOSPITAL INFECTION

In many hospitals the responsibility for investigating hospital infection falls on the infection control committee (including an infection control officer who may be a physician or microbiologist, and at least one nurse). The roles of the infection control committee include the surveillance of hospital infection, establishment and monitoring of policies and procedures designed to prevent infection (e.g. catheter care policy, antibiotic policy, disinfectant policy), and investigation of outbreaks.

Surveillance

Although hospital infection has been recognized for many years, accurate records of incidence and prevalence were not initiated until the late 1950s. Since 1960 several national surveys both in the UK and USA have highlighted the prevalence and importance of hospital infection. By maintaining surveillance, the infection control team can establish the normal trends in their hospital and thus recognize any change in numbers or types of infections early on. Sources of surveillance data are:

- Microbiology laboratory reports. These can be used for general surveillance or for monitoring 'alert' organisms such as *Staph. aureus, Strep. pyogenes, M. tuberculosis*, salmonellae, shigellae;
- Ward rounds. New cases of infection can be identified by direct inspection, plus previously identified cases of infection followed up. Surveys can also be carried out on the wards, e.g. of wound infections after different practices or procedures;
- Other sources, including autopsy reports, staff health records, surveys of patients after discharge from hospital, etc.

Investigation of outbreaks

When an outbreak (or epidemic) occurs, or when routine surveillance highlights an increase in the incidence of infection, the control of infection team should initiate an investigation. There is no universally applicable routine for finding the cause of an outbreak, but in principle each investigation has an epidemiological element and a microbiological element. There must be a definition of the situation in epidemiological terms; how many people are infected, when were they admitted, when did they develop their infection, are they all on the same ward, treated by the same medical or surgical team, and so on. It is the role of the microbiology laboratory to attempt to isolate the causative organisms and to show that all the patients in the outbreak are infected with the same strain (i.e. strains that are indistinguishable; see below). The identity of the infecting organism provides clues to the possible source; for example, an outbreak of wound infection with *Staph. aureus* is likely to be associated with contact spread from staff in theatre or on the ward, whereas an outbreak of salmonella gastroenteritis is more likely to originate in the kitchen.

While the investigation is proceeding, efforts must be made to contain the outbreak and prevent spread to other patients. Infected patients must be isolated and treated appropriately, and staff who are found to be infected or carriers must be suspended from duty until they have been treated. At the end of the investigation the relevant procedures must be reviewed to try and prevent a similar outbreak occurring again.

Epidemiological typing techniques

In epidemiological studies of the spread of infections and in the investigation of outbreaks both in hospital and in the community it is necessary to compare bacterial isolates to determine whether they belong to the same species, and if so, whether they are distinct or of the same strain (in fact it is not possible to say that two organisms are the same, only that they are indistinguishable). If the species is a regular member of the normal human flora, or if it is found frequently in the environment, it is necessary to distinguish the 'outbreak' strain from other strains of the same species not involved in the outbreak, but which may also be isolated during the course of the investigation. Various phenotypic and genotypic characters can be used to 'fingerprint' strains for epidemiological purposes.

A good typing technique must be discriminatory, i.e. able to show differences between strains of the same species; reproducible, i.e. the same strain gives the same result when tested on different occasions and in different places; and have a high degree of typability, i.e. capable of assigning a type to all strains.

Antibiotic susceptibility patterns

These tests are performed readily in the diagnostic laboratory (see Chapter 35), and are useful as a preliminary clue as to whether two isolates are indistinguishable. However, discrimination is poor; many susceptibility patterns are common and quite different strains may have the same pattern; conversely, during an outbreak, strains may gain or lose plasmids carrying antibiotic resistance markers.

Biotyping

This is a method of typing organisms by their ability to grow on different substrates or produce different enzymes. Ideally the biochemical test employed in a biotyping scheme should be different from those used to identify the organisms. Identification tests are chosen because they 'lump' similar organisms together; biotyping tests are chosen because they 'split' species into distinct strains. However, diagnostic laboratories often use the profiles from minaturized multi-test identifications systems as biotypes (Fig. 39.16).

Serotyping

This classical technique distinguishes between strains by difference in their antigenic structure, recognized by reaction with specific antisera. Thus the 'O' somatic antigens and 'H' flagellar antigens are used to divide salmonellae into types (sometimes referred to as species; see Chapter 25). *Streptococcus pneumoniae, Neisseria meningitidis* and *Klebsiella aerogenes* can be typed on the basis of their capsular (K) antigens and *Strep. pyogenes* on their M and T cell wall proteins. The established schemes use polyclonal antisera but newer schemes based on monoclonals are being developed. Serotyping requires the production and maintenance of appropriate banks of antisera which is both time-consuming and costly, and is thus usually restricted to reference laboratories.

Bacteriophage (phage) typing

This technique compares the pattern of lysis obtained when isolates (grown as lawns on agar plates) are exposed to a standard series of phage suspensions (Fig. 39.17). This method is important for typing *Staph. aureus, Staph. epidermidis* and *Salmonella typhi*, but has been applied to other species such as *Pseudomonas aeruginosa*. As with serotyping, phage typing requires the production, maintenance and testing of the standard phage suspensions and is usually carried out in reference laboratories rather than in the hospital diagnostic laboratory.

Bacteriocins

These are small protein molecules produced by species of bacteria and lethal to other strains of the same, or closely related, species. The pattern of inhibition of growth by the test strain of a standard set of indicator strains can be used to assign the strain to a type (Fig. 39.18). The method is potentially applicable to any species that produces bacteriocins (and most do). It has been most successfully applied to *Pseudomonas aeruginosa* (pyocine typing, from the old name for the organism; *Pseudomonas pyocyaneus*) and *Shigella sonnei* (colicine typing, so-named because the species is genetically very similar to *Escherichia coli* and sensitive to bacteriocins called colicines produced by that species).

Molecular typing techniques

With the development of techniques in molecular biology, there has been a trend away from the classical phenotypic methods towards characterization of an organism's DNA, either chromosome or plasmid (or total protein profile, i.e. all the proteins in the cell that are encoded by the DNA). Plasmid profiles are only useful for species that carry a variety of plasmids and they suffer from the drawback that what is actually being characterized is the plasmid and not the

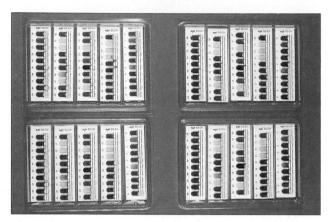

Fig. 39.16 Biotyping isolates of *Bacillus cereus* from an outbreak of infection in an intensive care unit. Biotyping schemes are based on the ability of different strains within a species to metabolize and grow on different substrates. Commercially-available multi-test systems are designed primarily for identification purposes, but can also be used for biotyping. The strips contain a series of different biochemical tests. The isolate is inoculated into each well and after incubation, a positive result is indicated by a colour change. Courtesy of S Dancer.

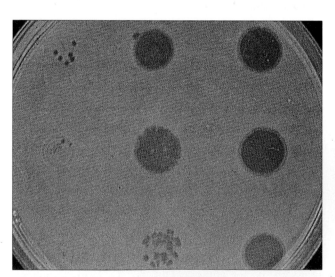

Fig. 39.17 Bacteriophage (phage) typing of staphylococci. After seeding the surface of an agar plate with the organism to be typed, suspensions of different phages are dropped onto the surface and the plate incubated. Phages that are able to lyse the strain will produce zones of clearing of the bacterial lawn. The patterns of lysis obtained with the same set of bacteriophages on different isolates of *Staph. aureus* collected, for example during an outbreak of wound infections, can be compared.

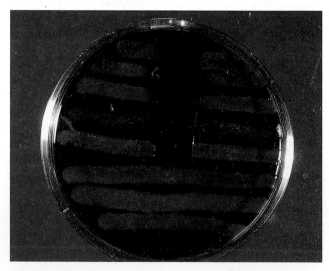

Fig. 39.18 Bacteriocin typing. Species that produce bacteriocins can be typed according to the pattern of inhibition produced by the bacteriocin on a standard set of indicator strains. The test isolate is grown in a band across the agar plate (during this time bacteriocins produced by the isolate diffuse into the agar). After overnight incubation, the macroscopic growth is removed and the surface of the plate exposed to chloroform to kill remaining organisms (bacteriocins are resistant to the action of chloroform). Indicator strains are streaked across the plate at right angles to the original line and the plate incubated a second time. The pattern of inhibition of growth of the indicator is recorded and the strain assigned to a type.

organism containing it. Different Gram-negative rods may acquire the same plasmids by conjugation between different species. However, this method has also been used to advantage to map the spread of antibiotic resistance plasmids among hospital pathogens (Fig. 39.19).

The total DNA of a cell can be analysed by extracting it and digesting it with restriction endonucleases. These enzymes cut the DNA at specific sites producing many short lengths of DNA which can be separated on a gel to give a pattern characteristic of the organism and the restriction enzyme (because different restriction enzymes cut the DNA at different sites they produce different fragment lengths from the same DNA). Comparison of the DNA from different isolates of the same species cut by the same restriction enzyme will show whether the isolates have the same pattern of bands and by implication, indistinguishable DNA (Fig. 39.20).

The advantage of DNA techniques for epidemiological fingerprinting is that all isolates can be typed (i.e. typability is 100%) and with choice of restriction enzyme, discrimination is also high. However the band patterns are fairly complex and isolates need to be run on the same gel for comparisons to be valid. Simpler patterns can be obtained by using DNA probes to identify gene sequences in isolates. Ribotyping, i.e. probing for the genes that encode ribosomal RNA, has been applied successfully to type some species. However discrimination between strains of the same species may be less because the rRNA genes tend to be highly conserved. Again, for valid results, the isolates to be compared should be run on the same gel.

Although antibacterial susceptibility patterns and simple biotyping can be carried out in most routine diagnostic laboratories, the specialized typing techniques are based in reference laboratories. This has the advantage that quality assurance can be optimized but also means that there is an inevitable delay in reporting the results and thus in learning whether an outbreak of hospital infection is caused by a single strain.

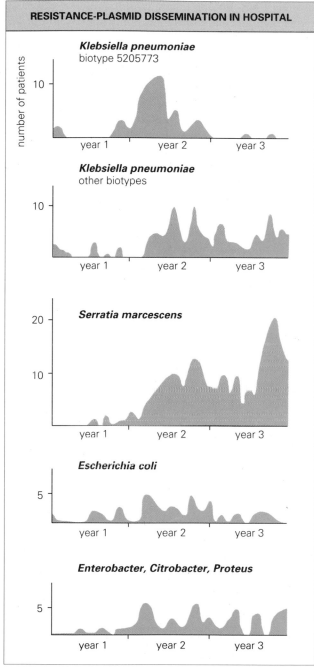

Fig. 39.19 Dissemination of a single resistance plasmid into several different strains and species of enterobacteria in one hospital. In year 1 in this hospital there were very few isolates of gentamicin-resistant enterobacteria. In the first 4 months of year 2, there was an outbreak of infection with a gentamicin-resistant *Klebsiella pneumoniae* belonging to a single biotype. Although this outbreak was contained, over subsequent months the same plasmid, coding for the same aminoglycoside-modifying enzyme, was found in other biotypes of the *Klebsiella* and in other Gram-negative species. Adapted from O'Brien et al., 1980.

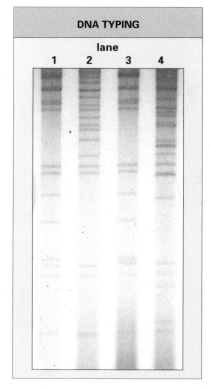

Fig. 39.20 DNA typing. The figure shows DNA from isolates of *Enterococcus faecalis* from four patients on the same ward. The DNA was extracted from each isolate and digested with the restriction endonuclease *Sst*1. After digestion the DNA fragments are separated by gel electrophoresis and stained with ethidium bromide. Comparison of the pattern of bands shows that isolates in lanes 1 and 3 are indistinguishable and different from those in lanes 2 and 4. Courtesy of L Hall.

STERILIZATION AND DISINFECTION

It is clear that the prevention of hospital infection depends in part on the availability of clean, and where necessary, sterile equipment, instruments, dressings, isolation facilities etc., and on the safe disposal of infected material. Sterilization and disinfection are often talked about by microbiologists in relation to the production of sterile culture media and other laboratory activities, but it must be stressed that the concept of sterility is central to almost all areas of medical practice. An understanding of the rationale of sterilization and disinfection will aid the intelligent use of the range of sterile equipment (from needles to protheses) and techniques (from surgery to handwashing) employed in medical practice.

Definitions

An item that is sterile is free from all viable organisms; in this sense viable means capable of reproducing. Sterilization is the process of killing or removing all viable organisms and it is achieved by physical or chemical means, either by the removal of organisms from an object or by killing the organisms *in situ*, sometimes leaving toxic breakdown products (pyrogens) in the object.

The term 'disinfection' is usually restricted to a process which removes or kills most, but not all, viable organisms. It employs either a chemical 'disinfectant' which kills pathogens but may not kill viruses or spores, or a physical process such as boiling water or low pressure steam, which reduces the bioburden (i.e. the load of viable organisms).

'Antisepsis' is the use of an antiseptic to reduce the number of viable organisms on the skin. Antiseptics are a particular group of disinfectants. Some act differentially, destroying the transient flora but leaving untouched the normal skin flora deep in the skin pores and hair follicles (Fig. 39.21). It is impossible to sterilize the skin (except by burning!) but thorough washing with antiseptic soaps can reduce considerably the numbers of organisms on the surface and thus reduce contact spread of infection (see above). However, the resident bacteria in the hair follicles and ducts of sweat glands can recolonize the skin surface within hours.

'Pasteurization' is a technique applied to eliminate pathogens and reduce the total numbers of viable microbes in bulk fluids such as milk, fruit juices etc., without destroying the flavour and palatability. It does not affect spores but is effective against intracellular organisms such as *Brucella* and mycobacteria and many viruses.

Since recorded history, various other techniques such as drying and salting of food have been used to prevent multiplication of microorganisms.

Sterilization and disinfection processes are costly and so it is important to choose the appropriate method and the one which causes the least damage to the material involved. The following considerations influence the choice of method:

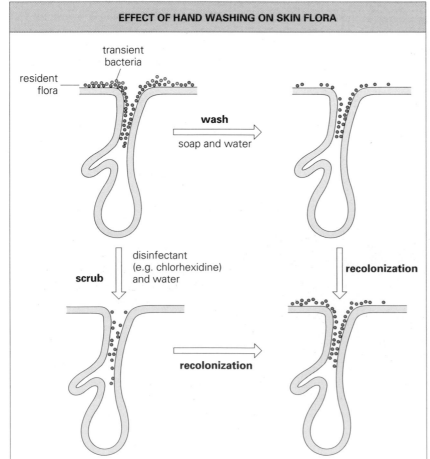

EFFECT OF HAND WASHING ON SKIN FLORA

transient bacteria

resident flora

wash
soap and water

scrub

disinfectant (e.g. chlorhexidine) and water

recolonization

recolonization

Fig. 39.21 Normal skin is colonized with bacteria both on the surface and deep in the pores and ducts of the sweat and sebaceous glands. In addition bacteria may be carried transiently on the skin surface and may be transmitted from a contaminated source to a susceptible patient. Careful hand washing with soap and water removes the transient flora and some of the superficial resident flora. Scrubbing the hands with disinfectants removes more of the resident flora but the skin surface is recolonized within hours from the normal flora deep in the skin pores.

- It is easier to sterilize a clean object than a (physically) dirty one (organic matter protects microbes and hinders penetration of heat or chemicals and may inactivate certain chemicals). In other words, a low bioburden is a prerequisite for cost-effective sterilization.
- The rate of killing of microorganisms depends on the concentration of the killing agent and time of exposure. The number of survivors can be expressed by the equation:

$$N \propto 1/CT$$

where N is the number of survivors, C is the concentration of agent and T is time of exposure to the agent. If a population of microbes is exposed to a sterilizing technique and the number of survivors, expressed as a logarithm, is plotted against time, the slope of the graph defines the death rate (Fig. 39.22) These lines may be sigmoid or have shoulders, indicating that individual cells

respond slightly differently, some being killed more easily than others. In the case of bacteria, the physiological state of the organisms influences the shape of the killing curve; young, replicating cells are usually more vulnerable than stationary or decline-phase organisms, or those that are sporing.

- Graphs like those shown in figure 39.22 can be used to predict the conditions necessary to achieve sterility. However these experimental data are usually based on pure cultures in the laboratory (bacterial spores are often used as model systems) whereas in real life the bioburden is mixed. Thus predictions from such data may be inappropriate to mixed populations.
- The detailed mechanisms of the death process of microorganisms may vary with the sterilizing technique used, but the net effect is similar in that essential cell constituents (nucleic acids or proteins) are inactivated.

TECHNIQUES FOR STERILIZATION

Sterilization may be achieved by:
- Heat
- Irradiation (gamma and ultraviolet)
- Filtration
- Chemicals, in liquid or gaseous phase.

Other techniques of doubtful efficiency include freezing and thawing, lysis, dessication, ultrasonication and the use of electrical discharges, but these are not applied in hospital practice. Ultraviolet irradiation is inefficient as a sterilant; its important uses in the hospital setting are in inhibiting growth of bacteria in water in complex apparatus such as auto-analyzers and in air in safety hoods in virology laboratories. The potential for damage to the cornea and skin also precludes wider use of ultraviolet irradiation.

Heat

Heat, as a way to transfer energy, is the preferred choice for sterilization on the grounds of ease of use, controllability, cost and efficiency. Sufficient heat, applied correctly, will sterilize even the agents of Creutzfeld-Jacob disease and scrapie, but it cannot be applied to living tissues or to materials that are damaged by high temperatures.

Dry heat

The sterilizing mechanism of dry heat is basically the oxidation of the cell components. Incineration and the use of the laboratory Bunsen burner are examples of sterilization by dry heat. Glassware can be sterilized in a hot air oven at 160–180°C for 1 hour.

Moist heat

The most effective agent for sterilization is saturated steam under pressure, as in an autoclave. The destruction of enzymes and membranes is influenced by the availability of water which disrupts hydrogen bonds. Steam under pressure aids penetration of heat into the material to be sterilized (such as dressings) and there is a direct relationship between temperature and steam pressure. Steam

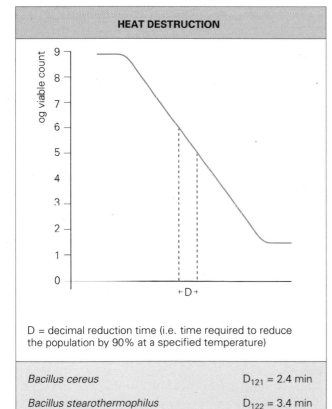

HEAT DESTRUCTION

D = decimal reduction time (i.e. time required to reduce the population by 90% at a specified temperature)

Bacillus cereus	$D_{121} = 2.4$ min
Bacillus stearothermophilus	$D_{122} = 3.4$ min
Clostridium botulinum	$D_{104} = 5.5$ min
Clostridium perfringens	$D_{104} = 2.3$ min

Fig. 39.22 Theoretically there is a straight line relationship between the log viable count of a bacterial population and time when the population is exposed to a lethal temperature. In practice these lines are usually sigmoid. The D value is the time required to reduce the population by 90% at a specified temperature. *Bacillus stearothermophilus* spores are used as biological indicators of effective heat sterilization by including filter paper strips carrying a standard number of spores into the autoclave cycle. The strips are then incubated to attempt to recover viable organisms. The usual autoclave cycle of 121°C for 15 minutes is adequate to kill *B. stearothermophilus* with a margin of safety.

under pressure has a temperature in excess of 100°C which gives increased killing of microbes.

Sterilizing efficiency is improved by evacuating all the air from the autoclave chamber. The subsequent introduction of high pressure steam rapidly penetrates to all parts of the chamber and its load, and results in predictable rises in temperature in the centre of articles to be sterilized. The length of an autoclave cycle is determined by the holding time plus a margin of safety, and is derived from the thermal death curves for heat-resistant pathogens such as clostridia. Thus the usual cycle of 121°C for 15 minutes is sufficient to kill the spores of *Clostridium botulinum* with an adequate margin of safety. However the spores of some bacterial species, especially soil organisms, are able to withstand even this temperature. The safety margin is reduced in the presence of large numbers of organisms (because there is a greater probability of more heat-resistant individuals existing in a large population) and hence the importance of cleaning instruments etc., whenever possible, before sterilization.

Moist heat in an autoclave is used to sterilize surgical instruments and dressings and heat-resistant pharmaceuticals. A method for the sterilization of heat-sensitive instruments such as endoscopes uses a combination of low temperature (sub-atmospheric) steam and formaldehyde. All these processes need to be carried out in a suitable pressure vessel and are therefore usually available in the hospital central sterile supply department.

Moist heat disinfection

Immersion in boiling water for a few minutes will kill vegetative bacteria and many, but not all, spores, and can be used as a rapid emergency measure for instruments. The addition of 2% sodium carbonate to the water potentiates the sporicidal effect.

Pasteurization

This technique was devised by Pasteur to prevent the spoilage of wine by heating it to 50–60°C. It is now used for fluids such as milk to reduce the numbers of bacteria. This helps to eliminate pathogens present in small numbers and to improve the shelf-life of milk. The fluid is held at a temperature of 62.8–65.6°C for 30 minutes or may be 'flash' pasteurized at 71.7°C for 15 seconds. After either process the fluid should be held at a temperature below 10°C in order to minimize subsequent bacterial growth.

Irradiation

The use of gamma irradiation energy is now the method of choice to sterilize large batches of small volume items such as needles, syringes, intravenous lines, catheters and gloves. It can also be used for vaccines and for the prevention of food spoilage. Although the capital cost of the equipment is very high, the process is continuous and 100% efficient. Articles are sterilized, without any heat gain, sealed in their final packaging. The process must be conducted in a suitably constructed building, usually at a location distinct from the hospital (and usually outside the hospital administration). It is not a technique applicable to 'one-off' use. The killing mechanism involves the produc-

tion of free radicals which are effective in breaking the bonds in DNA. Irradiation kills spores, but at a higher dose than vegetative cells because of the relative lack of water in spores. The recommended dose is 4.5 megarads.

Sterilization using ultraviolet irradiation is discussed above.

Filtration

Solutions that are heat-sterilized will contain pyrogens. These heat-stable breakdown products of microbes are capable of inducing fever and are therefore undesirable in products such as intravenous fluids. Filtration or separation of the product from the contamination has a long history in the clarification of water and wine. Modern filters are composed of nitrocellulose and work by electrostatic attraction and physical pore size to retain organisms or other particles. The resulting fluid should be particle-free. Filtration is used in some parts of the world to purify drinking water.

Filtration techniques are also used to recover very small numbers of organisms from very large volumes of fluid e.g. *Legionella* from cooling tower water and can be used as a method for quantitating bacteria in fluids.

Chemical agents

Gases

The need for sterilization by gaseous chemicals has been greatly reduced by the success of gamma irradiation (see above) but two gasses, ethylene oxide and formaldehyde, are still used. Both are alkylating agents and kill by damaging proteins and nucleic acids.

Ethylene oxide is used in some centres to sterilize single-use medical requisites such as heart valves. However, it is toxic and potentially explosive.

Formaldehyde is not explosive but has an extremely unpleasant odour and is an irritant to mucous membranes. It is used as a disinfectant to decontaminate rooms (such as isolation rooms), and in the laboratory to disinfect exhaust-protective cabinets. A high relative humidity is essential for effective killing.

Liquids

Gluteraldehyde is less toxic than formaldehyde and can be stabilized in solution to remain active for up to 4 weeks at in-use concentration. It is used for the disinfection (but it does not sterilize) heat-sensitive articles such as endoscopes and for inanimate surfaces.

Other chemical agents

A wide range of antimicrobial chemicals is available. Some, like the derivatives of pine and turpentine, have been known since ancient times; chloride of lime and coal-tar fluids were in use before the germ theory of disease was established. Most fall into the category of disinfectant or antiseptic, but a few are capable of rendering articles sterile. Factors which affect their efficacy include:
- physical environment (e.g. porous or cracked surfaces);
- presence of moisture;
- temperature and pH;

DISINFECTANTS FOR HOSPITAL USE		
group	**examples**	**advantages and disadvantages**
Phenolics	clear-soluble phenolic compounds, white fluids	good general-purpose disinfectants, not readily inactivated by organic matter, active against wide range of organisms including mycobacteria, not sporicidal
	chloroxylenols	inactivated by hard water and organic matter, *Pseudomonas* grows readily in chloroxylenol solutions, limited activity against other Gram-negatives
Halogens	hypochlorites (chloramine)	cheap, effective, act by release of free chlorine, active against viruses and therefore recommended for disinfection of equipment soiled with blood (because of hepatitis risk), inactivated by organic material, corrode metals
	iodine and iodophors	useful skin disinfectants, sporicidal
Other heavy metals	mercuric chloride	used as topical skin preparation
Quaternary ammonium compounds	benzalkonium chloride, cetavlon	have detergent properties, activity against Gram-negative << Gram-positive, improved by combination with diguanide, e.g. chlorhexidine, useful as skin disinfectants, inactivated by hard water and organic materials, contamination of stock solutions with Gram-negative rods can be a problem
Diguanides	chlorhexidine	useful disinfectant for skin and mucous membranes, inactivated by many materials and too expensive for environmental use, alcoholic solutions are less easily contaminated, combinations of chlorhexidine and detergent highly effective for disinfection of hands
Alcohols	ethyl alcohol, isopropyl alcohol	good choice for skin disinfection and for clean surfaces, sometimes used in combination with iodine or chlorhexidine (see above), water must be present for bacterial killing (i.e. 70% ethanol best), isopropyl preferred for skin and articles in contact with patient
Aldehydes	formaldehyde/formalin	too irritant for use as general disinfectant
	glutaraldehyde	kills vegetative organisms including mycobacteria slowly but effectively, more active, less toxic than formaldehyde, sporicidal (within 6 hours when fresh), slightly irritant, used in alkaline solution which is stable for 1–2 weeks, expensive, limited use, e.g. disinfection of endoscopes
Hexachlorophane		activity against Gram-positive >> Gram-negative, used in soap or dusting powder as skin disinfectant (use restricted after potentially toxic blood levels found in infants who had hexachlorophane emulsion spread over whole body)
	irgasan	introduced as substitute for hexachlorophane in soap, considerable antibacterial effect on repeated use

Fig. 39.23 Disinfectants for use in hospitals. Note that no one group of disinfectant has all the properties desirable for use both on skin and on inanimate surfaces.

- concentration of the agent;
- hardness of water;
- the bioburden on the object to be disinfected;
- the nature and state of the microbes in the bioburden;
- the ability of the microbes to inactivate the chemical agent.

It is obvious that the above factors are difficult to control in every circumstance. The main groups of chemical agents are shown in figure 39.23. They act by causing chemical damage to proteins or nucleic acids, or to cell membrane lipids. The activity of a given disinfectant may result from more than one pathway of damage.

CONTROLLING STERILIZATION AND DISINFECTION

In general it is preferable to control the process rather than the product, i.e. to run checks on the technique while it is in operation rather than attempting to recognize process failure by isolating microorganisms from the product. Trying to discover whether one or a few viable organisms remain is analogous to trying to find a needle in haystack. It is known that damaged bacteria can recover given time and special nutrient recovery media but it may not be feasible to hold back a batch of product for such tests. How many samples of the product should be tested? If too few are examined, the likelihood of missing a failed sample is high; if too many are examined, too much of the batch is used up in quality control to be economically sensible.

The usual process controls are either physical or chemical checks on the technique. In other word, tests which tell you that, for example, the autoclave reached the desired temperature for the desired time. They do not show that there are no viable organisms remaining after the process but this is assumed if the process satisfies the controls. However, the stringency of the controls can be altered intentionally or accidentally to give an under- or over-sensitive test.

Disinfectants can be monitored by microbiological 'in-use' tests in which the solution is challenged with a bacterial suspension, samples are withdrawn, treated to prevent carryover of the disinfectant and cultured. However these tests are rarely performed in the hospital setting where the use of disinfectants is guided largely by the manufacturers' recommendations.

SUMMARY

Hospital infections often have serious consequences for the individual, for the hospital community and for the community at large. They may be caused by almost any organism but a few species cause the vast majority of infections. However the hospital environment favours the survival of resistant strains and thus infections are often caused by organisms with limited antibiotic susceptibility. Because of the serious consequences of infection, control and prevention of infection should have a high priority and depend on education of staff in proper procedures as well as on the provision of a clean environment and sterile equipment. Sterility cannot be demonstrated unequivocally, i.e. it is not possible to prove that no viable organisms remain. Nonetheless it is a cornerstone on which much of modern medicine and surgery depends.

Further Reading

Bennet JV, Brachman PS, eds. *Hospital infections*. Baltimore/Toronto: Little Brown & Co., 1986.

Casewell MW, Phillips I. Hands as route of transmission for *Klesiella* sp. *Br Med J* 1977; **2:** 1315.

Lowbury EJL, Ayliffe GAJ, Geddes AM, Williams JD, eds. *Control of hospital infection*. 3rd edition. London: Chapman and Hall, 1992.

Maurer IM. *Hospital hygeine*. London: Edward Arnold, 1974.

O'Brien TE *et al*. Dissemination of an antibiotic resistance plasmid in hospital patient flora. *Antimicrob Ag Chemother* 1980: **17:** 537.

Williams REO, Blowers R, Garrod LP, Shooter RA. *Hospital infection*. London: Lloyd Luke, 1966.

section 5

APPENDIX

VIRUSES					
PARVOVIRUSES					

Characteristics	Virus Family	Type	Envelope	Shape	Size (nm)	Nucleocapsid
	Papovaviridae	ssDNA	–	Icosahedral	22	Icosahedral
	The family contains human parvovirus B19 (single serotype), and the adeno-associated viruses (4 serotypes). The latter are defective, requiring concurrent infection of the cell with 'helper' adenovirus or herpesvirus; positive DNA strands and negative DNA strands are carried in separate particles. The former are autonomous, with negative strand DNA in particles.					

Replication	Occurs in the nucleus. Viral DNA replication takes place only when cell DNA replication is occuring, i.e. during the S phase of the cell cycle. Cellular transcriptase forms a cDNA strand to give dsDNA, and transcripts produce mRNAs.
Laboratory identification	Detection of parvovirus-specific IgM antibody or viral nucleic acid sequences.
Diseases	Bl9 parvovirus causes a mild disease, erythema infectiosum, in children, with a 'slapped cheek' rash. Aplastic crisis may occur in those with sickle cell anaemia. Arthropathy common in infected adults. Intrauterine infection may result in foetal death with hydrops foetalis. The adeno-associated viruses are not known to cause disease.
Transmission	Via respiratory droplets.
Pathogenesis	Virus spreads from respiratory tract and can infect haemopoetic cells in bone marrow.
Treatment and prevention	There is no specific treatment and no vaccine.

PAPOVAVIRUSES					

Characteristics	Virus Family	Type	Envelope	Shape	Size (nm)	Nucleocapsid
	Papovaviridae	dsDNA (circular)	–	Icosahedral	45–55	Icosahedral

Replication	Virus attaches via unknown receptor to epithelial cell; viral mRNA is transcribed in the nucleus by a cellular transcriptase; early gene products initiate viral DNA replication, transcription, transformation; late gene products are structural proteins. Only the early genes (for T antigens) are expressed in tranformed cells. The papovaviridae include PApillomaviruses, POlyomaviruses and simian VAcuolating viruses (e.g. SV40), with at least 65 types of human papillomavirus and two polyomaviruses (BK and JC). These viruses persist in latent form and can reactivate.
Laboratory identification	Serological methods are unsatisfactory. Vacuolated or inclusion-bearing cells (koilocytosis) seen on Papanicolau staining; virus particles visible (urine or tissues) by electron microscope. Virus culture either difficult (polyomaviruses) or impossible (papillomaviruses). In special laboratories viral antigens or viral DNA sequences (southern blotting, *in situ* hybridization, polymerase chain reaction) can be tested for.
Diseases	Papillomaviruses cause warts on skin and genital regions. Sexually transmitted warts can cause laryngeal papilloma in children (infected via birth canal) and types HPV16, HPV18 strongly associated with carcinoma of cervix (also carcinoma of penis, vulva, rectum). Polyomaviruses on primary infection cause mild upper respiratory illness. In immunocompromised patients JC virus causes PML (progressive multifocal leukoencephalopathy), and BK virus is excreted in urine but only rarely with pathological consequences.
Transmission	Papillomaviruses: from skin to skin by direct or indirect contact, and between mucosae by sexual intercourse. Polyomaviruses: from the upper respiratory tract by droplets and perhaps by contact with infected urine.

PAPOVAVIRUSES (CONT.)	
Pathogenesis	Papillomaviruses infection of epithelial cells and local multiplication results in wart after incubation period of up to 1–2 months. The wart regresses over the course of many months; no spread to deeper tissues but viral DNA remains in basal epithelial cells and can reactivate. When genital warts undergo malignant change, viral genome remains in cell; cofactors are involved. Polyomaviruses spread from the upper respiratory tract and localize in tubular epithelium in the kidney (excretion in urine) or in oligodendrocytes to cause PML.
Treatment and prevention	No effective antivirals or vaccines available. Skin warts can be destroyed by freezing (liquid nitrogen) and areas of cervical dysplasia (genital warts) by laser treatment. Many slower methods are used (podophylin, salicylic acid). Preventive measures include shoes (plantar warts) and condoms etc. for genital warts.

HERPESVIRUSES						
Characteristics	Virus Family	Type	Envelope	Shape	Size (nm)	Nucleocapsid
	Herpesviridae	dsDNA	+	Icosahedral	180–200	Icosahedral
Replication	Virus attaches to specific receptor on cell and enters by fusion of envelope with plasma membrane. Nucleocapsid moves to nucleus, viral DNA is uncoated at nuclear pores and then transcribed by cellular RNA polymerase so that the 5 sets of viral genes are sequentially activated. 'Immediate-early' gene products stimulate synthesis of second wave of 'early' gene products that are involved in genome replication and include the DNA polymerases. After DNA replication the remaining 'late' gene products are expressed and are involved in assembly. In the nucleus viral DNA is inserted into capsids and resulting nucleocapsids attach to sites on inner nuclear membrane where envelope proteins are present and budding takes place between inner and outer nuclear membranes. Enveloped virus particles are transported through the cytoplasm and released by reverse phagocytosis. Replication cycle about 36 hours. Generally persist for long periods in body, often in latent form, and can reactivate.					
Laboratory identification	Isolation of virus in cell culture (HSV, CMV); multinucleated cells (HSV,VZV) or intranuclear inclusions (CMV) in smears, tissues. Rise in antibody titre (all). Lymphocytosis, atypical lymphocytes, and heterophil antibody (Monospot) for EBV.					

Diseases	Type	Clinical Features
	HHV1(HSV1)	Gingivostomatitis, cold sores
	HHV2(HSV2)	Genital herpes, cutaneous herpes, encephalitis, meningo-encephalitis
	HHV3(VZV)	Varicella, zoster
	HHV4 (EBV)	Mononucleosis (glandular fever), hepatitis, encephalitis, BL, NPC
	HHV5(CMV)	Mononucleosis, hepatitis, pneumonitis, congenital CMV.
	HHV6	Exanthem subitum
	HHV7	??

Transmission	HSV: saliva, vesical fluid, sexual contact, birth canal in neonate. VZV: respiratory droplets, vesical fluid. EBV: saliva. CMV: saliva, urine, semen, cervical secretions, milk; also via transplanted tissues and across placenta.
Pathogenesis	HSV: vesicular lesions on mouth, skin, genitals. Axonal travel to latency sites in sensory ganglia. Reactivation (cold sores). VZV: respiratory infection, systemic spread to skin, axonal travel to latency sites sensory ganglia. Reactivation (zoster). EBV: pharyngeal infection, systemic spread, latency in B cells, epithelium. Subclinical reactivation. CMV: pharyngeal infection, systemic spread, latency in mononuclear cells. Reactivation.
Treatment and prevention	Acyclovir (HSV,VZV); Ganciclovir (CMV). Varicella-zoster immune globulin (VZIG) is used to prevent disease when immunocompromised are exposed to infection. No vaccines yet available for herpes viruses.

ADENOVIRUSES

Characteristics	Virus Family	Type	Envelope	Shape	Size (nm)	Nucleocapsid
	Adenoviridae	dsDNA	–	Icosahedral	60–70	Icosahedral

41 types, sharing a common group-specific antigen. Rod-like structures (fibres) topped with knobs project from the vertices of particles, and function by attaching virus to the cell.

Replication	After attachment, endocytosis and uncoating, viral DNA is transcribed within the nucleus by cellular DNA-dependent RNA polymerase. RNA transcripts corresponding to several genes (less than the whole genome) undergo cleavage and splicing to form monocistronic mRNA. Early mRNA codes for enzymes needed for replication; late mRNA (after viral DNA synthesis) for structural proteins. Particles are assembled in the nucleus and released from the damaged cell.
Laboratory identification	Rise in CF antibody titre. Demonstation of the virus in mouth washings, throat swabs, faeces etc., using HEL or Hela cells and looking for cpe, for antigen by FA staining, or for virions by EM.
Diseases	Cause pharyngoconjunctival fever; epidemics of acute respiratory disease, including pneumonia (especially types 3,4,7,14,21); intestinal illness (mesenteric adenitis, intususception); keratoconjunctivitis . Very occasionally cause haemorrhagic cystitis or CNS disease. Some are oncogenic in laboratory animals, but not in humans.
Transmission	Via respiratory droplets, via faeces, and sometimes from eye to eye via contaminated hands, towels, eyedrops, etc.
Pathogenesis	Adenoviruses infect epithelium of respiratory tract and eyes, and probably intestine. Spread to involve lymphoid tissues and can persist for long periods in tonsils and adenoids of children (types 1,2,5,6).
Treatment and prevention	No specific treatment. Live oral vaccine (types 3, 4, 7, in enteric-coated capsules) has been used in military recruits.

HEPADNAVIRUSES (HEPATITIS B)

Characteristics	Virus Family	Type	Envelope	Shape	Size (nm)	Nucleocapsid
	Hepadnaviridae	dsDNA (circular)	+	Spherical	42	Icosahedral

Particles consist of an envelope (HBs antigen) surrounding a core containing HBc (core antigen) and HBe antigen. Infected blood contains 22nm particles of HBs, outnumbering by at least 100 to 1 the 42 nm infectious (Dane) particles. One serotype (minor antigenic variants such as adn, adw, give complete cross; protection).

Replication	After attachment to hepatocytes, particles are endocytosed and uncoated. In the nucleus, viral DNA polymerase converts viral DNA into a complete circular dsDNA. Negative strand DNA is transcribed by cellular RNA polymerase to form a single positive RNA strand, which is encapsulated into cores together with viral DNA polymerase. The positive RNA strand is then used to synthesize negative strand DNA. A small fragment from the 5' end of the positive RNA strand primes synthesis of all but about one third of the positive DNA strand. Hence complete particles contain dsDNA with a ssDNA region. Release from cell is by budding.
Laboratory identification	The virus cannot be grown in cell culture. HBs antigen in blood (detectable during incubation period), indicates either acute or persistent infection. Presence of HBe antigen means blood is highly infectious. Presence of anti-HBs, anti-HBc (latter occurs early in the disease before anti-HBs), and anti-HBe indicates recent or past infection and immunity.
Diseases	Causes hepatitis, often severe in adults; important immunopathological contribution to disease. Incubation period 10–12 weeks. Persistent infection common, especially after infection in infancy or early childhood, when blood remains infectious, possibly for life; this can lead to chronic hepatitis, cirrhosis, liver cancer.
Transmission	Spread via blood (contaminated needles etc.), by sexual routes and from mother to offspring.

HEPADNAVIRUSES (CONT.)	
Pathogenesis	Virus spreads via blood to liver, replicates in hepatocytes. Immune complex formation can cause initial rash, arthritis; hepatitis is probably largely due to immune destruction of infected liver cells.
Treatment and prevention	No specific treatment. Carriage of virus can be terminated by massive doses of alpha and beta interferon. The excellent vaccine consists of genetically engineered HBs antigen. Post-exposure treatment is possible with human hyperimmune immunoglobulin.

POXVIRUSES

Characteristics						
	Virus Family	Type	Envelope	Shape	Size (nm)	Nucleocapsid
	Poxviridae	dsDNA	+/−	Brick or ovoid	200–300	complex structure
	The largest viruses; dermatotrophic, causing 'pocks' on the skin.					

Replication	Takes place in the cytoplasm (unlike other DNA viruses) and viral DNA-dependent RNA polymerase is used to synthesize mRNA. Transcripts are translated directly into proteins, some of which undergo post-translational cleavage to give functional molecules. After assembly, infectious virions are released as the cell disintegrates, some of them acquiring an envelope in the Golgi complex.
Laboratory identification	Characteristic poxvirus particles are seen on electron microscope examination of scrapings or biopsies of skin lesions. Neither cell culture methods for virus isolation nor antibody tests are routinely available.
Diseases	Molluscum contagiosum causes a mild infection with nodular skin lesions. Cowpox or milkers nodules virus lesions on cow udders can cause vesicular lesions on the skin of milkers. Orfvirus is responsible for contagious pustular dermatitis in sheep, and those in contact with infected animals (e.g. shepherds) may develop vesicular skin lesions. After exposure to monkeys infected with monkeypox virus (monkeys are a favourite food in some parts of the Ivory Coast), humans develop a smallpox-like disease, which is distinguishable from smallpox by laboratory tests.
Transmission	By direct contact with virus from skin lesions. Molluscum contagiosum is transmitted between humans, but monkeypox, cowpox, orf, and milkers nodules viruses are zoonoses, transmissible from the animal host to humans. Smallpox was eradicated in 1980.
Pathogenesis	Infection generally initiated in skin with local replication to form virus-rich vesicles, and limited spread to local lymph nodes. Smallpox, however, infected via respiratory tract, and spread via blood to cause severe disease with disseminated skin and mucosal lesions.
Treatment and prevention	In the past methisazone was used to treat the serious side effects very occasionally caused by vaccination against smallpox with live vaccinia virus. Vaccination was the principal method used to eradicate smallpox but is no longer necessary.

PICORNAVIRUSES

Characteristics						
	Virus Family	Type	Envelope	Shape	Size (nm)	Nucleocapsid
	Picornaviridae	ssDNA	−	Icosahedral	25–30	Icosahedral

Replication	Virus binds to cell via receptor molecule ICAM-1, resulting in endocytosis and uncoating. The positive sense viral ssRNA acts as mRNA which is translated into a single polyprotein, cleaved by virus-coded protease into separate proteins. These include the RNA polymerase that makes negative-strand cRNA, which in turn acts as template for positive strands of viral RNA. RNA and capsid proteins assemble in the cytoplasm to form nucleocapsids which are released on death of the cell. General features: four viral capsid proteins (VPI-VP4). There is no envelope.
Laboratory identification	Rhinoviruses cannot be routinely cultivated. Enteroviruses recoverable from throat, faeces, CSF etc. by cultivation in monkey kidney or human embryo lung cells, where they cause cytopathic effect and cell death. Significance of isolations needs thought because these viruses are ubiquitous in children. Tests for antibody not useful in view of multiple serotypes, but rise in titre to specific serotype (e.g. Coxsackievirus B in myocarditis) may be useful.

PICORNAVIRUSES (CONT.)

Diseases	Rhinoviruses: more than 100 serotypes; common cold viruses. Enteroviruses: polioviruses, types 1-3; aseptic meningitis, paralytic poliomyelitis. Echoviruses (enterocytopathic human orphans):32 types; aseptic meningitis, rashes. Coxsackieviruses: 29 types; aseptic meningitis, herpangina, myopericarditis (Coxsackievirus B). Enteroviruses 68-72: conjunctivitis (enterovirus 70), polio-like illness (enterovirus 71), hepatitis type A (enterovirus 72).
Transmission	Respiratory (droplet) spread for rhinoviruses and certain group A Coxsackieviruses. Other enteroviruses faecal–oral spread.
Pathogenesis	Rhinoviruses replicate in upper respiratory tract. Enteroviruses replicate in pharynx and gastrointestinal tract, often with spread to lymph nodes and blood, and then to CNS (polio, echoviruses etc.), heart and muscle (Coxsackie B), or liver (hepatitis A).
Treatment and prevention	No specific treatment. Poliomyelitis prevented by vaccination with live attenuated (Sabin) or killed (Salk) vaccine. Hepatitis A prevented by immunoglobulins or inactivated virus vaccine. No vaccines for other picornaviruses.

ORTHOMYXOVIRUSES (INFLUENZA VIRUSES)

Characteristics	Virus Family	Type	Envelope	Shape	Size (nm)	Nucleocapsid
	Orthomyxoviridae	ssDNA, linear 8 segments −ve sense	+	Spherical	80–120	Helical

	Envelope glycoproteins: haemagglutinin (H) attaches virus to sialic acid-containing receptor on cell; Neuraminidase (N) cleaves sialic acid from glycoproteins; involved in release of virus from cell surface.
Replication	Virus binds to cell via its H, enters a vesicle. its envelope fusing with vesicle wall. After uncoating, viral polymerase transcribes genome into 8 mRNAs which are translated in the cytoplasm. Progeny RNA is synthesized in nucleus and nucleocapsids assembled in cytoplasm. Viral matrix protein joins nucleocapsid to viral envelope components in the cell wall and maturation takes place by budding. Influenza A: widespread in birds, and in horses, pigs, humans. Genetic reassortments between animal and human strains produce subtypes with novel combinations of H and N genes, i.e. antigenic 'shift'; new strains can cause pandemics. Antigenic 'drift' also occurs, i.e. point mutations occur in HA to generate new strains. Influenza B: occurs only in humans; undergoes antigenic drift and can cause epidemics. Influenza C: of doubtful pathogenicity in humans.
Laboratory identification	Serology: CF tests with S (soluble) antigen, and H inhibition tests. Isolation of virus in monkey kidney cells. Detection of viral antigen by immunofluorescence.
Diseases	Incubation period 1-2 days. Fever, myalgia, malaise, nasal discharge, sore throat, cough, pneumonia.
Transmission	Via respiratory droplets.
Pathogenesis	Infection limited to respiratory tract. Cytokines contibute to symptoms and secondary bacterial infection quite common.
Treatment and prevention	Amantidine can be used (also in prophylaxis). A killed vaccine containing current A and B strains prevents disease in susceptible individuals (e.g. the elderly).

PARAMYXOVIRUSES (MEASLES, MUMPS ETC.)

Characteristics	Virus Family	Type	Envelope	Shape	Size (nm)	Nucleocapsid
	Paramyxoviridae	ssDNA non-segmented −ve sense	+	Pleomorphic	45–55	helical

	Envelope glycoproteins are H and N (often combined) and fusion protein, which can cause multinucleated giant cell formation.

PARAMYXOVIRUSES (CONT.)

Replication	Virus particle binds via its H to cell surface, penetrates and is uncoated. Viral polymerase transcribes genome into mRNAs which are translated into viral proteins. Nucleocapsid is assembled and matrix protein joins it to the envelope proteins forming on the plasma membrane of the infected cell. Release then occurs by budding.
Laboratory ientification	Serology of limited value for in parainfluenza, measles; CF tests for RSV, mumps. Demonstration of viral antigen by immunofluorescence in nasal aspirates (RSV, measles).
Diseases	Measles: fever, nasal discharge, rash (very rarely encephalitis, SSPE). Incubation period 10–14 days; Mumps: parotitis, aseptic meningitis (rarely orchitis, encephalitis). Incubation period 18–24 days; Parainfluenzaviruses: common cold, bronchiolitis, pneumonia. Incubation period 3–6 days. Respiratory syncytial virus: common cold (adults), bronchiolitis, pneumonia (infants). Incubation period 2–8 days.
Transmission	Respiratory droplets.
Pathogenesis	Initial infection via respiratory tract. RSV and parainfluenzavirus infections – local replication and disease. Measles and mumps – no lesions at site of initial infection, spread to local lymph nodes, blood and invasion of skin and mucosa (measles) or salivary glands, CNS etc. (mumps).
Treatment and prevention	Aerosolized ribavirin for infants with severe RSV infections. Nil available for other paramyxoviruses. Measles and mumps prevented by live attenuated virus vaccines. No vaccines in routine use for RSV and parainfluenzaviruses.

TOGAVIRUSES (RUBELLA, YELLOW FEVER ETC.)

Characteristics	Virus Family	Type	Envelope	Shape	Size (nm)	Nucleocapsid
	Togaviridae	ssDNA +sense	+	Spherical	60–70	Icosahedral

	Human togaviruses include rubella (genus rubivirus), and more than 80 serologically distinct arthropod-transmitted viruses. The latter occur in all parts of the world, often have exotic names (Kyasanur Forest disease virus, India; Omsk haemorrhagic fever virus, Russia), and replicate in the arthropod vector as well as in the vertebrate host. Most have animal reservoirs. The alphaviruses (WEE, EEE, Ross River) are distinguished from the flaviviruses (yellow fever, dengue, St Louis Encephalitis).
Replication	The plus strand RNA is translated into structural -and non structural proteins, the latter including the RNA-dependent RNA–polymerase which replicates the viral genome by directing the formation of a negative-strand template and thus giving rise to positive strand progeny. Full length and subgenomic length RNA is formed (full length only in flaviviruses*). After assembly the virus exits from the cell, budding from the plasma membrane (or endoplasmic reticulum in the case of flaviviruses*).
Laboratory diagnosis	Rubella can be isolated in cell culture and specific IgM antibody (H inhibition, ELISA) indicates recent infection. Serological methods and to a lesser extent virus isolation are used to diagnose the arthropod-borne togavirus infections.
Diseases	Rubella causes a mild exanthematous disease, in adults sometimes complicated by arthralgia, and in pregnant women by foetal infection, with congenital malformations. The remaining togaviruses cause febrile illnesses which may be severe when there is involvement of liver (yellow fever) or CNS (equine encephalitides), or when there are immunopathological complications (dengue haemorrhagic fever).
Transmission	Rubella is transmitted between humans by the respiratory droplets; the rest are transmitted by the bite of infected arthropods, but *not* directly from human to human.

*Flaviviruses are now placed in a separate group, but are included with togaviruses for convenience. Arboviruses include not only togaviruses but bunyaviruses (Californian encephalitis, Rift Valley fever) and reoviruses (Colorado tick fever).

TOGAVIRUSES (CONT.)	
Pathogenesis	Initial infection via respiratory tract (rubella) or skin (arthropod-borne viruses) causes no detectablelocal lesion.Virus spreads to local lymph nodes and blood, multiplying in respiratory tract,placenta and foetus (rubella), liver (yellow fever), or CNS (equine encephalitides). Mononuclear cells often infected (rubella, dengue). Immunopathology important in dengue haemorrhagic fever and probably in the equine encephalitides.
Treatment and prevention	There is no antiviral therapy. A live attenuated virus vaccine prevents rubella and congenital rubella, and a live attenuated (17D) vaccine is highly effective against yellow fever. Vaccines are not available for the other arthropod-transmitted togaviruses, but horses can be protected from WEE and EEE with veterinary vaccines.

RETROVIRUSES

Characteristics	Virus Family	Type	Envelope	Shape	Size (nm)	Nucleocapsid
	Retroviridae	ssDNA diploid +ve sense	+	Spherical	80–120	Icosahedral

Family includes: HIV1, HIV2 (lentiviruses); HTLV1, HTLV2 (oncoviruses); human foamy virus-causes foamy change in cells, but little else known; endogenous retroviruses exist as sequences in human genome.

Replication	HIV: binds to CD4 on cell surface, enters and is uncoated. Virion RNA-dependent DNA polymerase (reverse transcriptase) transcribes viral genome into dsDNA, which is then integrated into host cell DNA by viral integrase. Viral mRNA is transcribed by host RNA polymerase and translated into structural and regulatory proteins. Viral genes *gag, pol, env* code for structural proteins, and five other gene products have regulatory functions. Nucleocapsids assemble in cytoplasm and released by budding.
Laboratory identification	HIV: antibodies to envelope antigens gp120 (CD4-binding), gp41 (fusion protein), p24 (group-specific antigen in core) are tested by ELISA, latex agglutination, western blotting (similar tests for HTLV1 antibodies). p24 antigen may be detected in serum. Virus isolation in cultured T cells, but only in specialized laboratories.
Diseases	HIV: mild early illness with mononucleosis, sometimes aseptic meningitis; later: 1) AIDS-related complex (ARC), leading to AIDS, with multiple opportunistic infections, Kaposi's sarcoma; 2) HIV-specific CNS disease (AIDS neuropathy, AIDS-related dementia); 3) intestinal syndrome, with diarrhoea, weight loss ('slim' disease in Africa). HTLV1: tropical spastic paraparesis, T cell leukaemia. HTLV2: hairy cell leukaemia.
Transmission	HIV: via blood, semen, transplacental transfer. HIV1 world-wide, HIV2 mainly W Africa. HTLV1: via milk and blood; occurs in certain islands in Caribbean and Japan, and in parts of S America, Africa. HTLV2: via blood.
Pathogenesis	HIV: initial entry via mucosal route with infection of CD4-positive cells (helper T cells, dendritic cells,monocytes, macrophages). Spread through body including CNS, placenta. Action on immune cells results in severe immunosuppression leading to opportunist infections and reactivations (viral, bacterial, protozoal). Also Kaposi's sarcoma, possibly of separate infectious origin. HTLV1: pathogenesis of CNS disease not clear. Leukaemia (mean 30 years after infection) results from multistage process initiated by *tat* gene product in infected T cells stimulating transcription of host genes that control cell division.
Treatment and prevention	HIV: Azidothymidine (AZT) inhibits virus replication and arrests disease progress without eliminating virus from body (viral DNA transcripts remain in infected cells). Treatment of opportunist infections. Various vaccines are undergoing clinical trials. Prevention by avoiding blood-borne virus (needle exchange programmes, treatment of blood and blood products, etc.) and practising safe sex (education, condoms, etc.). HTLV1 and 2: AZT presumably effective.

RHABDOVIRUS (RABIES)

Characteristics	Virus Family	Type	Envelope	Shape	Size (nm)	Nucleocapsid
	Rhabdoviridae	ssDNA	+	Bullet shaped	180	Helical

Replication	Virus attaches to cell (via acetylcholine receptor or other molecules), is endocytosed and uncoated. Virion RNA polymerase synthesizes five mRNAs, and virus-coded RNA polymerase replicates viral RNA. After assembly of nucleocapsid the envelope is acquired by budding from the plasma membrane without detectable cell damage. Rabies virus can infect all mammals. Present in wild animals in all continents except Australia and Antarctica. Only one serotype.
Laboratory identification	Brain tissue (at autopsy), corneal scrapings, or biopsy of hair-bearing skin, examined for presence of inclusions (Negri bodies) or rabies antigen (by FA staining). Virus isolation is not necessary.
Diseases	Incubation period 2–10 weeks. CNS symptoms and signs (excitement, confusion, lethargy, hydrophobia progress to seizures, paralysis, coma and death.
Transmission	Via bite of infected dog, cat, skunk, raccoon, bat. Human to human transmission not a feature.
Pathogenesis	Virus replicates at site of bite, ascends axons to CNS where it spreads, and then descends peripheral nerves to skin, salivary glands.
Treatment and prevention	No specific treatment. Post-exposure prophylaxis by washing wound, giving human rabies-specific immune serum, and vaccine. Disease prevented by inactivated vaccine produced in human diploid cells.

ARENAVIRUSES (LCM, LASSA FEVER)

Characteristics	Virus Family	Type	Envelope	Shape	Size (nm)	Nucleocapsid
	Arenaviridae	ssDNA		Spherical	50–300	Helical

	Virions are pleomorphic, containing 2 segments of negative strand DNA and in addition host ribosomes, visible as granules inside the envelope; Latin *arena*, sand.
Replication	Viral RNA-dependant RNA polymerase produces plus strand RNA which is translated to form a nucleoprotein and two glycoproteins. Maturation by budding with no cytopathic effect on the cell
Laboratory identification	Detection of specific antibody (CF, ELISA, immunofluorescence tests) or virus isolation.
Diseases	Febrile illness, sometimes complicated by aseptic meningitis (LCM), or by severe haemorrhagic disease (Lassa fever, Argentinian and Bolivian haemorrhagic fevers).
Transmission	Cause inapparent persistent infections in the natural rodent host and spread to humans via contact with rodent excreta. Lymphocytic choriomeningitis (LCM) virus occurs world-wide, comes from mice and hamsters; Lassa fever virus in West Africa from the bush rat *Mastomys natalensis*; Junin and Machupo viruses from bush mice *(Calomys* sp.) in S America causing Argentinian and Bolivian haemorrhagic fevers.
Pathogenesis	Natural rodent host is infected *in utero* or neonatally, and virus (noncytopathic) remains in all tissues throughout life. In human host, virus spreads systemically causing meningitis or haemorrhagic disease by local or general replication plus immunopathology.
Treatment and prevention	Ribavirin may be useful in Lassaa fever and the S American haemorrhagic fevers. Vaccines for routine use are not available.

REOVIRUSES (COLORADO TICK FEVER, ROTAVIRUSES)

Characteristics	Virus Family	Type	Envelope	Shape	Size (nm)	Nucleocapsid
	Reoviridae	dsDNA	–	Icosahedral	75	Icosahedral (double layered)

Replication	Virus attaches to cells via receptor, enters phagocytic vacuole which fuses with lysosome; uncoating in lysosome.Viral RNA-dependent RNA polymerase (one molecule for each genome segment) synthesizes 10–11 mRNAs (not polyadenylated) which direct synthesis of proteins, one of which is an RNA polymerase. The latter produces negative-strand viral RNA; positive strands are formed, and the assembled virus is released by cell lysis.
Laboratory identification	Detection of antibody rise or of antiviral IgM (Colorado tick fever). Serology not useful for rotaviruses. Virus particles visible in stool by EM (rotaviruses). Detection of viral antigens by immunofluorescence (Colorado tick fever) or by ELISA, latex agglutination (rotaviruses). Virus isolation not generallly used.
Diseases	Orthoreovirus (3 types): few if any symptoms; the word reovirus derives from respiratory enteric orphan virus (orphan because initially not associated with any disease). Rotaviruses (types A-D): diarrhoeal illness, especially in infancy and childhood, and sometimes respiratory symptoms Colorado tick fever virus (orbivirus group): acute febrile illness .
Transmission	Orthoreoviruses: faecal-oral and possibly respiratory spread. Rotaviruses: faecal-oral spread (virus survives drying and stomach acid). Colorado tick fever virus: by bite of an infected tick.
Pathogenesis	Orthoreoviruses: entry via respiratory or gastrointestinal tract and spread to local lymphoid tissue. Rotaviruses: infection of enterocytes with no spread to deeper tissues; causes gastrointestinal illness (shortening of villi, interference with transport mechanisms). Colorado tick fever: virus enters skin via tick bite, spreads to local lymph nodes and blood, infects erythrocytes, and causes febrile illness.
Treatment and prevention	No antiviral agents and no vaccines routinely available. Rotavirus diarrhoea (prevented by improved hygiene) is treated by replacing water and electrolytes. Antitick measures protect against Colorado tick fever.

CORONAVIRUSES

Characteristics	Virus Family	Type	Envelope	Shape	Size (nm)	Nucleocapsid
	Coronaviridae	ssRNA +ve sense	+	Spherical (corona)	80–160	Helical

Replication	Viral RNA-dependent RNA polymerase uses genomic positive strand to produce negative-strand RNA, which acts as template for new positive strands. Nucleocapsids bud into endoplasmic reticulum from which they are released by exocytosis.
Laboratory identification	Antibody tests, EM examination (clubs, project from envelope and from 'Corona'), viral isolation (difficult) not routinely available and rarely necessary.
Diseases	Common cold type illness (possibily gastroenteritis).
Transmission	Respiratory droplets.
Pathogenesis	Replication in cells lining upper respiratory tract. Optimum growth temperature 33–35°C.
Treatment and prevention	No antivirals or vaccines are available.

SCRAPIE-TYPE AGENTS (SLOW VIRUSES)	
Characteristics	Probably not viruses. Structure and mode of replication unknown. Contain little or no nucleic acid. Host-coded prion protein, in slightly altered form (protease-resistant), is closely associated with infectivity. Highly resistant to heat (special autoclaving procedures required for destruction), chemical agents, and irradiation. Very slow replication, very long incubation period (up to 20 years in humans). Infect a variety of mammals and can be transmitted to cows, mink, cats, mice etc. when food contains infected material.
Laboratory identification	Intracellular vacuoles (spongiform change) visible histologically in brain. Altered prion protein detectable in brain but test not routinely available. Isolation of agent requires experimental animals, is lengthy, difficult and not undertaken. No specific immune (e.g. antibody) responses.
Diseases	'Spongiform encephalopathies', 'prion diseases'. Kuru: fatal neurological disease in Papua New Guinea; no longer seen. Creutzfeld-Jakob disease (CJD): rare, chronic encephalopathy, occurs world-wide; 10% cases familial, with mutated prion protein gene.
Transmission	Kuru: from infected human brain by cannibalism. CJD: in most cases unknown. Occasionally transmitted from infected human brain by medical and surgical procedures. Familial cases possibly genetically transmitted.
Pathogenesis	Infectious agent replicates inexorably in lymphoid tissues, and then in brain cells, where it produces intracellular vacuoles and deposition of altered host prion protein.
Treatment and prevention	No treatment or vaccine. Kuru died out when cannibalism ceased. Iatrogenic transfer of CJD preventable, e.g. when genetically engineered growth hormone became available.

BACTERIA

GRAM-POSITIVE COCCI

Genus *Staphylococcus*

Genus contains at least 15 different species, of which three are of medical importance:
Staphylococcus aureus
Staphylococcus epidermidis
Staphylococcus saprophyticus

Major distinguishing features of medically-important staphylococci

Test	*Staphylococcus*		
	aureus	*epidermidis*	*saprophyticus*
Coagulase production	+	−	−
Protein A on cell surface	+	−	−
Production of recognized exotoxins	+	−	−
Haemolysin production	+*	−*	−
Resistance to novobiocin	−	−	+

* usual result but not for all strains

Staphylococcus aureus

Characteristics	Gram-positive coccus; cells in clusters (reflecting ability to divide in more than one plane); individual cells approximately 1 μm in diameter. Some strains produce capsules. Non-fastidious; capable of aerobic and anaerobic respiration.
Laboratory identification	White or golden colonies on blood agar. Catalase positive, coagulase positive; most strains ferment mannitol anaerobically. Kits available for biochemical characterization.

Staphylococcus aureus (cont.)	
Diseases	Boils; skin sepsis; post-operative wound infection; scalded skin syndrome; catheter-associated infection; food-borne infection; septicaemia; endocarditis; toxic shock syndrome; osteomyelitis; pneumonia.
Transmission	Normal habitat: humans (and animals associated with them); skin, especially nose and perineum (carriage rates higher in hospital patients and staff). Spread is by contact and airborne routes. Organism survives drying; tolerant of salt and nitrites.
Epidemiological markers	Bacteriophage typing.

Pathogenesis	Virulence multifactorial; most factors shown below are present in some but not all strains. Present in all strains:
	Mucopeptide
	Coagulase
	
	Present in some strains:
	
	Cell-associated **Extracellular products**
	capsule enterotoxins
	protein A* epidermolytic toxin
	fibronectin-binding protein toxic shock syndrome toxin
	collagen-binding proteins membrane-damaging toxins (haemolysins)
	       leucocidin
	       staphylokinase
	
	* many strains have protein A bound to the mucopeptide of the cell wall. This protein interacts non-specifically with host IgG antibodies reducing opsonisation and causing local activation of complement

Treatment and prevention	Antibiotics of choice are beta-lactamase stable penicillins (> 80% hospital isolates beta-lactamase producers). Methicillin resistance is a local problem and vancomvcin is indicated. Mupirocin can be used for topical treatment of carriage. Prevention of spread by isolation and/or treatment of carriers in high risk areas in hospital. No vaccine available.

Staphylococcus epidermidis	
Characteristics	As for *Staph. aureus.*
Laboratory identification	White colonies on blood agar; Catalase positive, coagulase negative, mannitol not fermented anaerobically. Kits available for biochemical characterization.
Diseases	Opportunist pathogen associated with device-related sepsis, e.g. catheter-related sepsis; prosthetic valve endocarditis; infection of artificial joints; shunt infections; urinary tract infection; sternal wound osteomyelitis.
Transmission	Normal habitat: Skin (carriage rate approx. 100%). Spread by contact with self, other patients or hospital personnel. Infections almost all acquired in hospital but may be endogenous. Survives drying; salt tolerant.
Epidemiological markers	Bacteriophage typing.
Pathogenesis	Extracellular slime production thought to be marker of virulence and may account for ability to colonize plastic implants (e.g. intravenous catheters and prostheses).
Treatment and prevention	Antibiotic resistance: often multi-resistant (including penicillin and methicillin); susceptible to novobiocin (5µg); useful characteristic for distinguishing between *Staph. epidermidis* and *Staph. saprophyticus*. Prevention of infection: catheter care; no vaccine available.

Staphylococcus saprophyticus	
Characteristics	As for *Staph. aureus*.
Laboratory identification	White colonies on blood agar; catalase negative, coagulase negative, mannitol not fermented anaerobically. Kits available for biochemical characterization.
Diseases	Urinary tract infection in previously healthy women (associated with intercourse).
Transmission	Normal habitat: skin, and genitourinary mucosa. Endogenous spread to urinary tract in colonized women.
Epidemiological markers	None in common use.
Pathogenesis	Virulence factors unknown, but organism has the ability to colonize periurethral skin and mucosa.
Treatment and prevention	Resistant to nalidixic acid and to novobiocin (5μg); useful charactersitic for distingushing between *Staph. saprophyticus* and *Staph. epidermidis*. Urination after intercourse helps to wash organisms out of the bladder and prevent infection.

Genus *Streptococcus*

A large group of Gram-positive cocci distributed widely in man and animals, mostly forming part of the normal flora but some species responsible for some major infection problems. Individual cells 0.5-1 μm in diameter and, because they divide in one plane only, occur in pairs and chains. The medically significant streptococci may be conveniently divided either the basis of haemolysis on blood agar:

Complete haemolysis   Beta
Partial haemolysis   Alpha
No haemolysis   Gamma
or by presence or absence of a group specific carbohydrate antigen,i.e. the Lancefield Group labelled alphabetically A to S.

Beta-Haemolytic Streptococci

Streptococcus pyogenes (group A streptococci)	
Characteristics	Gram-positive cocci in chains, cells <1 μm diameter, non-motile, non-sporing.
Laboratory identification	Grow on blood agar. Pronounced haemolytic activity (enhanced anaerobically). Catalase negative. Bacitracin (0.04 units) used as an identifier, all strains are susceptible.
Lancefield grouping	Acid extraction of antigen from cell wall reacting with specific antisera (rabbit) either in a precipitin or latex agglutination reaction. In addition to this Group-specific polysaccharide, type-specific M and T antigens can be detected and are used as a typing scheme for epidemiologic purposes.
Diseases	Infections of upper respiratory tract and of skin and soft tissue e.g. pharyngitis, cellulitis, erysipelas, lymphadenitis. Toxic manifestations include scarlet fever. Non-suppurative sequelae (acute glomerulonephritis and rheumatic fever) important complications of both skin and throat infections.
Transmission	Normal habitat is the human upper respiratory tract and skin. Spread by airborne droplets and by contact. Survival in dust may be important. Epidemiological typing of strains (based on M and T proteins; see above) useful in outbreaks.
Pathogenesis	*Strep. pyogenes* elaborates many enzymes and exotoxins which may play a role in infection: erythrogenic toxin (lysogenic phage mediated); streptolysins; streptokinase A & B (therapeutic applications); deoxyribonuclease; hyaluronidase ('spreading factor').
Treatment and prevention	Penicillin is drug of choice. Erythromycin is an alternative for penicillin-allergic patients. Vaccines not available.

Streptococcus agalactiae (group B streptococci)	
Characteristics	Gram-positive cocci in chains.
Laboratory identification	Beta haemolytic on blood agar, colonies larger than Strep. pyogenes frequently pigmented after anaerobic incubation on Columbia agar (Islam's medium). Grow in the presence of bile on MacConkey agar. Biochemical tests include: hippurate hydrolysis (positive), aesculin hydrolysis (negative). Possesses Group B Lancefield capsular antigen.
Diseases	Neonatal meningitis and septicaemia. Mastitis in bovines.
Transmission	Normal habitat; gut and vagina. Babies acquire organism from colonized mother at birth or by contact spread between babies in nursery after birth.
Pathogenesis	Virulence factors not clearly identified.
Treatment and prevention	Susceptible to penicillin but less so than Strep. pyogenes; combination of penicillin and gentamicin for serious infections. Screening pregnant women not reliable but prophylactic antibiotics may be given to babies (especially premature) of carriers.

Other Beta-Haemolytic Streptococci of Medical Importance

Streptococci of Lancefield groups C and G may sometimes cause pharyngitis;
Group D streptococci now reclassified in the genus *Enterococcus* (see below)

Streptococcus milleri

A microaerophilic streptococcus which often forms small colonies and carries Lancefield Group F or G antigen.
Has a propensity for abscess formation (especially in liver and brain).

Alpha-Haemolytic Streptococci

Streptococcus pneumoniae

Characteristics	Gram-positive coccus characteristically appearing in pairs (diplococci) in Gram films. Cells approx. $1\mu m$, often capsulate. Requires blood or serum for growth. Capable of aerobic and anaerobic respiration; growth may be enhanced in CO_2.
Laboratory diagnosis	On blood agar alpha-haemolytic 'draughtsman' colonies that may autolyse within 48 hours at 35°C. Catalase negative. Susceptible to bile (bile solubility test) and optochin (ethyl hydrocuprein hydrochloride; available in paper discs). Polysaccharide capsules can be demonstrated by appropriate staining techniques. They are antigenic and in the presence of specific antiserum appear to swell (Quellung reaction).
Diseases	Pneumonia, septicaemia and meningitis. Otitis and related infections in children. Capsular type III frequently associated with pneumonia.
Transmission	Normal habitat is the human respiratory tract; up to 4% of population may carry in small numbers. Transmission via droplet spread.
Pathogenesis	Capsule protects the organism from phagocytosis. Pneumolysin may have a role as a virulence factor but to date no known exotoxins. Splenectomy appears to predispose to infection. Viral infection may be a precursor to pneumonia.
Treatment and prevention	Penicillin remains the antibiotic of choice but penicillin resistance has been noted in some countries. A vaccine is available (Pneumovax) composed of antigens of the most common serotypes; does not confer protection against other serotypes.

Oral Streptococci

There are several other species of alpha-haemolytic streptococci which in the past have been lumped together under the colloquial heading 'viridans streptococci'. These and some of the non-haemolytic streptococci have now been reclassified. Most species are commensals in the mouth. *Strep. mutans* is strongly associated with dental caries. Several species are capable of causing bacterial endocarditis. They are all susceptible to penicillin. It is important to distinguish these streptococci from *Strep. pneumoniae* in cultures from the respiratory tract.

Genus *Enterococcus* (Faecal Streptococci)

Formerly classified in the genus *Streptococcus* with which they share many characteristics; there are currently 15 species of which two, *E. faecalis* and *E. faecium* are of medical importance and are considered together.

Characteristics	Gram-positive cocci, cells often in pairs and chains; more ovate appearance than streptococci. Non-fastidious; capable of aerobic and anaerobic respiration.
Laboratory identification	On blood agar may produce alpha, beta or no haemolysis. Bile tolerant (grow on MacConkey agar and in 40% bile); relatively heat tolerant (grow at 45°C), and salt tolerant (grow in 6.5% NaCl). Hydrolyse aesculin and arginine. Kits available for complete biochemical identification. Carry Lancefield's Group D antigen but extraction of the antigen is more difficult than with streptococci (it is teichoic acid rather than polysaccharide).
Diseases	Urinary tract infection, endocarditis, infrequent but severe septicaemia after surgery and in the immunocompromised.
Transmission	Normal habitat is the gut of humans and animals. Most infections thought to be endogenously acquired but cross-infection may occur in hospitalized patients
Pathogenesis	No toxins or other virulence factors convincingly demonstrated. Plasmid-mediated haemolysin may play a role.
Treatment and prevention	Susceptible to penicillins but less so than streptococci. Penicillins used in combination with aminoglycosides for synergy in severe infections. Resistant to cephalosporins. Patients with known heart defects should be given prophylactic antibiotics to prevent endocarditis prior to dentistry or surgery on gut or urinary tract.

GRAM-POSITIVE RODS

Genus *Corynebacterium*

This genus contains many species, is widely distributed in nature and is part of a spectrum, with *Mycobacterium* and *Nocardia*, of similar cell wall structure containing mycolic acids. The species of major importance is *C. diphtheriae*. This and other pathogens within the genus need to be distinguished from commensal corynebacteria.

Corynebacterium diphtheriae

Characteristics	Gram-positive, non-capsulate, non-sporing, non-motile rods, 2–6 μm in length. In Gram-stained films cells arranged as 'Chinese letters' or pallisades and showing irregular staining or granule formation are characteristic. Non-fastidious, but growth enhanced by inspissated serum (Loefflers medium). Capable of aerobic and anaerobic respiration.
Laboratory diagnosis	Grows on blood agar but identification aided by a selective medium (e.g. blood tellurite) on which characteristic black colonies form within 48 hours at 35°C (but many other organisms may produce black colonies). Three biotypes of *C. diphtheriae* are recognized: *mitis*, *intermedius* and *gravis*, and they have characteristic colony morphology. *C. diphtheriae* is catalase positive and reduces nitrate. Species identification on the basis of carbohydrate fermentation tests should be performed in serum base *not* peptone. Toxin production is demonstrated by the Elek test. (Important to demonstrate toxigenicity to confirm a diagnosis of diphtheria because non-toxigenic strains may be carried as part of the normal skin or throat flora.)

Corynebacterium diphtheriae (cont.)	
Diseases	Diphtheria caused by toxigenic strains of *C. diphtheriae*. Focus of infection may be the throat or, increasingly commonly, the skin.
Transmission	Normal habitat: usually nasopharynx, occasionally skin of humans. Infection is usually spread by aerosol. Patients may carry toxigenic organisms for up to 2–3 months after infection.
Pathogenesis	Disease is due to production of diphtheria toxin controlled by the *tox* gene, which is integrated into the bacterial chromosome on a lysogenic phage. When concentration of exogenous inorganic iron (Fe^{3+}) is very low, toxin production is maximal; the selective advantage to the organism is unknown. The mode of action of the toxin is to block protein synthesis of the host cells by inactivating an elongation factor.
Treatment and prevention	Urgent supportive therapy to maintain airway essential in throat diphtheria. Antitoxin neutralizes toxin, penicillin kills organisms; antibiotics have little effect since diffusion of toxin not influenced by inhibition of organisms at local site. In outbreak, carriers treated with penicillin or erythromycin. Immunization effective in prevention of diphtheria; in areas where immunization rates reach 85%, herd immunity sufficient to protect whole population. Circulating antibody after immunization neutralizes test dose of standardized toxin (Schick test). Positive result equates with insufficient antibody. Babies acquire immunity from immune mothers for a few months.

Other *Corynebacteria*

C. ulcerans has been found in diphtheria-like disease. It produces two toxins, one of which is neutralized by diphtheria antitoxin, the other is similar to that produced by *C. pseudotuberculosis*. *C. jeikeium* is being isolated increasingly from blood cultures and wounds in immunosuppressed patients. It is usually detected by its relative resistance to all antibiotics other than vancomycin and teicoplanin. *C. pseudotuberculosis* is a significant pathogen of horses and sheep. *C. xerosis* and *C. pseudodiphtheriticum* are skin inhabitants and many other coryneforms may also be found on skin. These, and other related genera such as *Brevibacterium* and *Rhodococcus,* are lipophilic and require lipids for optimal growth.

Genus *Bacillus*

This genus contains nearly 50 species, most of which are soil organisms.
There are two species of major medical importance: *B. anthracis* and *B. cereus.*

Characteristics	Large (4-10 μm) Gram-positive, spore-forming, encapsulated rods. Spores are formed only after the organism is shed from the body. Respires aerobically.
Laboratory identification	In smears of body fluids the capsule can be stained with polychrome methylene blue (McFadyean reaction). This is diagnostic of *B. anthracis.* The species is non-fastidious; grows well on simple media. Characteristic colonies (Medusa head) are probably related to chaining of the long rods. Non-haemolytic on horse blood agar (many of the other species are haemolytic). Growth in CO_2 encourages the formation of the capsule and smooth colonies. Biochemical reactions are unhelpful except in expert hands.
Diseases	Anthrax is a significant disease in animals both domesticated and in the wild. It is a zoonosis and humans are usually infected by contact with infected hides or bones. Woolsorters disease i.e. respiratory or inhalation anthrax, is now rare. Intestinal anthrax is rare in humans but remains a possibility which attracts interest as an aspect of biological warfare.
Transmission	Soil organisms; *B. anthracis* can survive in competition with other organisms for many years depending on the temperature and humidity. The carcasses of animals dying with anthrax are buried 6 feet deep to prevent organisms being carried to the surface. Humans are accidental hosst and infection is usually acquired when spores enter abrasions on the skin or are inhaled.
Pathogenesis	The polyglutamic acid capsule is antiphagocytic. In addition an exotoxin encoded on a temperature-sensitive plasmid is produced. Toxin has three components: oedema factor, lethal factor and protective antigen. Individually the components have no biologic effect but toxicity is produced by either of the first two factors together with the antigen. The toxin acts locally in the skin and lung. Pasteur used heat attenuation to produce a virulent strainthat could be used as an attenuated vaccine.

Genus *Bacillus* (cont.)	
Treatment and prevention	Penicillin is the drug of choice. Prevention includes control measures such as formalin disinfection of hides, strict control of infected domestic animals and the immunization of veterinarians and laboratory workers at risk.

Bacillus cereus	
Characteristics	Large Gram-positive, spore-forming rod. This and many other *Bacillus* species are similar to *B. anthracis* in many respects except most are motile and non-capsulate. Respires aerobically.
Laboratory identification	Non-fastidious. Produces haemolysis on horse and sheep blood agar. Lecithinase production and inability to utilize mannitol are used as distinguishing features on a specially-designed selective medium.
Diseases	*B. cereus* causes food poisoning, the commonest association being with reheated cooked rice and pulses. Two different syndromes are recognized, due to different toxins (see below). The organism is also a rare cause of bacteraemia in immunocompromised hosts.
Transmission	*B. cereus* spores are found on many foods, especially rice, pulses and vegetables. Infection is acquired by ingestion of organisms or toxin.
Pathogenesis	Some strains produce heat-stable toxin in food which is associated with spore germination; gives rise to a syndrome of vomiting with 1–5 hours of ingestion. Others produce a heat-labile enterotoxin after ingestion which causes diarrhoea within 10-15 hours.
Treatment and prevention	The majority of illness is short-lived and self-limiting and antibiotic treatment is not indicated. Bacteraemia in immunocompromised patients should be treated promptly with penicillin or vancomycin. As with other food-borne infections, hygienic preparation of food is paramount. Cooked food should be stored in a refrigerator and re-heated thoroughly before serving.

Genus *Listeria*

These organisms were included with the genus *Corynebacterium* in earlier classifications. They share antigenic relationships also with enterococci and lactobacilli. *Listeria monocytogenes* is the species of major medical importance.

Characteristics	Short Gram-positive rods, often coccobacillary in clinical material (must avoid confusion with streptococci in chains); frequently gram variable. Motile at 25°C with a characteristic 'tumbling' movement; non-motile at 37°C.
Laboratory identification	Haemolytic on sheep or horse blood agar. Selective medium aids recovery of these organisms especially from food samples (fish, chicken and cheeses). Cold enrichment at +4°C for several weeks is also an effective selective technique. On translucent, non-blood containing agar colonies appear green–blue in oblique light. Catalase-positive, nitrate reduction negative; coupled with motility at room temperature these results are useful identifying features.
Diseases	Meningitis and sepsis in neonates. Infections in the immunocompromised (particularly meningitis) and in pregnant women.
Transmission	Widely distributed in nature, survives well in cold. Reaches food chain via silage as well as more directly via vegetables etc. Excreted in large numbers in cows' milk. Humans may carry *Listeria* in gut as normal flora. Infection may be acquired by ingestion or, transplacentally to the baby *in utero*. Serotyping has been used to investigate outbreaks but not practicable except for reference laboratories. Many serotypes exist, but 4b appears to be associated with outbreaks.
Pathogenesis	Virulence factors unknown but organism can survive in phagocytes.

Genus *Listeria* (cont.)	
Treatment and prevention	Treatment with penicillin or ampicillin, often in combination with gentamicin. Widespread distribution of organism in nature makes prevention of acquisition difficult. Pregnant women have been advised against eating uncooked food which is thought to be of particular risk (e.g. coleslaw, paté, soft cheese, unpasteurized milk).

Genus *Clostridium*
This genus contains many species of Gram-positive anaerobic spore-forming rods; a few are aerotolerant. Widely distributed in soil and in the gut of man and animals. The spores are resistant to environmental conditions. The major diseases associated with species of the genus are gangrene, tetanus, botulism, food poisoning and pseudomembranous colitis. In each of these the production of potent protein exotoxins is an important cause of pathology and in several species the toxins are carried by plasmids or bacteriophages.

Clostridium perfringens	
Characteristics	Anaerobic Gram-positive rods, spore-forming but spores rarely seen in infected material. More tolerant of oxygen than other clostridia.
Laboratory diagnosis	Haemolytic colonies on blood agar incubated anaerobically. Identification confirmed by demonstration of alpha-toxin (lecithinase) production in the Nagler test. Heat resistant spores may be responsible for food poisoning (see specimen processing section). Five types of *Cl. perfringens* (A–E) identified on the basis of toxins produced; type A strains can be further divided into several serotypes.
Diseases	Gas gangrene resulting from infection of dirty ischaemic wounds. Food poisoning following ingestion of food contaminated with enterotoxin-producing strains.
Transmission	Spores and vegetative organisms widespread in soil and normal flora of man and animals. Infection acquired by contact; may be endogenous, e.g. wound contaminated from patient's own faecal flora, or exogenous e.g. contamination of a wound with soil, ingestion of contaminated food.
Pathogenesis	In ischaemic wounds, production of various (at least 12) toxins and tissue-destroying enzymes allows organism to establish itself and multiply in wound. Local action of toxins produce necrosis thereby further impairing blood supply and keeping conditions anaerobic, and aiding spread of organism into adjacent tissues. Food poisoning results from the ingestion of large numbers of vegetative cells which sporulate in the gut and release enterotoxin.
Treatment and prevention	Gangrene requires rapid intervention with extensive debridement of the wound. Penicillin or metronidazole are the antibiotics of choice. Anti-alpha-toxin may be given. The role of hyperbaric oxygen treatment is debated. Food poisoning does not usually require specific treatment.

Clostridium tetani	
Characteristics	Gram-positive spore-forming rod with terminal round spore (drumstick). Strict anaerobe.
Laboratory identification	Grows on blood agar in anaerobic conditions as a fine spreading colony ; 'ground glass' appearance (hand lens inspection of all cultures essential). Has very little biochemical activity useful for identification purposes. Demonstration of toxin in a specimen is possible in a two-mouse model in which one animal is protected with antitoxin, the other unprotected. Injection of suspect material is via the root of the tail.
Diseases	Tetanus (lockjaw). Severe disease characterized by tonic muscle spasms and hyperflexia, trismus, opisthotonus and convulsions.
Transmission	Organism widespread in soil. Acquired by man by implantation of contaminated soil into wound. Wound may be major, e.g. in war, in road traffic accident, or minor, e.g. a rose thorn puncture while gardening. No person-to-person spread.

Clostridium tetani (cont.)	
Pathogenesis	Tetanus results from neurotoxin (tetanospasmin) produced by organisms in wound. Toxin genes are plasmid-encoded. The organism is non-invasive but the toxin spreads from site of infection via bloodstream and acts by binding to ganglioside receptors and inhibiting release of inhibitory neurotransmitter glycine. Causes convulsive contractions of voluntary muscles.
Treatment and prevention	Antitoxin is available (hyperimmune human gamma globulin). Penicillin and spasmolytic drugs indicated. Prevention readily available and effective in form of immunization with toxoid. Usually given in childhood but if immunization status of injured patient is unknown, toxoid is given in addition to antitoxin.

Clostridium botulinum	
Characteristics	Anaerobic Gram-positive rods. Not easily cultivated in competition with other organisms. Produces most potent toxins known to man. Eight immunologically-distinct toxins (A, B, Cα, Cβ, D, E and F) produced by different strains of *Cl. botulinum*. Three are most commonly associated with human disease: serotypes A and B associated with meat, E with fish.
Laboratory identification	Requires strictly anaerobic conditions for isolation. Grows on blood agar but very rarely isolated from human cases of disease. Detection of the toxin in the food or serum from the patient is the way of confirming the diagnosis.
Diseases	Major pathogen of birds and mammals but very rare in humans. Botulism acquired by ingesting preformed toxin. Disease entirely due to effects of toxin. Infant botulism results from ingestion of organisms and production of toxin in infant's gut. Associated with feeding honey contaminated with spores of *Cl. botulinum*. Extremely rare. Wound botulism: toxin produced by organisms infecting a wound. Extremely rare.
Transmission	Soil is the normal habitat. Intoxication most often by ingestion of toxin in foods that have not been adequately sterilized, e.g. home-preserved foods and improperly processed cans of food. Toxin is associated with germination of spores. There is no person-to-person spread.
Pathogenesis	Toxin released from organism as inactive protein and cleaved by proteases to uncover active site. It is acid-stable and survives passage through stomach. Taken up through stomach and intestinal mucosa into bloodstream. Acts at neuromuscular junctions inhibiting acetylcholine release. Results in muscle paralysis and death from respiratory failure.
Treatment and prevention	Supportive therapy is paramount. Antitoxin is available from reference centres. In the rare cases of infant and wound botulism, i.e. when the organism is growing *in vivo*, penicillin is effective. Prevention relates to good manufacturing practice. The toxin is not heat stable therefore adequate cooking of food before consumption will destroy it.

Clostridium difficile	
Characteristics	Slender Gram-positive anaerobic rod; spore-former; motile.
Laboratory identification	Difficult to isolate in ordinary culture because of overgrowth by other organisms, selective medium containing cefoxitin, cycloserine and fructose is effective. The mere presence of this organism is not indicative of infection, but a marker to note. Diagnosis by detection of toxin in faeces is practicable.
Diseases	Pseudomembranous colitis (antibiotic-associated diarrhoea). Can be rapidly fatal especially in the compromised host.
Transmission	Component of normal gut flora, flourishes under selective pressure of antibiotics. May also be spread from person-to-person by the faecal-oral route.
Pathogenesis	Toxin-mediated damage to gut wall. More than one toxin involved, at least one is a cytotoxin.
Treatment and prevention	Oral vancomycin or metronidazole. Other antibiotics should be withheld if possible. Prevention of cross-infection in hospitals depends on scrupulous attention to hygiene.

Genus *Mycobacterium*

Mycobacteria are widespread both in the environment and in animals. The major human pathogens are *Mycobacterium tuberculosis* and *M. leprae* but awareness of the importance of other species is increasing with their recognition as pathogens in AIDS patients.

Characteristics	Aerobic rods which have a Gram-positive cell wall structure but stain with difficulty because of the long-chain fatty acids (mycolic acids) in the cell wall. Acid fastness can be demonstrated by resistance to decolourization by mineral acid and alcohol (Ziehl-Neelsen stain). Mycobacteria grow more slowly than many other bacteria of medical importance, but the genus can be divided into: rapid growers (form visible colonies within 7 days); slow growers (form visible colonies only after 14 or more days incubation).
Laboratory identification	Staining and microscopic examination of specimens for acid-fast rods is important because of the time required for culture results. All species except *M. leprae* can be grown in artificial culture but they require complex media. Identification is based on rate of growth (rapid or slow), optimum temperature of growth and pigment production. Scotochromogens produce pigment in the absence of light whereas photochromogens require exposure to light before pigment becomes apparent. Further biochemical tests are required for full specification. DNA probes are being developed for identification purposes.
Diseases	*M. tuberculosis* causes tuberculosis in human and animals. *M. leprae* is a human pathogen and causes leprosy. Mycobacteria other than tuberculosis (MOTT) are associated with a range of conditions, usually in immunocompromised hosts. The *M. avium-intracellulare* complex has important associations with AIDS patients.
Transmission	Droplet spread aided by ability of organisms to survive in the environment (*M. tuberculosis*, *M. leprae*). Leprosy requires close and prolonged contact for spread. Milk-borne spread to humans from infected cattle has been important in the past. Social and environmental factors and genetic predisposition all have a role.
Pathogenesis	Both *M. tuberculosis* and *M. leprae* are intracellular parasites surviving within neutrophils. They give rise to slowly developing, chronic conditions in which much of the pathology is attributable to host immune responsiveness rather than to direct bacterial toxicity.
Treatment and prevention	Prolonged treatment with combinations of anti-mycobacterial drugs is required. BCG vaccination is valuable for prevention (in people who are not environmentally exposed to heavy loads of mycobacteria early in life). Isoniazid prophylaxis used for contacts of cases of tuberculosis. Pasteurization of milk and improvement of living conditions have played a major role in prevention.

Genus *Actinomyces*

The Actinomycetes are true bacteria, although they have in the past been considered to resemble fungi because they form branching filaments. They are related to the corynebacteria and mycobacteria in the chemical structure of their cell walls and some are acid-fast. It is important to differentiate them from fungi because infections with actinomycetes should respond to antibacterial agents whereas similar clinical presentations caused by fungi are extremely refractory to treatment by antifungal agents. This genus contains many species, some of which are important to man as producers of antimicrobial agents. A few are pathogenic to man and animals; *A. israelii* causes actinomycosis.

Actinomyces israelii

Characteristics	Gram-positive, anaerobic, filamentous branching rods. Non-sporing non-acid fast.

Actinomyces israelii (cont.)	
Laboratory identification	Forms 'sulphur granules' composed of a mass of bacterial filaments in pus. These can be identified by washing pus, squashing granules and observing in stained microscopic preparations. Gram-positive branching rods also visible in stained pus. Forms characteristic breadcrumb or 'molar tooth' colonies on blood agar after 3-7 days anaerobic incubation at 35°C.
Diseases	Actinomycosis follows local trauma and invasion from normal flora. Hard non-tender swellings develop which drain pus through sinus tracts. Cervicofacial lesions are most common, but abdominal lesions after surgery and infection related to intrauterine contraceptive devices (IUDs) occur.
Transmission	*A. israelii* forms part of normal flora in mouth, gut and vagina. Infection is endogenous. There is no person-to-person spread.
Pathogenesis	Virulence factors not described.
Treatment and prevention	Penicillin is the drug of choice. Prolonged treatment is required, accompanied by surgical drainage.

Genus *Nocardia*

Characteristics	Aerobic Gram-positive rods which form thin, branching filaments. Widespread in the environment. *Nocardia asteroides* is the important human pathogen, although other species can cause infection.
Laboratory diagnosis	Gram stains of pus may reveal Gram-positive filaments or rods. Sulphur granules not seen. Grow as 'breadcrumb' colonies on blood agar within 2-10 days incubation. Often acid-fast.
Diseases	*N. asteroides* is an opportunist pathogen infecting immunocompromised patients; primarily a pulmonary infection but secondary spread to form abscesses in brain or kidney is common. *N. brasiliensis* is the cause of actinomycetoma in Central and South America.
Transmission	Infection is acquired from the soil by the airborne route. Outbreaks of infection in renal transplant units have been associated with local building work. Actinomycetoma is acquired by implantation of organisms into wounds and progressive destruction of skin, fascia, bone and muscle
Pathogenesis	Appears to be related to organism's ability to survive the host's inflammatory responses Infection is controlled by cell-mediated immunity but this may be defective in immunocompromised patients.
Treatment and prevention	Nocardiosis is often difficult to treat but most regimens include sulphonamides as the drug of choice.

ENTEROBACTERIACEAE

Most numerous facultative anaerobes in the human gut, comprising approx. 10^9 per g of faeces. Outnumbered only by Gram-negative anaerobes (e.g. *Bacteroides*) which are present in numbers approx. 10x Enterobacteria.
Genera of the family Enterobacteriaceae share features which distinguish them from other families; can be distinguished from each other by biochemical tests.

Genus *Escherichia*

Genus contains only one species of medical importance: *Escherichia coli*.

Escherichia coli	
Characteristics	Gram-negative rod; motile; +/- capsule. Non-fastidious, facultative anaerobe; bile tolerant; capable of growth at 44°C.

Escherichia coli (cont.)	
Laboratory identification	Grows readily on routine laboratory media and on bile-containing selective media. Lactose fermenter. Kits available for full identification.
Diseases	Urinary tract infection; diarrhoeal diseases; neonatal meningitis; septicaemia.
Transmission	Normal habitat is gut of man and animals, may colonize lower end of urethra and vagina. Spread is by contact and ingestion (faecal–oral route); may be food-associated; may be endogenous. Possesses O (somatic), H (flagellar), K (capsular) and F (fimbrial) antigens which can be used to characterize strains by serotyping. Colicin (bacteriocin) typing also available.
Pathogenesis	A variety of virulence factors have been identified particularly in strains associated with diarrhoeal disease: (a) Endotoxin: present in all strains; (b) Adhesins: p fimbriae associated with urinary tract infection; colonization factors (e.g. CFA I and II, K 88, K 99) associated with gastrointestinal tract infection in humans and animals; (c) Capsule present in some strains; may be associated with adhesion. K1 capsular type associated with neonatal meningitis; (d) Enterotoxins associated with diarrhoeal disease: ETEC (enterotoxigenic *E. coli*) produce cholera-like heat-labile (LT) toxin; EIEC (enteroinvasive *E. coli*) produce shiga-like cytotoxin; EHEC (enterhaemorrhagic *E. coli*) produce verotoxin; associated with haemolytic uraemic syndrome.
Treatment and prevention	Wide range of antibacterial agents potentially available but incidence of resistance variable, often plasmid-mediated; must be determined by susceptibility testing. Specific treatment of diarrhoeal disease usually not required. No vaccine available currently.

Genus *Proteus*

Genus contains several species of which two are of medical importance: *Proteus mirabilis* and *Proteus vulgaris*.

Characteristics	Gram-negative rod; non-fastidious; facultative anaerobe; bile tolerant; likes alkaline pH; characteristic unpleasant odour; highly motile and swarms on some media.
Laboratory identification	Lactose non-fermenter; produces urease ; kits available for full identification. Species can be distinguished by indole test; *Pr. mirabilis*, indole -ve; *Pr. vulgaris*, indole +ve. O (somatic) and H (flagellar) antigens characterized. *Pr. vulgaris* strains OX-19, OX-2 and OX-K share antigens with Rickettsia in the typhus and spotted fever groups and are agglutinated by antibodies produced by patients with these rickettsial infections (Weil-Felix test). Serological response to *Proteus* infection not useful diagnostically.
Diseases	Urinary tract infection; hospital-acquired wound infection, septicaemia, pneumonia in the compromised host.
Transmission	Normal habitat is human gut, soil and water. Contact spread; infection often endogenous.
Pathogenesis	Characterized virulence factors include endotoxin, urease; possible role for bacteriocins.
Treatment and prevention	Range of agents available but *Pr. vulgaris* usually more resistant to antibacterials than *Pr. mirabilis*. Prevention is by good aseptic technique in hospitals. No vaccine available.

Genus *Klebsiella* and Related Enterobacteria *Serratia* and *Enterobacter*

Unlike *Escherichia coli*, species of the genera *Klebsiella*, *Serratia* and *Enterobacter* are rarely associated with infection except as opportunists in compromised patients.

Characteristics	Gram-negative rods, sometimes capsulate (usual in *Klebsiella*), non-fastidious growth requirements. Capable of aerobic and anaerobic respiration.
Laboratory identification	Lactose-fermenting, bile-tolerant organisms. Grow readily on routine laboratory media. Oxidase negative. Full identification based on biochemical reactions (commercial kits available).

Genus *Klebsiella* (cont.)	
Diseases	Opportunist infections in the compromised (usually hospitalized) host. Urinary and respiratory tracts most common sites of infection. Distinction between colonization and infection can be difficult.
Transmission	Normal habitat is gut of man and animals and moist inanimate environments, especially soil and water. Infection may be endogenous or acquired by contact spread. Klebsiella have remarkable capacity for survival on hands. Various methods of epidemiological fingerprinting available for investigation of outbreaks of hospital-acquired infection.
Pathogenesis	All possess endotoxin and fimbriae or other adhesins. Capsules, where present, are important in inhibiting phagocytosis.
Treatment and prevention	Multiple antibiotic resistance, usually plasmid-mediated, is common and susceptibility must be determined by laboratory tests if treatment is indicated. Prevention depends on scrupulous attention to aseptic techniques and to handwashing in hospitals.

Salmonella and *Shigella*

Unlike other members of the Enterobacteriaceae, *Salmonella* and *Shigella* are not normal inhabitants of the human gut (except in post-infection carriers). Both genera are responsible for diarrhoeal disease which may be severe; Salmonella typhi is also invasive and gives rise to systemic infection.

Genus *Salmonella*

Has been classified into >2000 species on basis of serological differences; more recent studies suggest such divisions are below the level of species and that three, or fewer, species exist. Distinction on basis of infection is between *S. typhi* (also *S. paratyphi* A and B) which cause enteric fevers and *S. enteritidis* (many other serotypes) which cause diarrhoeal disease.

Characteristics	Gram-negative, motile, non-sporing rods. All except S. typhi are non-capsulate. Capable of aerobic and anaerobic respiration.
Laboratory identification	Bile tolerant. Non-fastidious. Oxidase negative. Lactose non-fermenters. Produce acid and gas from glucose (except *S. typhi* which is anaerogenic). Combination of biochemistry (commercial kits available) and serotyping required for full identification; important to distinguish enteric fever salmonellae from others. Detection of circulating antibody (Widal test) may aid diagnosis of enteric fevers. Serotyping (and phage typing of most important serotypes) useful for investigation of outbreaks.
Diseases	Vast majority cause diarrhoeal disease; very occasionally invasive (particularly *S. cholerae-suis*). Sickle cell disease predisposes to osteomyelitis. *S. typhi* and *S. paratyphi* cause systemic disease, typhoid and paratyphoid (enteric fevers).
Transmission	Widespread in animals; encountered in food chain (especially in poultry, eggs, meat, milk and cream). Acquired by ingestion of contaminated food or person-to-person via faecal-oral route. *S. typhi* human pathogen only. Spread via faecal–oral route, usually via contaminated water or food. Carriers are important source of organisms.

Salmonella taxonomy

Kauffmann-White classification recognizes each serologically distinct salmonella (of which there are >2000) as a species. These are then arranged in groups. Ewing classification restricts genus to 3 species only. Further serologic distinctions recognized as sub-types. Recently proposed that genus contains only a single species, *Salmonella enterica*, within which 6 subgroups can be distinguished. Future DNA hybridization studies may reveal yet different groups.

Kauffmann-White classification:

Group	Name	Somatic (O) antigen	Flagella (H) antigen	
			Phase I	Phase II
A	*S. paratyphi* A	1, 2, 12	a	—
B	*S. paratyphi* B	1, 4, 5, 12	b	1, 2
	S. typhimurium	1, 4, 5, 12	i	1, 2
C1	*S. paratyphi* C	6, 7, Vi	c	1, 5
	S. cholerae-suis	6, 7	c	1, 5
	S. virchow	6, 7	r	1, 2
D	*S. typhi*	9, 12, Vi	d	—
	S. enteritidis	1, 9, 12	g,m	—

Ewing classification:

Three species:

Salmonella cholerae-suis (one serotype)

Salmonella typhi (one serotype)

Salmonella enteritidis (>2000 serotypes).

Genus *Shigella*

Contains four species of importance to man as causes of bacillary dysentery: *Shigella dysenteriae*, *Sh. boydii*, *Sh. flexneri* and *Sh. sonnei* (in descending order of severity of symptoms).

Characteristics	Gram-negative rods. Non-motile (in contrast to salmonellae). Non-capsulate. Capable of aerobic and anaerobic respiration.
Laboratory identification	Non-fastidious, bile-tolerant. Lactose non-fermenters. Full identification requires use of biochemistry (commercial kits available) and serological tests for O antigens. Serodiagnosis not applicable.
Diseases	Bacillary dysentery. Very rarely invasive.
Transmission	Human pathogens spread by faecal–oral route, especially in crowded conditions. Small infective dose.
Pathogenesis	Invasion of ileum and colon causes damage which results in diarrhoea. Intense inflammatory response involving PMNs and macrophages characteristic. Enterotoxins have not been identified but *Sh. dysenteriae* produces a neurotoxin.
Treatment and prevention	Antibiotic therapy should be avoided if possible; usually not required and many strains carry multiple antibiotic resistances, usually on plasmids. Prevention depends on interrupting faecal–oral spread; hand hygiene important. No vaccine available.

Genus *Pseudomonas*

This genus contains a large number of species, a few of which are human pathogens, some are animal pathogens and others are important pathogens of plants. Species also widely distributed in the environment and may contaminate the hospital environment and cause opportunist infections. Most important species in humans are *P. aeruginosa*, important opportunist in compromised patients, and *P. mallei*, cause of melioidosis, a disease of restricted geographical distribution.

Pseudomonas aeruginosa

Characteristics	Aerobic Gram-negative rod, motile by means of polar flagella. Able to utilize a very wide range of carbon and energy sources and to grow over a wide temperature range. Does not grow anaerobically (except when nitrate is provided as a terminal electron acceptor).

Pseudomonas aeruginosa (cont.)	
Laboratory identification	Grows readily on routine media including bile-containing selective media. Produces irregular irridescent colonies and a characteristic smell. Most strains produce a blue–green pigment (pyocyanin; unique to *P. aeruginosa*) and a yellow–green pigment (pyoverdin). Pigment production is enhanced on special media (King's A and B). Oxidase positive and oxidative in the Hugh and Liefson O/F test.
Diseases	*P. aeruginosa* is an opportunist pathogen which can infect almost any body site given the right predisposing conditions. It causes infections of skin and burns, it is a major lung pathogen in cystic fibrosis patients and can cause pneumonia in intubated patients. It can also cause urinary tract infections, septicaemia, osteomyelitis and endocarditis.
Transmission	Carriage as part of the normal gut flora occurs in a small percentage of normal healthy people and in a higher proportion of hospital inpatients. Thus endogenous infection may occur in compromised patients. *P. aeruqinosa* is widespread in moist areas in the environment; patients usually become infected by contact spread, directly or indirectly, from these environmental sites.
Pathogenesis	A number of virulence factors have been identified, including endotoxin, and exotoxin A which acts as an inhibitor of elongation factor in eucaryotic protein synthesis. Extracellular proteases and elastases contribute to destruction of tissue at sites of infection; extracellular slime (particularly massive amount of alginate produced by strains specifically in cystic fibrosis patients) helps to prevent phagocytosis. Pigments may have a role in pathogenicity and pyoverdin acts as a siderophore.
Treatment and prevention	Resistant to antibacterial agents, *P. aeruginosa* susceptible only to aminoglycosides and newer beta-lactams (carbenicillin and acylureidopenicillins; third generation cephalosporins and imipenem). Strains within the species may also acquire resistance to these agents. Immunotherapy with anti-endotoxin monoclonal antibodies may have a role in the future in severe infections. Prevention depends on good aseptic practice in hospitals. Avoidance of unnecessary or prolonged broad-spectrum antibiotic treatment and prophylaxis. Experimental vaccines have been tested in burned patients but have doubtful usefulness

CURVED GRAM-NEGATIVE RODS

There are several genera of curved Gram-negative rods that contain species that occur in humans as pathogens or as part of the normal flora:

Vibrio	aerobic	Campylobacter ⎤	microaerophilic
Wolinella ⎤		Helicobacter ⎦	
Anaerobiospirillum ⎦	anaerobic		

Aerobes and microaerophiles cause infection of gastrointestinal tract; anaerobic curved rods form part of normal flora of mouth and vagina. Role in endogenous infection unclear; unusual growth requirements (for formate and fumarate) means they often fail to grow in routine culture conditions.

Genus *Vibrio*	
Most important species, *Vibrio cholerae*, causes cholera. *V. parahaemolyticus* also causes diarrhoeal disease.	
Characteristics	Curved Gram-negative rods, highly motile by means of single polar flagellum. Capable of aerobic and anaerobic respiration. Many species salt (NaCl) tolerant; some salt-requiring.
Laboratory identification	Grow in alkaline conditions (can be selected from other gut flora in alkaline peptone water). Oxidase positive. Grow on thiosulphate citrate bile salt sucrose (TCBS) medium to form yellow colonies (*V. cholerae*) or green colonies (other species). *V. cholerae* susceptible to 0129 (vibriostatic agent), *V. parahaemolyticus* usually resistant. Biochemical tests and use of specific antisera required for complete identification.

Genus Vibrio (cont.)	
Diseases	Cholera caused by *V. cholerae*. *V. parahaemolyticus* causes diarrhoeal disease. Other species (e.g. *V. vulnificus, V. alginolyticus*) may cause wound infections.
Transmission	*V. cholerae* is a human pathogen; no animal reservoir, but El Tor biotype survives better in the inanimate environment than classical V. cholerae. Infection is acquired from contaminated water (usually) or food (sometimes). *V. parahaemolyticus* infection acquired from consumption of contaminated fish and seafood.
Pathogenesis	*V. cholerae* possesses several virulence factors (e.g. motility, mucinase, adhesins, and most importantly, enterotoxin). Chromosomally encoded subunit toxin, produced after cells bind to enterocytes, enters cells and binds to ganglioside receptors, activating adenylyl cyclase and causing fluid loss resulting in massive watery diarrhoea. *V. parahaemolyticus* produces a cytotoxin (which also haemolyses human RBC – the Kanagawa test).
Treatment and prevention	For cholera, fluid replacement (oral rehydration therapy, ORT) of prime importance. Tetracycline shortens symptoms and duration of carriage. Specific treatment not indicated for *V. parahaemolyticus* diarrhoea. Prevention of cholera depends on provision of a clean (chlorinated) water supply and adequate sewage disposal. A whole cell vaccine is available but of limited use (new vaccines are under development). *V. parahaem*olyticus infection can be prevented by adequate cooking of seafood.

Genus *Campylobacter*

Curved Gram-negative rods, once classified as vibrios. More recently *Campylobacter pylori*, organism associated with gastritis and duodenal ulcers, has been moved into a new genus as *Helicobacter pylori*. Campylobacters are primarily pathogens of animals but several species also cause infections in man. The most important is *C. jejuni*.

Campylobacter jejuni	
Characteristics	Slender curved (seagull-shaped) Gram-negative rods. Motile by means of a polar flagellum at one or both ends. Microaerophiles. Do not utilize carbohydrates.
Laboratory identification	Require enriched media and moist microaerophilic environment (10% O_2) for growth. Incubation at 42° C for 24-48 hr. Colonies resemble water drops. Full identification by biochemical tests and antibiotic susceptibility pattern.
Diseases	Diarrhoea. Can invade to give septicaemia.
Transmission	Animal reservoir. Organisms acquired from contaminated food and milk (but do not multiply in these vehicles). Person-to-person spread rare.
Pathogenesis	Little known but cytotoxin implicated. Also invasion and local destruction of gut mucosa.
Treatment and prevention	No specific treatment necessary for diarrhoea. Erythromycin for invasive disease. Prevention depends on good food hygiene. No vaccine.

GRAM-NEGATIVE NON-SPORING ANAEROBES

Historically, all short Gram-negative anaerobic rods or cocco-bacilli have been classified in the genus *Bacteroides* and longer rods with tapering ends in the genus *Fusobacterium*. Recent applications of new techniques to the *Bacteroides* have resulted in the definition of two additional genera: *Porphyromonas* and *Prevotella*. The genus *Bacteroides* now restricted to species found among the normal gut flora. *Prevotella* contains saccharolytic oral and genitourinary species, including *Pr. melaninocenica* (formerly *Bacteroides melaninogenicus)* which produces a characteristic black–brown pigment. The genus *Porphyromonas* contains assacharolytic pigmented species which form part of the normal mouth flora (*P. gingivalis*) and may be involved in endogenous infection within the oral cavity. Most important non-sporing anaerobe causing infection is *Bacteroides fragilis* (although others are much more common e.g. in gingivitis and other endogenous oral infections).

Bacteroides fragilis	
Characteristics	Small pleomorphic Gram-negative rod. Capable only of anaerobic respiration. Non-spore forming, non-motile.
Laboratory identification	Grows on blood agar incubated anaerobically and in other media designed for isolation of anaerobes. Plates may require up to 48hrs. Incubation at 35°C for colonies to become visible. Cultures have a foul odour due to the fatty acid end-products of metabolism. These can be used as identifying characteristics by analysis of culture supernates by gas–liquid chromatography (GLC). The major products of *Bacteroides* are acetate and succinate. Full identification in the diagnostic laboratory is based on biochemical tests and antibiogram. Commercial kits are available.
Diseases	Intra-abdominal sepsis, liver abscesses, aspiration pneumonia, brain abscesses, wound infections. Infections often mixed with aeobic and microaerophilic bacteria.
Transmission	Endogenous infection arising from contamination by gut contents or faeces is most common route of acquisition.
Pathogenesis	Little is known about the virulence factors of *B. fragilis*. A polysaccharide capsule and production of extracellular enzymes are probably important features. An anaerobic environment is essential and in mixed infections, growth of aerobic organisms probably helps the growth of *Bacteroides* by using up available oxygen.
Treatment and prevention	Metronidazole well-established as the drug of choice for *Bacteroides* infections in UK, but only recently licensed for this indication in USA. Many strains produce beta-lactamases and thus susceptibility to penicillin and ampicillin in unreliable. Augmentin or cefoxitin are beta-lactams in common use. Chloramphenicol used for treatment of abscesses as it penetrates very well. Prevention of endogenous infection difficult; good surgical technique and appropriate use of prophylactic antibiotics important in abdominal surgery.

Genus *Neisseria*	
The genus contains several more or less fastidious species of which two, *Neisseria gonorrhoeae* and *N. meningitidis* are important human pathogens.	
Characteristics	Non-motile Gram-negative diplococci with fastidious growth requirements, capnophilic. *N. meningitidis* is capsulate, *N. gonorrhoeae* is not.
Laboratory identification	Gram stains of pus or CSF may reveal Gram-negative kidney-shaped diplococci, often intracellular (in polymorphs). Require supplemented media for growth (chocolate agar). *N. gonorrhoeae* easier to isolate on enriched media containing antibiotics to inhibit otherorganisms of normal flora from sample sites. The two species are differentiated by sugar utilization pattern.
Diseases	*N. gonorrhoeae* : gonorrhoea, and pelvic inflammatory disease and salpingitis in females; ophthalmia neonatorum in infants born to infected mothers. *N. meningitidis* : meningitis (occasionally septicaemia in absence of meningitis).
Transmission	Human pathogens; no animal reservoir. *N. gonorrhoeae* may be carried in genital tract, nasopharynx and anus. Spread by sexual or intimate contact. *N. meningitidis* carried in pharynx. Carriage rate in population increases during epidemics. Droplet spread. Several immunologically distinct capsular types (A,B,C,).
Pathogenesis	Several virulence factors have been identified: In *N. gonorrhoeae* pili or fimbriae acts as adhesins; endotoxin; outer membrane proteins, protease production, resistance to lytic activity of serum, IgA proteases. In *N. meningitidis* the polysaccharide capsule is antiphagocytic; endotoxin and IgA protease also implicated.

Genus *Neisseria* (cont.)	
Treatment and prevention	*N. gonorrhoeae*: resistance to first line drugs now widespread; usual choice is beta-lactamase stable cephalosporin. Spectinomycin for beta-lactam resistant strains. *N. meningitidis*: Penicillin or cefotaxime (or equivalent cephalosporin). Can be combined with chloramphenicol. Prevention of gonorrhoea requires education, contact tracing. No vaccine available. Rifampicin is used for prophylaxis of close contacts of *N. meningitidis* meningitis. Vaccine is available for type A and C but ineffective in preventing infection with type B strains.

Genus *Branhamella (Moraxella)*
Branhamella catarrhalis, now reclassified by some into the genus *Moraxella*, is a Gram-negative coccus morphologically similar to *Neisseria* but with less fastidious growth requirements. Formerly regarded as a commensal in the respiratory tract, it has been associated with severe infections including endocarditis. The majority of strains produce β-lactamase and may be involved in the 'protection' of more obvious pathogens, especially in the respiratory tract, by destroying penicillin or ampicillin administered as treatment.

Genus *Haemophilus*
The genus contains many species; *H. influenzae* and *H. ducreyi* are of medical importance.

Haemophilus influenzae	
Characteristics	Small Gram-negative rods, frequently coccobacillary. Non-motile. Fastidious, capnophilic, facultative anaerobe. May be capsulate when isolated from site of infection.
Laboratory identification	Requires both haematin (TX factor) and NADP (V factor) for growth (other species require one factor only). Grows on blood containing enriched media. Larger colonies around colonies of other organisms that secrete V factor e.g. *Staph. aureus* (satellitism). Dependence on X and V used as indicator of identity. *H. influenzae* can also be distinguished from other species by its inability to produce porphyrin. Six antigenically distinct capsular types recognized (a–f) of which type b is most frequently found in disease. Capsulate organisms can be agglutinated by specific antisera and detected (by e.g. latex agglutination) directly in specimens.
Diseases	Capsular type b *H. influenzae* causes meningitis, osteomyelitis, epiglottitis, otitis. All are more common in children than older age groups. Non-capsulate strains associated with acute exacerbations of chronic bronchitis.
Transmission	Normal habitat is upper respiratory tract in humans and associated animals. Transmitted from person to person by airborne route. Osteomyelitis probably follows septicaemia from respiratory focus.
Pathogenesis	Polysaccharide capsule is important virulence factor. Outer membrane proteins and endotoxin may play a part but no known exotoxin.
Treatment and prevention	Ampicillin (or amoxycillin) if non-beta-lactamase producing strain. Third-generation cephalosporin (e.g. Cefotaxime, ceftriaxone or cefixime) or chloramphenicol are usual alternatives. Hib vaccine now being introduced for all children in USA and UK. Rifampicin prophylaxis recommended for close contacts of haemophilus meningitis.

Haemophilus ducreyi
Cause of the genital tract infection 'soft chancre'. Slender Gram-negative rods appearing in pairs or chains. Direct microscopical examination of smear from chancre can be diagnostic. Organism very susceptible to dehydration; inoculate plates in clinic. Requires enriched medium (as for *H. influenzae* but with addition of antibiotics to inhibit growth of other genital tract organisms).

Genus *Bordetella*
There are three species of which one *B. pertussis* is of medical importance.

Bordetella pertussis	
Characteristics	Small Gram-negative rod. Slow growing and fastidious in its growth requirements.
Laboratory identification	Requires enriched medium, e.g. Bordet-Gengou or blood charcoal agar. Intolerant of fatty acids in medium. Fails to grow on routine blood agar (i.e. 5–7% blood). Requires 3–5 days incubation in moist atmosphere. Irridescent bisected pearl colony type characteristic on Bordet–Gengou. Further identification by reaction with specific antisera.
Diseases	Whooping cough (pertussis).
Transmission	Human pathogen spread by airborne route from cases of disease (healthy carriage not documented).
Pathogenesis	Tracheal cytotoxin, fimbrial antigen and endotoxin all implicated as virulence factors. Stimulates a lymphocytic response.
Treatment and prevention	Erythromycin is the drug of choice for cases and close contacts of whooping cough. Antibacterial therapy has little effect on clinical course but may reduce infectivity and incidence of superinfection. Whole-cell inactivated vaccine administered to young children in three doses together with diphtheria and tetanus toxoids. New subunit vaccines currently undergoing trials.

Genus *Brucella*	
There are several species of the genus *Brucella*, each characteristically associated with an animal species. Three species: *B. abortus* from cattle, *B. suis* from pigs, and *B. melitensis* from goats are the species most often found causing human zoonotic infections.	
Characteristics	Small Gram-negative rods. Intracellular pathogens. Growth enhanced by erythritol in placenta of animals (not in man).
Laboratory identification	Some strains slow-growing and fastidous, requiring complex growth media. Isolation from blood cultures improved by use of biphasic systems (e.g. Castenada bottles). Usually require 3–5 days incubation in CO_2-enriched environment, but some strains of *B. abortus* may take up to 4 weeks (important in investigation of PUO). Identification is by biochemical reactions, patterns of resistance to certain dyes, and serological tests. The disease may be diagnosed by examination of patient's serum for antibodies.
Diseases	Undulant fever (brucellosis). Patients frequently present with PUO. Infection may become chronic if not adequately treated.
Transmission	Zoonotic infections transmitted to man through consumption of contaminated milk or other unpasteurized dairy products (increasingly seen in 'health freaks' who prefer untreated products) and by direct contact (occupational hazard for veterinarians, abbatoir workers and farmers).
Pathogenesis	Virulence associated with ability to survive intracellularly especially in bone marrow, liver and spleen, and thus 'hide' from host defences. Erythritol is a growth stimulant for the organism in animals and accounts for the tropism of the organisms to the placenta and foetus. This is not true in humans.
Treatment and prevention	Erythromycin or tetracycline; the latter may be tolerated during long treatment courses required. Recrudescence of infection is common. Prevention depends on eliminating the disease from domestic animals by vaccination (SV19 live attenuated vaccine) and pasteurization of milk. Vaccination is available for persons at risk in some countries but is not used in USA and UK.

Genus *Legionella*
A relatively recent discovery in microbiological history. Originally demonstrated by techniques used for virus isolation (e.g. growth in embryonated hens eggs). In free-living state can grow in water but difficult to cultivate on routine laboratory media. Large number of species (distinguished mainly on the basis of their DNA restriction patterns), but *L. pneumophila* is the pathogen of greatest medical importance.

Legionella pneumophila	
Characteristics	Gram-negative rods but stain poorly by Gram's stain (and therefore easily missed). Fastidious growth requirements in laboratory.
Laboratory identification	Direct fluorescent antibody tests performed on sputum samples have the advantage of specificity, distinguishing *L. pneumophila* from environmental contaminants. However relatively few organisms may be present in expectorated sputum. Silver staining techniques better than standard Gram staining method. Require enriched media containing iron and cysteine and absorbants to remove fatty acids. Moist incubation for 3–5 days required for growth. Produces tenacious colony. Further identification based on requirement for cysteine and serological characteristics. Diagnosis is often based on antibody detection rather than culture.
Diseases	Legionnaire's disease; one of the causes of atypical pneumonia. Pontiac fever (may be caused by other species) is a less severe, flu-like illness.
Transmission	Environmental saprophyte acquired by inhalation of contaminated water from showers, air conditioning systems, cooling towers.
Pathogenesis	Virulence factors unclear, but intracellular survival in alveolar macrophages important. Host predisposition (e.g. immunocompromise, chronic lung disease) important.
Treatment and prevention	Erythromycin (may be combined with rifampicin or ciprofloxacin). No vaccine available; prevention depends on maintenance of hot water and air conditioning systems, particularly in large buildings such as offices, hospitals and hotels.

SPIRAL BACTERIA

There are three genera of medical importance: *Treponema*, *Leptospira* and *Borrelia*.

Genus *Treponema*
Regularly coiled spirochaetes with a longer wavelength than Leptospira. Several species and subspecies important human pathogens; others are members of the normal flora, especially in the mouth. *Treponema pallidum* and its subspecies *pertenue* and *T. carateum* are most important species.

Characteristics	Individual cells too small to visualize by direct light microscopy; can be seen with dark ground illumination, or after silver impregnation or immunofluorescent staining. Cells are actively motile by means of flagella contained within the periplasmic sheath.
Laboratory identification	*T. pallidum* and closely related species cannot be grown in artificial media; diagnosis of infection depends on microscopic examination of fluid from primary lesions and on serology.
Diseases	*T. pallidum*: syphilis. *T. pallidum-pertenue* and *T. carateum*: the non-sexually transmitted treponematoses, yaws and pinta.
Transmission	Very susceptible to heat and drying, so successful transmission depends on very close contact. *T. pallidum* is spread by close sexual contact and may also be vertically transmitted *in utero*. Yaws and pinta spread by direct contact from infected skin lesions. No animal reservoir.
Pathogenesis	Study of virulence factors hampered by the inability to grow *T. pallidum* in artificial culture media. Disease presents characteristically in three phases: after local primary infection, organisms widely disseminated in the body and may become quiescent for months or years. Immunopathology plays a major role in causing damage to the host particularly in the tertiary stage of disease.

Genus Treponoma (cont.)	
Treatment and prevention	Penicillin is the treatment of choice for syphilis. Tetracycline may be given to penicillin-allergic patients. Prevention depends on detection and treatment of cases, contact tracing and serological testing of pregant women. Possible cross-reactions between *T. pallidum* and the species causing yaws and pinta must be noted.

Genus *Leptospira*

Two species: *L. interrogans* and *L. biflexa*; the former is parasitic, the latter contains freeliving species. Within the species interrogans there are several different serogroups and serovars responsible for disease in humans and animals.

Leptospira interrogans

Characteristics	Finely coiled spirochaetes with hooked ends. Cells 0.1–0.2 μm in diameter, up to 20 μm in length. Not visible by direct light microscopy unless stained by sliver impregnation or immunofluorescent methods. Dark ground microscopy reveals rotational and directional motility by means of periplasmic flagella.
Laboratory identification	Direct microscopy of blood and urine possible but difficult to interpret. Leptospira can be grown, with difficulty, in special serum-containing media. Serological diagnosis is usual.
Diseases	Leptospirosis or Weil's disease in humans and animals.
Transmission	Leptospirosis in humans is a zoonosis, usual hosts being rodents, bats, cattle, sheep, goats and other domestic animals. Leptospires excreted in urine contaminate food and water. Infection occurs by contact either through occupation (e.g. sewer workers, farmers, abbatoir workers) or recreation (e.g. canoeing, wind-surfing etc. on inland waters). Organisms may penetrate unabraded skin and conjunctiva.
Pathogenesis	After initial invasion there is haematogenous spread before the organisms localize in various organs including the liver and kidney. Subclinical infection common in endemic areas.
Treatment and prevention	Penicillin; tetracycline or erythromycin in penicillin-allergic patients. Disease may be prevented after exposure by penicillin or doxycycline.

Genus *Borrelia*

Two species of *Borrelia* of importance in humans. *Borrelia recurrentis* causes relapsing fever (now rare). *Borrelia burgdorferi* recognized recently as cause of Lyme disease.

Characteristics	Less finely coiled than the Leptospires. Cells 0.2 0.5 μm in diameter; stain readily, so are visible by light microscopy.
Laboratory identification	*B. recurrentis* demonstrated in blood smears by staining with Giemsa or acridine orange. *B. burgdorferi* much more difficult to visualize. Culture from biopsy material possible but difficult; diagnosis usually by serology.
Diseases	In relapsing fever the relapsing element may be due to antigen switching. Lyme disease slowly progressive rather than relapsing. Characteristic skin lesion 'erythema chronicum migrans' occurs in approx. 50% of cases. Joint pains and fatigue common and later, in untreated cases, neurologic and cardiac manifestations.
Transmission	*B. recurrentis* spread from person to person by lice. Lyme disease is a zoonosis transmitted to humans by hard ticks (*Ixodes* spp.) associated with deer. Ticks are found on bracken and undergrowth and attach to exposed skin. Tick bite is often unnoticed but less than a minute is required for the organisms to enter the host.
Pathogenesis	Little known about pathogenesis of either disease. Antigen switching in *B. recurrentis* presumably allows evasion of host's antibody response.
Treatment and prevention	Tetracycline; but erythromycin and penicillin have both been used successfully. Prevention depends on avoiding contact with vectors, e.g. protective clothing for walkers and forestry workers.

Mycoplasmas	
Characteristics	Distinguished from other procaryotes and placed in the class mollicutes because they lack a true cell wall and consequent rigidity. This is a stable characteristic exhibited by the genera *Mycoplasma*, *Ureaplasma* and *Acholeplasma* and is distinct from cell wall deficient and L-forms of other species. The outer membrane, the outermost layer, functions as the major antigenic interface. It is flexible triple-layered structure of proteins and lipids. Many species also contain cholesterol in the membrane which is absent from other bacterial cells. The important species is *Mycoplasma pneumoniae*, but *M. hominis* and *Ureaplasma urealyticum* may cause genital tract infections.
Laboratory identification	Many species are fastidious, and complex media and soft agar may be required for satisfactory culture. Cultures incubated for at least 7 days although some species (e.g. *M. hominis*) grow readily on moist blood agar plates within 48 hours. Cells very variable in size (up to 100μm) and morphology; cannot be stained by Gram's stain (no cell wall) but impressions of colonies can be stained with Dienes' or Romanowsky stains. Diagnosis of infection based on serology due to difficulties of culture,
Diseases	*M. pneumoniae* important cause of 'atypical pneumonia'. Mycoplasmas also associated with genital infections (e.g. non-gonococcal urethritis) and with joint and other inflammatory infections. Other mycoplasmas important pathogens of animals and birds.
Transmission	Transmission of *M. pneumonia* from person to person by airborne route. Other mycoplasmas and ureaplasmas can be transmitted by sexual contact.
Pathogenesis	Surface protein adhesin binds *M. pneumoniae* to sialogycolipids on respiratory epithelium of host. Other virulence factors are not yet clearly understood.
Treatment and prevention	Tetracycline or erythromycin (N.B. lack of cell wall target means lack of susceptibility to beta-lactams). No vaccine currently available. Prevention by interruption of spread is difficult.
Rickettsiae	
Characteristics	These organisms have requirement for coenzyme A, NAD and ATP which they cannot supply themselves, and are therefore obligate intracellular parasites; with rare exceptions need to be grown in cell cultures or experimental animals.
Laboratory identification	Small (0.7–2μm diameter), Gram-negative bacteria. Isolation in laboratory is difficult for the reasons outlined above (and may carry a high risk of laboratory-acquired infection); therefore rarely attempted outside specialized facilities. Diagnosis of infection based on serology.
Diseases	Typhus; Rocky Mountain, Mediterranean and other spotted fevers; Q fever.
Transmission	*Coxiella burnetii* survives drying and is transmitted in aerosols from animals or materials contaminated by infected animals and inhaled. All other rickettsiae maintained in animal reservoirs and transmitted by bites of tricks, fleas, mites and lice.
Pathogenesis	Mechanisms unclear but organisms have a predilection for endothelial cells, giving rise to characteristic primary skin lesion (in spotted fevers) and vasculitis. The intracellular habitat is important to the organisms survival in the face of host defences.
Treatment and prevention	Tetracycline, erythromycin, chloramphenicol. The newer fluoroquinolones may be useful in treatment. Beta-lactams ineffective. Infection prevented by avoiding contact with vectors. Vaccines available for at risk groups (e.g. vets, farm workers).
Chlamydiae	
Characteristics	Obligate intracellular parasites with distinct life cycle involving elementary bodies and reticulate bodies. Small cells with genome approx. 25% of that of *E. coli*. Important species are *Chlamydia trachomatis*, *C. psittaci* and *C. pneumoniae*.

Chlamydiae (cont.)	
Laboratory identification	Chlamydiae must be grown in cell culture, so cultural techniques limited to specialized laboratories. In cell cultures, *C. trachomatis* forms characteristic, glycogen-containing inclusion bodies which can be stained with iodine. Both *C. psittaci* and *C. trachomatis* contain specific surface antigens that allow detection by immunofluourescent antibody techniques. *C. pneumoniae* currently detectable only by serology.
Diseases	*C. trachomatis* causes trachoma (eye infection), urethritis and other infections of the genital tract, and pneumonitis in newborns, acquired during birth from infected mothers. *C. pneumoniae*, described more recently, now recognized as important cause of atypical pneumonia. *C. psittaci* causes the atypical pneumonia, psittacosis.
Transmission	*C. pneumoniae* and *C. psittaci* acquired by inhalation, the latter from infected birds or contaminated bird litter. *C. trachomatis* spread by direct contact and is sexually-transmitted.
Pathogenesis	Virulence factors remain unclear but the intracellular habitat and different life cycle forms help organisms to evade host defences. Uptake into cells may be by parasite-encoded mechanisms.
Treatment and prevention	Tetracyclines and erythromycin (tetracycline should not be used in children). The new fluoroquinolones may be useful. Vaccines not available and are unlikely to be useful because of the immunopathological element of the infections.

FUNGI

SUPERFICIAL MYCOSES

Dermatophytes

General term for species invading superficial layers of skin. Of the many species involved,
those belonging to *Epidermophyton*, *Microsporum* and *Trichophyton* are of greatest importance .

Characteristics	Filamentous fungi invading surface keratinized structures–skin, hair, nails. Hyphae penetrate between cells.
Laboratory identification	Examination of KOH-treated skin scrapings for hyphae; fluorescence under Wood's lamp. Culture on media useful in identifying species. Both Sabouraud dextrose agar (SDA) and dermatophyte test medium (DTM) can be used.
Diseases	Tinea, ringworm, athlete's foot etc.
Transmission	By fungal material on skin scales.
Pathogenesis	Skin inflammation, pruritus - sometimes localized hypersensitivity reactions.
Treatment and prevention	Topical antifungal agents. Improved skin care and hygiene.

Sporothrix schenckii

Characteristics	Dimorphic fungus (capable of growing as both single-celled yeast and multicelled hyphae). Occurs in external environment. Invades subcutaneous tissues.
Laboratory identification	Budding cells in inflammatory exudate from lesions. Culture on SDA.
Diseases	Sporotrichosis.
Transmission	Direct fungal contamination of wounds in skin (e.g. those made by thorns).
Pathogenesis	Ulceration or abcess formation in draining lymphatics.
Treatment and prevention	Potassium iodide, Ketoconazole. Protection of skin.

DEEP MYCOSES	
Aspergillus	
A. fumigatus is the most important of 3 common species, the others being _A. flavus_ and _A. niger_.	
Characteristics	Filamentous fungi causing opportunistic infections in immunocompromised patients. Occur widely in external environment. Invade lungs and blood vessels.
Laboratory identification	Presence of hyphae in tissues. Culture on SDA. Serology.
Diseases	Aspergillosis.
Transmission	Inhalation of airborne stages (conidia).
Pathogenesis	Causes thrombosis and infarction when blood vessels invaded. Partial blockage of airways from fungal mass. Allergic broncho-pulmonary reactions.
Treatment and prevention	Amphotericin B.
Blastomycoses dermatitidis	
Characteristics	Dimorphic fungus. Invades through lungs, can become widely disseminated in body.
Laboratory identification	Yeast cells in sputum or skin lesions. Culture on SDA.
Diseases	Blastomycosis.
Transmission	Inhalation of airborne spores.
Pathogenesis	Fungal infection in lungs may present as tuberculosis. Can produce abcesses.
Treatment and prevention	Ketoconazole.
Candida albicans	
Characteristics	Dimorphic fungus, occurring as yeast on mucosal surfaces as component of normal flora, but forms hyphae when invasive. Produces opportunistic infections in stressed, suppressed and antibiotic-treated individuals. _Paracocidioides brasiliensis_ in central and S America has many similarities.
Laboratory identification	Fungal stages in tissues. Culture on SDA.
Diseases	Candidiasis, thrush.
Transmission	Part of normal flora on skin, in mouth and intestine.
Pathogenesis	Localized mucocutaneous lesions; invasion of all major organs in the disseminated condition.
Treatment and prevention	Oral and topical antifungals (e.g. Nystatin, Miconazole). Ketoconazole, Amphotericin B and Flucytosine for disseminated disease.
Coccidioides immitis	
Characteristics	Dimorphic fungus, growing as hyphae in soils, but as yeast-like endospores within capsules (spherules) in tissues. Invasion through lungs, can become widely disseminated in body.
Laboratory identification	In sputum or tissues. Culture on SDA. Serology.
Diseases	Coccidiomycosis. Indigenous to the Americas.

Coccidioides immitis (cont.)	
Transmission	Inhalation of airborne stages (arthroconidia).
Pathogenesis	Lung infections give mild, influenza-like condition, but serious illness may follow dissemination.
Treatment and prevention	Amphotericin B, Ketoconazole.

Cryptococcus neoformans	
Characteristics	Encapsulated yeast-like fungus common in soils where there are bird-droppings. Invades through lungs, can spread to CNS.
Laboratory identification	Encapsulated yeast cells in sputum or cerebrospinal fluid. Culture on SDA. Serology.
Diseases	Cryptococcosis.
Transmission	Inhalation of airborne cells.
Pathogenesis	Lung infection may result in influenza-like condition or pneumonia. In immunocompromised patients CNS involvement leads to meningitis.
Treatment and prevention	Amphotericin B and Flucytosine.

Histoplasma capsulatum	
Characteristics	Dimorphic fungus, growing in as hyphae in soil where there are bird droppings. Invades through lungs and grows as yeast cells, which can survive intracellularly after phagocytosis. Can become widely disseminated in body.
Laboratory identification	Yeast cells in sputum or tissues. Culture on SDA. Serology.
Diseases	Histoplasmosis.
Transmission	Inhalation of airborne spores.
Pathogenesis	Can produce acute and chronic pulmonary disease. Serious illness results from dissemination into other organs.
Treatment and prevention	Amphotericin, B7 Ketoconazole.

Pneumocystis carinii	
Characteristics	Respiratory organism previously classed as a sporozoan protozoan, now classified as a fungus. Lives extracellularly within alveoli.
Laboratory identification	Histological identification of organism in tissues.
Diseases	Pneumonia-like condition, severe in immunocompromised patients. World-wide distribution.
Transmission	Assumed to be by droplets.
Pathogenesis	Inflammation in lung.
Treatment and prevention	Trimethoprin plus sulphamethoxazole.

PROTOZOA	
Cryptosporidium parvum	
Characteristics	Intestinal sporozoan, invades and reproduces in epithelial cells of small intestine. Forms oocysts which are passed in faeces.
Laboratory identification	Small (5μm) oocysts in faeces, detected by flotation and acid-fast staining.
Diseases	Cryptosporidiosis. World-wide distribution.
Transmission	Faecal-oral. Swallowing infective oocysts, usually in contaminated water. Animal reservoirs of infection.
Pathogenesis	Invasion of epithelial cells causes diarrhoea, can be profuse in immunocompromised patients.
Treatment and prevention	No routine treatment yet available. Improved sanitation.
Entamoeba histolytica	
Characteristics	Intestinal amoeba, lives in intestine as trophozoite, produces resistant cysts, which are passed in faeces.
Laboratory identification	Motile trophozoites or 4-nucleate cysts in faeces, detected in fresh or fixed-stained smears.
Diseases	Amoebic dysentery, liver abcess. World-wide distribution, commonest in tropical/subtropical countries.
Transmission	Faecal-oral. Swallowing cysts in contaminated water or food.
Pathogenesis	Invasion of large bowel mucosa causes ulceration and diarrhoea, often bloody. Spread to liver causes formation of sterile abcess.
Treatment and prevention	Metronidazole, Tinidazole; Hygiene and sanitation.
Giardia lamblia	
Characteristics	Intestinal flagellate, lives on mucosa of small bowel. Produces cysts, which are passed in faeces.
Laboratory diagnosis	4-nucleate cysts in faeces, detected in fixed-stained smears. Direct recovery of bi-nucleate trophozoites from bowel.
Diseases	Giardiasis. World-wide distribution.
Transmission	Faecal-oral. Swallowing cysts, usually in contaminated water. Animal reservoirs of infection.
Pathogenesis	Large numbers of trophozoites can cause severe diarrhoea and impaired absorption. Most severe in immunocompromised patients.
Treatment and prevention	Metronidazole, Tinidazole; Improved sanitation, water treatment.
Genus Leishmania	
Genus contains several species, of which *L. brasiliensis*, *L. donovani* and *L. tropica* cause major disease.	
Characteristics	Sporozoa living intracellularly in macrophages as amastigote stage. Transmitted by phlebotomine sandflies.

Genus *Leishmania* (cont.)	
Laboratory identification	Clinical signs, presence of amastigotes in stained biopsy material, *in vitro* culture of tissue specimens to obtain promastigotes.
Diseases	Visceral (*donovani*), cutaneous (*tropica*) and muco-cutaneous (*brasiliensis*) leishmaniasis. Disease also known by many local names, e.g. Kala Azar, Oriental Sore, Espundia. Commonest in trophical/subtropical countries.
Transmission	By bite of infected sandfly.
Pathogenesis	Visceral: hepato-splenomegaly from invasion of macrophages in liver and spleen, allergic reactions after treatment causing dermal nodules; Cutaneous: localized ulcers, which resolve; Muco-cutaneous: progressive invasion of mucocutaneous tissues in nose and mouth.
Treatment and prevention	Antimonials, pentamidine. Avoidance of vectors.

Genus *Plasmodium*	
Genus contains four species causing disease, *P. falciparum, P. malariae, P. ovale,* and *P. vivax. Falciparum* and *vivax* are commonest.	
Characteristics	Sporozoa living intracellularly in liver and, primarily, in red blood cells.
Laboratory identification	Parasites in red blood cells in stained blood smear.
Diseases	Malaria. Commonest in tropical/subtropical countries.
Transmission	By bite of infected anopheline mosquito.
Pathogenesis	Bursting of infected red cells causes periodic fevers. In *falciparum* malaria, sequestration of infected cells in brain capillaries can cause fatal cerebral malaria; this infection is sometimes associated with intravascular haemolysis. Infection with *P. malariae* can lead to nephritis from immune complex deposition.
Treatment and prevention	Many antimalarial drugs, but parasites show considerable drug resistance. Avoidance of vectors. Mosquito control.

Toxoplasma gondii	
Characteristics	Sporozoan living intracellularly, forming large tissue cysts. Natural host is cat, where parasite has enteric cycle, producing oocysts in faeces. In humans organisms can invade many tissues.
Laboratory diagnosis	Serology; need repeated tests to establish current infection.
Diseases	Toxoplasmosis. World-wide distribution.
Transmission	Swallowing oocysts passed by cats; ingestion of tissue cysts in raw or undercooked meat; transplacental.
Pathogenesis	In adults causes mild influenza-like disease, lymph nodes may be enlarged. Symptoms more severe in immunocompromised patients. Congenital infections can damage eye or brain and prove fatal .
Treatment and prevention	Pyrimethamine, Sulphadiazine; hygiene, cooking of meat.

Trichomonas vaginalis

Characteristics	Flagellate living in urogenital system of females and, occasionally, males. Trophozoite form only, no cyst.
Laboratory identification	Identification of trophozoites in stained material from vaginal smears.
Diseases	Trichomoniasis. World-wide distribution.
Transmission	Venereal.
Pathogenesis	Mild in males, causes vaginitis with discharge in females
Treatment and prevention	Metronidazole, Tinidazole. Use of condoms.

Genus Trypanosoma

Genus contains 3 species causing disease: *T. gambiense, T. rhodesiense* (African trypanosomiasis) and *T. cruzi* (American trypanosomiasis)

Characteristics	Flagellates living in blood and tissues. *T. cruzi* has intracellular stages.
Laboratory identification	Organisms in blood or cerebrospinal fluid (African) or blood, biopsy or culture (American). Serology.
Diseases	African trypanosomiasis (sleeping sickness): sub-Saharan Africa. American trypanosomiais(Chagas' disease): S America.
Transmission	By bite of infected insect vector: Tsetse fly (African) or Reduviid Bug (American).
Pathogenesis	African: infection of CNS causing meningoencephalitis. American: destruction of infected cells, especially neurons, megacolon, megaoesophagus, cardiac failure.
Treatment and prevention	Chemotherapy. Avoidance of vectors. Vector control .

HELMINTHS

TAPEWORMS

Diphyllobothrium latum

Characteristics	Large adult tapeworm in intestine. Scolex with sucking grooves not suckers. Eggs released and passed in faeces.
Laboratory identification	Faecal smears, fresh or stained. Eggs in faeces have characteristic operculum (lid).
Diseases	Diphyllobothriasis (fish tapeworm). World-wide distribution. Commonest where fish eaten raw.
Transmission	Larval stages in fish. Adult worm acquired when infected fish eaten raw or undercooked.
Pathogenesis	Usually harmless, may be associated with vitamin B_{12} deficiency.
Treatment and prevention	Niclosamide, Praziquantel; Cooking of fish, sanitation.

Echinococcus granulosus

Characteristics	Large fluid-filled (hydatid) cysts, the larval stages of the tapeworm, in abdomen, liver, lungs, CNS.

Echinococcus granulosus (cont.)	
Laboratory identification	Scans, serology.
Diseases	Hydatidosis, hydatid disease. World-wide distribution, commonest in sheep-rearing countries.
Transmission	Swallowing eggs released from adult tapeworms in dogs. Natural cycle is adult (dog), larval cysts (sheep).
Pathogenesis	Cysts exert pressure on internal organs. Release of cyst fluid can cause anaphylaxis.
Treatment and prevention	Mebendazole. Surgical removal of cysts. Prevention of dogs eating infected viscera from sheep. Hygiene after handling dogs.
Hymenolepis nana	
Characteristics	Small (2-4 cm) adult tapeworms in intestine. Scolex with suckers and hooks. Eggs passed in faeces. Life cycle can be direct or via insect intermediate host.
Laboratory identification	Faecal smears, fresh or stained. Thin-shelled eggs in faeces.
Diseases	Hymenolepiasis (dwarf tapeworm). World-wide distribution.
Transmission	Swallowing eggs, accidental ingestion of larvae in insects.
Pathogenesis	Usually harmless. Numbers of worms can build up by autoinfection (direct hatching of eggs from adult worms in intestine) and enteritis may result.
Treatment and prevention	Niclosamide, Praziquantel. Hygiene and sanitation
Genus *Taenia*	
Two species of this genus infect humans, *T. saginata* and *T. solium*.	
Characteristics	Large (metres) adult tapeworms in intestine. Scolices with suckers (*saginata*) or suckers and hooks (*saginata* and *solium*). Proglottids (segments) passed in faeces. Small cysts (larval stages of solium) in muscles CNS and eyes.
Laboratory identification	Proglottids in faeces. Species identifiable on basis of number of branches to uterus (saginata 15/20; *solium* 5/10).
Diseases	Taeniasis (beef and pork tapeworms). Cysticercosis (solium only). World-wide distribution.
Transmission	Adult worms acquired by eating raw or undercooked meat (beef , *saginata*, pork *solium*) from animals infected with larval stages. T. solium eggs can hatch in humans, allowing cysts to develop.
Pathogenesis	Adult worms essentially harmless. In cysticercosis, cysts in brain can result in neurological symptoms.
Treatment and prevention	Niclosamide, Praziquantel. Adequate cooking of meat. Prevention of human faeces contaminating grazing/feeding areas of cattle and pigs.
FLUKES	
Clonorchis sinensis	
Characteristics	Liver fluke. Narrow, elongate worms in bile ducts.
Laboratory identification	Faecal smears, fresh or stained. Eggs in faeces.

Clonorchis sinensis (cont.)	
Diseases	Clonorchiasis (Asia).
Transmission	Larval stages in fish; adult flukes acquired when infected fish eaten raw or undercooked.
Pathogenesis	Damage to liver, inflammation of bile ducts.
Treatment and prevention	Praziquantel. Cooking of fish. Sanitation.
Paragonimus westermanii	
Characteristics	Lung fluke, thick fleshy worms living as pairs in cysts.
Laboratory identification	Eggs in sputum or faeces.
Diseases	Paragonimiasis (Asia).
Transmission	Larval stages in crabs; adult flukes acquired when infected crab meat eaten raw or undercooked.
Pathogenesis	Inflammation of lungs, secondary bacterial infections.
Treatment and prevention	Praziquantel. Cooking of crab meat. Sanitation.
Genus _Schistosoma_	
Genus contains several species able to infect humans. Three are of major importance _S. haematobium_, _S. japonicum_ and _S. mansoni_.	
Characteristics	Blood flukes, adult worms in blood vessels around intestine (japonicum, mansoni.) or bladder (_haematobium_). Eggs in tissues.
Laboratory identification	Faecal smears, fresh or stained. Spined eggs in faeces (_japonicum_ - small lateral spine; _mansoni_, - large lateral spine). Eggs in urine (_haematobium_, - terminal spine).
Diseases	Schistosomiasis. Widely distributed in tropical/subtropical countries (_mansoni_, Africa, S. America; _haematobium_, Africa, Middle East; _japonicum_, Asia).
Transmission	Larvae released from eggs infect aquatic snails. These release infective cercaria larvae which actively penetrate human skin.
Pathogenesis	Hypersensitivity responses to eggs cause inflammation, granuloma formation, fibrosis and obstructive disease in intestine, bladder and liver.
Treatment and prevention	Praziquantel. Avoidance of infected waters. Removal of snails. Sanitation.
NEMATODES	
Ascaris lumbricoides	
Characteristics	Large (up to 30cm) intestinal roundworm, migratory stages pass through liver and lungs.
Laboratory identification	Faecal smears, fresh or stained. Thick-shelled eggs in faeces, worms occasionally also passed.
Diseases	Ascariasis (world-wide distribution, commonest in tropical/subtropical countries).
Transmission	Swallowing infective eggs in contaminated soil, food or water.

Ascaris lumbricoides (cont.)	
Pathogenesis	Migrating larvae cause pneumonia-like symptoms. Adults can obstruct intestine, interfere with digestion/absorption of food, migrate in bile duct. Allergic symptoms common.
Treatment and prevention	Mebendazole, Pyrantel, Piperazine. Hygiene and sanitation.

Enterobius vermicularis	
Characteristics	Small (1cm) roundworm in large bowel. Worms emerge from anus at night to lay eggs.
Laboratory identification	Eggs recovered from perianal skin, adult worms in faeces.
Diseases	Enterobiasis, Pinworm. World-wide distribution. commonest in children.
Transmission	Swallowing eggs, which can be carried on fingers and in dust. Eggs infective when laid, so direct reinfection is common.
Pathogenesis	Perianal pruritis.
Treatment and prevention	Mebendazole, Pyrantel, Piperazine. Hygiene.

Filarial Nematodes	
Large group. Most important species living in lymphatic tissues (*Wuchereria bancrofti, Brugia malayi*) or in skin (*Onchocerca volvulus*).	
Characteristics	Adults very long, thin worms, living in lymphatics, with microfilaria larvae in blood (*Wuchereria, Brugia*), or in subcutaneous nodules with microfilaria in skin (*Onchocerca*).
Laboratory identification	Detection of microfilaria in stained blood smear or fresh skin nip.
Diseases	Lymphatic filariasis (*Wuchereria, Brugia*): onchocerciasis or river blindness (*Onchocerca*).
Transmission	Microfilaria taken up by blood-feeding insects (mosquitoes, *Wuchereria, Brugia*; *Simulium* blackflies, *Onchocerca*), develop to infective stage and reintroduced into humans at next blood meal. Widely distributed in tropical/subtropical countries.
Pathogenesis	In lymphatic filariasis, adult worms cause inflammation of lymph nodes and blockage of lymphatics, sometimes causing elephantiasis (big-leg). In onchocerciasis, hypersensitivity to microfilaria larvae leads to skin and eye lesions.
Treatment and prevention	Diethyl carbamazine (lymphatic) and Ivermectin (onchocerciasis). Avoidance of vectors. Vector control

Hookworms	
General term for intestinal blood-sucking worms. Two major species *Ancylostoma duodenale* and *Necator americanus*.	
Characteristics	Small (1cm) intestinal roundworms, migratory stages pass through skin and lungs. Adult worms have expanded mouths for attachment to intestilnal mucosa.
Laboratory identification	Faecal smears, fresh or stained. Thin-shelled eggs in faeces. Culture of faeces, eggs hatching after 24 hours to release larvae.
Diseases	Hookworm disease (ancylostomiasis, necatoriasis). Widespread in tropical/subtropical countries.
Transmission	Infective larvae penetrate skin (both species) or mucous membranes after ingestion (*Ancylostoma*).

Hookworms (cont.)	
Pathogenesis	Blood-sucking of worms can lead to anaemia and protein loss. Larval penetration associated with dermatitis.
Treatment and prevention	Mebendazole. Pyrantel. Hygiene and sanitation.

Strongyloides stercoralis	
Characteristics	Minute (2mm) intestinal roundworm, living in humans only as larvae and parthenogenetic females. Migratory stages pass through skin and (possibly) lungs. Eggs hatch in intestine, larvae in faeces may become infective directly or initiate a free-living generation in soil, from which infective larvae develop.
Laboratory identification	Larvae in fresh faecal specimens.
Diseases	Strongyloidiasis. Widespread in tropical/subtropical countries.
Transmission	Infective larvae penetrate skin.
Pathogenesis	In immunocompromised patients, repeated autoinfection (development of larvae released from females in the intestine) can lead to hyperinfection (disseminated strongyloidiasis.) with larvae invading all body tissues Hyperinfection can be fatal. Diarrhoea and malabsorption accompany heavy intestinal infections.
Treatment and prevention	Thiabendazole. Hygiene and sanitation.

Toxocara canis	
Characteristics	Invasion by larvae of roundworm species normally maturing in intestine of dogs.
Laboratory identification	Serology.
Diseases	Toxocariasis, visceral larva migrans. World-wide distribution.
Transmission	Swallowing infective eggs passed by dogs, in contaminated soil, food or water.
Pathogenesis	Invasion of body tissues causing granulomatous inflammatory responses. Larvae in CNS may cause epilepsy-like condition, in the eye granulomata may cause blindness.
Treatment and prevention	Thiabendazole. Hygiene. Routine deworming of puppies and pregnant bitches.

Trichinella spiralis	
Characteristics	Minute (2–3mm) roundworms, living as adults in the intestine. Coiled larvae in muscles. Low host specificity, infects and matures in wide variety of mammals.
Laboratory identification	Clinical signs, serology, muscle biopsy.
Diseases	Trichinellosis (trichinosis). World-wide distribution.
Transmission	Acquired by eating raw or undercooked meat (usually pork) containing infective larvae.
Pathogenesis	Diarrhoea during intestinal phase. Allergic symptoms, muscle pain, cardiac effects during muscle invasion, latter phase can be fatal.
Treatment and prevention	Mebendazole. Cooking of meat.

Trichuris trichiura	
Characteristics	Medium size (0.75 cm) roundworms in large bowel. Body of characteristic 'whipworm' form, with long, thin anterior and short, thicker posterior.
Laboratory identification	Faecal smears, fresh or stained. Eggs in faeces have characteristic shape, oval with plugs at each pole. Endoscopy.
Diseases	Trichuriasis. World-wide distribution, commonest in tropical/subtropical countries.
Transmission	Swallowing infective eggs in contaminated soil, food or water.
Pathogenesis	Diarrhoea, intestinal inflammation, occasionally rectal prolapse.
Treatment and prevention	Mebendazole. Hygiene and sanitation.

APPENDIX II: PROTOCOLS FOR SPECIMEN PROCESSING

PROTOCOLS FOR SPECIMEN PROCESSING

Subsequent sections of this Appendix are devoted to the basic protocols used in the diagnostic laboratory for processing specimens. These protocols describe the processing of specimens for isolation of bacteria, and pathogenic fungi where relevant. Isolation of viruses from clinical specimens as a method of diagnosis is generally slower, more difficult and costly and viral infections are usually diagnosed by antigen detection or serological methods (see Chapter 18). The following types of specimens are considered:

Urine
Faeces
Genital tract specimens
Skin and soft tissue specimens
Respiratory tract specimens (including
  nose, throat eye and, ear swabs, and
sputum)
Cerebrospinal fluid (CSF)
Pus
Other fluids such as pleural, pericardial
  fluids and joint aspirates
Blood
Bone marrow
Biopsy samples
Autopsy samples
Forensic samples

ABBREVIATIONS:

Culture media

BA	Blood agar (different species of blood may be specified)
Mac	MacConkey agar
CLED	Cysteine lactose electrolyte deficient agar
EMB	Eosin methylene blue agar
TM	Thayer-Martin agar
WC	Wilkins Chalgren agar
CA	Chocolate agar
TcBs	Thiosulphate citrate bite salt sucrase agar
Sab	Sabouraud agar

Incubation conditions

CO_2	air enriched with 7–10% carbon dioxide
AnO_2	anaerobic environment; one in which oxygen has been removed and replaced by nitrogen and hydrogen. These conditions can be achieved in 'gas jars' with commercially available gas generating sachets.

The duration and temperature of incubation are also stated.

URINE	
Specimen type	Mid-stream urine (MSU) Catheter urine (CSU) Supra-pubic aspirate (SPA) Early morning urine (EMU)
Examination of specimens	Macroscopically: note appearance (e.g. cloudy, bloodstained) Microscopically: examine drop of urine (wet preparation; unstained) note presence and numbers of WBC (normal < 10-50/cm^3) note presence of: RBC epithelial cells* bacteria crystals Commercial test kits available to detect WBC and RBC.
Culture	Numbers of bacteria important so quantitative/semiquantitative methods used. Media: BA, Mac or CLED. Incubation: air for 18 hrs at 35–37°C.
Likely pathogens (basic method)	*E. coli, Proteus, Staph. saprophyticus, Enterococcus, Klebsiella, Pseudomonas, Salmonella, Candida* (N.B. growth of yeasts improved on Sabouraud agar). Growth significant if >10^5 organisms/ml isolated from a MSU; presence of any number of bacteria in CSU or SPA specimens may be significant; any number of mycobacteria in EMU specimens may be significant.

Important pathogens (not isolated by above technique)

Mycobacteria
EMU specimens best for isolation of mycobacteria; prior to culture, decontaminate with NaOH or HCl, centrifuge, neutralize deposit.
Microscopy: not recommended; other non-pathogenic mycobacteria from water or environment may be detected.
Culture: inoculate centrifuged deposit on to Lowenstein-Jensen or Middlebrook agar (in screw-capped bottles to prevent dessication and reduce hazard).
Incubation: Air for 4–12 weeks at 35-37°C

Leptospira
Can be demonstrated in urine in weeks 2–3 of infection by dark ground microscopy; urine must be very fresh (<15min); culture possible but difficult; diagnosis usually serological.

Schistosoma
Ova of *Schistosoma haematobium* can be seen by microscopy; urine usually contains RBCs.

FAECES	
Specimen type	Samples of faeces preferable to rectal swabs; swabs from soiled diapers acceptable; because of random distribution of organisms in sample, take three sequential samples.
Examination of specimens	Macroscopically: note appearance, gross blood, mucus, parasites Microscopically: note WBC and RBC in wet prep; ova, cysts and parasites in concentrated suspension. Electron microscopy can be useful for rapid detection of some viruses.
Culture	Media/inoculum: Mac or EM/lightly for discrete colonies Deoxycholate citrate agar/heavy* Bismuth sulphite agar/heavy* Selenite F broth/ >1g faeces (subculture to DCA after 18 hrs incubation) Incubation: air for 18–48 hr at 35–37°C. *because these selective media inhibit pathogens but to a lesser extent than commensals.

FAECES (CONT).	
Likely pathogens (basic method)	*Salmonella* spp., *Shigella* spp., *E. coli* (see below for verotoxin-producers).

Important pathogens (not isolated by above technique)	History/presentation of patient dictates culture type.
	
	Pathogens demonstrated by special culture techniques:
	Campylobacter
	  Medium: Columbia BA (rich BA) made selective by addition of antibiotic cocktail
	  Incubation: microaerophilic (10% O_2) for 24-48 hrs at 43°C (for *C. jejuni*; lower temperature
	    for other species).
	
	Verotoxin-producing *E. coli*
	  Medium: sorbitol Mac (verotoxin producers do not usually ferment sorbitol;
	    other *E. coli* do).
	  Incubation: As basic method above.
	
	Yersinia enterocolitica
	  Medium: CIN (cefsulodin, irgasan, novobiocin) agar.
	  Incubation: air for 48-96 hrs at 30°C.
	
	Clostridium perfringens
	  Medium: Robertson's cooked meat medium (x2); heat one at 80°C for 10 min
	    prior to incubation.
	  Incubation: air (anaerobic conditions provided in depths of medium) for 18 hrs at 35-37°C.
	  Subculture to:
	  Medium: neomycin BA (NB haemolysis differs on horse and sheep blood).
	  Incubation: AnO_2 for 18 hrs at 35-37°C.
	
	Vibrio cholerae
	  Medium: TCBS.
	  Incubation: air for 18 hrs at 35°C.
	  Medium for enrichment: alkaline peptone water (pH 9).
	  Incubation: air for 3-6 hrs at 35°C.
	  Subculture to TCBS and incubate as above.
	
	Pathogens demonstrated microscopically
	  Ova; cysts; helminth parasites; *Entamoeba histolytica* (mobile form visible if specimen
	    examined early on); *Giardia lamblia* trophozoites (acute diarrhoea) or cysts; rotaviruses
	    (and certain other viruses) visible by EM.

GENITAL TRACT SPECIMENS

Specimen type	Swabs transported in buffered medium essential due to fastidiousness and multiplicity of species causing genital infections

Examination of specimens	Microscopically:
	Wet preparation (for *Trichomonas vaginalis, Candida*);
	Acridine orange stain: view by fluorescence microscopy (*T. vaginalis*); obviates need for
	  expensive, time-consuming culture;
	Gram stain: note WBC, Gram-negative intracellular diplococci (*N. gonorrhoeae*);
	  presence of WBC in absence of any of above species, consider *Chlamydia trachomatis*;
	  clue cells characteristic of bacterial vaginosis.

Culture	Media: BA, TM (or other medium selective for gonococci), Mac, WC, Sab, human BA
	  (if diagnosis of vaginal discharge/pelvic inflammatory disease).
	Incubation: BA
	      TM $\big]$ CO_2
	      Mac: air $\big]$ for 18-72 hrs at 35-37°C
	      WC
	      Human BA $\big]$ AnO_2
	      Sab: air for 18-48 hrs at 30°C

GENITAL TRACT SPECIMENS (CONT.)	
Likely pathogens (basic method)	*Neisseria gonorrhoeae, Candida albicans, Strep. agalactiae* (group B streptococcus), *Bacteroides* spp., *Gardnerella vaginalis* (enhanced growth on human blood agar), *Mycoplasma* and *Ureaplasma* spp., *Listeria monocytogenes.*
Important pathogens (not isolated by above technique)	*Chlamydia trachomatis* Culture: inoculate specimen onto monolayer of irradiated McCoy cells; examine after 48hrs for characteristic inclusions; alternatively direct examination of specimen by immunofluorescent staining techniques. *Haemophilus ducreyi* Medium: culture on CA + isovitalex 1%. Incubation: CO_2 for 2-9 days at 30-34°C. *Treponema pallidum* Cannot be cultured *in vitro*; demonstrated in primary and secondary lesions by dark ground microscopy of exudate; otherwise diagnosis depends on serology.

SKIN AND SOFT TISSUE SPECIMENS	
Specimen type	Sampling of skin lesions problematic; of doubtful value in absence of obvious lesion; serum-coated swabs or swabs soaked in broth or peptone helpful in sampling and conserving skin flora; sellotape effective for sampling skin for carriage; skin scrapings, required to establish dermatophyte fungal infections, must include apparently uninfected tissue from periphery of lesion. Soft tissue lesions, e.g. bites , traumatic injuries, often polymicrobic and anaerobes must be sought. Viral infections: electron microscopy of vesicle fluid and/or culture, but superficial bacterial contamination of open lesions presents serious interpretive problems.
Examination of specimens	**Skin scrapings** Microscopically: treat portion of scrapings with KOH (24 hr) to dissolve keratin; examine in wet preparation for fungal hyphae.
Culture	Use untreated portion of sample. Medium: Saboraud agar. Incubation: air for 1-10 days at ambient temp (~25°C).
Likely pathogens (basic method)	*Trichophyton, Epidermophyton* and *Microsporum* spp., *Candida* spp., and other skin yeasts (important in immunocompromised, e.g. *Trichosporon beigelii, Cryptococcus neoformans;* also *Sporothrix schenkii*)
Examination of specimens	**Skin and soft tissue samples** Microscopically: Gram-stain (N.B. of limited value except for grossly infected open lesions)
Culture	Media: BA, WC Incubation: air (BA)or AnO_2(WC) for 18-48 hrs at 35-37°C.
Likely pathogens (basic method)	Frequent: *Staph. aureus, Strep. pyogenes, Propionibacterium acnes,* enterobacteria and pseudomonads (in warmer climates or after exposure to detergents), *Candida.* Infrequent: *Corynebacterium diphtheriae* (from cutaneous diphtheria), *C. ulcerans, Erysipelothrix rhusiopathiae, Bacillus anthracis.*

SKIN AND SOFT TISSUES SPECIMENS (CONT.)	
Important pathogens (not isolated by above technique)	*Mycobacterium* spp. particularly *M. marinum* (see section on sputum for technique). *Treponema pallidum* cannot be cultivated *in vitro*; examine fluid from primary and secondary lesions by dark ground microscopy. Pathogens demonstrated microscopically: *Leichmania tropica*, *L. mexicana* (amastigotes in smear from skin lesion); *Draculunculus medinensis* (adult, or in fluid from vesicle); *Onchocerca volvulus* (microfilariae in skin snips from nodule); *Sarcoptes scabei* (mites in skin scrapings or hooked out from burrow). *Mycobacterium leprae* Cannot be cultivated *in vitro* Stain samples from skin lesion or nasal scrapings by Ziehl-Neelsen or auramine. In lepromatous leprosy organisms are readily seen; in tuberculoid leprosy, few if any organisms are seen.

RESPIRATORY TRACT SAMPLES

The upper respiratory tract flora is liable to alter as a result of environmental conditions, e.g. moist atmospheres encourage Gram-negative rods.

Specimen type	**Throat swabs**
Examination of specimens	Microscopy of no value, unless Ludwig's angina (a mixed infection caused by a spirochaete and a Gram-negative anaerobic fusiform) suspected.
Culture	Media: BA, CA, Tellurite BA (if *C. diphtheriae* suspected) Incubation: BA: AnO_2* CA: CO_2 } for 18-48 hrs at 35-37°C * (better for streptococcal haemolysis)
Likely pathogens (basic method)	*Strep. pyogenes* (also beta-haemolytic streptococci of groups C and G), *C. diphtheriae*, *Candida* (important in immunosuppressed).
Specimen type	**Nasal swabs (usually to detect carriage of pathogens not to sample site of infection)**
Culture	As for throat swabs with addition of Mac agar.
Likely pathogens (basic method)	*Staph. aureus*, *Strep. pyogenes*, *Neisseria meningitidis*, *C. diphtheriae*.
Specimen type	**Pernasal swabs (can be used to sample the nasopharynx)**
Culture	Bordet-Gerngou, or charcoal BA for *Bordetella pertussis*. BA or CA to detect carriage of *Neisseria meningitidis*.
Specimen type	**Outer ear swabs**
Culture	As for throat swabs with addition of Mac agar.
Likely pathogens (basic method)	*Strep. pneumoniae*, *H. influenzae*, *Staph. aureus*, Gram-negative rods, especially *P. aeruginosa* .
Specimen type	**Eye swabs**
Examination of specimens	Microscopically: Gram-stained smears: note WBC and bacteria Direct immunofluorescence (DFA) for *C. trachomatis* if clinical history suggestive.
Culture	Media: BA, CA. Incubation: CO_2 for 18-48 hrs at 35-37°C.

RESPIRATORY TRACT SPECIMENS (CONT.)	
Likely pathogens (basic method)	*Strep. pneumoniae, Staph. aureus, H. influenzae, Acinetobacter lwoffi, N. gonorrhoeae.*
Important pathogens (special techniques)	*Chlamydia trachomatis* (for methods see genital tract specimens).
Specimen type	**Sputum**
Examination of specimens	Macroscopically: note appearance (purulent, mucoid, salivary), volume. Microscopically: Gram stain: note polymorphs bacteria (numbers, different types, predominant morphotype) epithelial cells (contamination with mouth flora)
Culture	Media: BA, CA. Incubatlon: CO_2 for 24–48 hrs for 35–37°C.
Likely pathogens (basic method)	*Strep pneumoniae, H. influenzae, Staph. aureus, K. pneumoniae, Pseudomonas* spp., *Branhamella catarrhalis, Candida* spp., *Aspergillus* spp.
Important pathogens (not isolated by above technique)	(N.B. laboratory needs to be warned if these pathogens are suspected) Anaerobes If lung abscess suspected, follow basic method and inoculate additional BA and incubate anaerobically for 48 hrs. *Legionella pneumophila* Medium: blood charcoal yeast agar supplemented with cysteine. Incubation: CO_2 for 3–7 days for 35–37°C. *Bordetella pertussis* Medium: Bordet-Gengou or charcoal blood agar + cephalexin. Incubation: CO_2 for 2–4 days at 35–37°C. Mycobacteria If mycobacteria suspected, handle sputum in safety cabinet. Prior to culture: decontaminate sputum with an equal volume of 4% NaOH to kill other bacteria. Neutralize with HCl or dilute. Microscopy: ZN or auramine stain; observe for acid-fast rods. Culture: Lowenstein Jensen or Middlebrook agar (in screw capped bottles to prevent dessication). Incubation: air* for up to 12 weeks at 35°C for *M. tuberculosis*, 25, 35 & 43°C for *M. avium-intracellulare* *for mycobacteria other than tuberculosis (MOTT) incubation in dark and in continous light may reveal pigments. (Alternatively use radiometric growth detection system: Add sputum homogenate and antibiotic cocktail to suppress other respiratory organisms to commerical medium containing radioisotope. Incubation: air for 2–12 days at 35°C. Growth detected by automated detection of radiolabelled CO_2.) Important pathogens (serology only) *Mycoplasma pneumonia, Chlamydia pneumoniae* and *Chlamydia psittaci, Coxiella burnetti.* Other important pathogens Viruses (RSV), influenza virus etc.) detected by immunofluorescence imaging of nasopharyngeal washings; *Pneumocystis carlnii* (sputum); *Paragonimus westermanii* (eggs in sputum).

CEREBROSPINAL FLUID	
Specimen type	This specimen is irreplaceable and must be processed as soon as possible after collection, with utmost care.

Examination of specimens	Macroscopically:
	  note volume, colour (presence of xanthochromia); presence of clot (will invalidate attempts at accurate cell count).
	Microscopically:
	  Wet preparations (in counting chambers) for accurate counts of WBC and RBC
	  Gram stain
	  Cytological stain (aids recognition of eosinophils indistinguishable in Gram-stained smears)
	  Ziehl-Neelsen or auramine stain for acid-fast rods (when indicated by history)
	Chemically: analysis of protein and sugar content.
	Antigen detection techniques may aid rapid diagnosis.

Culture	Media: BA ($\times$2); CA; fluid enrichment medium (e.g. thioglycollate); Saboraud (if *Crytococcus* suspected from microscopy or history); Lowenstein-Jensen, Middlebrook or other suitable for mycobacteria (if suspected from microscopy or history); Radiometric growth detection systems incorporating Middlebrook medium. Incubation: BA $\}$ CO$_2$ CA $\}$ $\}$ for 18-48 hrs at 35-37°C BA: AnO$_2$ $\}$ Saboraud: air for 18-48 hrs at 30°C Fluid enrichment medium: subculture to BA ($\times$2) after 48 hrs and incubate as for BA above. Lowenstein-Jensen (or equivalent): air for up to 6 weeks at 37°C.
Likely pathogens (basic method)	*N. meningitidis, H. influenzae, Strep. pneumoniae, E. coli* and other Gram-negative rods, *Strep. agalactiae* (group B streptococcus), *Listeria monocytogenes, Crytococcus neoformans, M. tuberculosis.*
Likely pathogens (not isolated by above technique)	*Heptospira interrogens;* viruses (cell culture to isolate enteroviruses, mumps virus, HSV); *Naegleria* (amoeboe, plus leucocytes and RBC's maybe visible).
PUS	
Specimen type	Pus, rather than a swab dipped in the exudate, should be sent for culture whenever possible. Bacteria survive less well on swabs and because recovery in culture depends among other things, on the number of organisms present in the sample, the larger the volume the better.

Examination of specimens	Microscopically:
	  Gram stain: note polymorphs, bacteria and fungi (numbers, different types, predominant type).
	  If mycobacteria are suspected: Ziehl-Neelsen or auramine stain.
	  If actinomycetes are suspected: examine pus for sulphur granules.
	  If anaerobes are suspected: examine pus directly by gas-liquid chromatography for volatile fatty acid end-products of metabolism.

Culture	Media: BA, WC, CA, Mac, fluid enrichment medium. Incubation: BA $\}$ Mac $\}$ air $\}$ Fluid enrichment $\}$ 35-37°C for 1–5 days CA: CO$_2$ $\}$ WC (or equivalent): AnO$_2$ $\}$ NB. many fastidious anaerobes particularly susceptible to oxygen in early stages of colony formation, so one set of anaerobic plates should be incubated undisturbed for 48 hrs unless examined in an anaerobic cabinet.

PUS (CONT.)	
Likely pathogens (basic method)	*Staph. aureus, Strep. pyogenes*, enterococci, peptococci, *Listeria, Pasteurella* spp., *Yersinia* spp, *Neisseria* spp., enterobacteria and pseudomonads, anaerobes including *Clostridium* spp., *Bacteroides* spp., and *Fusobacterium* spp., *Nocardia* spp., and *Actinomyces* spp. (the last two may require >48 hrs incubation). Any bacteria or fungi isolated in pure culture or in heavy growth considered significant if specimen collected carefully from lesion.
Important pathogens (not isolated by above technique)	*Mycobacterium* spp. Pus from which no organisms recovered should be examined microscopically and cultured for mycobacteria (using methods for sputum above); from some lesions, e.g. injection abscesses, mycobacteria other than *M. tuberculosis* may be isolated and significant

OTHER FLUIDS	
Specimen type	e.g. pleural, pericardial, ascitic, joint fluids. In health, amount of fluid is small but large volumes may accumulate in disease; transudates result from stasis or obstruction; exudates from inflammation.; specimens should be collected aseptically by aspiration into two sterile containers, one of which contains anticoagulant

Examination of specimens	Macroscopically: note appearance and volume
	Centrifuge fluid and examine deposit (use supernatant for serology and chemical analysis).
	
	Microscopically:
	  Gram stain: note polymorphs
	              lymphocytes (if present, suspect mycobacteria)
	              bacteria (numbers, different types, predominant type)
	  Cytological stain

Culture	Use deposit. Media: BA, WC or BA (with additions suitable for anaerobes), fluid enrichment medium (e.g. thioglycollate).
Likely pathogens (basic method)	Wide range of pathogens may be found; any isolate from specimen collected aseptically considered significant.
Important pathogens (not isolated by above technique)	Examine microscopically and culture for mycobacteria if indicated (see sputum section).

BLOOD	
Specimen type	Volume of blood collected, ratio of blood to culture medium and presence of antibiotics all affect this important diagnostic process; scrupulous adherence to aseptic collection of samples is essential; inoculate blood directly into culture medium at bedside; use two bottles of culture medium: one contains a good broth medium, the other a broth medium formulated to support growth of anaerobes; dilute at least 1 part blood to 15 parts culture medium; distribute at least 20ml of blood between the two culture bottles; Some blood culture systems include a third bottle with broth medium containing liquoid (sodium polyanethol sulphonate, 0.05%) which helps to neutralize antibiotics and antibacterial activity of blood; some commercial systems do not require subculture but use automated techniques to detect bacterial growth.
Examination of specimens	Transport blood cultures rapidly to the laboratory, incubate at 37°C, and examine 6, 24 and 48 hours after collection; prolonged incubation (up to 21 days) may be required for growth of some organisms (e.g. *Brucella* spp.). Detection of positive cultures: Unless alternative commercial systems used, bacterial and fungal growth detected microscopically. Gram stain: note bacteria (Gram-negative organisms may be difficult to see as RBC and protein debris also stain pink).

BLOOD (CONT.)	
Culture	Media: BA, WC or BA (with additions suitable for anaerobes), Mac (if Gram-negative rods seen by microscopy). Incubation: BA: CO_2 Mac: air — for 24–48 hr at 35–37°C WC: AnO_2
Likely pathogens (basic method)	Any isolate from more than one blood culture considered significant; blood culture system can support growth of any bacterial species which can grow *in vitro* without specific growth requirements; polymicrobic infections may be found and isolation of one species does not preclude possibility of a second; normal skin commensals such as coagulase-negative staphylococci are common contaminants of blood cultures.

BONE MARROW	
Specimen type	Usually only available for microbiological evaluation when collected for haematological reasons; if collected and manipulated aseptically, bone marrow can be processed as for blood culture
Likely pathogens (basic method)	*Salmonella typhi*, *Brucella* spp., mycobacteria, *Leishmania donovani* can be demonstrated in stained smears.

BIOPSY SAMPLES
As with CSF, process biopsy samples with care as are irreplacable; processing protocol dictated by patient history; divide sample into 3 parts for histology, bacteriology and virology; (N.B. Specimens for bacteriology and virology must not be placed in histological fixatives). Lymph nodes and other tissues may require maceration; this process may produce aerosols and should be carried out with appropriate precautions.

AUTOPSY SAMPLES
Collection of samples requires collaborative effort; superficial contaminants may be eliminated by searing outer surface with hot iron before cutting or by washing the sample several times in sterile broth or saline.

FORENSIC SAMPLES
All samples must be retained for legal purposes, precluding any destructive processing; it is imperative that all samples and slides are clearly labelled; staff should sign for custody of samples.

INDEX